MOSBY'S

GUIDE TO
# NURSING
# DIAGNOSIS

## MOSBY'S

# GUIDE TO
# NURSING
# DIAGNOSIS

*Gail B. Ladwig*
MSN, RN, HNC

*Betty J. Ackley*
MSN, EdS, RN

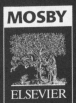

**MOSBY**

ELSEVIER

## MOSBY
### ELSEVIER

11830 Westline Industrial Drive
St. Louis, Missouri 63146

MOSBY'S GUIDE TO NURSING DIAGNOSIS

ISBN-13 978-0-323-03665-8
ISBN-10 0-323-03665-1

**Copyright © 2006 by Mosby, Inc.**

### NOTICE

Knowledge and best practice in this field are constantly changing. As new research and experience broaden our knowledge, changes in practice, treatment and drug therapy may become necessary or appropriate. Readers are advised to check the most current information provided (i) on procedures featured or (ii) by the manufacturer of each product to be administered, to verify the recommended dose or formula, the method and duration of administration, and contraindications. It is the responsibility of the practitioner, relying on their own experience and knowledge of the patient, to make diagnoses, to determine dosages and the best treatment for each individual patient, and to take all appropriate safety precautions. To the fullest extent of the law, neither the Publisher nor the Authors assume any liability for any injury and/or damage to persons or property arising out of or related to any use of the material contained in this book.

**International Standard Book Number 0-323-03665-1**

*Acquisitions Editor:* Sandra Clark Brown
*Senior Developmental Editor:* Cindi Anderson
*Publishing Services Manager:* Deborah L. Vogel
*Project Manager:* Katherine Hinkebein
*Designer:* Paula Ruckenbrod

Printed in the United States of America

Last digit is the print number: 9 8 7 6 5 4 3 2 1

# Acknowledgments

We would like to thank Cindi Anderson, Senior Developmental Editor, for the excellent work she did in making this "pocket guide" a reality. Cindi is always a joy to work with. We treasure our association with her. And a special thank-you to Katherine Hinkebein for project management of this text.

The authors would also like to thank the following individuals for their contributions to *Nursing Diagnosis Handbook: A Guide to Planning Care*, Seventh Edition, by Betty Ackley and Gail Ladwig, from which this book has been developed:

Donna Algase, PhD, RN, FAAN
Sharon Baranoski, MSN, RN, CWOCN
Lisa Burkhart, MPH, PhD, RN
Mary DeWys, RN, BS
Terri Ellis, RN, MSN
Brenda Emick-Herring, RN, MSN, CRRN
Arlene T. Farren, RN, MA, AOCN
Judith A. Floyd, PhD, RN, FAAN
Terri Foster, RN, BSN, CNOR
Judith Gentz, RN, CS, NP
Barbara A. Given, RN, PhD, FAAN
Mikel Gray Jr., PhD, CUNP, CCCN, FAAN
Elizabeth Henneman, RN, PhD
T. Heather Herdman, RN, PhD
Kimberly Hickey, MSN, RN
Teresa Howell, MSN, ARHP
Linda Hutson, RN, SANE-A
Ann C. Keeley, RN, MN, CNS/PMH
Marcia LaHaie, MSN, RN, OCN
Scott Chisholm Lamont, BSN, RN, CCRN, CFRN, ENC(C)
Margaret Lunney, RN, PhD
Margo McCaffrey, RN, MS, FAAN
Graham J. McDougall Jr., PhD, RN, APRN, BC, FAAN

Pamela H. Mitchell, PhD, RN, CNRN, FAAN
Leslie H. Nicoll, PhD, MBA, RN, BC
Chris Pasero, MS, RN, FAAN
Paula R. Sherwood, RN, PhD, CNRN
P. Ann Solari-Twadell, RN, PhD, MPA, FAAN
Michelle Walters, RN, MSN, ARNP
Linda S. Williams, MSN, RNBC
Kathleen L. Patusky, PhD, APRN-BC
Marina Martinez-Kratz, RN, MS
Beth Ann Swann, PhD, CRNP

## Consultants to previous editions of *Nursing Diagnosis Handbook: A Guide to Planning Care*

Elizabeth L. Foster, MS, RN
Ann F. Jacobson, PhD, RN
Debra Martinez, BSW
Brenda J. Wagner, PhD, RN
Elizabeth H. Winslow, PhD, RN, FAAN
Jill Barnes, MS, RNCS
Victoria L. Cole-Schonlau, DNSc, MPA, RN
Sandra Cunningham, MS, RN, CCRN, CS
Jane Maria Curtis, MSN, CAN, RN
Gwethalyn B. Edwards, MSN, RN
Pamela M. Emery, BS, RNFA, CNOR, RN
Nancy English, PhD, RN
Roslyn Fine, MS, CCC, SLP
J. Keith Hampton, MSN, RN, CS
Mary Henrikson, MN, RNC, ARNP
Kathie D. Hesnan, BSN, RN, CETN
Constance Hollman, MA, EdS
Leslie Kalbach, MN, RN, CETN
Helen Kelley, MSN, RN, CHTP, HNC, NP
Diane Krasner, PhD, RN, CWOCN, CWS, FAAN
Carroll A. Lutz, MA, BSN, RN
Leslie Lysaght, RN, MS, CS
Mary Markle, MSN, RNC
Marty J. Martin, MSN, RN

Michelle Masta, RN, BSN
Cathy McClean, RN, BSN
Vicki McClurg, MN, RN
Beverly Pickett, MA, BS, RN, CHTP, HNC
Nancee B. Radtke, MSN, RN
Judith S. Rizzo, MS, RN, CS
Pam B. Schweitzer, MS, RN, CS
Suzanne Skowronski, MSN, RN
Teepa Snow, MS, OTR-L, FAOTA
Martha A. Spies, MSN, RN
Kathy A. Stimac O'Brien, MSN, RN
Linda Straight, MA, RN
Terry VandenBosch, PhD, RN, CS
Catherine Vincent, MSN, RN
Virginia Wall, RN, MN, IBCLC
Peggy A. Wetsch, RN, MSN, CNA
Fran Wistom, MSN, RN, CSW, CPN
Janet Woodruff, BSN, RN
Kathy Wyngarden, MSN, FNP, RN

# How to Use Mosby's Guide to Nursing Diagnosis

## ASSESS
Assess the client using the format provided by the clinical setting. Collect data including client's symptoms, clinical state, and known medical or psychiatric diagnoses.

## DIAGNOSIS
Using Section I, Guide to Nursing Diagnoses, locate the client's symptoms, clinical state, medical, surgical or psychiatric diagnoses, and anticipated or prescribed diagnostic studies or surgical interventions (listed in alphabetical order). Note suggestions for appropriate nursing diagnoses and select an appropriate diagnosis.

Use Section II, Guide to Planning Care, to evaluate each suggested nursing diagnosis and "related to" etiology statement. Section II contains a listing of care plans according to NANDA-I, arranged alphabetically by diagnostic concept, for each nursing diagnosis referred to in Section I. Determine the appropriateness of each nursing diagnosis by reading the definition and comparing the Defining Characteristics and Risk Factors to the client data collected.

## DETERMINE OUTCOMES
Use Section II, Guide to Planning Care, to find appropriate Client Outcomes for the client.

## PLAN INTERVENTIONS
Use Section II, Guide to Planning Care, to find appropriate interventions for the client.

## GIVE NURSING CARE
Administer nursing care following the plan of care based on the interventions.

## EVALUATE NURSING CARE
Evaluate nursing care administered using the Client Outcomes.

If the outcomes were not met, and the nursing interventions were not effective, it may be appropriate to reassess the client and determine if the appropriate nursing diagnoses were made.

## DOCUMENT

Document all of the previous steps using the format provided in the clinical setting.

# Contents

# Guide to Nursing Diagnoses

A

## ABDOMINAL DISTENTION

Acute **Pain** r/t retention of air, gastrointestinal secretions

**Constipation** r/t decreased activity, decreased fluid intake, decreased fiber intake, pathological process

Delayed **Surgical** recovery r/t pain, nausea

Imbalanced **Nutrition**: less than body requirements r/t nausea, vomiting

**Nausea** r/t irritation of gastrointestinal tract

## ABDOMINAL HYSTERECTOMY

*See Hysterectomy*

## ABDOMINAL PAIN

Acute **Pain** r/t injury, pathological process

Imbalanced **Nutrition**: less than body requirements r/t unresolved pain

*See cause of Abdominal Pain*

## ABDOMINAL PERINEAL RESECTION

Risk for perioperative positioning **Injury** r/t prolonged surgery, lithotomy position

*See Abdominal Surgery; Colostomy*

## ABDOMINAL SURGERY

Acute **Pain** r/t surgical procedure

**Constipation** r/t decreased activity, decreased fluid intake, anesthesia, narcotics

Imbalanced **Nutrition**: less than body requirements r/t high metabolic needs, decreased ability to ingest or digest food

Ineffective **Health** maintenance r/t knowledge deficit regarding self-care after surgery

Ineffective **Tissue** perfusion: peripheral r/t immobility, abdominal surgery resulting in stasis of blood flow

Risk for **Infection** r/t invasive procedure

*See Surgery, Perioperative Care; Surgery, Postoperative Care; Surgery, Preoperative Care*

## ABDOMINAL TRAUMA

Acute **Pain** r/t abdominal trauma

Deficient **Fluid** volume r/t hemorrhage

Disturbed **Body** image r/t scarring, change in body function, need for temporary colostomy

Ineffective **Breathing** pattern r/t abdominal distention, pain

Risk for **Infection** r/t possible perforation of abdominal structures

## ABORTION, INDUCED

Acute **Pain** r/t surgical intervention

Chronic low **Self-esteem** disturbance r/t feelings of guilt

Chronic **Sorrow** r/t loss of potential child

Compromised family **Coping** r/t unresolved feelings about decision

Ineffective **Health** maintenance r/t deficient knowledge regarding self-care following abortion

Risk for delayed **Development** r/t unplanned or unwanted pregnancy

Risk for imbalanced **Fluid** volume r/t possible hemorrhage

Risk for **Infection** r/t open uterine blood vessels, dilated cervix

Risk for **Post-trauma** syndrome r/t psychological trauma of abortion

Risk for **Spiritual** distress r/t perceived moral implications of decision

Spiritual distress r/t perceived moral implications of decision

## ABORTION, SPONTANEOUS

Acute **Pain** r/t uterine contractions, surgical intervention

Chronic **Sorrow** r/t loss of potential child

Disabled family **Coping** r/t unresolved feelings about loss

Disturbed **Body** image r/t perceived inability to carry pregnancy, produce child

**Fear** r/t implications for future pregnancies

**Grieving** r/t loss of fetus

Ineffective **Coping** r/t personal vulnerability

Ineffective **Health** maintenance r/t deficient knowledge regarding self-care following abortion

Interrupted **Family** processes r/t unmet expectations for pregnancy and childbirth

Risk for deficient **Fluid** volume r/t hemorrhage

Risk for **Infection** r/t septic or incomplete abortion of products of conception, open uterine blood vessels, dilated cervix

Risk for **Post-trauma** syndrome r/t psychological trauma of abortion

Risk for **Spiritual** distress r/t loss of fetus

**Self-esteem** disturbance r/t feelings of failure, guilt

## ABRUPTIO PLACENTAE <36 WEEKS

Acute **Pain** r/t irritable uterus, hypertonic uterus

**Anxiety** r/t unknown outcome, change in birth plans

Death **Anxiety** r/t unknown outcome, hemorrhage/pain

**Fear** r/t threat to well-being of self and fetus

Impaired **Gas** exchange: placental r/t decreased uteroplacental area

Impaired **Tissue** integrity: maternal r/t possible uterine rupture

Interrupted **Family** process r/t unmet expectations for pregnancy/childbirth

Ineffective **Health** maintenance r/t deficient knowledge regarding self-care with disorder

Risk for deficient **Fluid** volume r/t hemorrhage

Risk for disproportionate **Growth** r/t uteroplacental insufficiency

Risk for ineffective **Tissue** perfusion: fetal r/t uteroplacental insufficiency

Risk for **Infection** r/t partial separation of placenta

## ABSCESS FORMATION

Impaired **Tissue** integrity r/t altered circulation, nutritional deficit/excess

Ineffective **Health** maintenance r/t deficient knowledge regarding self-care with abscess

Ineffective **Protection** r/t inadequate nutrition, abnormal blood profile, drug therapy, depressed immune function

## ABUSE, CHILD

*See Child Abuse*

## ABUSE, SPOUSE, PARENT, OR SIGNIFICANT OTHER

**Anxiety** r/t threat to self-concept, situational crisis of abuse

**Caregiver** role strain r/t chronic illness, self-care deficits, lack of respite care, extent of caregiving required

Compromised family **Coping** r/t abusive patterns

Defensive **Coping** r/t low self-esteem

A

Disturbed **Sleep** pattern r/t psychological stress

Impaired verbal **Communication** r/t psychological barriers of fear

Interrupted **Family** process: alcoholism r/t inadequate coping skills

**Post-trauma** syndrome r/t history of abuse

**Powerlessness** r/t lifestyle of helplessness

Risk for **Post-trauma** syndrome r/t inadequate social support

Risk for self-directed **Violence** r/t history of abuse

**Self-esteem** disturbance r/t negative family interactions

## ACCESSORY MUSCLE USE (TO BREATHE)

Ineffective **Breathing** pattern r/t compromised lung function, neuromuscular impairment, pain, musculoskeletal impairment, perception/cognitive impairment, anxiety, decreased energy, fatigue

*See Asthma; Bronchitis; COPD; Respiratory Infections, Acute Childhood*

## ACCIDENT PRONE

Acute **Confusion** r/t altered level of consciousness

Adult **Failure** to thrive r/t fatigue

Ineffective **Coping** r/t personal vulnerability, situational crises

Risk for **Injury** r/t history of accidents

## ACHALASIA

Acute **Pain** r/t stasis of food in esophagus

Impaired **Swallowing** r/t neuromuscular impairment

Ineffective **Coping** r/t chronic disease

Risk for **Aspiration** r/t nocturnal regurgitation

## ACIDOSIS, METABOLIC

Acute **Pain**: headache r/t neuromuscular irritability

Decreased **Cardiac** output r/t dysrhythmias from hyperkalemia

Disturbed **Thought** processes r/t central nervous system depression

Imbalanced **Nutrition**: less than body requirements r/t inability to ingest, absorb nutrients

Impaired **Memory** r/t electrolyte imbalance

Ineffective **Tissue** perfusion: cardiopulmonary r/t progressive shock

Risk for **Injury** r/t disorientation, weakness, stupor

## ACIDOSIS, RESPIRATORY

**Activity** intolerance r/t imbalance between oxygen supply and demand

Disturbed **Thought** processes r/t central nervous system depression

Impaired **Gas** exchange r/t ventilation perfusion imbalance

Impaired **Memory** r/t hypoxia

Risk for decreased **Cardiac** output r/t dysrhythmias associated with respiratory acidosis

## ACNE

Disturbed **Body** image r/t biophysical changes associated with skin disorder

Impaired **Skin** integrity r/t hormonal changes (adolescence, menstrual cycle)

Ineffective management of **Therapeutic** regimen r/t deficient knowledge (medications, personal care, cause)

## ACQUIRED IMMUNODEFICIENCY SYNDROME

*See AIDS (Acquired Immunodeficiency Syndrome)*

## ACROMEGALY

Disturbed **Body** image r/t changes in body function and appearance

Impaired physical **Mobility** r/t joint pain

Ineffective **Airway** clearance r/t airway obstruction by enlarged tongue

**Sexual** dysfunction r/t changes in hormonal secretions

## ACTIVITY INTOLERANCE

**Activity** intolerance r/t bedrest/immobility, generalized weakness, sedentary lifestyle, imbalance between oxygen supply/demand, pain

## ACTIVITY INTOLERANCE, POTENTIAL TO DEVELOP

Risk for **Activity** intolerance r/t deconditioned status, presence of circulatory/respiratory problems, inexperience with activity

## ACUTE ABDOMEN

Acute **Pain** r/t pathological process

Deficient **Fluid** volume r/t air and fluids trapped in bowel, inability to drink

*See cause of Acute Abdomen*

## ACUTE ALCOHOL INTOXICATION

Disturbed **Thought** processes r/t central nervous system depression

Dysfunctional **Family** processes: alcoholism r/t abuse of alcohol

Ineffective **Breathing** pattern r/t depression of the respiratory center

Risk for **Aspiration** r/t depressed reflexes with acute vomiting

Risk for **Infection** r/t impaired immune system from altered nutrition

## ACUTE BACK

Acute **Pain** r/t back injury

**Anxiety** r/t situational crisis, back injury

**Constipation** r/t decreased activity

Impaired physical **Mobility** r/t pain

Ineffective **Coping** r/t situational crisis, back injury

Ineffective **Health** maintenance r/t deficient knowledge regarding self-care with painful back

## ACUTE CONFUSION

*See Confusion, Acute*

## ACUTE RESPIRATORY DISTRESS SYNDROME

*See ARDS (Acute Respiratory Distress Syndrome)*

## ADAMS-STOKES SYNDROME

*See Dysrhythmia*

## ADDICTION

*See Alcoholism; Drug Abuse*

## ADDISON'S DISEASE

**Activity** intolerance r/t weakness, fatigue

Deficient **Fluid** volume r/t failure of regulatory mechanisms

Disturbed **Body** image r/t increased skin pigmentation

Imbalanced **Nutrition**: less than body requirements r/t chronic illness

Ineffective **Health** maintenance r/t deficient knowledge

Risk for **Injury** r/t weakness

## ADENOIDECTOMY

Acute **Pain** r/t surgical incision

Impaired **Comfort** r/t effects of anesthesia, nausea, vomiting

Ineffective **Airway** clearance r/t hesitation/reluctance to cough secondary to pain

Ineffective **Health** maintenance r/t deficient knowledge of postoperative care

**Nausea** r/t anesthesia effects, drainage from surgery

A

A

Risk for **Aspiration** r/t postoperative drainage, impaired swallowing

Risk for deficient **Fluid** volume r/t decreased intake secondary to painful swallowing, effects of anesthesia

Risk for imbalanced **Nutrition**: less than body requirements r/t hesitation/reluctance to swallow

## ADHESIONS, LYSIS OF

*See Abdominal Surgery*

## ADJUSTMENT DISORDER

**Anxiety** r/t inability to cope with psychosocial stressor

Disturbed personal **Identity** r/t psychosocial stressor (specific to individual)

Impaired **Adjustment** r/t assault to self-esteem

Impaired **Social** interaction r/t absence of significant others or peers

Situational low **Self-esteem** r/t change in role function

## ADJUSTMENT IMPAIRMENT

Impaired **Adjustment** r/t disability requiring change in lifestyle, inadequate support systems, impaired cognition, sensory overload assault to self-esteem, altered locus of control, incomplete grieving

## ADOLESCENT, PREGNANT

**Anxiety** r/t situational and maturational crisis, pregnancy

Decisional **Conflict**: keeping child vs. giving up child vs. abortion r/t lack of experience with decision-making, interference with decision-making, multiple or divergent sources of information, lack of support system

Deficient **Knowledge** r/t pregnancy, infant growth and development, parenting

Delayed **Growth** and development r/t pregnancy

Disabled family **Coping** r/t highly ambivalent family relationships, chronically unresolved feelings of guilt, anger, despair

Disturbed **Body** image r/t pregnancy superimposed on developing body

**Fear** r/t labor and delivery

**Health**-seeking behaviors r/t desire for optimal maternal and fetal outcome

Imbalanced **Nutrition**: less than body requirements r/t lack of knowledge of nutritional needs during pregnancy and as growing adolescent

Impaired **Social** interaction r/t self-concept disturbance

Ineffective **Coping** r/t situational and maturational crisis, personal vulnerability

Ineffective **Denial** r/t fear of consequences of pregnancy becoming known

Ineffective **Health** maintenance r/t deficient knowledge with denial of pregnancy, desire to keep pregnancy secret, fear

Ineffective **Role** performance r/t pregnancy

Interrupted **Family** processes r/t unmet expectations for adolescent, situational crisis

**Noncompliance** r/t denial of pregnancy

Risk for **Constipation** r/t hormone effect, inadequate fiber in diet, inadequate fluid in diet

Risk for delayed **Development** r/t unplanned or unwanted pregnancy

Risk for impaired parent-infant **Attachment** r/t anxiety associated with the parent role

Risk for impaired **Parenting** r/t adolescent parent, unplanned or unwanted pregnancy, single parent

Risk for urge urinary **Incontinence** r/t pressure on bladder by growing uterus

Situational low **Self-esteem** r/t feelings of shame and guilt about becoming/being pregnant

**Social** isolation r/t absence of supportive significant other(s)

## ADOPTION, GIVING CHILD UP FOR

Chronic **Sorrow** r/t loss of relationship with child

Decisional **Conflict** r/t unclear personal values or beliefs, perceived threat to value system, support system deficit

Disturbed **Sleep** pattern r/t depression or trauma of relinquishment of child

Ineffective **Coping** r/t final decision

Interrupted **Family** processes r/t conflict within family regarding relinquishment of child

**Grieving** r/t loss of child, loss of role of parent

Readiness for enhanced **Spiritual** well-being r/t harmony with self, regarding final decision

Risk for **Post-trauma** syndrome r/t psychological trauma of relinquishment of child

Risk for **Spiritual** distress r/t perceived moral implications of decision

**Social** isolation r/t making choice that goes against values of significant other(s)

## ADRENAL CRISIS

Deficient **Fluid** volume r/t insufficient ability to reabsorb water

Delayed **Surgical** recovery r/t inability to respond to stress

Ineffective **Protection** r/t inability to tolerate stress

*See Addison's Disease; Shock*

## ADVANCE DIRECTIVES

Anticipatory **Grieving** r/t possible loss of self, significant other

Death **Anxiety** r/t planning for end-of-life health decisions

Decisional **Conflict** r/t unclear personal values or beliefs, perceived threat to value system, support system deficit

Readiness for enhanced **Spiritual** well-being r/t harmonious interconnectedness with self, others, higher power/God

## AFFECTIVE DISORDERS

Adult **Failure** to thrive r/t altered mood state

Chronic low **Self-esteem** r/t repeated unmet expectations

Chronic **Sorrow** r/t chronic mental illness

**Constipation** r/t inactivity, decreased fluid intake

Disturbed **Sleep** pattern r/t inactivity

Dysfunctional **Grieving** r/t lack of previous resolution of former grieving response

**Fatigue** r/t psychological demands

**Hopelessness** r/t feeling of abandonment, long-term stress

Ineffective **Coping** r/t dysfunctional grieving

Ineffective **Health** maintenance r/t lack of ability to make good judgments regarding ways to obtain help

Risk for **Loneliness** r/t pattern of social isolation, feelings of low self-esteem

Risk for **Suicide** r/t panic state

**Self-care** deficit: specify r/t depression, cognitive impairment

**Sexual** dysfunction r/t loss of sexual desire

**Social** isolation r/t ineffective coping

*See specific disorder: Depression; Dysthymic Disorder; Manic Disorder, Bipolar I*

A

## AGE-RELATED MACULAR DEGENERATION

*See Macular Degeneration*

## AGGRESSIVE BEHAVIOR

**Fear** r/t real or imagined threat to own well-being

Risk for other-directed **Violence** r/t antisocial character, battered woman, catatonic excitement, child abuse, manic excitement, organic brain syndrome, panic states, rage reactions, suicidal behavior, temporal lobe epilepsy, toxic reactions to medication

Risk for self-directed **Violence** r/t antisocial character, battered woman, catatonic excitement, child abuse, manic excitement, organic brain syndrome, panic states, rage reactions, suicidal behavior, temporal lobe epilepsy, toxic reactions to medication

## AGING

Adult **Failure** to thrive r/t depression, apathy, fatigue

Anticipatory **Grieving** r/t multiple losses, impending death

Chronic **Sorrow** r/t multiple losses

Death **Anxiety** r/t fear of unknown, loss of self, impact on significant others

Disturbed **Sensory** perception: visual or auditory r/t aging process

Functional urinary **Incontinence** r/t impaired vision, impaired cognition, neuromuscular limitations, altered environmental factors

**Health**-seeking behaviors r/t knowledge about medication, nutrition, exercise, coping strategies

Impaired **Dentition** r/t ineffective oral hygiene; barriers to self-care, professional care; nutritional deficits; dietary habits; selected prescription medications; chronic use of tobacco, coffee, tea, red wine; lack of knowledge regarding dental health

Impaired **Memory** r/t fluid and electrolyte imbalance, neurological disturbances, excessive environmental disturbances, anemia, acute or chronic hypoxia, decreased cardiac output

Ineffective management of **Therapeutic** regimen r/t deficient knowledge: medication, nutrition, exercise, coping strategies

Ineffective **Thermoregulation** r/t aging

Readiness for enhanced community **Coping** r/t providing social support and other resources identified as needed for elderly client

Readiness for enhanced family **Coping** r/t ability to gratify needs, address adaptive tasks

Readiness for enhanced **Knowledge** of: specify r/t need to improve health

Readiness for enhanced **Nutrition** r/t need to improve health

Readiness for enhanced **Sleep** r/t need to improve sleep

Readiness for enhanced **Spiritual** well-being r/t one's experience of life's meaning, harmony with self, others, higher power/God, environment

Readiness for enhanced **Urinary** elimination r/t need to improve health

Risk for **Caregiver** role strain r/t inability to handle increasing needs of significant other

Risk for **Injury** r/t disturbed sensory perception

Risk for **Loneliness** r/t inadequate support system, role transition, health alterations, depression, fatigue

**Sleep** deprivation r/t aging-related sleep stage shifts

## AGITATION

Acute **Confusion** r/t side effects of medication, hypoxia, decreased cerebral perfusion, alcohol abuse or withdrawal, substance abuse or withdrawal, sensory deprivation, sensory overload

**Sleep** deprivation r/t sundown syndrome

## AGORAPHOBIA

**Anxiety** r/t real or perceived threat to physical integrity

**Fear** r/t leaving home, going out in public places

Impaired **Social** interaction r/t disturbance in self-concept

Ineffective **Coping** r/t inadequate support systems

**Social** isolation r/t altered thought process

## AGRANULOCYTOSIS

Delayed **Surgical** recovery r/t abnormal blood profile

Ineffective **Health** maintenance r/t deficient knowledge of protective measures to prevent infection

Ineffective **Protection** r/t abnormal blood profile

## AIDS (ACQUIRED IMMUNODEFICIENCY SYNDROME)

Anticipatory **Grieving**: family/parental r/t potential/impending death of loved one

Anticipatory **Grieving**: individual r/t loss of physiopsychosocial well-being

Disturbed **Body** image r/t chronic contagious illness, cachexia

**Caregiver** role strain r/t unpredictable illness course, presence of situation stressors

Chronic **Pain** r/t tissue inflammation and destruction

Chronic **Sorrow** r/t living with long-term chronic illness

Death **Anxiety** r/t fear of premature death

**Diarrhea** r/t inflammatory bowel changes

Disturbed **Energy** field r/t chronic illness

**Fatigue** r/t disease process, stress, poor nutritional intake

**Fear** r/t powerlessness, threat to well-being

**Hopelessness** r/t deteriorating physical condition

Imbalanced **Nutrition**: less than body requirements r/t decreased ability to eat and absorb nutrients secondary to anorexia, nausea, diarrhea; pathology in gastrointestinal tract

Ineffective **Health** maintenance r/t deficient knowledge regarding transmission of infection, lack of exposure to information, misinterpretation of information

Ineffective **Protection** r/t risk for infection secondary to inadequate immune system

Ineffective **Sexuality** pattern r/t possible transmission of disease

Interrupted **Family** processes r/t distress about diagnosis of human immunodeficiency virus (HIV) infection

Risk for deficient **Fluid** volume r/t diarrhea, vomiting, fever, bleeding

Risk for impaired **Oral** mucous membranes r/t immunological deficit

Risk for impaired **Skin** integrity r/t immunological deficit, diarrhea

Risk for **Infection** r/t inadequate immune system

Risk for **Loneliness** r/t social isolation

Risk for **Spiritual** distress r/t physical illness

Situational low **Self-esteem** r/t crisis of chronic contagious illness

A

**Social** isolation r/t self-concept disturbance, therapeutic isolation

**Spiritual** distress r/t challenged beliefs or moral system

*See AIDS, Child; Cancer; Pneumonia*

## AIDS DEMENTIA

Chronic **Confusion** r/t viral invasion of nervous system

Disturbed **Thought** processes r/t viral infection in the brain

*See Dementia*

## AIDS, CHILD

Impaired **Parenting** r/t congenital acquisition of infection secondary to intravenous (IV) drug use, multiple sexual partners, history of contaminated blood transfusion

**Parental** role conflict r/t interruption of family life due to home care regimen, intimidation with invasive or restrictive modalities

Risk for delayed **Development** r/t chronic illness

Risk for disproportionate **Growth** r/t chronic illness

*See AIDS (Acquired Immunodeficiency Syndrome); Child with Chronic Condition; Hospitalized Child; Terminally Ill Child, Adolescent; Terminally Ill Child, Infant/Toddler; Terminally Ill Child, Preschool Child; Terminally Ill Child, School-Age Child/Preadolescent; Terminally Ill Child, Death of Child, Parent*

## AIRWAY OBSTRUCTION/SECRETIONS

Ineffective **Airway** clearance r/t decreased energy; fatigue; tracheobronchial infection, obstruction, secretions; perceptual/cognitive impairment; trauma; decreased force of cough because of aging

## ALCOHOL WITHDRAWAL

Acute **Confusion** r/t effects of alcohol withdrawal

**Anxiety** r/t situational crisis, withdrawal

Chronic low **Self-esteem** r/t repeated unmet expectations

Disturbed **Sensory** perception: visual, auditory, kinesthetic, tactile, olfactory r/t neurochemical imbalance in brain

Disturbed **Sleep** pattern r/t effect of depressants, alcohol withdrawal, anxiety

Disturbed **Thought** processes r/t potential delirium tremors

Dysfunctional **Family** processes: alcoholism r/t abuse of alcohol

Imbalanced **Nutrition**: less than body requirements r/t poor dietary habits

Ineffective **Coping** r/t personal vulnerability

Ineffective **Health** maintenance r/t deficient knowledge regarding chronic illness or effects of alcohol consumption

Risk for deficient **Fluid** volume r/t excessive diaphoresis, agitation, decreased fluid intake

Risk for other-directed **Violence** r/t substance withdrawal

Risk for self-directed **Violence** r/t substance withdrawal

## ALCOHOLISM

Acute **Confusion** r/t alcohol abuse

**Anxiety** r/t loss of control

Chronic **Confusion** r/t neurological effects of chronic alcohol intake

Defensive **Coping** r/t alcoholism

Ineffective **Denial** r/t refusal to acknowledge alcoholism

Disturbed **Sleep** pattern r/t irritability, nightmares, tremors

Dysfunctional family **Coping:** alcoholism r/t codependency issues

Imbalanced **Nutrition:** less than body requirements r/t anorexia

Impaired **Adjustment** r/t lack of motivation to change behaviors

Impaired **Home** maintenance r/t memory deficits, fatigue

Impaired **Memory** r/t alcohol abuse

Ineffective **Coping** r/t use of alcohol to cope with life events

Ineffective **Protection** r/t malnutrition, sleep deprivation

Interrupted **Family** process: alcoholism r/t alcohol abuse

**Powerlessness** r/t alcohol addiction

Risk for **Injury** r/t alteration in sensory/perceptual function

Risk for **Loneliness** r/t unacceptable social behavior

Risk for other-directed **Violence** r/t reactions to substances used, impulsive behavior, disorientation, impaired judgment

Risk for self-directed **Violence** r/t reactions to substances used, impulsive behavior, disorientation, impaired judgment

**Self-esteem** disturbance r/t failure at life events

**Social** isolation r/t unacceptable social behavior, values

## ALCOHOLISM, DYSFUNCTIONAL FAMILY PROCESSES

Dysfunctional **Family** processes: alcoholism r/t abuse of alcohol, genetic predisposition, lack of problem-solving skills, inadequate coping skills, family history of alcoholism, resistance to treatment, biochemical influences, addictive personality

## ALKALOSIS

*See Metabolic Alkalosis*

## ALLERGIES

Ineffective **Health** maintenance r/t deficient knowledge regarding allergies

Latex **Allergy** r/t hypersensitivity to natural rubber latex

Risk for latex **Allergy** r/t repeated exposure to products containing latex

## ALOPECIA

Deficient **Knowledge** r/t self-care needed to promote hair growth

Disturbed **Body** image r/t loss of hair, change in appearance

## ALTERED MENTAL STATUS

*See Confusion, Acute; Confusion, Chronic; Impaired Memory*

## ALS (AMYOTROPHIC LATERAL SCLEROSIS)

*See Amyotrophic Lateral Sclerosis*

## ALZHEIMER'S TYPE DEMENTIA

Adult **Failure** to thrive r/t difficulty in reasoning, judgment, memory, concentration

Disturbed **Thought** processes r/t chronic organic disorder

**Caregiver** role strain r/t duration and extent of caregiving required

Chronic **Confusion** r/t Alzheimer's disease

Compromised family **Coping** r/t interrupted family processes

Disturbed **Sleep** pattern r/t neurological impairment, daytime naps

**Fear** r/t loss of self

**Hopelessness** r/t deteriorating condition

Impaired **Environmental** interpretation syndrome r/t Alzheimer's disease

A

Impaired **Home** maintenance r/t impaired cognitive function, inadequate support systems

Impaired **Memory** r/t neurological disturbance

Impaired physical **Mobility** r/t severe neurological dysfunction

Ineffective **Health** maintenance r/t deficient knowledge of caregiver regarding appropriate care

**Powerlessness** r/t deteriorating condition

Risk for **Injury** r/t confusion

Risk for **Loneliness** r/t potential social isolation

Risk for other-directed **Violence** r/t frustration, fear, anger

Risk for **Relocation** stress syndrome r/t impaired psychosocial health, decreased health status

**Self-care** deficit: specify r/t psychological-physiological impairment

**Social** isolation r/t fear of disclosure of memory loss

**Wandering** r/t cognitive impairment, frustration, physiological state

*See Dementia*

## AMD (AGE-RELATED MACULAR DEGENERATION)

*See Macular Degeneration*

## AMENORRHEA

Imbalanced **Nutrition**: less than body requirements r/t inadequate food intake

Risk for **Sexual** dysfunction r/t altered body function

*See Sexuality, Adolescent*

## AMI (ACUTE MYOCARDIAL INFARCTION)

*See MI (Myocardial Infarction)*

## AMNESIA

Acute **Confusion** r/t alcohol abuse, delirium, dementia, drug abuse

Dysfunctional **Family** processes: alcoholism r/t alcohol abuse, inadequate coping skills

Impaired **Memory** r/t excessive environmental disturbance, neurological disturbance

**Post-trauma** syndrome r/t history of abuse, catastrophic illness, disaster, accident

## AMNIOCENTESIS

**Anxiety** r/t threat to self and fetus, unknown future

Decisional **Conflict** r/t choice of treatment pending results of test

Risk for **Infection** r/t invasive procedure

## AMNIONITIS

*See Chorioamnionitis*

## AMNIOTIC MEMBRANE RUPTURE

*See Premature Rupture of Membranes*

## AMPUTATION

Acute **Pain** r/t surgery, phantom limb sensation

Chronic **Pain** r/t surgery, phantom limb sensation

Chronic **Sorrow** r/t grief associated with loss of body part

Disturbed **Body** image r/t negative effects of amputation, response from others

**Grieving** r/t loss of body part, future lifestyle changes

Impaired physical **Mobility** r/t musculoskeletal impairment, limited movement

Impaired **Skin** integrity r/t poor healing, prosthesis rubbing

Ineffective **Health** maintenance r/t deficient knowledge of care of stump, rehabilitation

Ineffective **Tissue** perfusion: peripheral r/t impaired arterial circulation

Risk for deficient **Fluid** volume: hemorrhage r/t vulnerable surgical site

## AMYOTROPHIC LATERAL SCLEROSIS (ALS)

Chronic **Sorrow** r/t chronic illness

Death **Anxiety** r/t impending progressive loss of function leading to death

Decisional **Conflict**: ventilator therapy r/t unclear personal values or beliefs, lack of relevant information

Impaired spontaneous **Ventilation** r/t weakness of muscles of respiration

Impaired **Swallowing** r/t weakness of muscles involved in swallowing

Impaired verbal **Communication** r/t weakness of muscles of speech, deficient knowledge of ways to compensate and alternative communication devices

Ineffective **Breathing** pattern r/t compromised muscles of respiration

Risk for **Aspiration** r/t impaired swallowing

Risk for **Spiritual** distress r/t chronic debilitating condition

*See Neurological Disorders*

## ANAL FISTULA

*See Hemorrhoidectomy*

## ANAPHYLACTIC SHOCK

Impaired spontaneous **Ventilation** r/t acute airway obstruction

Ineffective **Airway** clearance r/t laryngeal edema, bronchospasm

Latex **Allergy** response r/t abnormal immune mechanism response

*See Shock*

## ANASARCA

Excess **Fluid** volume r/t excessive fluid intake, cardiac/renal dysfunction, loss of plasma proteins

Risk for impaired **Skin** integrity r/t impaired circulation to skin

*See cause of Anasarca*

## ANEMIA

**Anxiety** r/t cause of disease

Delayed **Surgical** recovery r/t decreased oxygen supply to body, increased cardiac workload

**Fatigue** r/t decreased oxygen supply to the body, increased cardiac workload

Impaired **Memory** r/t anemia

Ineffective **Health** maintenance r/t deficient knowledge regarding nutritional and medical treatment of anemia

Ineffective **Protection** r/t bleeding disorder

Risk for **Injury** r/t alteration in peripheral sensory perception

## ANEMIA, IN PREGNANCY

**Anxiety** r/t concerns about health of self and fetus

**Fatigue** r/t decreased oxygen supply to the body, increased cardiac workload

Ineffective **Health** maintenance r/t deficient knowledge regarding nutrition in pregnancy

Risk for delayed **Development** r/t reduction in the oxygen-carrying capacity of blood

Risk for **Infection** r/t reduction in oxygen-carrying capacity of blood

## ANEMIA, SICKLE CELL

*See Anemia; Sickle Cell Anemia/Crisis*

## ANENCEPHALY

*See Neurotube Defects*

A

## ANEURYSM, ABDOMINAL SURGERY

Risk for deficient **Fluid** volume: hemorrhage r/t potential abnormal blood loss

Risk for ineffective **Tissue** perfusion: peripheral or renal r/t impaired arterial circulation

Risk for **Infection** r/t invasive procedure

*See Abdominal Surgery*

## ANEURYSM, CEREBRAL

*See Craniectomy/Craniotomy; Subarachnoid Hemorrhage (if aneurysm has ruptured)*

## ANGER

**Anxiety** r/t situational crisis

Defensive **Coping** r/t inability to acknowledge responsibility for actions and results of actions

**Fear** r/t environmental stressor, hospitalization

**Grieving** r/t significant loss

Impaired **Adjustment** r/t assault to self-esteem, disability requiring change in lifestyle, inadequate support system

**Powerlessness** r/t health care environment

Risk for other-directed **Violence** r/t history of violence, rage reaction

Risk for **Post-trauma** syndrome r/t inadequate social support

Risk for self-directed **Violence** r/t history of violence, history of abuse, rage reaction

## ANGINA PECTORIS

**Activity** intolerance r/t acute pain, dysrhythmias

Acute **Pain** r/t myocardial ischemia

Ineffective **Sexuality** pattern r/t disease process, medications, loss of libido

**Anxiety** r/t situational crisis

Decreased **Cardiac** output r/t myocardial ischemia, medication effect, dysrhythmia

**Grieving** r/t pain, lifestyle changes

Ineffective **Coping** r/t personal vulnerability to situational crisis of new diagnosis, deteriorating health

Ineffective **Denial** r/t deficient knowledge of need to seek help with symptoms

Ineffective **Health** maintenance r/t deficient knowledge of care of angina condition

## ANGIOCARDIOGRAPHY (CARDIAC CATHETERIZATION)

*See Cardiac Catheterization*

## ANGIOPLASTY, CORONARY

Decreased **Cardiac** output r/t ventricular ischemia, dysrhythmias

**Fear** r/t possible outcome of interventional procedure

Ineffective **Health** maintenance r/t deficient knowledge regarding care following procedures, measures to limit coronary artery disease

Risk for deficient **Fluid** volume r/t possible damage to coronary artery, hematoma formation, hemorrhage

Risk for ineffective **Tissue** perfusion: peripheral/cardiopulmonary r/t vasospasm, hematoma formation

## ANOMALY, FETAL/NEWBORN (PARENT DEALING WITH)

**Anxiety** r/t threat to role functioning, situational crisis

Chronic **Sorrow** r/t loss of ideal child

Decisional **Conflict**: interventions for fetus/newborn r/t lack of relevant information, spiritual distress, threat to value system

Deficient **Knowledge** r/t limited exposure to situation

Effective **Therapeutic** regimen management r/t verbalized intent to reduce risk factors for progression of illness and sequelae associated with anomaly

**Fear** r/t real or imagined threat to baby, implications for future pregnancies, powerlessness

**Hopelessness** r/t long-term stress, deteriorating physical condition of child, lost spiritual belief

Disabled family **Coping** r/t chronically unresolved feelings about loss of perfect baby

Ineffective **Coping** r/t personal vulnerability in situational crisis

Impaired **Parenting** r/t interruption of bonding process

Interrupted **Family** processes r/t unmet expectations for perfect baby, lack of adequate support systems

Parental role **Conflict** r/t separation from newborn, intimidation with invasive or restrictive modalities, specialized care center policies

**Powerlessness** r/t complication threatening fetus/newborn

Risk for dysfunctional **Grieving** r/t loss of perfect child

Risk for disorganized **Infant** behavior r/t congenital disorder

Risk for impaired parent/infant/child **Attachment** r/t ill infant who is unable to effectively initiate parental contact as result of altered behavioral organization

Risk for impaired **Parenting** r/t interruption of bonding process; unrealistic expectations for self, infant, or partner; perceived threat to own emotional survival; severe stress; lack of knowledge

Risk for **Spiritual** distress r/t lack of normal child to raise and carry on family name

**Self-esteem** disturbance r/t perceived inability to produce a perfect child

**Social** isolation r/t alterations in child's physical appearance, altered state of wellness

**Spiritual** distress r/t test of spiritual beliefs

## ANORECTAL ABSCESS

Acute **Pain** r/t inflammation of perirectal area

Disturbed **Body** image r/t odor and drainage from rectal area

Risk for **Constipation** r/t fear of painful elimination

## ANOREXIA

Deficient **Fluid** volume r/t inability to drink

Delayed **Surgical** recovery r/t inadequate nutritional intake

Imbalanced **Nutrition**: less than body requirements r/t loss of appetite, nausea, vomiting

## ANOREXIA NERVOSA

**Activity** intolerance r/t fatigue, weakness

Chronic low **Self-esteem** r/t repeated unmet expectations

**Constipation** r/t lack of adequate food, fiber, and fluid intake

Defensive **Coping** r/t psychological impairment, eating disorder

**Diarrhea** r/t laxative abuse

Disabled family **Coping** r/t highly ambivalent family relationships

Disturbed **Body** image r/t misconception of actual body appearance

Disturbed **Thought** processes r/t anorexia, impaired nutrition

Imbalanced **Nutrition**: less than body

A

requirements r/t inadequate food intake

Ineffective **Denial** r/t fear of consequences of therapy, possible weight gain

Ineffective family **Therapeutic** regimen management r/t family conflict, excessive demands on family associated with complexity of condition and treatment

Ineffective **Sexuality** pattern r/t loss of libido from malnutrition

Interrupted **Family** processes r/t situational crisis

Risk for **Infection** r/t malnutrition resulting in depressed immune system

Risk for **Spiritual** distress r/t low self-esteem

*See Maturational Issues, Adolescent*

## ANOSMIA (SMELL, LOSS OF ABILITY TO)

Disturbed **Sensory** perception: olfactory r/t altered sensory reception, transmission, integration

Imbalanced **Nutrition**: less than body requirements r/t loss of appetite associated with loss of smell

## ANTEPARTUM PERIOD

*See Pregnancy, Normal; Prenatal Care, Normal*

## ANTERIOR REPAIR, ANTERIOR COLPORRHAPHY

Risk for urge urinary **Incontinence** r/t trauma to bladder

**Urinary** retention r/t edema of urinary structures

*See Vaginal Hysterectomy*

## ANTICOAGULANT THERAPY

**Anxiety** r/t situational crisis

Ineffective **Health** maintenance r/t deficient knowledge regarding precautions to take with anticoagulant therapy

Ineffective **Protection** r/t altered clotting function from anticoagulant

Risk for deficient **Fluid** volume: hemorrhage r/t altered clotting mechanism

## ANTISOCIAL PERSONALITY DISORDER

Defensive **Coping** r/t excessive use of projection

Disturbed **Thought** processes r/t internal turmoil and conflict (intrusive thinking)

**Hopelessness** r/t abandonment

Impaired **Social** interaction r/t sociocultural conflict, chemical dependence, inability to form relationships

Ineffective **Coping** r/t frequently violating the norms and rules of society

Ineffective family **Therapeutic** regimen management r/t excessive demands on family

Risk for impaired **Parenting** r/t inability to function as parent or guardian, emotional instability

Risk for **Loneliness** r/t inability to interact appropriately with others

Risk for other-directed **Violence** r/t history of violence

Risk for **Self-mutilation** r/t self-hatred, depersonalization

**Spiritual** distress r/t separation from religious/cultural ties

## ANURIA

*See Renal Failure*

## ANXIETY

**Anxiety** r/t threat to or change in role status, unmet needs, interpersonal transmission/contagion, situational/maturational crisis, threat of death, threat to or change in health status, threat to or change in interaction patterns, threat to or change in role function, threat to self-concept, unconscious conflict regarding essential values/goals of life, threat to or change in environment, stress, threat to or change in economic status, substance abuse

Risk for **Powerlessness** r/t anxiety

Risk for situational low **Self-esteem** r/t anxiety

## ANXIETY DISORDER

**Anxiety** r/t unmet security and safety needs

Death **Anxiety** r/t fears of unknown, powerlessness

Decisional **Conflict** r/t low self-esteem, fear of making a mistake

Defensive **Coping** r/t overwhelming feelings of dread

Disabled family **Coping** r/t ritualistic behavior, actions

Disturbed **Energy** field r/t hopelessness, helplessness, fear

Disturbed **Sleep** pattern r/t psychological impairment, emotional instability

Disturbed **Thought** processes r/t anxiety

Ineffective **Coping** r/t inability to express feelings appropriately

Ineffective **Denial** r/t overwhelming feelings of hopelessness, fear, threat to self

**Powerlessness** r/t lifestyle of helplessness

Risk for **Spiritual** distress r/t psychological distress

**Self-care** deficit r/t ritualistic behavior, activities

**Sleep** deprivation r/t prolonged psychological discomfort

## AORTIC ANEURYSM REPAIR (ABDOMINAL SURGERY)

*See Abdominal Surgery; Aneurysm, Abdominal Surgery*

## AORTIC VALVULAR STENOSIS

*See Congenital Heart Disease/Cardiac Anomalies*

## APHASIA

**Anxiety** r/t situational crisis of aphasia

Impaired verbal **Communication** r/t decrease in circulation to brain

Ineffective **Coping** r/t loss of speech

Ineffective **Health** maintenance r/t deficient knowledge regarding information on aphasia and alternative communication techniques

## APLASTIC ANEMIA

**Activity** intolerance r/t imbalance between oxygen supply and demand

**Anxiety** r/t deficient knowledge of disease process and treatment

Delayed **Surgical** recovery r/t risk for infection

Impaired **Protection** r/t inadequate immune function

Risk for **Infection** r/t inadequate immune function

## APNEA IN INFANCY

*See Premature Infant (Child); Premature Infant (Parent); SIDS*

## APNEUSTIC RESPIRATIONS

Impaired **Breathing** pattern r/t perception/cognitive impairment, neurological impairment

*See cause of Apneustic Respirations*

## APPENDECTOMY

Acute **Pain** r/t surgical incision

Deficient **Fluid** volume r/t fluid restriction, hypermetabolic state, nausea, vomiting

Ineffective **Health** maintenance r/t deficient knowledge regarding self-care following appendectomy

Risk for **Infection** r/t perforation/rup-

A

ture of appendix, surgical incision, peritonitis

*See Hospitalized Child; Surgery, Postoperative*

## APPENDICITIS

Acute **Pain** r/t inflammation

Deficient **Fluid** volume r/t anorexia, nausea, vomiting

Delayed **Surgical** recovery r/t risk for infection

Risk for **Infection** r/t possible perforation of appendix

## APPREHENSION

**Anxiety** r/t threat to self-concept, threat to health status, situational crisis

Death **Anxiety** r/t apprehension over loss of self, consequences to significant others

## AMD (AGE-RELATED MACULAR DEGENERATION)

*See Macular Degeneration*

## ARDS (ACUTE RESPIRATORY DISTRESS SYNDROME)

Death **Anxiety** r/t seriousness of physical disease

Delayed **Surgical** recovery r/t complications associated with respiratory pathology

Impaired **Gas** exchange r/t damage to alveolar-capillary membrane, change in lung compliance

Impaired spontaneous **Ventilation** r/t damage to alveolar capillary membrane

Ineffective **Airway** clearance r/t excessive tracheobronchial secretions

*See Child with Chronic Condition; Ventilator Client*

## ARRHYTHMIA

*See Dysrhythmia*

## ARTERIAL INSUFFICIENCY

Delayed **Surgical** recovery r/t ineffective tissue perfusion

Ineffective **Tissue** perfusion: peripheral r/t interruption of arterial flow

## ARTHRITIS

**Activity** intolerance r/t chronic pain, fatigue, weakness

Chronic **Pain** r/t progression of joint deterioration

Chronic **Sorrow** r/t presence of chronic condition

Disturbed **Body** image r/t ineffective coping with joint abnormalities

Impaired physical **Mobility** r/t musculoskeletal impairment

Ineffective **Health** maintenance r/t deficient knowledge regarding care of arthritis

Risk for **Spiritual** distress r/t presence of chronic condition

**Self-care** deficit: specify r/t pain, musculoskeletal impairment

*See JRA (Juvenile Rheumatoid Arthritis)*

## ARTHROCENTESIS

Acute **Pain** r/t invasive procedure

## ARTHROPLASTY (TOTAL HIP REPLACEMENT)

Acute **Pain** r/t tissue trauma associated with surgery

**Constipation** r/t immobility

Impaired physical **Mobility** r/t decreased muscle strength, surgery

Impaired **Walking** r/t decreased muscle strength, surgery

Risk for **Infection** r/t invasive surgery, foreign object in body, anesthesia, immobility with stasis of respiratory secretions

Risk for **Injury** r/t interruption of arterial blood flow, dislocation of prosthesis

Risk for perioperative positioning **Injury** r/t immobilization, muscle weakness

Risk for **Peripheral** neurovascular dysfunction r/t orthopedic surgery

*See Surgery, Perioperative; Surgery, Postoperative; Surgery, Preoperative*

## ARTHROSCOPY

Ineffective **Health** maintenance r/t deficient knowledge regarding procedure, postoperative restrictions

## ASCITES

Chronic **Pain** r/t altered body function

Imbalanced **Nutrition**: less than body requirements r/t loss of appetite

Ineffective **Breathing** pattern r/t increased abdominal girth

Ineffective **Health** maintenance r/t deficient knowledge of care with condition of ascites

*See cause of Ascites; Cancer; Cirrhosis*

## ASPHYXIA, BIRTH

Anticipatory **Grieving** r/t loss of "perfect" child, concern of loss of future abilities

**Fear** (parental) r/t concern over safety of infant

Impaired **Gas** exchange r/t poor placental perfusion, lack of initiation of breathing by newborn

Impaired spontaneous **Ventilation** r/t brain injury

Ineffective **Breathing** pattern r/t depression of breathing reflex secondary to anoxia

Ineffective **Coping** r/t uncertainty of child outcome

Ineffective **Tissue** perfusion: cerebral r/t poor placental perfusion or cord compression resulting in lack of oxygen to brain

Risk for delayed **Development** r/t lack of oxygen to brain

Risk for disorganized **Infant** behavior r/t lack of oxygen to brain

Risk for disproportionate **Growth** r/t lack of oxygen to brain

Risk for impaired parent/infant **Attachment** r/t ill infant who is unable to initiate parental contact, hospitalization in critical care environment

Risk for **Injury** r/t lack of oxygen to brain

Risk for **Post-trauma** syndrome: parental r/t psychological trauma of sudden potential for loss of newborn

## ASPIRATION, DANGER OF

Risk for **Aspiration** r/t reduced level of consciousness; depressed cough or gag reflexes; presence of tracheostomy or endotracheal tube; incomplete lower esophageal sphincter; presence of gastrointestinal tubes or tube feedings; medication administration; situations hindering elevation of upper body; increased intragastric pressure; increased gastric residual; decreased gastrointestinal motility; delayed gastric emptying; impaired swallowing; facial, oral, or neck surgery or trauma; wired jaws

## ASSAULT VICTIM

**Post-trauma** syndrome r/t assault

**Rape-trauma** syndrome r/t rape

Risk for **Post-trauma** syndrome r/t perception of event, inadequate social support, nonsupportive environment, diminished ego strength, duration of event

Risk for **Spiritual** distress r/t physical, psychological stress

## ASSAULTIVE CLIENT

Disturbed **Thought** process r/t use of hallucinogenic substance, psychological disorder

A

Ineffective **Coping** r/t lack of control of impulsive actions

Risk for **Injury** r/t confused thought process, impaired judgment

Risk for other-directed **Violence** r/t paranoid ideation, anger

## ASTHMA

**Activity** intolerance r/t fatigue, energy shift to meet muscle needs for breathing to overcome airway obstruction

**Anxiety** r/t inability to breathe effectively, fear of suffocation

Disturbed **Body** image r/t decreased participation in physical activities

Impaired **Home** maintenance r/t deficient knowledge regarding control of environmental triggers

Ineffective **Airway** clearance r/t tracheobronchial narrowing, excessive secretions

Ineffective **Breathing** pattern r/t anxiety

Ineffective **Coping** r/t personal vulnerability to situational crisis

Ineffective **Health** maintenance r/t deficient knowledge regarding physical triggers, medications, treatment of early warning signs

**Sleep** deprivation r/t ineffective breathing pattern

*See Child with Chronic Condition; Hospitalized Child*

## ATAXIA

**Anxiety** r/t change in health status

Disturbed **Body** image r/t staggering gait

Impaired physical **Mobility** r/t neuromuscular impairment

Risk for **Injury** r/t gait alteration

## ATELECTASIS

Impaired **Gas** exchange r/t decreased alveolar-capillary surface

Ineffective **Breathing** pattern r/t loss of functional lung tissue, depression of respiratory function or hypoventilation because of pain

## ATHLETE'S FOOT

Impaired **Skin** integrity r/t effects of fungal agent

Ineffective **Health** maintenance r/t deficient knowledge regarding treatment and prevention of athlete's foot

*See Itching*

## ATN (ACUTE TUBULAR NECROSIS)

*See Renal Failure*

## ATRIAL FIBRILLATION

*See Dysrhythmia*

## ATRIAL SEPTAL DEFECT

*See Congenital Heart Disease/ Cardiac Anomalies*

## ATTENTION DEFICIT DISORDER

Disabled family **Coping** r/t significant person with chronically unexpressed feelings of guilt, anxiety, hostility, and despair

Impaired **Adjustment** r/t intense emotional state

Risk for delayed **Development** r/t behavior disorders

Risk for impaired **Parenting** r/t lack of knowledge of factors contributing to child's behavior

Risk for **Loneliness** r/t social isolation

Risk for **Spiritual** distress r/t poor relationships

**Self-esteem** disturbance r/t difficulty in participating in expected activities

**Social** isolation r/t unacceptable social behavior

## AUTISM

Compromised family **Coping** r/t parental guilt over etiology of disease, inability to accept or adapt to child's condition, inability to help child and other family members seek treatment

Delayed **Growth** and development r/t inability to develop relations with other human beings, inability to identify own body as separate from those of other people, inability to integrate concept of self

Disturbed personal **Identity** r/t inability to distinguish between self and environment, inability to identify own body as separate from those of other people, inability to integrate concept of self

Disturbed **Thought** processes r/t inability to perceive self or others, cognitive dissonance, perceptual dysfunction

Impaired **Social** interaction r/t communication barriers, inability to relate to others

Impaired verbal **Communication** r/t speech and language delays

Risk for delayed **Development** r/t autism

Risk for **Loneliness** r/t health alterations, change in cognition

Risk for other-directed **Violence** r/t frequent destructive rages toward others secondary to extreme response to changes in routine, fear of harmless things

Risk for self-directed **Violence** r/t frequent destructive rages toward self, secondary to extreme response to changes in routine, fear of harmless things

Risk for **Self-mutilation** r/t autistic state

*See Child with Chronic Condition; Mental Retardation*

## AUTONOMIC DYSREFLEXIA

**Autonomic** dysreflexia r/t bladder distention, bowel distention, noxious stimuli

Risk for **Autonomic** dysreflexia r/t bladder distention, bowel distention, noxious stimuli

## AUTONOMIC HYPERREFLEXIA

*See Autonomic Dysreflexia*

# B

## BACK PAIN

Acute **Pain** r/t back injury

**Anxiety** r/t situational crisis, back injury

Chronic **Pain** r/t back injury

Disturbed **Energy** field r/t chronic pain

Impaired physical **Mobility** r/t pain

Ineffective **Coping** r/t situational crisis, back injury

Ineffective **Health** maintenance r/t deficient knowledge regarding prevention of further injury, proper body mechanics

Risk for **Constipation** r/t decreased activity, side effect of pain medication

Risk for **Disuse** syndrome r/t severe pain

## BACTEREMIA

Ineffective **Protection** r/t compromised immune system

*See Infection; Infection, Potential for*

## BARREL CHEST

*See Aging (if appropriate); COPD (Chronic Obstructive Pulmonary Disease)*

## BATHING/HYGIENE PROBLEMS

Bathing/hygiene **Self-care** deficit r/t intolerance to activity, decreased strength and endurance, pain, discomfort, perceptual or cognitive impairment, neuromuscular impair-

B

ment, musculoskeletal impairment, depression, severe anxiety

Impaired bed **Mobility** r/t chronic physically limiting condition

## BATTERED CHILD SYNDROME

Acute **Pain** r/t physical injuries

Chronic low **Self-esteem** r/t lack of positive feedback, excessive negative feedback

Chronic **Sorrow** r/t situational crises

Deficient **Diversional** activity r/t diminished/absent environmental or personal stimuli

Delayed **Growth** and development: regression vs. delayed r/t diminished/absent environmental stimuli, inadequate caretaking, inconsistent responsiveness by caretaker

Disturbed **Sleep** pattern r/t hypervigilance, anxiety

Dysfunctional **Family** processes: alcoholism r/t inadequate coping skills

**Fear** r/t threat of punishment for perceived wrongdoing

Imbalanced **Nutrition**: less than body requirements r/t inadequate caretaking

Impaired **Skin** integrity r/t altered nutritional state, physical abuse

**Post-trauma** syndrome r/t physical abuse, incest, rape, molestation

Risk for delayed **Development** r/t shaken baby, abuse

Risk for disproportionate **Growth** r/t abuse

Risk for **Aspiration** r/t propped bottle

Risk for **Poisoning** r/t inadequate safeguards, lack of proper safety precautions, accessibility of illicit substances secondary to impaired home maintenance

Risk for **Post-trauma** syndrome r/t physical abuse, incest, rape, molestation

Risk for **Self-mutilation** r/t feelings of rejection, dysfunctional family

Risk for **Suffocation** r/t unattended child, unsafe environment

Risk for **Trauma** r/t inadequate precautions, cognitive or emotional difficulties

**Sleep** deprivation r/t prolonged psychological discomfort

**Social** isolation: family imposed r/t fear of disclosure of family dysfunction and abuse

## BATTERED PERSON

*See Abuse, Spouse, Parent, or Significant Other*

## BED MOBILITY, IMPAIRED

Impaired bed **Mobility** r/t intolerance to activity, decreased strength and endurance, pain or discomfort, perceptual or cognitive impairment, neuromuscular impairment, musculoskeletal impairment, depression, severe anxiety

## BEDBUGS, INFESTATION

Impaired **Home** maintenance r/t deficient knowledge regarding prevention of bedbug infestation

Impaired **Skin** integrity r/t bites of bedbugs

*See Itching*

## BEDREST, PROLONGED

Deficient **Diversional** activity r/t prolonged bedrest

Impaired bed **Mobility** r/t neuromuscular impairment

Risk for **Disuse** syndrome r/t prolonged immobility

Risk for **Loneliness** r/t prolonged bedrest

**Social** isolation r/t prolonged bedrest

## BEDSORES

*See Pressure Ulcer*

## BEDWETTING

*See Enuresis; Toilet Training*

## BELL'S PALSY

Acute **Pain** r/t inflammation of facial nerve

Disturbed **Body** image r/t loss of motor control on one side of face

Imbalanced **Nutrition**: less than body requirements r/t difficulty with chewing

Risk for **Injury** (eye) r/t dysfunction of facial nerve

## BENIGN PROSTATIC HYPERTROPHY

*See BPH (Benign Prostatic Hypertrophy); Prostatic Hypertrophy*

## BEREAVEMENT

Chronic **Sorrow** r/t death of loved one, chronic illness, disability

Disturbed **Sleep** pattern r/t grief

Dysfunctional **Grieving** r/t death of a loved one

**Grieving** r/t loss of significant person

Risk for **Spiritual** distress r/t death of a loved one

## BILIARY ATRESIA

**Anxiety** r/t surgical intervention, possible liver transplantation

Imbalanced **Nutrition**: less than body requirements r/t decreased absorption of fat and fat-soluble vitamins, poor feeding

Impaired **Comfort** r/t pruritus, nausea

Risk for impaired **Skin** integrity r/t pruritus

Risk for ineffective **Breathing** pattern r/t enlarged liver, development of ascites

Risk for **Injury**: bleeding r/t vitamin K deficiency, altered clotting mechanisms

*See Child with Chronic Condition; Cirrhosis (as complication); Hospitalized Child; Terminally Ill Child, Adolescent; Terminally Ill Child, Infant/Toddler; Terminally Ill Child, Preschool Child; Terminally Ill Child, School-Age-Child/Preadolescent; Terminally Ill Child, Death of Child, Parent*

## BILIARY CALCULUS

*See Cholelithiasis*

## BILIARY OBSTRUCTION

*See Jaundice*

## BIOPSY

**Fear** r/t outcome of biopsy

Ineffective **Health** maintenance r/t deficient knowledge regarding biopsy site, further needed health care

## BIOTERRORISM

Risk for **Infection** r/t exposure to harmful biological agent

Risk for **Injury** r/t harmful chemical agent exposure

Risk for **Post-Trauma** syndrome r/t perception of event of bioterrorism

## BIPOLAR DISORDER I (MOST RECENT EPISODE, DEPRESSED OR MANIC)

Chronic low **Self-esteem** r/t repeated unmet expectations

Disturbed **Energy** field r/t disharmony of mind, body, spirit

Dysfunctional **Grieving** r/t lack of previous resolution of former grieving response

**Fatigue** r/t psychological demands

Impaired **Adjustment** r/t low state of optimism

Ineffective **Coping** r/t dysfunctional grieving

B

Ineffective **Health** maintenance r/t lack of ability to make good judgments regarding ways to obtain help

Risk for **Loneliness** r/t stress, conflict

Risk for **Spiritual** distress r/t mental illness

**Self-care** deficit: specify r/t depression, cognitive impairment

**Social** isolation r/t ineffective coping

*See Depression; Manic Disorder, Bipolar I*

## BIRTH ASPHYXIA

*See Asphyxia, Birth*

## BIRTH CONTROL

*See Contraceptive Method*

## BLADDER CANCER

**Urinary** retention r/t clots obstructing urethra

*See Cancer; TURP*

## BLADDER DISTENTION

**Urinary** retention r/t high urethral pressure caused by weak detrusor, inhibition of reflex arc, blockage, strong sphincter

## BLADDER TRAINING

Disturbed **Body** image r/t difficulty in maintaining control of urinary elimination

Functional urinary **Incontinence** r/t altered environment; sensory, cognitive, mobility deficit

Ineffective **Health** maintenance r/t deficient knowledge regarding incontinence self-care

Stress urinary **Incontinence** r/t degenerative change in pelvic muscles and structural supports

Urge urinary **Incontinence** r/t decreased bladder capacity, increased urine concentration, overdistention of bladder

## BLEEDING TENDENCY

Ineffective **Protection** r/t abnormal blood profile, drug therapies

Risk for delayed **Surgical** recovery r/t bleeding tendency

## BLEPHAROPLASTY

Disturbed **Body** image r/t effects of surgery

Ineffective **Health** maintenance r/t deficient knowledge regarding postoperative care of surgical area

## BLINDNESS

Disturbed **Sensory** perception: visual r/t altered sensory reception, transmission, integration

Impaired **Home** maintenance r/t decreased vision

Ineffective **Role** performance r/t alteration in health status (change in visual acuity)

Interrupted **Family** processes r/t shift in health status of family member (change in visual acuity)

Risk for delayed **Development** r/t vision impairment

Risk for **Injury** r/t sensory dysfunction

**Self-care** deficit r/t inability to see to be able to perform activities of daily living

*See Vision Impairment*

## BLOOD DISORDER

Ineffective **Protection** r/t abnormal blood profile

*See cause of Blood Disorder*

## BLOOD PRESSURE ALTERATION

*See Hypertension; Hypotension; HTN*

## BLOOD TRANSFUSION

**Anxiety** r/t possibility of harm from transfusion

*See Anemia*

## BODY DYSMORPHIC DISORDER

Disturbed **Body** Image r/t over involvement in physical appearance

## BODY IMAGE CHANGE

Disturbed **Body** image r/t psychosocial, biophysical, cognitive/perceptual, cultural, spiritual, developmental changes; illness; trauma or injury; surgery; illness treatment

## BODY TEMPERATURE, ALTERED

Risk for imbalanced **Body** temperature r/t extremes of age or weight, exposure to cold or hot environment, dehydration, change in activity, effects of medication, dysfunction of body temperature regulation center

## BONE MARROW BIOPSY

Acute **Pain** r/t bone marrow aspiration

**Fear** r/t unknown outcome of results of biopsy

Ineffective **Health** maintenance r/t deficient knowledge of expectations following procedure, disease treatment following biopsy

*See disease necessitating bone marrow biopsy (e.g., Leukemia)*

## BORDERLINE PERSONALITY DISORDER

**Anxiety** r/t perceived threat to self-concept

Defensive **Coping** r/t difficulty with relationships, inability to accept blame for own behavior

Disturbed **Thought** processes r/t poor reality testing

Ineffective **Coping** r/t use of maladjusted defense mechanisms (e.g., projection, denial)

Ineffective family **Therapeutic** regimen management r/t manipulative behavior of client

**Powerlessness** r/t lifestyle of helplessness

Risk for **Caregiver** role strain r/t inability of care receiver to accept criticism, care receiver taking advantage of others to meet own needs or having unreasonable expectations

Risk for self-directed **Violence** r/t feelings of need to punish self, manipulative behavior

Risk for **Self-mutilation** r/t ineffective coping, feelings of self-hatred

Risk for **Spiritual** distress r/t poor relationships associated with behaviors attributed to borderline personality disorder

**Social** isolation r/t immature interests

## BOREDOM

Deficient **Diversional** activity r/t environmental lack of diversional activity

**Social** isolation r/t altered state of wellness

## BOTULISM

Deficient **Fluid** volume r/t profuse diarrhea

Ineffective **Health** maintenance r/t deficient knowledge regarding prevention of botulism, care following episode

## BOWEL INCONTINENCE

**Bowel** incontinence r/t decreased awareness of need to defecate, loss of sphincter control, fecal impaction

## BOWEL OBSTRUCTION

Acute **Pain** r/t pressure from distended abdomen

**Constipation** r/t decreased motility, intestinal obstruction

Deficient **Fluid** volume r/t inadequate fluid volume intake, fluid loss in bowel

Imbalanced **Nutrition**: less than body requirements r/t nausea, vomiting

B

B

## BOWEL RESECTION
*See Abdominal Surgery*

## BOWEL SOUNDS, ABSENT OR DIMINISHED

**Constipation** r/t decreased or absent peristalsis

Deficient **Fluid** volume r/t inability to ingest fluids, loss of fluids in bowel

Delayed **Surgical** recovery r/t inability to obtain adequate nutritional status

## BOWEL SOUNDS, HYPERACTIVE

**Diarrhea** r/t increased gastrointestinal motility

## BOWEL TRAINING

**Bowel** incontinence r/t loss of control of rectal sphincter

Ineffective **Health** maintenance r/t deficient knowledge regarding treatment of bowel incontinence

## BPH (BENIGN PROSTATIC HYPERTROPHY)

Disturbed **Sleep** pattern r/t nocturia

Ineffective **Health** maintenance r/t deficient knowledge regarding self-care with prostatic hypertrophy

Risk for **Infection** r/t urinary residual postvoiding, bacterial invasion of bladder

Risk for urge urinary **Incontinence** r/t detrusor muscle instability with impaired contractility, involuntary sphincter relaxation

**Urinary** retention r/t obstruction

*See Prostatic Hypertrophy*

## BRADYCARDIA

Decreased **Cardiac** output r/t slow heart rate supplying inadequate amount of blood for body function

Ineffective **Health** maintenance r/t deficient knowledge of condition, effects of cardiac medications

Ineffective **Tissue** perfusion: cerebral r/t decreased cardiac output secondary to bradycardia, vagal response

Risk for **Injury** r/t decreased cerebral tissue perfusion

## BRADYPNEA

Ineffective **Breathing** pattern r/t neuromuscular impairment, pain, musculoskeletal impairment, perception/cognitive impairment, anxiety, fatigue/decreased energy, effects of drugs

*See cause of Bradypnea*

## BRAIN INJURY
*See Intracranial Pressure, Increased*

## BRAIN SURGERY
*See Craniectomy/Craniotomy*

## BRAIN TUMOR

Acute **Pain** r/t pressure from tumor

Anticipatory **Grieving** r/t potential loss of physiopsychosocial well-being

Decreased **Intracranial** adaptive capacity r/t presence of brain tumor

Disturbed **Sensory** perception: specify r/t tumor growth compressing brain tissue

Disturbed **Thought** processes r/t altered circulation, destruction of brain tissue

**Fear** r/t threat to well-being

Risk for **Injury** r/t sensory-perceptual alterations, weakness

*See Cancer; Chemotherapy; Child with Chronic Condition; Craniectomy/Craniotomy; Hospitalized Child; Radiation Therapy; Terminally Ill Child, Adolescent; Terminally Ill Child, Infant/Toddler; Terminally Ill Child, Preschool Child; Terminally Ill Child, School-Age Child/Preadolescent; Terminally Ill Child, Death of Child, Parent*

## BRAXTON HICKS CONTRACTIONS

**Activity** intolerance r/t increased perception of contractions with increased gestation

**Anxiety** r/t uncertainty about beginning labor

Disturbed **Sleep** pattern r/t contractions when lying down

**Fatigue** r/t lack of sleep

Ineffective **Sexuality** patterns r/t fear of contractions

Stress urinary **Incontinence** r/t increased pressure on bladder with contractions

## BREAST BIOPSY

**Fear** r/t potential for diagnosis of cancer

Ineffective **Health** maintenance r/t deficient knowledge regarding appropriate postoperative care of breasts

Risk for **Spiritual** distress r/t fear of diagnosis of cancer

## BREAST CANCER

Chronic **Sorrow** r/t diagnosis of cancer, loss of body integrity

Death **Anxiety** r/t diagnosis of cancer

**Fear** r/t diagnosis of cancer

Ineffective **Coping** r/t treatment, prognosis

Risk for **Spiritual** distress r/t fear of diagnosis of cancer

**Sexual** dysfunction r/t loss of body part, partner's reaction to loss

*See Cancer; Chemotherapy; Mastectomy; Radiation Therapy*

## BREAST LUMPS

**Fear** r/t potential for diagnosis of cancer

Ineffective **Health** maintenance r/t deficient knowledge regarding appropriate care of breasts

## BREAST PUMPING

**Anxiety** r/t interrupted breastfeeding

Decisional **Conflict** r/t infant feeding method

Disturbed **Body** image r/t individual response to breastfeeding process

Ineffective **Health** maintenance r/t deficient knowledge regarding breast milk expression and storage

Risk for impaired **Skin** integrity r/t high suction

Risk for **Infection** r/t contaminated breast pump parts, incomplete emptying of breast

## BREASTFEEDING, EFFECTIVE

Effective **Breastfeeding** r/t basic breastfeeding knowledge, normal breast structure, normal infant oral structure, infant gestational age >34 weeks, support sources, maternal confidence

## BREASTFEEDING, INEFFECTIVE

Impaired **Swallowing** r/t prematurity of infant

Ineffective **Breastfeeding** r/t prematurity, infant anomaly, maternal breast anomaly, previous breast surgery, previous history of breastfeeding failure, infant receiving supplemental feedings with artificial nipple, poor infant sucking reflex, nonsupportive partner/family, deficient knowledge, interruption in breastfeeding, maternal anxiety or ambivalence

Ineffective **Infant** feeding pattern r/t prematurity of infant

*See Painful Breasts, Sore Nipples; Painful Breasts, Engorgement*

B

B

## BREASTFEEDING, INTERRUPTED

Interrupted **Breastfeeding** r/t maternal or infant illness, prematurity, maternal employment, contraindications to breastfeeding (e.g., drugs, true breast milk jaundice), need to abruptly wean infant

## BREATH SOUNDS, DECREASED OR ABSENT

*See Atelectasis; Pneumothorax*

## BREATHING PATTERN ALTERATION

Ineffective **Breathing** pattern r/t neuromuscular impairment, pain, musculoskeletal impairment, perception/cognitive impairment, anxiety, decreased energy/fatigue

## BREECH BIRTH

**Anxiety**: maternal r/t threat to self, infant

**Fear**: maternal r/t danger to infant, self

Impaired **Gas** exchange: fetal r/t compressed umbilical cord

Ineffective **Tissue** perfusion: cerebral r/t compressed umbilical cord

Risk for **Aspiration**: fetal r/t birth of body before head

Risk for delayed **Development** r/t compressed umbilical cord

Risk for impaired **Tissue** integrity: fetal r/t difficult birth

Risk for impaired **Tissue** integrity: maternal r/t difficult birth

## BRONCHITIS

**Anxiety** r/t potential chronic condition

**Health**-seeking behavior r/t wish to stop smoking

Ineffective **Airway** clearance r/t excessive thickened mucus secretion

Ineffective **Health** maintenance r/t deficient knowledge regarding care of condition

## BRONCHOPULMONARY DYSPLASIA

**Activity** intolerance r/t imbalance between oxygen supply and demand

Excess **Fluid** volume r/t sodium and water retention

Imbalanced **Nutrition**: less than body requirements r/t poor feeding, increased caloric needs secondary to increased work of breathing

*See Child with Chronic Condition; Hospitalized Child; Respiratory Conditions of the Neonate*

## BRONCHOSCOPY

Risk for **Aspiration** r/t temporary loss of gag reflex

Risk for **Injury** r/t complication of pneumothorax, laryngeal edema, hemorrhage (if biopsy done)

## BRUITS, CAROTID

Ineffective **Tissue** perfusion: cerebral r/t interruption of carotid blood flow

Risk for **Injury** r/t loss of motor, sensory, visual function

## BRYANT'S TRACTION

*See Traction and Casts*

## BUCK'S TRACTION

*See Traction and Casts*

## BUERGER'S DISEASE

*See Peripheral Vascular Disease*

## BULIMIA

Chronic low **Self-esteem** r/t lack of positive feedback

Defensive **Coping** r/t eating disorder

Disturbed **Body** image r/t misperception about actual appearance, body weight

**Fear** r/t food ingestion, weight gain

Imbalanced **Nutrition**: less than body requirements r/t induced vomiting

Compromised family **Coping** r/t chronically unresolved feelings of guilt, anger, hostility

**Noncompliance** r/t negative feelings toward treatment regimen

**Powerlessness** r/t urge to purge self after eating

*See Maturational Issues, Adolescent*

## BUNION

Ineffective **Health** maintenance r/t deficient knowledge regarding appropriate care of feet

## BUNIONECTOMY

Impaired physical **Mobility** r/t sore foot

Impaired **Walking** r/t pain associated with surgery

Ineffective **Health** maintenance r/t deficient knowledge regarding postoperative care of feet

Risk for **Infection** r/t surgical incision, advanced age

## BURNS

Acute **Pain** r/t burn injury, treatments

Anticipatory **Grieving** r/t loss of bodily function, loss of future hopes and plans

Deficient **Diversional** activity r/t long-term hospitalization

Delayed **Surgical** recovery r/t ineffective tissue perfusion

Disturbed **Body** image r/t altered physical appearance

**Fear** r/t pain from treatments, possible permanent disfigurement

**Hypothermia** r/t impaired skin integrity

Imbalanced **Nutrition**: less than body requirements r/t increased metabolic needs, anorexia, protein and fluid loss

Impaired physical **Mobility** r/t pain, musculoskeletal impairment, contracture formation

Impaired **Skin** integrity r/t injury of skin

Ineffective **Tissue** perfusion: peripheral r/t circumferential burns, impaired arteriovenous circulation

**Post-trauma** syndrome r/t life-threatening event

Risk for deficient **Fluid** volume r/t loss from skin surface, fluid shift

Risk for ineffective **Airway** clearance r/t potential tracheobronchial obstruction, edema

Risk for **Infection** r/t loss of intact skin, trauma, invasive sites

Risk for **Peripheral** neurovascular dysfunction r/t eschar formation with circumferential burn

Risk for **Post-trauma** syndrome r/t perception, duration of event that caused burns

*See Hospitalized Child; Safety, Childhood*

## BURSITIS

Acute **Pain** r/t inflammation in joint

Impaired physical **Mobility** r/t inflammation in joint

## BYPASS GRAFT

*See Coronary Artery Bypass Grafting*

## CACHEXIA

Adult **Failure** to thrive r/t imbalanced nutrition: less than body requirements

Imbalanced **Nutrition**: less than body requirements r/t inability to ingest food because of biological factors

Ineffective **Protection** r/t inadequate nutrition

## CALCIUM ALTERATION

*See Hypercalcemia; Hypocalcemia*

## CANCER

**Activity** intolerance r/t side effects of treatment, weakness from cancer

Anticipatory **Grieving** r/t potential loss of significant others, high risk for infertility

Chronic **Pain** r/t metastatic cancer

Chronic **Sorrow** r/t chronic illness of cancer

Compromised family **Coping** r/t prolonged disease or disability progression that exhausts supportive ability of significant others

**Constipation** r/t side effects of medication, altered nutrition, decreased activity

Death **Anxiety** r/t unresolved issues regarding dying

Decisional **Conflict** r/t selection of treatment choices, continuation/discontinuation of treatment, "do not resuscitate" decision

Disturbed **Body** image r/t side effects of treatment, cachexia

Disturbed **Sleep** pattern r/t anxiety, pain

**Fear** r/t serious threat to well-being

**Hopelessness** r/t loss of control, terminal illness

Imbalanced **Nutrition**: less than body requirements r/t loss of appetite, difficulty swallowing, side effects of chemotherapy, obstruction by tumor

Impaired physical **Mobility** r/t weakness, neuromusculoskeletal impairment, pain

Impaired **Skin** integrity r/t immunological deficit, immobility

Impaired **Oral** mucous membranes r/t chemotherapy, effects of radiation, oral pH changes, decreased oral secretions

Ineffective **Coping** r/t personal vulnerability in situational crisis, terminal illness

Ineffective **Denial** r/t dysfunctional grieving process

Ineffective **Health** maintenance r/t deficient knowledge regarding prescribed treatment

Ineffective **Protection** r/t cancer suppressing immune system

Ineffective **Role** performance r/t change in physical capacity, inability to resume prior role

**Powerlessness** r/t treatment, progression of disease

Readiness for enhanced **Spiritual** well-being r/t desire for harmony with self, others, higher power/God when faced with serious illness

Risk for **Disuse** syndrome r/t severe pain, change in level of consciousness

Risk for impaired **Home** maintenance r/t lack of familiarity with community resources

Risk for **Infection** r/t inadequate immune system

Risk for **Injury** r/t bleeding secondary to bone marrow depression

Risk for **Spiritual** distress r/t physical illness of cancer

**Self-care** deficit: specify r/t pain, intolerance to activity, decreased strength

**Social** isolation r/t hospitalization, lifestyle changes

**Spiritual** distress r/t test of spiritual beliefs

*See Chemotherapy; Child with Chronic Condition; Hospitalized Child; Radiation Therapy; Terminally Ill Child, Adolescent; Terminally Ill Child, Infant/Toddler; Terminally Ill Child, Preschool Child;*

*Terminally Ill Child, School-Age Child/Preadolescent; Terminally Ill Child, Death of Child, Parent*

## CANDIDIASIS, ORAL

Impaired **Oral** mucous membranes r/t overgrowth of infectious agent, depressed immune function

Ineffective **Health** maintenance r/t deficient knowledge regarding care of infected mouth

## CAPILLARY REFILL TIME, PROLONGED

Impaired **Gas** exchange r/t ventilation perfusion imbalance

Ineffective **Tissue** perfusion: peripheral r/t interruption of arterial or venous flow

*See Shock*

## CARDIAC ARREST

**Post-trauma** syndrome r/t sustaining serious life event

*See cause of Cardiac Arrest*

## CARDIAC CATHETERIZATION

**Anxiety** r/t invasive procedure, uncertainty of outcome of procedure

Decreased **Cardiac** output r/t ventricular ischemia, dysrhythmia

Impaired **Comfort** r/t postprocedure restrictions, invasive procedure

Ineffective **Health** maintenance r/t deficient knowledge regarding procedure, postprocedure care, treatment and prevention of coronary artery disease

Risk for ineffective **Tissue** perfusion r/t impaired arterial or venous circulation

Risk for **Injury**: hematoma r/t invasive procedure

Risk for **Peripheral** neurovascular dysfunction r/t vascular obstruction

## CARDIAC DISORDERS

Decreased **Cardiac** output r/t cardiac disorder

*See specific cardiac disorder*

C

## CARDIAC DISORDERS IN PREGNANCY

**Activity** intolerance r/t cardiac pathophysiology, increased demand secondary to pregnancy, weakness, fatigue

**Anxiety** r/t unknown outcomes of pregnancy, family well-being

Compromised family **Coping** r/t prolonged hospitalization/maternal incapacitation that exhausts supportive capacity of significant others

Death **Anxiety** r/t potential danger of condition

**Fatigue** r/t metabolic demands, psychological and emotional demands

**Fear** r/t potential maternal effects, potential poor fetal/maternal outcome

Ineffective **Coping** r/t personal vulnerability

Ineffective **Health** maintenance r/t deficient knowledge regarding treatment, restrictions with cardiac disorder

Ineffective **Role** performance r/t changes in lifestyle, expectations secondary to disease process with superimposed pregnancy

Interrupted **Family** processes r/t hospitalization, maternal incapacitation, changes in roles

**Powerlessness** r/t illness-related regimen

Risk for delayed **Development** r/t poor maternal oxygenation

Risk for disproportionate **Growth** r/t poor maternal oxygenation

Risk for excess **Fluid** volume r/t compromised regulatory mechanism with increased afterload, preload, circulating blood volume

C

Risk for imbalanced **Fluid** volume r/t sudden changes in circulation following delivery of placenta

Risk for impaired **Gas** exchange r/t pulmonary edema

Risk for ineffective **Tissue** perfusion: fetal r/t poor maternal oxygenation

Risk for **Spiritual** distress r/t fear of diagnosis for self and infant

Situational low **Self-esteem** r/t situational crisis, pregnancy

**Social** isolation r/t limitations of activity, bedrest/hospitalization, separation from family and friends

## CARDIAC DYSRHYTHMIA

*See Dysrhythmia*

## CARDIAC OUTPUT DECREASE

Decreased **Cardiac** output r/t cardiac dysfunction

## CARDIAC TAMPONADE

Decreased **Cardiac** output r/t fluid in pericardial sac

*See Pericarditis*

## CARDIOGENIC SHOCK

Decreased **Cardiac** output r/t decreased myocardial contractility, dysrhythmia

*See Shock*

## CAREGIVER ROLE STRAIN

**Caregiver** role strain r/t pathophysiological factors, developmental factors, psychosocial factors, situational factors

Risk for **Caregiver** role strain r/t pathophysiological factors, developmental factors, psychosocial factors, situational factors

## CARIOUS TEETH

*See Cavities in Teeth*

## CAROTID ENDARTERECTOMY

**Fear** r/t surgery in vital area

Ineffective **Health** maintenance r/t deficient knowledge regarding postoperative care

Risk for ineffective **Airway** clearance r/t hematoma compressing trachea

Risk for ineffective **Tissue** perfusion: cerebral r/t hemorrhage, clot formation

Risk for **Injury** r/t possible hematoma formation

## CARPAL TUNNEL SYNDROME

Chronic **Pain** r/t unrelieved pressure on median nerve

Impaired physical **Mobility** r/t neuromuscular impairment

**Self-care** deficit: bathing/hygiene, dressing/grooming, feeding r/t pain

## CARPOPEDAL SPASM

*See Hypocalcemia*

## CASTS

Deficient **Diversional** activity r/t physical limitations from cast

Ineffective **Health** maintenance r/t deficient knowledge regarding cast care, personal care with cast

Impaired physical **Mobility** r/t limb immobilization

Impaired **Walking** r/t cast(s) on lower extremities, fracture of bones

Risk for impaired **Skin** integrity r/t unrelieved pressure on skin

Risk for **Peripheral** neurovascular dysfunction r/t mechanical compression from cast(s)

**Self-care** deficit: bathing/hygiene, dressing/grooming, feeding r/t presence of cast(s) on upper extremities

**Self-care** deficit: toileting r/t presence of cast(s) on lower extremities

## CATARACT EXTRACTION

**Anxiety** r/t threat of permanent vision loss, surgical procedure

Disturbed **Sensory** perception: vision r/t edema from surgery

Ineffective **Health** maintenance r/t deficient knowledge regarding postoperative restrictions

Risk for **Injury** r/t increased intraocular pressure, accommodation to new visual field

*See Vision Impairment*

## CATARACTS

Disturbed **Sensory** perception: vision r/t altered sensory input

*See Vision Impairment*

## CATATONIC SCHIZOPHRENIA

Imbalanced **Nutrition**: less than body requirements r/t decrease in outside stimulation, loss of perception of hunger, resistance to instructions to eat

Impaired **Memory** r/t cognitive impairment

Impaired physical **Mobility** r/t cognitive impairment, maintenance of rigid posture, inappropriate/bizarre postures

Impaired verbal **Communication** r/t muteness

**Social** isolation r/t inability to communicate, immobility

*See Schizophrenia*

## CATHETERIZATION, URINARY

Ineffective **Health** maintenance r/t deficient knowledge of normal sensation of catheter in place, care of catheter

Risk for **Infection** r/t invasive procedure

## CAVITIES IN TEETH

Impaired **Dentition** r/t ineffective oral hygiene, barriers to self-care, economic barriers to professional care, nutritional deficits, dietary habits

Ineffective **Health** maintenance r/t lack of knowledge regarding prevention of dental disease secondary to high-sugar diet, giving infants/toddlers with erupted teeth bottles of milk at bedtime, lack of fluoride treatments, inadequate or improper brushing of teeth

## CELLULITIS

Acute **Pain** r/t inflammatory changes in tissues from infection

Impaired **Skin** integrity r/t inflammatory process damaging skin

Ineffective **Health** maintenance r/t lack of knowledge regarding prevention of further incidences of infection

Ineffective **Tissue** perfusion: peripheral r/t edema

## CELLULITIS, PERIORBITAL

Acute **Pain** r/t edema and inflammation of skin/tissues

Disturbed **Sensory** perception: visual r/t decreased visual fields secondary to edema of eyelids

**Hyperthermia** r/t infectious process

Impaired **Skin** integrity r/t inflammation/infection of skin/tissues

*See Hospitalized Child*

## CENTRAL LINE INSERTION

Ineffective **Health** maintenance r/t deficient knowledge regarding precautions to take when central line in place

Risk for **Infection** r/t invasive procedure

C

## CEREBRAL ANEURYSM

*See Craniectomy/Craniotomy; Intracranial Pressure, Increased; Subarachnoid Hemorrhage*

## CEREBRAL PALSY

Chronic **Sorrow** r/t presence of chronic disability

Deficient **Diversional** activity r/t physical impairments, limitations on ability to participate in recreational activities

Imbalanced **Nutrition**: less than body requirements r/t spasticity, feeding or swallowing difficulties

Impaired physical **Mobility** r/t spasticity, neuromuscular impairment/weakness

Impaired **Social** interaction r/t impaired communication skills, limited physical activity, perceived differences from peers

Impaired verbal **Communication** r/t impaired ability to articulate/speak words secondary to facial muscle involvement

Risk for delayed **Development** r/t chronic illness

Risk for disproportionate **Growth** r/t chronic illness

Risk for **Falls** r/t impaired physical mobility

Risk for impaired **Parenting** r/t caring for child with overwhelming needs resulting from chronic change in health status

Risk for **Injury** r/t muscle weakness, inability to control spasticity

Risk for **Spiritual** distress r/t psychic and psychological stress associated with chronic illness

**Self-care** deficit: specify r/t neuromuscular impairments, sensory deficits

*See Child with Chronic Condition*

## CEREBROVASCULAR ACCIDENT

*See CVA (Cerebrovascular Accident)*

## CERVICITIS

Ineffective **Health** maintenance r/t deficient knowledge regarding care and prevention of condition

Ineffective **Sexuality** patterns r/t abstinence during acute stage

Risk for **Infection** r/t spread of infection, recurrence of infection

## CESAREAN DELIVERY

Acute **Pain** r/t surgical incision, decreased or absent peristalsis secondary to anesthesia, manipulation of abdominal organs during surgery

**Anxiety** r/t unmet expectations for childbirth, unknown outcome of surgery

Disturbed **Body** image r/t surgery, unmet expectations for childbirth

**Fear** r/t perceived threat to own well-being

Impaired **Comfort**: nausea, vomiting, pruritus r/t side effects of systemic or epidural narcotics

Impaired physical **Mobility** r/t pain

Ineffective **Health** maintenance r/t deficient knowledge regarding postoperative care

Ineffective **Role** performance r/t unmet expectations for childbirth

Interrupted **Family** processes r/t unmet expectations for childbirth

Risk for deficient **Fluid** volume r/t increased blood loss secondary to surgery

Risk for imbalanced **Fluid** volume r/t loss of blood

Risk for **Infection** r/t surgical incision, stasis of respiratory secretions secondary to general anesthesia

Risk for **Post-trauma** syndrome r/t emergency condition to save life of mother or baby

Risk for **Urinary** retention r/t regional anesthesia

Situational low **Self-esteem** r/t inability to deliver child vaginally

## CHEMICAL DEPENDENCE

*See Alcoholism; Drug Abuse*

## CHEMOTHERAPY

Death **Anxiety** r/t chemotherapy not accomplishing desired results

Delayed **Surgical** recovery r/t compromised immune system

Disturbed **Body** image r/t loss of weight, loss of hair

**Fatigue** r/t disease process, anemia, drug effects

Imbalanced **Nutrition**: less than body requirements r/t side effects of chemotherapy

Impaired **Oral** mucous membranes r/t effects of chemotherapy

Ineffective **Health** maintenance r/t deficient knowledge regarding action, side effects, way to integrate chemotherapy into lifestyle

Ineffective **Protection** r/t suppressed immune system, decreased platelets

**Nausea** r/t effects of chemotherapy

Risk for deficient **Fluid** volume r/t vomiting, diarrhea

Risk for ineffective **Tissue** perfusion r/t anemia

Risk for **Infection** r/t immunosuppression

*See Cancer*

## CHEST PAIN

Acute **Pain** r/t myocardial injury, ischemia

Decreased **Cardiac** output r/t ventricular ischemia

**Fear** r/t potential threat of death

*See Angina Pectoris; MI (Myocardial Infarction)*

## CHEST TUBES

Acute **Pain** r/t presence of chest tubes, injury

Impaired **Gas** exchange r/t decreased functional lung tissue

Ineffective **Breathing** pattern r/t asymmetrical lung expansion secondary to pain

Risk for **Injury** r/t presence of invasive chest tube

## CHEYNE-STOKES RESPIRATION

Ineffective **Breathing** pattern r/t critical illness

*See cause of Cheyne-Stokes Respiration*

## CHF (CONGESTIVE HEART FAILURE)

**Activity** intolerance r/t weakness, fatigue

**Constipation** r/t activity intolerance

Decreased **Cardiac** output r/t impaired cardiac function

Excess **Fluid** volume r/t impaired excretion of sodium and water

**Fatigue** r/t disease process

**Fear** r/t threat to one's own well-being

Impaired **Gas** exchange r/t excessive fluid in interstitial space of lungs, alveoli

Ineffective **Health** maintenance r/t deficient knowledge regarding care of disease

**Powerlessness** r/t illness-related regimen

*See Child with Chronic Condition; Congenital Heart Disease/ Cardiac Anomalies; Hospitalized Child*

## CHICKENPOX

*See Communicable Diseases, Childhood*

C

## CHILD ABUSE

Acute **Pain** r/t physical injuries

Chronic low **Self-esteem** r/t lack of positive feedback, excessive negative feedback

Deficient **Diversional** activity r/t diminished or absent environmental/personal stimuli

Delayed **Growth** and development: regression vs. delayed r/t diminished/absent environmental stimuli, inadequate caretaking, inconsistent responsiveness by caretaker

Disturbed **Sleep** pattern r/t hypervigilance, anxiety

**Fear** r/t threat of punishment for perceived wrongdoing

Imbalanced **Nutrition**: less than body requirements r/t inadequate caretaking

Impaired **Parenting** r/t psychological impairment, physical or emotional abuse of parent, substance abuse, unrealistic expectations of child

Impaired **Skin** integrity r/t altered nutritional state, physical abuse

Ineffective community **Therapeutic** regimen management r/t deficits in community regarding prevention of child abuse

Interrupted **Family** process: alcoholism r/t inadequate coping skills

**Post-trauma** syndrome r/t physical abuse, incest, rape, molestation

Risk for delayed **Development** r/t shaken baby, abuse

Risk for disproportionate **Growth** r/t abuse

Risk for **Poisoning** r/t inadequate safeguards, lack of proper safety precautions, accessibility of illicit substances secondary to impaired home maintenance

Risk for **Suffocation** r/t unattended child, unsafe environment

Risk for **Trauma** r/t inadequate precautions, cognitive or emotional difficulties

**Social** isolation: family imposed r/t fear of disclosure of family dysfunction and abuse

## CHILD NEGLECT

*See Child Abuse; Failure to Thrive, Nonorganic*

## CHILD WITH CHRONIC CONDITION

**Activity** intolerance r/t fatigue associated with chronic illness

Chronic low **Self-esteem** r/t actual or perceived differences; peer acceptance; decreased ability to participate in physical, school, and social activities

Chronic **Pain** r/t physical, biological, chemical, or psychological factors

Chronic **Sorrow** r/t developmental stages and missed opportunities or milestones that bring comparisons with social or personal norms, unending caregiving as reminder of loss

Compromised family **Coping** r/t prolonged overconcern for child; distortion of reality regarding child's health problem, including extreme denial about its existence or severity

Decisional **Conflict** r/t treatment options, conflicting values

Deficient **Diversional** activity r/t immobility, monotonous environment, frequent/lengthy treatments, reluctance to participate, self-imposed social isolation

Deficient **Knowledge** r/t knowledge/skill acquisition regarding health practices, acceptance of limitations, promotion of maximal potential of child, self-actualization of rest of family

Delayed **Growth** and development r/t regression or lack of progression toward developmental milestones secondary to frequent or prolonged hospitalization, inadequate or inappropriate stimulation, cerebral insult, chronic illness, effects of physical disability, prescribed dependence

Disabled family **Coping** r/t prolonged disease or disability progression that exhausts supportive capacity of significant people

Disturbed **Sleep** pattern: child or parent r/t time-intensive treatments, exacerbation of condition, 24-hour care needs

**Hopelessness**: child r/t prolonged activity restriction, long-term stress, lack of involvement in or passively allowing care secondary to parental overprotection

Imbalanced **Nutrition**: less than body requirements r/t anorexia, fatigue secondary to physical exertion

Imbalanced **Nutrition**: more than body requirements r/t effects of steroid medications on appetite

Impaired **Home** maintenance r/t overtaxed family members (e.g., exhausted, anxious)

Impaired **Social** interaction r/t developmental lag/delay, perceived differences

Ineffective **Coping**: child r/t situational or maturational crises

Ineffective **Health** maintenance r/t exhausting family resources (finances, physical energy, support systems)

Ineffective **Sexuality** patterns: parental r/t disrupted relationship with sexual partner

Interrupted **Family** processes r/t intermittent situational crisis of illness, disease, hospitalization

Parental role **Conflict** r/t separation from child as a result of chronic illness, home care of child with special needs, interruptions of family life resulting from home care regimen

**Powerlessness**: child r/t health care environment, illness-related regimen, lifestyle of learned helplessness

Readiness for enhanced family **Coping** r/t impact of crisis on family values, priorities, goals, or relationships; changes in family choices to optimize wellness

Risk for delayed **Development** r/t chronic illness

Risk for disproportionate **Growth** r/t chronic illness

Risk for impaired **Parenting** r/t impaired/disrupted bonding, caring for child with perceived overwhelming care needs

Risk for **Infection** r/t debilitating physical condition

**Social** isolation: family r/t actual or perceived social stigmatization, complex care requirements

## CHILDBIRTH

*See Labor, Normal; Postpartum, Normal Care*

## CHILLS

**Hyperthermia** r/t infectious process

## CHLAMYDIA INFECTION

*See STD (Sexually Transmitted Disease)*

## CHOKING/COUGHING WITH FEEDING

Impaired **Swallowing** r/t neuromuscular impairment

Risk for **Aspiration** r/t depressed cough and gag reflexes

C

## CHOLASMA

Disturbed **Body** image r/t change in skin color

## CHOLECYSTECTOMY

Acute **Pain** r/t trauma from surgery

Imbalanced **Nutrition**: less than body requirements r/t high metabolic needs, decreased ability to digest fatty foods

Ineffective **Health** maintenance r/t deficient knowledge regarding postoperative care

Risk for deficient **Fluid** volume r/t restricted intake, nausea, vomiting

Risk for ineffective **Breathing** pattern r/t proximity of incision to lungs resulting in pain with deep breathing

*See Abdominal Surgery*

## CHOLELITHIASIS

Acute **Pain** r/t obstruction of bile flow, inflammation in gallbladder

Imbalanced **Nutrition**: less than body requirements r/t anorexia, nausea, vomiting

Ineffective **Health** maintenance r/t deficient knowledge regarding care of disease

## CHORIOAMNIONITIS

Anticipatory **Grieving** r/t guilt about potential loss of ideal pregnancy and birth

**Anxiety** r/t threat to self and infant

**Hyperthermia** r/t infectious process

Risk for delayed **Growth** and development r/t risk of preterm birth

Risk for **Infection** transmission from mother to fetus r/t infection in fetal environment

Situational low **Self-esteem** r/t guilt about threat to infant's health

## CHRONIC CONFUSION

*See Confusion, Chronic*

## CHRONIC LYMPHOCYTIC LEUKEMIA

*See Cancer; Chemotherapy; Leukemia*

## CHRONIC OBSTRUCTIVE PULMONARY DISEASE

*See COPD (Chronic Obstructive Pulmonary Disease)*

## CHRONIC PAIN

*See Pain, Chronic*

## CHRONIC RENAL FAILURE

*See Renal Failure*

## CHVOSTEK'S SIGN

*See Hypocalcemia*

## CIRCUMCISION

Acute **Pain** r/t surgical intervention

Ineffective **Health** maintenance r/t deficient knowledge (parental) regarding care of surgical area

Risk for deficient **Fluid** volume r/t hemorrhage

Risk for **Infection** r/t surgical wound

## CIRRHOSIS

Chronic low **Self-esteem** r/t chronic illness

Chronic **Pain** r/t liver enlargement

Chronic **Sorrow** r/t presence of chronic illness

**Diarrhea** r/t dietary changes, medications

Disturbed **Thought** processes r/t chronic organic disorder with increased ammonia levels, substance abuse

**Fatigue** r/t malnutrition

Imbalanced **Nutrition**: less than body requirements r/t loss of appetite, nausea, vomiting

Ineffective **Health** maintenance r/t deficient knowledge regarding correlation between lifestyle habits and disease process

Ineffective management of **Therapeutic** regimen r/t denial of severity of illness

Ineffective **Protection** r/t risk of impaired blood coagulation, bleeding from portal hypertension

**Nausea** r/t irritation to gastrointestinal system

Risk for deficient **Fluid** volume: hemorrhage r/t abnormal bleeding from esophagus

Risk for impaired **Oral** mucous membranes r/t altered nutrition

Risk for impaired **Skin** integrity r/t altered nutritional state, altered metabolic state

Risk for **Injury** r/t substance intoxication, potential delirium tremors

## CJD (CREUTZFELDT-JAKOB DISEASE)

Acute **Pain** r/t neck (nuchal) rigidity, inflammation of meninges, headache, kinesthetic

Decreased **Intracranial** adaptive capacity r/t sustained increase in intracranial pressure

Delayed **Growth** and development r/t brain damage secondary to infectious process, increased intracranial pressure

Disturbed **Sensory** perception: hearing r/t central nervous system infection, ear infection

Disturbed **Sensory** perception: kinesthetic r/t central nervous system infection

Disturbed **Thought** processes r/t inflammation of brain, fever

Excess **Fluid** volume r/t increased intracranial pressure, syndrome of inappropriate secretion of antidiuretic hormone (SIADH)

Impaired **Comfort** r/t central nervous system inflammation

Impaired **Comfort**: photophobia r/t increased sensitivity to external stimuli secondary to central nervous system inflammation

Impaired physical **Mobility** r/t neuromuscular or central nervous system insult

Ineffective **Airway** clearance r/t seizure activity

Ineffective **Tissue** perfusion: cerebral r/t inflamed cerebral tissues and meninges, increased intracranial pressure

Risk for **Aspiration** r/t seizure activity

Risk for **Falls** r/t neuromuscular dysfunction

Risk for **Injury** r/t seizure activity

## CLEFT LIP/CLEFT PALATE

Acute **Pain** r/t surgical correction, elbow restraints

Chronic **Sorrow** r/t loss of perfect child, birth of child with congenital defect

**Fear**: parental r/t special care needs, surgery

**Grieving** r/t loss of perfect child, birth of child with congenital defect

Imbalanced **Nutrition**: less than body requirements r/t inability to feed with normal techniques

Impaired **Oral** mucous membranes r/t surgical correction

Impaired physical **Mobility** r/t imposed restricted activity, use of elbow restraints

Impaired **Skin** integrity r/t incomplete joining of lip, palate ridges

Impaired verbal **Communication** r/t inadequate palate function, possible hearing loss from infected eustachian tubes

Ineffective **Airway** clearance r/t common feeding and breathing passage, postoperative laryngeal, incisional edema

Ineffective **Breastfeeding** r/t infant anomaly

Ineffective **Health** maintenance r/t lack of parental knowledge regarding feeding techniques, wound care, use of elbow restraints

Ineffective **Infant** feeding pattern r/t cleft lip, cleft palate

Risk for **Aspiration** r/t common feeding and breathing passage

Risk for deficient **Fluid** volume r/t inability to take liquids in usual manner

Risk for delayed **Development** r/t inadequate nutrition resulting from difficulty feeding

Risk for disproportionate **Growth** r/t inability to feed with normal techniques

Risk for disturbed **Body** image r/t disfigurement, speech impediment

Risk for **Infection** r/t invasive procedure, disruption of eustachian tube development, aspiration

### CLOTTING DISORDER

**Fear** r/t threat to well-being

Ineffective **Health** maintenance r/t deficient knowledge regarding treatment of disorder

Ineffective **Protection** r/t clotting disorder

Risk for deficient **Fluid** volume r/t uncontrolled bleeding

*See Anticoagulant Therapy; DIC (Disseminated Intravascular Coagulation); Hemophilia*

### COCAINE ABUSE

Disturbed **Thought** processes r/t excessive stimulation of nervous system by cocaine

Ineffective **Breathing** pattern r/t drug effect on respiratory center

Ineffective **Coping** r/t inability to deal with life stresses

*See Substance Abuse*

### COCAINE BABY

*See Crack Baby*

### CODEPENDENCY

**Caregiver** role strain r/t codependency

Decisional **Conflict** r/t support system deficit

Ineffective **Denial** r/t unmet self-needs

Impaired verbal **Communication** r/t psychological barriers

Ineffective **Coping** r/t inadequate support systems

**Powerlessness** r/t lifestyle of helplessness

### COGNITIVE DEFICIT

Disturbed **Thought** processes r/t neurological impairment

### COLD, VIRAL

Impaired **Comfort**: sore throat, aching, nasal discomfort r/t viral infection

Ineffective **Health** maintenance r/t deficient knowledge regarding care of viral condition, prevention of further infections

### COLECTOMY

Acute **Pain** r/t recent surgery

**Constipation** r/t decreased activity, decreased fluid intake

Imbalanced **Nutrition**: less than body requirements r/t high metabolic needs, decreased ability to ingest/digest food

Ineffective **Health** maintenance r/t deficient knowledge regarding procedure, postoperative care

Risk for **Infection** r/t invasive procedure

*See Abdominal Surgery*

## COLITIS

Acute **Pain** r/t inflammation in colon

Deficient **Fluid** volume r/t frequent stools

**Diarrhea** r/t inflammation in colon

*See Crohn's Disease; Inflammatory Bowel Disease*

## COLLAGEN DISEASE

*See specific disease (e.g., Lupus Erythematosus; JRA)*

*See Congenital Heart Disease/ Cardiac Anomalies*

## COLOSTOMY

Disturbed **Body** image r/t presence of stoma, daily care of fecal material

Ineffective **Health** maintenance r/t deficient knowledge regarding care of stoma, integrating colostomy care into lifestyle

Ineffective **Sexuality** patterns r/t altered body image, self-concept

Risk for **Constipation** r/t inappropriate diet

Risk for **Diarrhea** r/t inappropriate diet

Risk for impaired **Skin** integrity r/t irritation from bowel contents

Risk for **Social** isolation r/t anxiety about appearance of stoma and possible leakage

## COLPORRHAPHY, ANTERIOR

*See Vaginal Hysterectomy*

## COMA

Death **Anxiety**: significant others r/t unknown outcome of coma state

Disturbed **Thought** processes r/t neurological changes

Ineffective family **Therapeutic** regimen management r/t complexity of therapeutic regimen

Interrupted **Family** processes r/t illness/disability of family member

Risk for **Aspiration** r/t impaired swallowing, loss of cough/gag reflex

Risk for **Disuse** syndrome r/t altered level of consciousness impairing mobility

Risk for impaired **Oral** mucous membranes r/t dry mouth

Risk for impaired **Skin** integrity r/t immobility

Risk for **Injury** r/t potential seizure activity

Risk for **Spiritual** distress: significant others r/t loss of ability to relate to loved one, unknown outcome of coma

**Self-care** deficit: specify r/t neuromuscular impairment

Total urinary **Incontinence** r/t neurological dysfunction

*See cause of Coma*

## COMFORT, LOSS OF

Impaired **Comfort** r/t injury agent

## COMMUNICABLE DISEASES, CHILDHOOD (MEASLES, MUMPS, RUBELLA, CHICKENPOX, SCABIES, LICE, IMPETIGO)

Acute **Pain** r/t impaired skin integrity, edema

Deficient **Diversional** activity r/t imposed isolation from peers, disruption in usual play activities, fatigue, activity intolerance

Impaired **Comfort** r/t hyperthermia secondary to infectious disease process, pruritus secondary to skin rash or subdermal organisms

Ineffective **Health** maintenance r/t nonadherence to appropriate immunization schedules, lack of prevention of transmission of infection

C

Risk for **Infection**: transmission to others r/t contagious organisms

*See Meningitis/Encephalitis; Respiratory Infections, Acute Childhood; Reye's Syndrome*

## COMMUNICATION

Readiness for enhanced **Communication** r/t expressed willingness to enhance communication; ability to speak or write a language; ability to form words, phrases, and language; ability to express thoughts and feelings; ability to use and interpret nonverbal cues appropriately; expression of satisfaction with ability to share information and ideas with others

## COMMUNICATION PROBLEMS

Impaired verbal **Communication** r/t decrease in circulation to brain, brain tumor, physical barrier (e.g., tracheostomy, intubation), anatomical defect, impaired hearing, cleft palate, psychological barriers (e.g., psychosis, lack of stimuli), cultural difference, developmentally related or age-related factors, side effects of medication, environmental barriers, absence of significant others, altered perceptions, lack of information, stress, alteration of self-esteem or self-concept, physiological conditions, alteration of central nervous system, weakening of musculoskeletal system, emotional conditions

## COMMUNITY COPING

Ineffective community **Coping** r/t natural or manmade disasters; ineffective or nonexistent community systems (e.g., lack of emergency medical, transportation, or disaster planning systems), deficits in community social support services and resources, inadequate resources for problem solving

Readiness for enhanced community **Coping** r/t community sense of power to manage stressors, social supports available, resources available for problem solving

## COMMUNITY MANAGEMENT OF THERAPEUTIC REGIMEN

Ineffective community **Therapeutic** regimen management r/t inadequate community resources

## COMPARTMENT SYNDROME

Acute **Pain** r/t pressure in compromised body part

**Fear** r/t possible loss of limb, damage to limb

Ineffective **Tissue** perfusion: peripheral r/t increased pressure within compartment

## COMPULSION

*See Obsessive-Compulsive Disorder*

## CONDUCTION DISORDERS (CARDIAC)

*See Dysrhythmia*

## CONFUSION, ACUTE

Acute **Confusion** r/t >70 years of age with hospitalization, alcohol abuse, delirium, dementia, drug abuse

Adult **Failure** to thrive r/t confusion

Impaired **Memory** r/t fluid and electrolyte imbalance, neurological disturbances, excessive environmental disturbances, anemia, acute or chronic hypoxia, decreased cardiac output

## CONFUSION, CHRONIC

Adult **Failure** to thrive r/t confusion

Chronic **Confusion** r/t Alzheimer's disease, Korsakoff's psychosis, multiinfarct dementia, cerebrovascular accident, head injury

Disturbed **Thought** processes r/t organic mental disorder, disruption of cerebral arterial blood flow, chemical imbalance, intoxication

Impaired **Memory** r/t fluid and electrolyte imbalance, neurological disturbances, excessive environmental disturbances, anemia, acute or chronic hypoxia, decreased cardiac output

## CONGENITAL HEART DISEASE/CARDIAC ANOMALIES

### ACYANOTIC

Patent ductus arteriosus, atrial/ventricular septal defect, pulmonary stenosis, endocardial cushion defect, aortic valvular stenosis, coarctation of aorta

### CYANOTIC

Tetralogy of Fallot, tricuspid atresia, transposition of great vessels, truncus arteriosus, total anomalous pulmonary venous return, hypoplastic left lung

**Activity** intolerance r/t fatigue, generalized weakness, lack of adequate oxygenation

Decreased **Cardiac** output r/t cardiac dysfunction

Delayed **Growth** and development r/t inadequate oxygen and nutrients to tissues

Excess **Fluid** volume r/t cardiac defect, side effects of medication

Imbalanced **Nutrition**: less than body requirements r/t fatigue, generalized weakness, inability of infant to suck and feed, increased caloric requirements

Impaired **Gas** exchange r/t cardiac defect, pulmonary congestion

Ineffective **Breathing** pattern r/t pulmonary vascular disease

Interrupted **Family** processes r/t ill child

Risk for deficient **Fluid** volume r/t side effects of diuretics

Risk for delayed **Development** r/t inadequate oxygen and nutrients to tissues

Risk for disproportionate **Growth** r/t inadequate oxygen and nutrients to tissues

Risk for disorganized **Infant** behavior r/t invasive procedures

Risk for ineffective **Thermoregulation** r/t neonatal age

Risk for **Poisoning** r/t potential toxicity of cardiac medications

*See Child with Chronic Condition; Hospitalized Child*

## CONGESTIVE HEART FAILURE

*See CHF (Congestive Heart Failure)*

## CONJUNCTIVITIS

Acute **Pain** r/t inflammatory process

Disturbed **Sensory** perception r/t change in visual acuity resulting from inflammation

Risk for **Injury** r/t change in visual acuity

## CONSCIOUSNESS, ALTERED LEVEL OF

Acute **Confusion** r/t alcohol abuse, delirium, dementia, drug abuse

Adult **Failure** to thrive r/t altered level of consciousness

Chronic **Confusion** r/t multiinfarct dementia, Korsakoff's psychosis, head injury, Alzheimer's disease, cerebrovascular accident

Decreased **Intracranial** adaptive capacity r/t brain injury

Disturbed **Thought** processes r/t neurological changes

Impaired **Memory** r/t neurological disturbances

Ineffective **Tissue** perfusion: cerebral r/t increased intracranial pressure, decreased cerebral perfusion

Risk for **Aspiration** r/t impaired swallowing, loss of cough/gag reflex

C

Risk for **Disuse** syndrome r/t impaired mobility resulting from altered level of consciousness

Risk for impaired **Oral** mucous membranes r/t dry mouth

Risk for impaired **Skin** integrity r/t immobility

**Self-care** deficit: specify r/t neuromuscular impairment

Total urinary **Incontinence** r/t neurological dysfunction

*See cause of Altered Level of Consciousness*

## CONSTIPATION

**Constipation** r/t decreased fluid intake, decreased intake of foods containing bulk, inactivity, immobility, deficient knowledge of appropriate bowel routine, lack of privacy for defecation

## CONSTIPATION, PERCEIVED

Perceived **Constipation** r/t cultural or family health beliefs, faulty appraisal, impaired thought processes

## CONSTIPATION, RISK FOR

Risk for **Constipation** r/t functional factors impeding defecation, inappropriate diet, psychological factors, physical factors, medications

## CONTINENT ILEOSTOMY (KOCK POUCH)

Imbalanced **Nutrition**: less than body requirements r/t malabsorption

Ineffective **Coping** r/t stress of disease, exacerbations caused by stress

Ineffective **Health** maintenance r/t deficient knowledge regarding postoperative care

Risk for **Injury** r/t failure of valve, stomal cyanosis, intestinal obstruction

*See Abdominal Surgery*

## CONTRACEPTIVE METHOD

Decisional **Conflict**: method of contraception r/t unclear personal values or beliefs, lack of experience or interference with decision-making, lack of relevant information, support system deficit

**Health-seeking** behaviors r/t requesting information about available and appropriate birth control methods

Ineffective **Sexuality** patterns r/t fear of pregnancy

## CONVERSION DISORDER

**Anxiety** r/t unresolved conflict

Disturbed personal **Identity** r/t overwhelming stress

**Hopelessness** r/t long-term stress

Impaired **Adjustment** r/t multiple stressors

Impaired physical **Mobility** r/t physical conversion symptom

Impaired **Social** interaction r/t altered thought process

Ineffective **Coping** r/t personal vulnerability

Ineffective **Role** performance r/t physical conversion system

**Powerlessness** r/t lifestyle of helplessness

Risk for **Injury** r/t physical conversion symptom

**Self-esteem** disturbance r/t unsatisfactory or inadequate interpersonal relationships

## CONVULSIONS

**Anxiety** r/t concern over controlling convulsions

Impaired **Memory** r/t neurological disturbance

Ineffective **Health** maintenance r/t deficient knowledge regarding need for medication and care during seizure activity

Risk for **Aspiration** r/t impaired swallowing

Risk for delayed **Development** r/t seizures

Risk for disturbed **Thought** processes r/t seizure activity

Risk for **Injury** r/t seizure activity

*See Seizure Disorders, Adult; Seizure Disorders, Childhood*

## COPD (CHRONIC OBSTRUCTIVE PULMONARY DISEASE)

**Activity** intolerance r/t imbalance between oxygen supply and demand

Interrupted **Family** processes r/t role changes

**Anxiety** r/t breathlessness, change in health status

Chronic low **Self-esteem** r/t chronic illness

Chronic **Sorrow** r/t presence of chronic illness

Death **Anxiety** r/t seriousness of medical condition, difficulty being able to "catch breath," feeling of suffocation

**Health-seeking** behaviors r/t wish to stop smoking

Imbalanced **Nutrition**: less than body requirements r/t decreased intake because of dyspnea, unpleasant taste in mouth left by medications

Impaired **Gas** exchange r/t ventilation-perfusion inequality

Impaired **Social** interaction r/t social isolation secondary to oxygen use, activity intolerance

Ineffective **Airway** clearance r/t bronchoconstriction, increased mucus, ineffective cough, infection

Ineffective **Health** maintenance r/t deficient knowledge regarding care of disease

**Noncompliance** r/t reluctance to accept responsibility for changing detrimental health practices

**Powerlessness** r/t progressive nature of disease

Risk for **Infection** r/t stasis of respiratory secretions

**Self-care** deficit: specify r/t fatigue secondary to increased work of breathing

**Sleep** deprivation r/t breathing difficulties when lying down

## COPING

Readiness for enhanced **Coping** r/t defining stressors as manageable; seeking social support; using a broad range of problem-oriented and emotion-oriented strategies; using spiritual resources; acknowledging power; seeking knowledge of new strategies; being aware of possible environmental changes

## COPING PROBLEMS

Defensive **Coping** r/t superior attitude toward others, difficulty establishing or maintaining relationships, hostile laughter or ridicule of others, difficulty in reality-testing perceptions, lack of follow-through or participation in treatment or therapy

Ineffective **Coping** r/t gender differences in coping strategies, inadequate level of confidence in ability to cope, uncertainty, inadequate social support created by characteristics of relationships, inadequate level of perception of control, inadequate resources available, high degree of threat, disturbance in pattern of tension release, inadequate opportunity to prepare for stressor, inability to conserve adaptive energies, disturbance in appraisal of threat

*See Community Coping; Family Problems*

## CORNEAL REFLEX, ABSENT

Risk for **Injury** r/t accidental corneal abrasion, drying of cornea

## CORNEAL TRANSPLANT

Risk for **Infection** r/t invasive procedure; surgery

Readiness for enhanced **Therapeutic** regimen management r/t describes need to rest and avoid strenuous activities during healing phase

## CORONARY ARTERY BYPASS GRAFTING

Acute **Pain** r/t traumatic surgery

Decreased **Cardiac** output r/t dysrhythmia, depressed cardiac function, increased systemic vascular resistance

Deficient **Fluid** volume r/t intraoperative fluid loss, use of diuretics in surgery

**Fear** r/t outcome of surgical procedure

Ineffective **Health** maintenance r/t deficient knowledge regarding postprocedure care, lifestyle adjustment after surgery

Risk for perioperative positioning **Injury** r/t hypothermia, extended supine position

## COSTOVERTEBRAL ANGLE TENDERNESS

*See Kidney Stone; Pyelonephritis*

## COUGH, EFFECTIVE/ INEFFECTIVE

Ineffective **Airway** clearance r/t decreased energy, fatigue, normal aging changes

*See Bronchitis; COPD (Chronic Obstructive Pulmonary Disease); Pulmonary Edema*

## CRACK ABUSE

*See Cocaine Abuse*

## CRACK BABY

Delayed **Growth** and development r/t effects of maternal use of drugs, neurological impairment, decreased attentiveness to environmental stimuli

**Diarrhea** r/t effects of withdrawal, increased peristalsis secondary to hyperirritability

Disorganized **Infant** behavior r/t prematurity, pain, lack of attachment

Disturbed **Sensory** perception: specify r/t hypersensitivity to environmental stimuli

Disturbed **Sleep** pattern r/t hyperirritability, hypersensitivity to environmental stimuli

Imbalanced **Nutrition**: less than body requirements r/t feeding problems; uncoordinated/ineffective suck and swallow; effects of diarrhea, vomiting, colic

Impaired **Parenting** r/t impaired/lack of attachment behaviors, inadequate support systems

Ineffective **Airway** clearance r/t pooling of secretions secondary to lack of adequate cough reflex

Ineffective **Infant** feeding pattern r/t prematurity, neurological impairment

Ineffective **Protection** r/t effects of maternal substance abuse

Risk for delayed **Development** r/t substance abuse

Risk for disproportionate **Growth** r/t substance abuse

Risk for impaired parent-infant **Attachment** r/t parent's inability to meet infant's needs, substance abuse

Risk for **Infection** (skin, meningeal, respiratory) r/t effects of withdrawal

## CRACKLES IN LUNGS, COARSE

Ineffective **Airway** clearance r/t excessive secretions in airways, ineffective cough

*See cause of Coarse Crackles*

## CRACKLES IN LUNGS, FINE

Ineffective **Breathing** pattern r/t fatigue, surgery, decreased energy

*See Bronchitis or Pneumonia (if from pulmonary infection); CHF (Congestive Heart Failure) (if cardiac in origin); Infection*

## CRANIECTOMY/CRANIOTOMY

Acute **Pain** r/t recent surgery, headache

Adult **Failure** to thrive r/t altered cerebral tissue perfusion

Decreased **Intracranial** adaptive capacity r/t brain injury, intracranial hypertension

**Fear** r/t threat to well-being

Impaired **Memory** r/t neurological surgery

Ineffective **Tissue** perfusion: cerebral r/t cerebral edema, decreased cerebral perfusion, increased intracranial pressure

Risk for disturbed **Thought** processes r/t neurophysiological changes

Risk for **Injury** r/t potential confusion

*See Coma (if relevant)*

## CREPITATION, SUBCUTANEOUS

*See Pneumothorax*

## CRISIS

Anticipatory **Grieving** r/t potential significant loss

**Anxiety** r/t threat to or change in environment, health status, interaction patterns, situation, self-concept, or role-functioning; threat of death of self or significant other

Compromised family **Coping** r/t situational or developmental crisis

Death **Anxiety** r/t feelings of hopelessness associated with crisis

Disturbed **Energy** field r/t disharmony caused by crisis

**Fear** r/t crisis situation

Ineffective **Coping** r/t situational or maturational crisis

Risk for **Spiritual** distress r/t physical or psychological stress, natural disasters, situational losses, maturational losses

Situational low **Self-esteem** r/t perception of inability to handle crisis

**Spiritual** distress r/t intense suffering

## CROHN'S DISEASE

Acute **Pain** r/t increased peristalsis

**Anxiety** r/t change in health status

**Diarrhea** r/t inflammatory process

Imbalanced **Nutrition**: less than body requirements r/t diarrhea, altered ability to digest and absorb food

Ineffective **Coping** r/t repeated episodes of diarrhea

Ineffective **Health** maintenance r/t deficient knowledge regarding management of disease

**Powerlessness** r/t chronic disease

Risk for deficient **Fluid** volume r/t abnormal fluid loss with diarrhea

## CROUP

*See Respiratory Infections, Acute Childhood*

## CRYOSURGERY FOR RETINAL DETACHMENT

*See Retinal Detachment*

C

## CUSHING'S SYNDROME

**Activity** intolerance r/t fatigue, weakness

Disturbed **Body** image r/t change in appearance from disease process

Excess **Fluid** volume r/t failure of regulatory mechanisms

Ineffective **Health** maintenance r/t deficient knowledge regarding needed care

Risk for **Infection** r/t suppression of immune system secondary to increased cortisol

Risk for **Injury** r/t decreased muscle strength, osteoporosis

**Sexual** dysfunction r/t loss of libido

## CVA (CEREBROVASCULAR ACCIDENT)

Adult **Failure** to thrive r/t neurophysiological changes

**Anxiety** r/t situational crisis, change in physical or emotional condition

**Caregiver** role strain r/t cognitive problems of care receiver, need for significant home care

Chronic **Confusion** r/t neurological changes

**Constipation** r/t decreased activity

Disturbed **Body** image r/t chronic illness, paralysis

Disturbed **Sensory** perception: visual, tactile, kinesthetic r/t neurological deficit

Disturbed **Thought** processes r/t neurophysiological changes

**Grieving** r/t loss of health

Impaired **Home** maintenance r/t neurological disease affecting ability to perform activities of daily living (ADLs)

Impaired **Memory** r/t neurological disturbances

Impaired physical **Mobility** r/t loss of balance and coordination

Impaired **Social** interaction r/t limited physical mobility, limited ability to communicate

Impaired **Swallowing** r/t neuromuscular dysfunction

Impaired **Transfer** ability r/t limited physical mobility

Impaired verbal **Communication** r/t pressure damage, decreased circulation to brain in speech center informational sources

Impaired **Walking** r/t loss of balance and coordination

Ineffective **Coping** r/t disability

Ineffective **Health** maintenance r/t deficient knowledge regarding self-care following CVA

Interrupted **Family** process r/t illness, disability of family member

Reflex **Incontinence** r/t loss of feeling to void

Risk for **Aspiration** r/t impaired swallowing, loss of gag reflex

Risk for **Disuse** syndrome r/t paralysis

Risk for impaired **Skin** integrity r/t immobility

Risk for **Injury** r/t disturbed sensory perception

**Self-care** deficit: specify r/t decreased strength and endurance, paralysis

Total urinary **Incontinence** r/t neurological dysfunction

Unilateral **Neglect** r/t disturbed perception from neurological damage

## CYANOSIS, CENTRAL WITH CYANOSIS OF ORAL MUCOUS MEMBRANES

Impaired **Gas** exchange r/t alveolar-capillary membrane changes

## CYANOSIS, PERIPHERAL WITH CYANOSIS OF NAIL BEDS

Ineffective **Tissue** perfusion r/t interruption of arterial flow, severe vasoconstriction, cold temperatures

Risk for **Peripheral** neurovascular dysfunction r/t condition causing disruption in circulation

## CYSTIC FIBROSIS

**Activity** intolerance r/t imbalance between oxygen supply and demand

**Anxiety** r/t dyspnea, oxygen deprivation

Chronic **Sorrow** r/t presence of chronic disease

Disturbed **Body** image r/t changes in physical appearance, treatment of chronic lung disease (clubbing, barrel chest, home oxygen therapy)

Imbalanced **Nutrition**: less than body requirements r/t anorexia; decreased absorption of nutrients, fat; increased work of breathing

Impaired **Gas** exchange r/t ventilation-perfusion imbalance

Impaired **Home** maintenance r/t extensive daily treatment, medications necessary for health, mist/oxygen tents

Ineffective **Airway** clearance r/t increased production of thick mucus

Risk for **Caregiver** role strain r/t illness severity of care receiver, unpredictable course of illness

Risk for deficient **Fluid** volume r/t decreased fluid intake, increased work of breathing

Risk for delayed **Development** r/t chronic illness

Risk for disproportionate **Growth** r/t chronic illness

Risk for **Infection** r/t thick, tenacious

mucus; harboring of bacterial organisms; debilitated state

Risk for **Spiritual** distress r/t presence of chronic disease

*See Child with Chronic Condition; Hospitalized Child; Terminally Ill Child, Adolescent; Terminally Ill Child, Infant/Toddler; Terminally Ill Child, Preschool Child; Terminally Ill Child, School-Age Child/Preadolescent; Terminally Ill Child, Death of Child, Parent*

## CYSTITIS

Acute **Pain**: dysuria r/t inflammatory process in bladder

Impaired **Urinary** elimination: frequency r/t urinary tract infection

Ineffective **Health** maintenance r/t deficient knowledge regarding methods to treat and prevent urinary tract infections

Risk for urge urinary **Incontinence** r/t infection in bladder

## CYSTOCELE

Ineffective **Health** maintenance r/t deficient knowledge regarding personal care, Kegel exercises to strengthen perineal muscles

Risk for urge urinary **Incontinence** r/t lack of bladder support

Stress urinary **Incontinence** r/t prolapsed bladder

Urge urinary **Incontinence** r/t prolapsed bladder

## CYSTOSCOPY

Ineffective **Health** maintenance r/t deficient knowledge regarding postoperative care

Risk for **Infection** r/t invasive procedure

**Urinary** retention r/t edema in urethra obstructing flow of urine

# D

## DEAFNESS

Disturbed **Sensory** perception: auditory r/t alteration in sensory reception, transmission, integration

Impaired verbal **Communication** r/t impaired hearing

Risk for delayed **Development** r/t impaired hearing

Risk for **Injury** r/t alteration in sensory perception

## DEATH

Risk for sudden infant **Death** syndrome (SIDS) r/t modifiable risk factors such as infants placed to sleep in the prone or side-lying position, prenatal and/or postnatal infant smoke exposure, infant overheating/overwrapping, soft underlayment/loose articles in the sleep environment, delayed or nonattendance of prenatal care; potentially modifiable risk factors such as low birth weight, prematurity, young maternal age; nonmodifiable risk factors such as male gender, ethnicity (e.g., African American, Native American race of mother), seasonality of SIDS deaths (higher in winter and fall months); peaking of SIDS mortality between infant ages of 2 and 4 months

## DEATH, ONCOMING

Anticipatory **Grieving** r/t loss of significant other

Compromised family **Coping** r/t client's inability to provide support to family

Death **Anxiety** r/t unresolved issues surrounding dying

**Fear** r/t threat of death

Ineffective **Coping** r/t personal vulnerability

**Powerlessness** r/t effects of illness, oncoming death

Readiness for enhanced **Spiritual** well-being r/t desire of client and family to be in harmony with each other and higher power/God

**Social** isolation r/t altered state of wellness

**Spiritual** distress r/t intense suffering

*See Terminally Ill Child, Adolescent; Terminally Ill Child, Infant/Toddler; Terminally Ill Child, Preschool Child; Terminally Ill Child, School-Age Child/Preadolescent; Terminally Ill Child, Death of Child, Parent*

## DECISIONS, DIFFICULTY MAKING

Decisional **Conflict** r/t support system deficit, perceived threat to value system, multiple or divergent sources of information, lack of relevant information, unclear personal values/beliefs

## DECUBITUS ULCER

*See Pressure Ulcer*

## DEEP VEIN THROMBOSIS

*See DVT (Deep Vein Thrombosis)*

## DEFENSIVE BEHAVIOR

Defensive **Coping** r/t nonacceptance of blame, denial of problems or weakness

Ineffective **Denial** r/t inability to face situation realistically

## DEHISCENCE, ABDOMINAL

Acute **Pain** r/t stretching of abdominal wall

Delayed **Surgical** recovery r/t altered circulation, malnutrition, opening in incision

**Fear** r/t threat of death, severe dysfunction

Impaired **Skin** integrity r/t altered circulation, malnutrition, opening in incision

Impaired **Tissue** integrity r/t exposure of abdominal contents to external environment

Risk for imbalanced **Fluid** volume r/t altered circulation associated with opening of wound and exposure of abdominal contents

Risk for **Infection** r/t loss of skin integrity

## DEHYDRATION

Deficient **Fluid** volume r/t active fluid volume loss

Impaired **Oral** mucous membranes r/t decreased salivation, fluid deficit

Ineffective **Health** maintenance r/t deficient knowledge regarding treatment and prevention of dehydration

*See cause of Dehydration*

## DELIRIUM

Acute **Confusion** r/t effects of medication, response to hospitalization, alcohol abuse, substance abuse, sensory deprivation or overload

Adult **Failure** to thrive r/t delirium

Disturbed **Thought** processes r/t head trauma, altered metabolic state, substance abuse, sleep deprivation, sensory deprivation or overload

Impaired **Memory** r/t delirium

Risk for **Injury** r/t altered level of consciousness

**Sleep** deprivation r/t nightmares

## DELIRIUM TREMENS (DT)

*See Alcohol Withdrawal*

## DELIVERY

*See Labor, Normal*

## DELUSIONS

Acute **Confusion** r/t alcohol abuse, delirium, dementia, drug abuse

Adult **Failure** to thrive r/t delusional state

**Anxiety** r/t content of intrusive thoughts

Disturbed **Thought** processes r/t mental disorder

Impaired verbal **Communication** r/t psychological impairment, delusional thinking

Ineffective **Coping** r/t distortion and insecurity of life events

Risk for self-directed **Violence** r/t delusional thinking

Risk for other-directed **Violence** r/t delusional thinking

## DEMENTIA

Adult **Failure** to thrive r/t depression, apathy

Chronic **Confusion** r/t neurological dysfunction

Chronic **Sorrow** r/t chronic mental illness

Disturbed **Sleep** pattern r/t neurological impairment, naps during the day

Imbalanced **Nutrition**: less than body requirements r/t psychological impairment

Impaired **Environmental** interpretation syndrome r/t dementia

Impaired **Home** maintenance r/t inadequate support system

Impaired physical **Mobility** r/t neuromuscular impairment

Interrupted **Family** process r/t disability of family member

Risk for **Caregiver** role strain r/t number of caregiving tasks, duration of caregiving required

Risk for **Falls** r/t diminished mental status

Risk for impaired **Skin** integrity r/t altered nutritional status, immobility

D

Risk for **Injury** r/t confusion, decreased muscle coordination

**Self-care** deficit: specify r/t psychological or neuromuscular impairment

Total urinary **Incontinence** r/t neuromuscular impairment

## DENIAL OF HEALTH STATUS

Ineffective **Denial** r/t lack of perception about health status effects of illness

Ineffective management of **Therapeutic** regimen r/t denial of seriousness of health situation

## DENTAL CARIES

Impaired **Dentition** r/t ineffective oral hygiene, barriers to self-care, economic barriers to professional care, nutritional deficits, dietary habits

Ineffective **Health** maintenance r/t lack of knowledge regarding prevention of dental disease secondary to high-sugar diet, giving infants or toddlers with erupted teeth bottles of milk at bedtime, lack of fluoride treatments, inadequate or improper brushing of teeth

## DENTITION PROBLEMS

*See Dental Caries*

## DEPRESSION (MAJOR DEPRESSIVE DISORDER)

Adult **Failure** to thrive r/t depression

Chronic low **Self-esteem** r/t repeated unmet expectations

Chronic **Sorrow** r/t unresolved grief

**Constipation** r/t inactivity, decreased fluid intake

Death **Anxiety** r/t feelings of lack of self-worth

Disturbed **Energy** field r/t disharmony

Disturbed **Sleep** pattern r/t inactivity

Dysfunctional **Grieving** r/t lack of previous resolution of former grieving response

**Fatigue** r/t psychological demands

**Hopelessness** r/t feeling of abandonment, long-term stress

Impaired **Environmental** interpretation syndrome r/t severe mental functional impairment

Ineffective **Coping** r/t dysfunctional grieving

Ineffective **Health** maintenance r/t lack of ability to make good judgments regarding ways to obtain help

**Powerlessness** r/t pattern of helplessness

Risk for **Suicide** r/t panic state

**Self-care** deficit: specify r/t depression, cognitive impairment

**Sexual** dysfunction r/t loss of sexual desire

**Social** isolation r/t ineffective coping

## DERMATITIS

**Anxiety** r/t situational crisis imposed by illness

Impaired **Comfort**: pruritus r/t inflammation of skin

Impaired **Skin** integrity r/t side effect of medication, allergic reaction

Ineffective **Health** maintenance r/t deficient knowledge regarding methods to decrease inflammation

## DESPONDENCY

**Hopelessness** r/t long-term stress

*See Depression*

## DESTRUCTIVE BEHAVIOR TOWARD OTHERS

Impaired **Adjustment** r/t intense emotional state

Ineffective **Coping** r/t situational crises, maturational crises, personal vulnerability

Risk for other-directed **Violence** r/t history of violence, neurological impairment, cognitive impairment, history of childhood abuse, history of witnessing family violence, cruelty to animals, firesetting, history of alcohol/drug abuse, pathological intoxication, psychotic symptomatology, motor vehicle offenses, impulsivity, availability or possession of weapon, body language

## DEVELOPMENTAL CONCERNS

Delayed **Growth** and development r/t prescribed dependence, indifference, separation from significant other(s), environmental and stimulation deficiencies, effects of physical disability, inadequate caretaking, inconsistent responsiveness, multiple caretakers

### INDIVIDUAL

Risk for delayed **Development** r/t prematurity, seizures, congenital or genetic disorders, positive drug screening test, brain damage (e.g., hemorrhage in post-natal period, shaken baby, abuse, accident), vision impairment, hearing impairment or frequent otitis media, chronic illness, technology dependence, failure to thrive, inadequate nutrition, foster or adopted child, lead poisoning, chemotherapy, radiation therapy, natural disaster, behavior disorders, substance abuse

### ENVIRONMENTAL

Risk for delayed **Development** r/t poverty, violence

### CAREGIVER

Risk for delayed **Development** r/t abuse, mental illness, mental retardation or severe learning disability

## DIABETES IN PREGNANCY

*See Gestational Diabetes*

## DIABETES INSIPIDUS

Deficient **Fluid** volume r/t inability to conserve fluid

Ineffective **Health** maintenance r/t deficient knowledge regarding care of disease, importance of medications

## DIABETES MELLITUS

Adult **Failure** to thrive r/t undetected disease process

Disturbed **Sensory** perception r/t ineffective tissue perfusion

Imbalanced **Nutrition**: less than body requirements r/t inability to use glucose (type I [insulin- dependent] diabetes)

Imbalanced **Nutrition**: more than body requirements r/t excessive intake of nutrients (type II diabetes)

Ineffective **Health** maintenance r/t deficient knowledge regarding care of diabetic condition

Ineffective management of **Therapeutic** regimen r/t complexity of therapeutic regimen

Ineffective **Tissue** perfusion: peripheral r/t impaired arterial circulation

**Noncompliance** r/t restrictive lifestyle; changes in diet, medication, exercise

**Powerlessness** r/t perceived lack of personal control

Risk for disturbed **Thought** processes r/t hypoglycemia, hyperglycemia

Risk for impaired **Skin** integrity r/t loss of pain perception in extremities

Risk for **Infection** r/t hyperglycemia, impaired healing, circulatory changes

Risk for **Injury**: hypoglycemia or hyperglycemia r/t failure to consume adequate calories, failure to take insulin

**Sexual** dysfunction r/t neuropathy associated with disease

## DIABETES MELLITUS, JUVENILE (IDDM TYPE I)

Acute **Pain** r/t insulin injections, peripheral blood glucose testing

Disturbed **Body** image r/t imposed deviations from biophysical and psy-

D

chosocial norm, perceived differences from peers

Imbalanced **Nutrition**: less than body requirements r/t inability of body to adequately metabolize and use glucose and nutrients, increased caloric needs of child to promote growth and physical activity participation with peers

Impaired **Adjustment** r/t inability to participate in normal childhood activities

Ineffective **Health** maintenance r/t parental/child deficient knowledge regarding dietary management, medication administration, physical activity, and interaction among the three; daily changes in diet, medications, activity associated with child's growth spurts and needs; need to instruct other caregivers and teachers regarding signs and symptoms of hypoglycemia or hyperglycemia and treatment

Risk for delayed **Development** r/t chronic illness

Risk for disproportionate **Growth** r/t chronic illness

Risk for **Noncompliance** r/t disturbed body image, impaired adjustment secondary to adolescent maturational crises

*See Diabetes Mellitus; Child with Chronic Condition; Hospitalized Child*

## DIABETIC COMA

Deficient **Fluid** volume r/t hyperglycemia resulting in polyuria

Disturbed **Thought** processes r/t hyperglycemia, presence of excessive metabolic acids

Ineffective management of **Therapeutic** regimen r/t lack of understanding of preventive measures, adequate blood sugar control

Risk for **Infection** r/t hyperglycemia, changes in vascular system

*See Diabetes Mellitus*

## DIABETIC KETOACIDOSIS

*See Ketoacidosis: Diabetic*

## DIABETIC RETINOPATHY

Disturbed **Sensory** perception r/t change in sensory reception

**Grieving** r/t loss of vision

Ineffective **Health** maintenance r/t deficient knowledge regarding preserving vision with treatment if possible, use of low-vision aids

*See Vision Impairment*

## DIALYSIS

*See Hemodialysis; Peritoneal Dialysis*

## DIAPHORESIS

Impaired **Comfort** r/t excessive sweating

## DIAPHRAGMATIC HERNIA

*See Hiatus Hernia*

## DIARRHEA

**Diarrhea** r/t infection, change in diet, gastrointestinal disorders, stress, medication effect, impaction

## DIC (DISSEMINATED INTRAVASCULAR COAGULATION)

Deficient **Fluid** volume: hemorrhage r/t depletion of clotting factors

**Fear** r/t threat to well-being

Ineffective **Protection** r/t abnormal clotting mechanism

Risk for ineffective **Tissue** perfusion: peripheral r/t hypovolemia from profuse bleeding, formation of microemboli in vascular system

## DIGITALIS TOXICITY

Decreased **Cardiac** output r/t drug toxicity affecting cardiac rhythm, rate

Ineffective management of **Therapeutic** regimen r/t deficient knowledge regarding action, appropriate method of administration of digitalis

## DILATION AND CURETTAGE (D & C)

Acute **Pain** r/t uterine contractions

Ineffective **Health** maintenance r/t deficient knowledge regarding postoperative self-care

Risk for deficient **Fluid** volume: hemorrhage r/t excessive blood loss during or after procedure

Risk for ineffective **Sexuality** patterns r/t painful coitus, fear associated with surgery on genital area

Risk for **Infection** r/t surgical procedure

## DISCHARGE PLANNING

Deficient **Knowledge** r/t lack of exposure to information for home care

Impaired **Home** maintenance r/t family member's disease or injury interfering with home maintenance

Ineffective **Health** maintenance r/t lack of material sources

## DISCOMFORTS OF PREGNANCY

Acute **Pain**: leg cramps r/t nerve compression, calcium/phosphorus/potassium imbalance

**Constipation** r/t decreased gastrointestinal tract motility, pressure from enlarged uterus, supplementary iron

Disturbed **Body** image r/t pregnancy-induced body changes

Disturbed **Sleep** pattern r/t psychological stress, fetal movement, muscular cramping, urinary frequency, shortness of breath

**Fatigue** r/t hormonal, metabolic, body changes

Impaired **Comfort** r/t hormonal

changes (nausea, ptyalism, leukorrhea, urinary frequency), enlarged uterus (shortness of breath, abdominal distention, pruritus, reduced bladder capacity), increased vascularization (nasal stuffiness, varicosities)

**Nausea** r/t hormone effect

Risk for **Constipation** r/t decreased intestinal motility, inadequate fiber in diet

Risk for **Injury** r/t faintness and/or syncope secondary to vasomotor lability or postural hypotension, venous stasis in lower extremities

Risk for urge urinary **Incontinence** r/t hormone effect, pressure on bladder from growing uterus

Stress urinary **Incontinence** r/t enlarged uterus, fetal movement

## DISLOCATION

Acute **Pain** r/t dislocation of a joint

Risk for **Injury** r/t unstable joint

**Self-care** deficit: specify r/t inability to use a joint

## DISSECTING ANEURYSM

**Fear** r/t threat to well-being

*See Abdominal Surgery; Aneurysm, Abdominal Surgery*

## DISSEMINATED INTRAVASCULAR COAGULATION

*See DIC (Disseminated Intravascular Coagulation)*

## DISSOCIATIVE IDENTITY DISORDER (NOT OTHERWISE SPECIFIED)

**Anxiety** r/t psychosocial stress

Disturbed personal **Identity** r/t inability to distinguish self caused by multiple personality disorder, depersonalization, disturbance in memory

D

Disturbed **Sensory** perception: kinesthetic r/t underdeveloped ego

Disturbed **Thought** processes r/t repressed anxiety

Impaired **Memory** r/t altered state of consciousness

Ineffective **Coping** r/t personal vulnerability in crisis of accurate self-perception

*See Multiple Personality Disorder*

### DISTRESS

**Anxiety** r/t situational crises, maturational crises

Death **Anxiety** r/t denial of one's own mortality or impending death

Disturbed **Energy** field r/t disruption in flow of energy as result of pain, depression, fatigue, anxiety, stress

### DISUSE SYNDROME, POTENTIAL TO DEVELOP

Risk for **Disuse** syndrome r/t paralysis, mechanical immobilization, prescribed immobilization, severe pain, altered level of consciousness

### DIVERSIONAL ACTIVITY, LACK OF

Deficient **Diversional** activity r/t environmental lack of diversional activity as in frequent hospitalizations, lengthy treatments

### DIVERTICULITIS

Acute **Pain** r/t inflammation of bowel

**Constipation** r/t dietary deficiency of fiber and roughage

Deficient **Knowledge** r/t diet needed to control disease, medication regimen

**Diarrhea** r/t increased intestinal motility secondary to inflammation

Imbalanced **Nutrition**: less than body requirements r/t loss of appetite

Risk for deficient **Fluid** volume r/t diarrhea

### DIZZINESS

Decreased **Cardiac** output r/t dysfunctional electrical conduction

Impaired physical **Mobility** r/t dizziness

Ineffective **Tissue** perfusion: cerebral r/t interruption of cerebral arterial blood flow

Risk for **Injury** r/t difficulty maintaining balance

### DOMESTIC VIOLENCE

**Anxiety** r/t threat to self-concept, situational crisis of abuse

**Caregiver** role strain r/t chronic illness, self-care deficits, lack of respite care, extent of caregiving required

Compromised family **Coping** r/t abusive patterns

Defensive **Coping** r/t low self-esteem

Disturbed **Sleep** pattern r/t psychological stress

Impaired verbal **Communication** r/t psychological barriers of fear

Interrupted **Family** processes: alcoholism r/t inadequate coping skills

**Post-trauma** syndrome r/t history of abuse

**Powerlessness** r/t lifestyle of helplessness

Risk for **Post-trauma** syndrome r/t inadequate social support

Risk for self-directed **Violence** r/t history of abuse

**Self-esteem** disturbance r/t negative family interactions

### DOWN SYNDROME

*See Child with Chronic Condition; Mental Retardation*

## DRESS SELF (INABILITY TO)

Dressing/grooming **Self-care** deficit r/t intolerance to activity, decreased strength and endurance, pain, discomfort, perceptual or cognitive impairment, neuromuscular impairment, musculoskeletal impairment, depression, severe anxiety

## DRIBBLING OF URINE

Stress urinary **Incontinence** r/t degenerative changes in pelvic muscles and structural supports

## DROOLING

Impaired **Swallowing** r/t neuromuscular impairment, mechanical obstruction

Risk for **Aspiration** r/t impaired swallowing

## DRUG ABUSE

**Anxiety** r/t threat to self-concept, lack of control of drug use

Disturbed **Sensory** perception: specify r/t substance intoxication

Disturbed **Sleep** pattern r/t effects of medications

Disturbed **Thought** processes r/t mind-altering effects of drugs

Imbalanced **Nutrition**: less than body requirements r/t poor eating habits

Impaired **Adjustment** r/t failure to intend to change behavior

Impaired **Social** interaction r/t disturbed thought processes from drug abuse

Ineffective **Coping** r/t situational crisis

**Noncompliance** r/t denial of illness

**Powerlessness** r/t feeling unable to change patterns of abuse

Risk for **Injury** r/t hallucinations, drug effects

Risk for **Violence** r/t poor impulse control

**Sexual** dysfunction r/t actions and side effects of drug abuse

**Sleep** deprivation r/t prolonged psychological discomfort

**Spiritual** distress r/t separation from religious, cultural ties

## DRUG WITHDRAWAL

Acute **Confusion** r/t effects of substance withdrawal

**Anxiety** r/t physiological withdrawal

Disturbed **Sensory** perception: specify r/t substance intoxication

Disturbed **Sleep** pattern r/t effects of medications

Imbalanced **Nutrition**: less than body requirements r/t poor eating habits

Ineffective **Coping** r/t situational crisis, withdrawal

**Noncompliance** r/t denial of illness

Risk for **Injury** r/t hallucinations

Risk for **Violence** r/t poor impulse control

*See Drug Abuse*

## DRY EYE

*See Conjunctivitis; Keratoconjunctivitis Sicca*

## DTS (DELIRIUM TREMENS)

*See Alcohol Withdrawal*

## DVT (DEEP VEIN THROMBOSIS)

Acute **Pain** r/t vascular inflammation, edema

**Constipation** r/t inactivity, bedrest

Delayed **Surgical** recovery r/t impaired physical mobility

Impaired physical **Mobility** r/t pain in extremity, forced bedrest

D

D

Ineffective **Health** maintenance r/t deficient knowledge regarding self-care needs, treatment regimen, outcome

Ineffective **Tissue** perfusion: peripheral r/t interruption of venous blood flow

*See Anticoagulant Therapy*

## DYING CLIENT

*See Terminally Ill Child, Adolescent; Terminally Ill Child, Infant/Toddler; Terminally Ill Child, Preschool Child; Terminally Ill Child, School-Age Child/Preadolescent; Terminally Ill Child, Death of Child, Parent*

## DYSFUNCTIONAL EATING PATTERN

Imbalanced **Nutrition**: less than body requirements r/t psychological factors

Risk for imbalanced **Nutrition**: more than body requirements r/t observed use of food as reward or comfort measure

*See Anorexia Nervosa; Bulimia; Maturational Issues, Adolescent*

## DYSFUNCTIONAL FAMILY UNIT

*See Family Problems*

## DYSFUNCTIONAL GRIEVING

Dysfunctional **Grieving** r/t actual or perceived loss

## DYSFUNCTIONAL VENTILATORY WEANING

Dysfunctional **Ventilatory** weaning response r/t physical, psychological, situational factors

## DYSMENORRHEA

Ineffective **Health** maintenance r/t deficient knowledge regarding prevention and treatment of painful menstruation

**Nausea** r/t prostaglandin effect

Acute **Pain** r/t cramping from hormonal effects

## DYSPAREUNIA

**Sexual** dysfunction r/t lack of lubrication during intercourse, alteration in reproductive organ function

## DYSPEPSIA

Acute **Pain** r/t gastrointestinal disease, consumption of irritating foods

**Anxiety** r/t pressures of personal role

Ineffective **Health** maintenance r/t deficient knowledge regarding treatment of disease

## DYSPHAGIA

Impaired **Swallowing** r/t neuromuscular impairment

Risk for **Aspiration** r/t loss of gag or cough reflex

## DYSPHASIA

Impaired **Social** interaction r/t difficulty in communicating

Impaired verbal **Communication** r/t decrease in circulation to brain

## DYSPNEA

**Activity** intolerance r/t imbalance between oxygen supply-demand

**Anxiety** r/t ineffective breathing pattern

Disturbed **Sleep** pattern r/t difficulty breathing, positioning required for effective breathing

**Fear** r/t threat to state of well-being, potential death

Impaired **Gas** exchange r/t alveolar-capillary damage

Ineffective **Breathing** pattern r/t compromised cardiac/pulmonary function, decreased lung expansion, neurological impairment affecting respiratory center, extreme anxiety

**Sleep** deprivation r/t ineffective breathing pattern

## DYSRHYTHMIA

**Activity** intolerance r/t decreased cardiac output

**Anxiety/fear** r/t threat of death, change in health status

Decreased **Cardiac** output r/t altered electrical conduction

Ineffective **Health** maintenance r/t deficient knowledge regarding self-care with disease

Ineffective **Tissue** perfusion: cerebral r/t interruption of cerebral arterial flow secondary to decreased cardiac output

## DYSTHYMIC DISORDER

Chronic low **Self-esteem** r/t repeated unmet expectations

Disturbed **Sleep** pattern r/t anxious thoughts

Ineffective **Coping** r/t impaired social interaction

Ineffective **Health** maintenance r/t inability to make good judgments regarding ways to obtain help

Ineffective **Sexuality** pattern r/t loss of sexual desire

**Social** isolation r/t ineffective coping

*See Depression*

## DYSTOCIA

**Anxiety** r/t difficult labor, deficient knowledge regarding normal labor pattern

**Fatigue** r/t prolonged labor

**Grieving** r/t loss of ideal labor experience

Ineffective **Coping** r/t situational crisis

Acute **Pain** r/t difficult labor, medical interventions

**Powerlessness** r/t perceived inability to control outcome of labor

Risk for deficient **Fluid** volume r/t hemorrhage secondary to uterine atony

Risk for delayed **Development** r/t difficult labor and birth

Risk for disproportionate **Growth** r/t difficult labor and birth

Risk for impaired **Tissue** integrity: maternal and fetal r/t difficult labor

Risk for ineffective **Tissue** perfusion: cerebral (fetal) r/t difficult labor and birth

Risk for **Infection** r/t prolonged rupture of membranes

Risk for **Post-trauma** syndrome r/t sudden emergency during delivery of infant

Situational low **Self-esteem** r/t perceived inability to have normal labor and delivery

## DYSURIA

Impaired **Urinary** elimination r/t urinary tract infection

Risk for urge urinary **Incontinence** r/t detrusor hyperreflexia from cystitis, urethritis

# E

## E. COLI INFECTION

Deficient **Knowledge** r/t how to prevent disease; care of self with serious illness

**Fear** r/t serious illness, unknown outcome

*See Gastroenteritis; Gastroenteritis, Child*

## EAR SURGERY

Acute **Pain** r/t edema in ears from surgery

Disturbed **Sensory** perception: hearing r/t invasive surgery of ears, dressings

Ineffective **Health** maintenance r/t deficient knowledge regarding postoperative restrictions, expectations, care

Risk for delayed **Development** r/t hearing impairment

Risk for **Injury** r/t dizziness from excessive stimuli to vestibular apparatus

*See Hospitalized Child*

### EARACHE

Acute **Pain** r/t trauma, edema, infection

Disturbed **Sensory** perception: auditory r/t altered sensory reception, transmission, integration

### ECLAMPSIA

**Fear** r/t threat of well-being to self and fetus

Interrupted **Family** processes r/t unmet expectations for pregnancy and childbirth

Risk for **Aspiration** r/t seizure activity

Risk for delayed **Development** r/t uteroplacental insufficiency

Risk for disproportionate **Growth** r/t uteroplacental insufficiency

Risk for excess **Fluid** volume r/t decreased urine output secondary to renal dysfunction

Risk for imbalanced **Fluid** volume r/t retained fluid, decreased renal activity

Risk for ineffective **Tissue** perfusion: fetal r/t uteroplacental insufficiency

Risk for **Injury**: maternal r/t seizure activity

### ECT (ELECTROCONVULSIVE THERAPY)

Decisional **Conflict** r/t lack of relevant information

**Fear** r/t real or imagined threat to well-being

Impaired **Memory** r/t effects of treatment

*See Depression*

### ECTOPIC PREGNANCY

Acute **Pain** r/t stretching or rupture of implantation site

Chronic **Sorrow** r/t loss of pregnancy, potential loss of fertility

Death **Anxiety** r/t emergency condition, hemorrhage

Deficient **Fluid** volume r/t loss of blood

Disturbed **Body** image r/t negative feelings about body and reproductive functioning

**Fear** r/t threat to self, surgery, implications for future pregnancy

Ineffective **Role** performance r/t loss of pregnancy

Risk for ineffective **Coping** r/t loss of pregnancy

Risk for **Infection** r/t traumatized tissue, blood loss

Risk for interrupted **Family** processes r/t situational crisis

Risk for **Spiritual** distress r/t grief process

Situational low **Self-esteem** r/t loss of pregnancy, inability to carry pregnancy to term

### ECZEMA

Acute **Pain**: pruritus r/t inflammation of skin

Disturbed **Body** image r/t change in appearance from inflamed skin

Impaired **Skin** integrity r/t side effect of medication, allergic reaction

Ineffective **Health** maintenance r/t deficient knowledge regarding how to decrease inflammation and prevent further outbreaks

### ED (ERECTILE DYSFUNCTION)

*See Erectile Dysfunction; Impotence*

## EDEMA

Excess **Fluid** volume r/t excessive fluid intake, cardiac dysfunction, renal dysfunction, loss of plasma proteins

Ineffective **Health** maintenance r/t deficient knowledge regarding treatment of edema

Risk for impaired **Skin** integrity r/t impaired circulation, fragility of skin

*See cause of Edema*

## ELDERLY

*See Aging*

## ELDERLY ABUSE

*See Abuse, Spouse, Parent, or Significant Other*

## ELECTROCONVULSIVE THERAPY

*See ECT*

## EMACIATED PERSON

Adult **Failure** to thrive r/t imbalanced nutrition: less than body requirements

Imbalanced **Nutrition**: less than body requirements r/t inability to ingest food, digest food, absorb nutrients because of biological, psychological, economic factors

## EMBOLECTOMY

**Fear** r/t threat of great bodily harm from embolus

Ineffective **Tissue** perfusion: specify r/t presence of embolus

Risk for deficient **Fluid** volume: hemorrhage r/t postoperative complication, surgical area

*See Surgery, Postoperative Care*

## EMBOLI

*See Pulmonary Embolism*

## EMESIS

**Nausea** r/t chemotherapy, irritation of gastrointestinal system, stimulation

of neuropharmacological mechanisms, viral infection

*See Vomiting*

## EMOTIONAL PROBLEMS

*See Coping Problems*

## EMPATHY

**Health**-seeking behaviors r/t desire to attain maximum level of health

Readiness for enhanced community **Coping** r/t social supports, being available for problem solving

Readiness for enhanced family **Coping** r/t basic needs met, desire to move to higher level of health

Readiness for enhanced **Spiritual** well-being r/t desire to establish interconnectedness through spirituality

## EMPHYSEMA

*See COPD (Chronic Obstructive Pulmonary Disease)*

## EMPTINESS

Chronic **Sorrow** r/t unresolved grief

**Social** isolation r/t inability to engage in satisfying personal relationships

**Spiritual** distress r/t separation from religious/cultural ties

## ENCEPHALITIS

*See Meningitis/Encephalitis*

## ENDOCARDIAL CUSHION DEFECT

*See Congenital Heart Disease/Cardiac Anomalies*

## ENDOCARDITIS

**Activity** intolerance r/t reduced cardiac reserve, prescribed bedrest

Acute **Pain** r/t biological injury, inflammation

Decreased **Cardiac** output r/t inflammation of lining of heart and change in structure of valve leaflets, increased myocardial workload

E

Ineffective **Health** maintenance r/t deficient knowledge regarding treatment of disease, preventive measures against further incidence of disease

Ineffective **Tissue** perfusion: cardiopulmonary/peripheral r/t high risk for development of emboli

Risk for imbalanced **Nutrition**: less than body requirements r/t fever, hypermetabolic state associated with fever

### ENDOMETRIOSIS

Acute **Pain** r/t onset of menses with distention of endometrial tissue

Anticipatory **Grieving** r/t possible infertility

Ineffective **Health** maintenance r/t deficient knowledge about disease condition, medications, other treatments

**Nausea** r/t prostaglandin effect

**Sexual** dysfunction r/t painful coitus

### ENDOMETRITIS

Acute **Pain** r/t infectious process in reproductive tract

**Anxiety** r/t prolonged hospitalization, fear of unknown

**Hyperthermia** r/t infectious process

Ineffective **Health** maintenance r/t deficient knowledge regarding condition, treatment, antibiotic regimen

### ENURESIS

Ineffective **Health** maintenance r/t unachieved developmental task, neuromuscular immaturity, diseases of urinary system, infections or illnesses such as diabetes mellitus or insipidus, regression in developmental stage secondary to hospitalization or stress, parental deficient knowledge regarding involuntary urination at night after age 6, fluid intake at bedtime, lack of control during sound sleep, male gender

*See Toilet Training*

### ENVIRONMENTAL INTERPRETATION PROBLEMS

Adult **Failure** to thrive r/t impaired environmental interpretation syndrome

Chronic **Confusion** r/t impaired environmental interpretation syndrome

Disturbed **Thought** processes r/t lack of orientation to person, place, time, circumstances

Impaired **Environmental** interpretation syndrome r/t dementia, Parkinson's disease, Huntington's disease, depression, alcoholism

Impaired **Memory** r/t environmental disturbances

Risk for **Injury** r/t lack of orientation to person, place, time, circumstances

### EPIDIDYMITIS

Acute **Pain** r/t inflammation in scrotal sac

**Anxiety** r/t situational crisis, pain, threat to future fertility

Ineffective **Health** maintenance r/t deficient knowledge regarding treatment for pain and infection

Ineffective **Sexuality** patterns r/t edema of epididymis and testes

### EPIGLOTTITIS

*See Respiratory Infections, Acute Childhood (Croup, Epiglottitis, Pertussis, Pneumonia, Respiratory Syncytial Virus)*

### EPILEPSY

**Anxiety** r/t threat to role functioning

Impaired **Memory** r/t seizure activity

Ineffective **Health** maintenance r/t deficient knowledge regarding seizures and seizure control

Ineffective **Therapeutic** regimen management r/t deficient knowledge regarding seizure control

Risk for **Aspiration** r/t impaired swallowing, excessive secretions

Risk for delayed **Development** r/t seizure disorder

Risk for disturbed **Thought** processes r/t excessive, uncontrolled neurological stimuli

Risk for **Injury** r/t environmental factors during seizure

*See Seizure Disorders, Adult; Seizure Disorders, Childhood*

### EPISIOTOMY

**Anxiety** r/t fear of pain

Disturbed **Body** image r/t fear of resuming sexual relations

Impaired physical **Mobility** r/t pain, swelling, tissue trauma

Impaired **Skin** integrity r/t perineal incision

Acute **Pain** r/t tissue trauma

Risk for **Infection** r/t tissue trauma

**Sexual** dysfunction r/t altered body structure, tissue trauma

### EPISTAXIS

**Fear** r/t large amount of blood loss

Risk for deficient **Fluid** volume r/t excessive fluid loss

### EPSTEIN-BARR VIRUS

*See Mononucleosis*

### ERECTILE DYSFUNCTION (ED)

Readiness for enhanced **Knowledge** of treatment information for erectile dysfunction

**Self-esteem** disturbance r/t physiological crisis, inability to practice usual sexual activity

**Sexual** dysfunction r/t altered body function

*See Impotence*

### ESOPHAGEAL VARICES

Deficient **Fluid** volume: hemorrhage r/t portal hypertension, distended variceal vessels that can easily rupture

**Fear** r/t threat of death

*See Cirrhosis*

### ESOPHAGITIS

Acute **Pain** r/t inflammation of esophagus

Ineffective **Health** maintenance r/t deficient knowledge regarding treatment of disease

### ETOH WITHDRAWAL

*See Alcohol Withdrawal*

### EVISCERATION

*See Dehiscence, Abdominal*

### EXPOSURE TO HOT OR COLD ENVIRONMENT

Risk for imbalanced **Body** temperature r/t exposure

### EXTERNAL FIXATION

Disturbed **Body** image r/t trauma, change to affected part

Risk for **Infection** r/t pressure of pins on skin surface

*See Fracture*

### EYE SURGERY

**Anxiety** r/t possible loss of vision

Disturbed **Sensory** perception: visual r/t surgical procedure

Ineffective **Health** maintenance r/t deficient knowledge regarding postoperative activity, medications, eye care

Risk for **Injury** r/t impaired vision

**Self-care** deficit r/t impaired vision

*See Hospitalized Child; Vision Impairment*

E

# F

## FAILURE TO THRIVE, ADULT

Adult **Failure** to thrive r/t depression, apathy, fatigue

## FAILURE TO THRIVE, NONORGANIC

Chronic low **Self-esteem**: parental r/t feelings of inadequacy, support system deficiencies, inadequate role model

Delayed **Growth** and development r/t parental deficient knowledge, lack of stimulation, nutritional deficit, long-term hospitalization

Disorganized **Infant** behavior r/t lack of boundaries

Disturbed **Sleep** pattern r/t inconsistency of caretaker, lack of quiet environment

Imbalanced **Nutrition**: less than body requirements r/t inadequate type/amounts of food for infant, inappropriate feeding techniques

Impaired **Parenting** r/t lack of parenting skills, inadequate role modeling

Risk for delayed **Development** r/t failure to thrive

Risk for disproportionate **Growth** r/t failure to thrive

Risk for impaired parent/infant **Attachment** r/t inability of parents to meet infant's needs

**Social** isolation r/t limited support systems, self-imposed situation

## FALLS, RISK FOR

Risk for **Falls** r/t history of falls, physiological factors, cognitive impairment, medication effect, unsafe environment, young child or older adult

## FAMILY PRESENCE

Family **Presence** r/t resuscitation or invasive procedures being performed on family member

## FAMILY PROBLEMS

Compromised family **Coping** r/t inadequate or incorrect information or understanding by primary person, temporary preoccupation by significant person who is trying to manage emotional conflicts and personal suffering and is unable to perceive or act effectively in regard to client's needs, temporary family disorganization and role changes, other situational or developmental crises the significant person may be facing, little support provided by client for primary person, prolonged disease or disability progression that exhausts supportive capacity of significant people

Disabled family **Coping** r/t significant person with chronically unexpressed feelings such as guilt, anxiety, hostility, despair; dissonant discrepancy of coping styles for dealing with adaptive tasks by significant person and client or among significant people; highly ambivalent family relationships; arbitrary handling of family's resistance to treatment, which tends to solidify defensiveness as it fails to deal adequately with underlying anxiety

Ineffective family **Therapeutic** regimen management r/t complexity of health care system, complexity of therapeutic regimen, decisional conflicts, economic difficulties, excessive demands made on individual or family, family conflict

Interrupted **Family** processes r/t situation transition and/or crises, developmental transition and/or crises

Readiness for enhanced family **Coping** r/t needs sufficiently gratified, adaptive tasks effectively addressed to enable goals of self-actualization to surface

## FAMILY PROCESS

Readiness for enhanced **Family** processes r/t expressed willingness to enhance family dynamics; family functioning that meets physical, social, and psychological needs of family members; activities that support the safety and growth of family members; adequate communication; relationships that are generally positive; interdependence with community; accomplishment of family tasks; family roles that are flexible and appropriate for developmental stages; evident respect for family members; adaptation of family to change; maintenance of boundaries of family members; energy level of family that supports activities of daily living; evident family resilience; balance between autonomy and cohesiveness

## FATIGUE

Disturbed **Energy** field r/t disharmony

**Fatigue** r/t decreased or increased metabolic energy production, overwhelming psychological or emotional demands, increased energy requirements to perform ADLs, excessive social and/or role demands, states of discomfort, altered body chemistry

## FEAR

Death **Anxiety** r/t fear of death

**Fear** r/t identifiable physical or psychological threat to person

## FEBRILE SEIZURES

*See Seizure Disorders, Childhood*

## FECAL IMPACTION

*See Impaction of Stool*

## FECAL INCONTINENCE

**Bowel** incontinence r/t neurological impairment, gastrointestinal disorders, anorectal trauma

## FEEDING PROBLEMS, NEWBORN

Disorganized **Infant** behavior r/t prematurity, immature neurological system

Impaired **Swallowing** r/t prematurity

Ineffective **Breastfeeding** r/t prematurity, infant anomaly, maternal breast anomaly, previous breast surgery, previous history of breastfeeding failure, infant receiving supplemental feedings with artificial nipple, poor infant sucking reflex, nonsupportive partner and family, deficient knowledge, maternal anxiety or ambivalence

Ineffective **Infant** feeding pattern r/t prematurity, neurological impairment or delay, oral hypersensitivity, prolonged NPO (nothing by mouth) status

Interrupted **Breastfeeding** r/t maternal or infant illness, prematurity, maternal employment, contraindications to breastfeeding, need to abruptly wean infant

Risk for delayed **Development** r/t inadequate nutrition

Risk for disproportionate **Growth** r/t feeding problems

Risk for imbalanced **Fluid** volume r/t inability to take in adequate amount of fluids

## FEMORAL POPLITEAL BYPASS

Acute **Pain** r/t surgical trauma, edema in surgical area

**Anxiety** r/t threat to or change in health status

Ineffective **Tissue** perfusion: peripheral r/t impaired arterial circulation

F

Risk for deficient **Fluid** volume: hemorrhage r/t abnormal blood loss

Risk for **Infection** r/t invasive procedure

Risk for **Peripheral** neurovascular dysfunction r/t vascular surgery, emboli

## FETAL ALCOHOL SYNDROME

*See Infant of Substance-Abusing Mother*

## FETAL DISTRESS/ NONREASSURING FETAL HEART RATE PATTERN

**Fear** r/t threat to fetus

Ineffective **Tissue** perfusion: fetal r/t interruption of umbilical cord blood flow

Ineffective **Tissue** perfusion: placental r/t small or old placenta, interference with gas exchange transplacentally

## FEVER

**Hyperthermia** r/t infectious process, damage to hypothalamus, exposure to hot environment, medications, anesthesia, inability or decreased ability to perspire

## FIBROCYSTIC BREAST DISEASE

*See Breast Lumps*

## FILTHY HOME ENVIRONMENT

Impaired **Home** maintenance r/t individual or family member disease or injury, insufficient family organization or planning, impaired cognitive or emotional functioning, lack of knowledge, economic factors

## FINANCIAL CRISIS IN THE HOME ENVIRONMENT

Impaired **Home** maintenance r/t insufficient finances

## FISTULECTOMY

*See Hemorrhoidectomy (same nursing care)*

## FLAIL CHEST

**Anxiety** r/t difficulty breathing

Impaired spontaneous **Ventilation** r/t paradoxical respirations

Ineffective **Breathing** pattern r/t chest trauma

## FLASHBACKS

**Post-trauma** syndrome r/t catastrophic event

Risk for **Post-trauma** syndrome r/t occupation (e.g., police, fire, rescue, corrections, emergency room staff, mental health), exaggerated sense of responsibility, perception of event, survivor's role in event, displacement from home, inadequate social support, nonsupportive environment, diminished ego strength, duration of event

## FLAT AFFECT

Adult **Failure** to thrive r/t apathy

**Hopelessness** r/t prolonged activity restriction creating isolation, failing or deteriorating physiological condition, long-term stress, abandonment, lost belief in transcendent values or higher power/God

Risk for **Loneliness** r/t social isolation, lack of interest in surroundings

*See Dysthymic Disorder*

## FLESH-EATING BACTERIA

*See Necrotizing Fasciitis*

## FLUID BALANCE

Readiness for enhanced **Fluid** balance r/t expressed willingness to enhance fluid balance; stable weight; moist mucous membranes; food and fluid intake adequate for daily needs; straw-colored urine with specific gravity within normal limits; good tissue turgor; no excessive thirst; urine output appropriate for intake; no evidence of edema or dehydration

## FLUID VOLUME DEFICIT

Deficient **Fluid** volume r/t active fluid loss, failure of regulatory mechanisms

## FLUID VOLUME EXCESS

Excess **Fluid** volume r/t compromised regulatory mechanism, excess sodium intake

## FLUID VOLUME IMBALANCE, RISK FOR

Risk for imbalanced **Fluid** volume r/t major invasive surgeries

## FOODBORNE ILLNESS

Deficient **Fluid** volume r/t active fluid loss

Deficient **Knowledge** r/t care of self with serious illness, prevention of further incidences of foodborne illness

**Diarrhea** r/t infectious material in gastrointestinal tract

**Nausea** r/t contamination irritating stomach

*See Gastroenteritis; Gastroenteritis, Child; E. coli Infection*

## FOREIGN BODY ASPIRATION

Impaired **Home** maintenance r/t insufficient family organization or planning, lack of resources or support systems, inability to maintain orderly and clean surroundings

Ineffective **Airway** clearance r/t obstruction of airway

Ineffective **Health** maintenance r/t parental deficient knowledge regarding small toys, pieces of toys, nuts, balloons

Risk for **Suffocation** r/t inhalation of small object

*See Safety, Childhood*

## FORMULA FEEDING

Decisional **Conflict**: maternal r/t multiple or divergent sources of information, values conflict, support system deficit

**Grieving**: maternal r/t loss of desired breastfeeding experience

Ineffective **Health** maintenance r/t maternal deficient knowledge regarding formula feeding

Risk for **Constipation**: infant r/t iron-fortified formula

Risk for imbalanced **Nutrition**: more than body requirements r/t composition of formula and bottle feeding, overuse of food for reward or comfort measures

Risk for **Infection**: infant r/t lack of passive maternal immunity, supine feeding position

## FRACTURE

Acute **Pain** r/t muscle spasm, edema, trauma

Deficient **Diversional** activity r/t immobility

Impaired physical **Mobility** r/t limb immobilization

Impaired **Walking** r/t limb immobility

Ineffective **Health** maintenance r/t deficient knowledge regarding care of fracture

Risk for impaired **Skin** integrity r/t immobility, presence of cast

Risk for ineffective **Tissue** perfusion r/t immobility, presence of cast

Risk for **Peripheral** neurovascular dysfunction r/t mechanical compression, treatment of fracture

## FRACTURED HIP

*See Hip Fracture*

F

## FREQUENCY OF URINATION

Impaired **Urinary** elimination r/t anatomical obstruction, sensory-motor impairment, urinary tract infection

Risk for urge urinary **Incontinence** r/t effects of medications, caffeine, alcohol, aging

Stress urinary **Incontinence** r/t degenerative change in pelvic muscles and structural support

Urge urinary **Incontinence** r/t decreased bladder capacity, irritation of bladder stretch receptors causing spasm, alcohol, caffeine, increased fluids, increased urine concentration, overdistended bladder

**Urinary** retention r/t high urethral pressure caused by weak detrusor, inhibition of reflex arc, strong sphincter, blockage

## FROSTBITE

Acute **Pain** r/t decreased circulation from prolonged exposure to cold

Impaired **Skin** integrity r/t freezing of skin

Impaired **Tissue** integrity r/t freezing of skin

Ineffective **Tissue** perfusion r/t damage to extremities from prolonged exposure to cold

*See Hypothermia*

## FROTHY SPUTUM

*See CHF (Congestive Heart Failure); Pulmonary Edema; Seizure Disorders, Adult; Seizure Disorders, Childhood*

## FUSION, LUMBAR

Acute **Pain** r/t discomfort at bone donor site, surgical operation

**Anxiety** r/t fear of surgical procedure, possible recurring problems

Impaired physical **Mobility** r/t limitations from surgical procedure, presence of brace

Ineffective **Health** maintenance r/t deficient knowledge regarding postoperative mobility restrictions, body mechanics

Risk for **Injury** r/t improper body mechanics

Risk for perioperative positioning **Injury** r/t immobilization

# G

## GAG REFLEX, DEPRESSED OR ABSENT

Impaired **Swallowing** r/t neuromuscular impairment

Risk for **Aspiration** r/t depressed cough/gag reflex

## GALLOP RHYTHM

Decreased **Cardiac** output r/t decreased contractility of heart

## GALLSTONES

*See Cholelithiasis*

## GANGRENE

Delayed **Surgical** recovery r/t obstruction of arterial flow

**Fear** r/t possible loss of extremity

Ineffective **Tissue** perfusion: peripheral r/t obstruction of arterial flow

## GAS EXCHANGE, IMPAIRED

Impaired **Gas** exchange r/t ventilation-perfusion imbalance

## GASTRIC SURGERY

Risk for **Injury** r/t inadvertent insertion of nasogastric tube through gastric incision line

*See Abdominal Surgery*

## GASTRIC ULCER

*See GI Bleed (Gastrointestinal Bleeding); Ulcer, Peptic*

## GASTRITIS

Acute **Pain** r/t inflammation of gastric mucosa

Imbalanced **Nutrition**: less than body requirements r/t vomiting, inadequate intestinal absorption of nutrients, restricted dietary regimen

Risk for deficient **Fluid** volume r/t excessive loss from gastrointestinal tract secondary to vomiting, decreased intake

## GASTROENTERITIS

Acute **Pain** r/t increased peristalsis causing cramping

Deficient **Fluid** volume r/t excessive loss from gastrointestinal tract secondary to diarrhea, vomiting

**Diarrhea** r/t infectious process involving intestinal tract

Imbalanced **Nutrition**: less than body requirements r/t vomiting, inadequate intestinal absorption of nutrients, restricted dietary intake

Ineffective **Health** maintenance r/t deficient knowledge regarding treatment of disease

**Nausea** r/t irritation to gastrointestinal system

*See Gastroenteritis, Child*

## GASTROENTERITIS, CHILD

Impaired **Skin** integrity: diaper rash r/t acidic excretions on perineal tissues

Ineffective **Health** maintenance r/t lack of parental knowledge regarding fluid and dietary changes

Risk for delayed **Development** r/t inadequate nutrition

*See Gastroenteritis; Hospitalized Child*

## GASTROESOPHAGEAL REFLUX

Acute **Pain** r/t irritation of esophagus from gastric acids

**Anxiety**: parental r/t possible need for surgical intervention (Nissen fundoplication, gastrostomy tube)

Deficient **Fluid** volume r/t persistent vomiting

Imbalanced **Nutrition**: less than body requirements r/t poor feeding, vomiting

Ineffective **Airway** clearance r/t reflux of gastric contents into esophagus and tracheal or bronchial tree

Ineffective **Health** maintenance r/t deficient knowledge regarding antireflux regimen (e.g., positioning, oral or enteral feeding techniques, medications), possible home apnea monitoring

Risk for **Aspiration** r/t entry of gastric contents in tracheal or bronchial tree

Risk for impaired **Parenting** r/t disruption in bonding secondary to irritable or inconsolable infant

*See Child with Chronic Condition; Hospitalized Child*

## GASTROINTESTINAL HEMORRHAGE

*See GI Bleed (Gastrointestinal Bleeding)*

## GASTROSCHISIS/ OMPHALOCELE

Anticipatory **Grieving** r/t threatened loss of infant, loss of perfect birth or infant secondary to serious medical condition

Impaired **Gas** exchange r/t effects of anesthesia, subsequent atelectasis

Ineffective **Airway** clearance r/t complications of anesthetic effects

Risk for deficient **Fluid** volume r/t inability to feed secondary to condition, subsequent electrolyte imbalance

Risk for **Infection** r/t disrupted skin integrity with exposure of abdominal contents

Risk for **Injury** r/t disrupted skin integrity, ineffective protection

## GASTROSTOMY

Risk for impaired **Skin** integrity r/t presence of gastric contents on skin

*See Tube Feeding*

## GENITAL HERPES

*See Herpes Simplex II*

## GENITAL WARTS

*See STD (Sexually Transmitted Disease)*

## GESTATIONAL DIABETES (DIABETES IN PREGNANCY)

**Anxiety** r/t threat to self and/or fetus

Impaired fetal **Nutrition**: more than body requirements r/t excessive glucose uptake

Impaired maternal **Nutrition**: less than body requirements r/t decreased insulin production and glucose uptake in cells

Ineffective **Health** maintenance: maternal r/t deficient knowledge regarding care of diabetic condition in pregnancy

**Powerlessness** r/t lack of control over outcome of pregnancy

Risk for delayed **Development**: fetal r/t endocrine disorder of mother

Risk for disproportionate **Growth**: fetal r/t endocrine disorder of mother

Risk for impaired **Tissue** integrity: fetal r/t macrosomia, congenital defects, birth injury

Risk for impaired **Tissue** integrity: maternal r/t delivery of large infant

*See Diabetes Mellitus*

## GI BLEED (GASTROINTESTINAL BLEEDING)

Acute **Pain** r/t irritated mucosa from acid secretion

Deficient **Fluid** volume r/t gastrointestinal bleeding

**Fatigue** r/t loss of circulating blood volume, decreased ability to transport oxygen

**Fear** r/t threat to well-being, potential death

Imbalanced **Nutrition**: less than body requirements r/t nausea, vomiting

Risk for ineffective **Coping** r/t personal vulnerability in crisis, bleeding, hospitalization

## GINGIVITIS

Impaired **Dentition** r/t ineffective oral hygiene, barriers to self-care

Impaired **Oral** mucous membrane r/t ineffective oral hygiene

## GLAUCOMA

Deficient **Knowledge** r/t treatment and self-care for disease

Disturbed **Sensory** perception: visual r/t increased intraocular pressure

*See Vision Impairment*

## GLOMERULONEPHRITIS

Acute **Pain** r/t edema of kidney

Excess **Fluid** volume r/t renal impairment

Imbalanced **Nutrition**: less than body requirements r/t anorexia, restrictive diet

Ineffective **Health** maintenance r/t deficient knowledge regarding care of disease

## GONORRHEA

Acute **Pain** r/t inflammation of reproductive organs

Ineffective **Health** maintenance r/t deficient knowledge regarding treatment and prevention of disease

Risk for **Infection** r/t spread of organism throughout reproductive organs

*See STD (Sexually Transmitted Disease)*

## GOUT

Chronic **Pain** r/t inflammation of affected joint

Impaired physical **Mobility** r/t musculoskeletal impairment

Ineffective **Health** maintenance r/t deficient knowledge regarding medications and home care

## GRAND MAL SEIZURE

*See Seizure Disorders, Adult; Seizure Disorders, Childhood*

## GRANDIOSITY

Defensive **Coping** r/t inaccurate perception of self and abilities

## GRANDPARENTS RAISING GRANDCHILDREN

**Anxiety** r/t change in role status

Compromised family **Coping** r/t family role changes

Decisional **Conflict** r/t support system deficit

Ineffective family **Therapeutic** regimen management r/t excessive demands on individual/family

Ineffective **Role** performance r/t role transition

Interrupted **Family** processes r/t family roles shift

Parental role **Conflict** r/t change in parental role

Readiness for enhanced **Parenting** r/t physical and emotional needs of children are met

Risk for impaired **Parenting** r/t role strain

Risk for **Powerlessness** r/t aging

Risk for **Spiritual** distress r/t life change

## GRAVES' DISEASE

*See Hyperthyroidism*

## GRIEVING

Anticipatory **Grieving** r/t anticipated significant loss

Chronic **Sorrow** r/t unresolved grief

Dysfunctional **Grieving** r/t actual or perceived significant loss

**Grieving** r/t actual significant loss; change in life status, style, or function

## GROOM SELF (INABILITY TO)

Dressing/grooming **Self-care** deficit r/t intolerance to activity, decreased strength and endurance, pain, discomfort, perceptual or cognitive impairment, neuromuscular impairment, musculoskeletal impairment, depression, severe anxiety

## GROWTH AND DEVELOPMENT LAG

Delayed **Growth** and development r/t inadequate caretaking, indifference, inconsistent responsiveness, multiple caretakers, separation from significant others, environmental and stimulation deficiencies, effects of physical disability, prescribed dependence

### PRENATAL

Risk for disproportionate **Growth** r/t congenital/genetic disorders, maternal nutrition, multiple gestation, teratogen exposure, substance abuse

### INDIVIDUAL

Risk for disproportionate **Growth** r/t infection, prematurity, malnutrition, organic and inorganic factors, caregiver and/or individual maladaptive feeding behaviors, anorexia, insa-

G

tiable appetite, infection, chronic illness, substance abuse

### ENVIRONMENTAL

Risk for disproportionate **Growth** r/t deprivation, teratogen exposure, lead poisoning, poverty, violence, natural disasters

*See Developmental Concerns*

## GUILLAIN-BARRÉ SYNDROME

Impaired spontaneous **Ventilation** r/t weak respiration muscles

*See Neurological Disorders*

## GUILT

Anticipatory **Grieving** r/t potential loss of significant person, animal, prized material possession

Chronic **Sorrow** r/t unresolved grieving

Dysfunctional **Grieving** r/t actual loss of significant person, animal, prized material possession

Readiness for enhanced **Spiritual** well-being r/t desire to be in harmony with self, others, higher power/God

Risk for **Post-trauma** syndrome r/t exaggerated sense of responsibility for traumatic event

**Self-esteem** disturbance r/t unmet expectations of self

# H

## HAIR LOSS

Disturbed **Body** image r/t psychological reaction to loss of hair

Imbalanced **Nutrition**: less than body requirements r/t inability to ingest food because of biological, psychological, economic factors

## HALITOSIS

Impaired **Dentition** r/t ineffective oral hygiene

Impaired **Oral** mucous membranes r/t ineffective oral hygiene

## HALLUCINATIONS

Acute **Confusion** r/t alcohol abuse, delirium, dementia, mental illness, drug abuse

Adult **Failure** to thrive r/t altered mental status

**Anxiety** r/t threat to self-concept

Disturbed **Thought** processes r/t inability to control bizarre thoughts

Ineffective **Coping** r/t distortion and insecurity of life events

Risk for other-directed **Violence** r/t catatonic excitement, manic excitement, rage/panic reactions, response to violent internal stimuli

Risk for self-directed **Violence** r/t catatonic excitement, manic excitement, rage/panic reactions, response to violent internal stimuli

Risk for **Self-mutilation** r/t command hallucinations

## HEAD INJURY

Acute **Confusion** r/t brain injury

Decreased **Intracranial** adaptive capacity r/t brain injury

Disturbed **Sensory** perception r/t pressure damage to sensory centers in brain

Disturbed **Thought** processes r/t pressure damage to brain

Ineffective **Breathing** pattern r/t pressure damage to breathing center in brain stem

Ineffective **Tissue** perfusion: cerebral r/t effects of increased intracranial pressure

*See Neurological Disorders*

## HEADACHE

Acute **Pain** r/t lack of knowledge of pain control techniques or methods to prevent headaches

Disturbed **Energy** field r/t disharmony

Ineffective management of **Therapeutic** regimen r/t lack of knowledge, identification and elimination of aggravating factors

## HEALTH MAINTENANCE PROBLEMS

Ineffective **Health** maintenance r/t significant alteration in communication skills, lack of ability to make deliberate and thoughtful judgments, perceptual or cognitive impairment, ineffective coping, dysfunctional grieving, unachieved developmental tasks, ineffective family coping, disabling spiritual distress, lack of material resources

## HEALTH-SEEKING PERSON

**Health-seeking** behaviors r/t expressed desire for increased control of own personal health

## HEARING IMPAIRMENT

Disturbed **Sensory** perception: auditory r/t altered state of auditory system

Impaired verbal **Communication** r/t inability to hear own voice

**Social** isolation r/t difficulty with communication

## HEART FAILURE

*See CHF (Congestive Heart Failure)*

## HEART SURGERY

*See Coronary Artery Bypass Grafting*

## HEARTBURN

Acute **Pain**: heartburn r/t gastroesophageal reflux

Ineffective **Health** maintenance r/t deficient knowledge regarding information about factors that cause esophageal reflex

**Nausea** r/t gastrointestinal irritation

Risk for imbalanced **Nutrition**: less than body requirements r/t pain after eating

## HEAT STROKE

Deficient **Fluid** volume r/t profuse diaphoresis

Disturbed **Thought** processes r/t hyperthermia, increased oxygen needs

**Hopelessness** r/t prolonged activity restriction creating isolation, failing or deteriorating physiological condition, long-term stress, abandonment, lost belief in transcendent values or higher power/God

**Hyperthermia** r/t vigorous activity, hot environment

**Powerlessness** r/t lifestyle of helplessness

## HEMATEMESIS

*See GI Bleed (Gastrointestinal Bleeding)*

## HEMATOLOGICAL DISORDER

Ineffective **Protection** r/t abnormal blood profile

*See cause of Hematological Disorder*

## HEMATURIA

Risk for deficient **Fluid** volume r/t excessive loss of blood through urinary system

## HEMIANOPIA

**Anxiety** r/t change in vision

Disturbed **Sensory** perception r/t altered sensory reception, transmission, integration

Risk for **Injury** r/t disturbed sensory perception

Unilateral **Neglect** r/t effects of disturbed perceptual abilities

## HEMIPLEGIA

**Anxiety** r/t change in health status

Disturbed **Body** image r/t functional loss of one side of body

H

Impaired physical **Mobility** r/t loss of neurological control of involved extremities

Impaired **Transfer** ability r/t partial paralysis

Impaired **Walking** r/t loss of neurological control of involved extremities

Risk for impaired **Skin** integrity r/t alteration in sensation, immobility

Risk for **Injury** r/t impaired mobility

Risk for unilateral **Neglect** r/t neurological impairment; loss of sensation, vision, movement

**Self-care** deficit: specify r/t neuromuscular impairment

Unilateral **Neglect** r/t effects of disturbed perceptual abilities

See CVA (Cerebrovascular Accident)

## HEMODIALYSIS

Excess **Fluid** volume r/t renal disease with minimal urine output

Ineffective **Coping** r/t situational crisis

Ineffective **Health** maintenance r/t deficient knowledge regarding hemodialysis procedure, restrictions, blood access care

Interrupted **Family** processes r/t changes in role responsibilities as a result of therapy regimen

**Noncompliance**: dietary restrictions r/t denial of chronic illness

**Powerlessness** r/t treatment regimen

Risk for **Caregiver** role strain r/t complexity of care receiver treatment

Risk for deficient **Fluid** volume r/t excessive removal of fluid during dialysis

Risk for **Infection** r/t exposure to blood products, risk for developing hepatitis B or C

Risk for **Injury**: clotting of blood access r/t abnormal surface for blood flow

See Renal Failure; Renal Failure, Acute/Chronic, Child

## HEMODYNAMIC MONITORING

Risk for **Infection** r/t invasive procedure

Risk for **Injury** r/t inadvertent wedging of catheter, dislodgement of catheter, disconnection of catheter with embolism

## HEMOLYTIC UREMIC SYNDROME

Deficient **Fluid** volume r/t vomiting, diarrhea

Impaired **Comfort**: nausea/vomiting r/t effects of uremia

Risk for impaired **Skin** integrity r/t diarrhea

Risk for **Injury** r/t decreased platelet count, seizure activity

See Hospitalized Child; Renal Failure, Acute/Chronic, Child

## HEMOPHILIA

Acute **Pain** r/t bleeding into body tissues

**Fear** r/t high risk for AIDS secondary to contaminated blood products

Impaired physical **Mobility** r/t pain from acute bleeds, imposed activity restrictions

Ineffective **Health** maintenance r/t knowledge and skill acquisition regarding home administration of intravenous clotting factors, protection from injury

Ineffective **Protection** r/t deficient clotting factors

Risk for **Injury** r/t deficient clotting factors, child's developmental level, age-appropriate play, inappropriate use of toys or sports equipment

See Child with Chronic Condition;

*Hospitalized Child; Maturational Issues, Adolescent*

## HEMOPTYSIS

**Fear** r/t serious threat to well-being

Risk for deficient **Fluid** volume r/t excessive loss of blood

Risk for ineffective **Airway** clearance r/t obstruction of airway with blood and mucus

## HEMORRHAGE

Deficient **Fluid** volume r/t massive blood loss

**Fear** r/t threat to well-being

*See cause of Hemorrhage; Hypovolemic Shock*

## HEMORRHOIDECTOMY

Acute **Pain** r/t surgical procedure

**Anxiety** r/t embarrassment, need for privacy

**Constipation** r/t fear of pain with defecation

Ineffective **Health** maintenance r/t deficient knowledge regarding pain relief, use of stool softeners, dietary changes

Risk for deficient **Fluid** volume: hemorrhage r/t inadequate clotting

**Urinary** retention r/t pain, anesthetic effect

## HEMORRHOIDS

**Constipation** r/t painful defecation, poor bowel habits

Impaired **Comfort**: pruritus r/t inflammation of hemorrhoids

Ineffective **Health** maintenance r/t deficient knowledge regarding care of condition

## HEMOTHORAX

Deficient **Fluid** volume r/t blood in pleural space

*See Pneumothorax*

## HEPATITIS

**Activity** intolerance r/t weakness or fatigue secondary to infection

Acute **Pain** r/t edema of liver, bile irritating skin

Deficient **Diversional** activity r/t isolation

**Fatigue** r/t infectious process, altered body chemistry

Imbalanced **Nutrition**: less than body requirements r/t anorexia, impaired use of proteins and carbohydrates

Ineffective **Health** maintenance r/t deficient knowledge regarding disease process and home management

Risk for deficient **Fluid** volume r/t excessive loss of fluids via vomiting and diarrhea

**Social** isolation r/t treatment-imposed isolation

## HERNIA

*See Hiatus Hernia; Inguinal Hernia Repair*

## HERNIATED DISK

*See Low Back Pain*

## HERNIORRHAPHY

*See Inguinal Hernia Repair*

## HERPES IN PREGNANCY

Acute **Pain** r/t active herpes lesion

**Fear** r/t threat to fetus, impending surgery

Impaired **Tissue** integrity r/t active herpes lesion

Impaired **Urinary** elimination r/t pain with urination

Ineffective **Health** maintenance r/t deficient knowledge regarding treatment of disease, protection of fetus

Risk for **Infection**: transmission r/t transplacental transfer during primary

H

herpes, exposure to active herpes during birth process

Situational low **Self-esteem** r/t threat to fetus secondary to disease process

## HERPES SIMPLEX I

Impaired **Dentition** r/t impaired oral mucous membranes

Impaired **Oral** mucous membranes r/t inflammatory changes in mouth

## HERPES SIMPLEX II

Acute **Pain** r/t active herpes lesion

Impaired **Tissue** integrity r/t active herpes lesion

Impaired **Urinary** elimination r/t pain with urination

Ineffective **Health** maintenance r/t deficient knowledge regarding treatment, prevention of spread of disease

**Sexual** dysfunction r/t disease process

Situational low **Self-esteem** r/t expressions of shame or guilt

## HERPES ZOSTER

*See Shingles*

## HHNC (HYPEROSMOLAR HYPERGLYCEMIC NONKETOTIC COMA)

*See Hyperosmolar Hyperglycemic Nonketotic Coma*

## HIATUS HERNIA

Acute **Pain** r/t gastroesophageal reflux

Imbalanced **Nutrition**: less than body requirements r/t pain after eating

Ineffective **Health** maintenance r/t deficient knowledge regarding care of disease

**Nausea** r/t effects of gastric contents in esophagus

## HIP FRACTURE

Acute **Confusion** r/t sensory overload, sensory deprivation, medication side effects

Acute **Pain** r/t injury, surgical procedure

**Constipation** r/t immobility, narcotics, anesthesia

**Fear** r/t outcome of treatment, future mobility, present helplessness

Impaired physical **Mobility** r/t surgical incision, temporary absence of weight bearing

Impaired **Transfer** ability r/t immobilization of hip

Impaired **Walking** r/t temporary absence of weight bearing

**Powerlessness** r/t health care environment

Risk for deficient **Fluid** volume: hemorrhage r/t postoperative complication, surgical blood loss

Risk for impaired **Skin** integrity r/t immobility

Risk for **Infection** r/t invasive procedure

Risk for **Injury** r/t dislodged prosthesis, unsteadiness when ambulating

Risk for perioperative positioning **Injury** r/t immobilization, muscle weakness, emaciation

**Self-care** deficit: specify r/t musculoskeletal impairment

## HIP REPLACEMENT

*See Total Joint Replacement*

## HIRSCHSPRUNG'S DISEASE

Acute **Pain** r/t distended colon, incisional postoperative pain

**Constipation**: bowel obstruction r/t inhibited peristalsis secondary to congenital absence of parasympathetic ganglion cells in distal colon

**Grieving** r/t loss of perfect child, birth of child with congenital defect even though child expected to be normal within 2 years

Imbalanced **Nutrition**: less than body

requirements r/t anorexia, pain from distended colon

Impaired **Skin** integrity r/t stoma, potential skin care problems associated with stoma

Ineffective **Health** maintenance r/t parental deficient knowledge regarding temporary stoma care, dietary management, treatment for constipation or diarrhea

*See Hospitalized Child*

## HIRSUTISM

Disturbed **Body** image r/t excessive hair

## HITTING BEHAVIOR

Acute **Confusion** r/t dementia, alcohol abuse, drug abuse, delirium

Impaired **Adjustment** r/t intense emotional state

Ineffective **Coping** r/t situational crises, maturational crises, personal vulnerability

Risk for other-directed **Violence** r/t history of violence, neurological impairment, cognitive impairment, history of childhood abuse, history of witnessing family violence, cruelty to animals, firesetting, history of alcohol/drug abuse, pathological intoxication, psychotic symptomatology, motor vehicle offenses, impulsivity, availability or possession of weapon, body language

## HIV (HUMAN IMMUNODEFICIENCY VIRUS)

**Fear** r/t possible death

Ineffective **Protection** r/t depressed immune system

*See AIDS (Acquired Immunodeficiency Syndrome)*

## HODGKIN'S DISEASE

*See Anemia; Cancer; Chemotherapy*

## HOME MAINTENANCE PROBLEMS

Impaired **Home** maintenance r/t individual or family member disease or injury, insufficient family organization or planning, insufficient finances, unfamiliarity with neighborhood resources, impaired cognitive or emotional functioning, lack of knowledge, lack of role modeling, inadequate support systems

## HOMELESSNESS

Impaired **Home** maintenance r/t impaired cognitive or emotional functioning, inadequate support system, insufficient finances

**Powerlessness** r/t interpersonal interactions

Risk for **Trauma** r/t being in high-crime neighborhood

## HOPELESSNESS

Chronic **Sorrow** r/t unresolved grief

**Hopelessness** r/t prolonged activity restriction creating isolation, failing or deteriorating physiological condition, long-term stress, abandonment, lost belief in transcendent values or higher power/God

**Powerlessness** r/t lifestyle of helplessness

## HOSPITALIZED CHILD

**Activity** intolerance r/t fatigue associated with acute illness

Acute **Pain** r/t treatments, diagnostic or therapeutic procedures

**Anxiety**: separation (child) r/t familiar surroundings and separation from family and friends

Compromised family **Coping** r/t possible prolonged hospitalization that exhausts supportive capacity of significant people

Deficient **Diversional** activity r/t immo-

H

bility, monotonous environment, frequent or lengthy treatments, reluctance to participate, therapeutic isolation, separation from peers

Delayed **Growth** and development r/t regression or lack of progression toward developmental milestones secondary to frequent or prolonged hospitalization, inadequate or inappropriate stimulation, cerebral insult, chronic illness, effects of physical disability, prescribed dependence

Disturbed **Sleep** pattern: child or parent r/t 24-hour care needs of hospitalization

**Fear** r/t deficient knowledge or maturational level with fear of unknown, mutilation, painful procedures, surgery

**Hopelessness**: child r/t prolonged activity restriction, uncertain prognosis

Ineffective **Coping**: parent r/t possible guilt regarding hospitalization of child, parental inadequacies

Interrupted **Family** processes r/t situational crisis of illness, disease, hospitalization

**Powerlessness**: child r/t health care environment, illness-related regimen

Readiness for enhanced family **Coping** r/t impact of crisis on family values, priorities, goals, relationships in family

Risk for impaired parent/child **Attachment** r/t separation

Risk for delayed **Growth** and development: regression r/t disruption of normal routine, unfamiliar environment or caregivers, developmental vulnerability of young children

Risk for imbalanced **Nutrition**: less than body requirements r/t anorexia, absence of familiar foods, cultural preferences

Risk for **Injury** r/t unfamiliar environment, developmental age, lack of parental knowledge regarding safety (e.g., side rails, IV site/pole)

## HOSTILE BEHAVIOR

Risk for other-directed **Violence** r/t antisocial personality disorder

## HTN (HYPERTENSION)

Disturbed **Energy** field r/t pain, discomfort

Imbalanced **Nutrition**: more than body requirements r/t lack of knowledge of relationship between diet and disease process

Ineffective **Health** maintenance r/t deficient knowledge regarding treatment and control of disease process

**Noncompliance** r/t side effects of treatments, lack of understanding regarding importance of controlling hypertension

## HUMAN IMMUNODEFICIENCY VIRUS (HIV)

*See AIDS (Acquired Immunodeficiency Syndrome); HIV (Human Immunodeficiency Virus)*

## HUNTINGTON'S DISEASE

Decisional **Conflict** r/t whether to have children

*See Neurological Disorders*

## HYDROCELE

Acute **Pain** r/t severely enlarged hydrocele

Ineffective **Sexuality** pattern r/t recent surgery on area of scrotum

## HYDROCEPHALUS

Decisional **Conflict** r/t unclear or conflicting values regarding selection of treatment modality

Delayed **Growth** and development r/t sequelae of increased intracranial pressure

Excess **Fluid** volume: cerebral ventricles r/t compromised regulatory mechanism

Imbalanced **Nutrition**: less than body requirements r/t inadequate intake secondary to anorexia, nausea, vomiting, feeding difficulties

Impaired **Skin** integrity r/t impaired physical mobility, mechanical irritation

Ineffective **Tissue** perfusion: cerebral r/t interrupted flow, hypervolemia of cerebral ventricles

Interrupted **Family** processes r/t situational crisis

Risk for delayed **Development** r/t sequelae of increased intracranial pressure

Risk for disproportionate **Growth** r/t sequelae of increased intracranial pressure

Risk for **Infection** r/t sequelae of invasive procedure (shunt placement)

*See Normal Pressure Hydrocephalus, Child with Chronic Condition; Hospitalized Child; Mental Retardation (if appropriate); Premature Infant (Child); Premature Infant (Parent)*

## HYGIENE, INABILITY TO PROVIDE OWN

Adult **Failure** to thrive r/t depression, apathy as evidenced by inability to perform self-care

**Self-care** deficit: bathing/hygiene r/t intolerance to activity, decreased strength and endurance, pain, discomfort, perceptual or cognitive impairment, neuromuscular impairment, musculoskeletal impairment, depression, severe anxiety

## HYPERACTIVE SYNDROME

Compromised family **Coping** r/t unsuccessful strategies to control excessive activity, behaviors, frustration, anger

Decisional **Conflict** r/t multiple or divergent sources of information regarding education, nutrition, medication regimens; willingness to change own food habits; limited resources

Impaired **Social** interaction r/t impulsive and overactive behaviors, concomitant emotional difficulties, distractibility and excitability

Ineffective **Role** performance: parent r/t stressors associated with dealing with hyperactive child, perceived or projected blame for causes of child's behavior, unmet needs for support or care, lack of energy to provide for those needs

Parental role **Conflict**: when siblings present r/t increased attention toward hyperactive child

Risk for delayed **Development** r/t behavior disorders

Risk for impaired **Parenting** r/t disruptive or uncontrollable behaviors of child

Risk for other-directed **Violence**: parent or child r/t frustration with disruptive behavior, anger, unsuccessful relationship(s)

**Self-esteem** disturbance r/t inability to achieve socially acceptable behaviors; frustration; frequent reprimands, punishment, or scoldings secondary to uncontrolled activity and behaviors; mood fluctuations and restlessness; inability to succeed academically; lack of peer support

## HYPERALIMENTATION

*See TPN (Total Parenteral Nutrition)*

## HYPERBILIRUBINEMIA

**Anxiety**: parent r/t threat to infant, unknown future

Disturbed **Sensory** perception: visual (infant) r/t use of eye patches for protection of eyes during phototherapy

Imbalanced **Nutrition**: less than body requirements (infant) r/t disinterest in feeding because of jaundice-related lethargy

Parental role **Conflict** r/t interruption of family life because of care regimen

Risk for disproportionate **Growth**: infant r/t disinterest in feeding because of jaundice-related lethargy

Risk for **Imbalanced** body temperature: infant r/t phototherapy

Risk for **Injury**: infant r/t kernicterus, phototherapy lights

## HYPERCALCEMIA

Decreased **Cardiac** output r/t brady-dysrhythmia

Disturbed **Thought** processes r/t elevated calcium levels that cause paranoia, decreased level of consciousness

Imbalanced **Nutrition**: less than body requirements r/t gastrointestinal manifestations of hypercalcemia (nausea, anorexia, ileus)

Impaired physical **Mobility** r/t decreased tone in smooth and striated muscle

Risk for **Trauma** r/t risk for fractures

## HYPERCAPNIA

**Fear** r/t difficulty breathing

Impaired **Gas** exchange r/t ventilation perfusion imbalance

## HYPEREMESIS GRAVIDARUM

**Anxiety** r/t threat to self and infant, hospitalization

Deficient **Fluid** volume r/t vomiting

Imbalanced **Nutrition**: less than body requirements r/t vomiting

Impaired **Home** maintenance r/t chronic nausea, inability to function

**Nausea** r/t hormonal changes of pregnancy

**Powerlessness** r/t health care regimen

**Social** isolation r/t hospitalization

## HYPERGLYCEMIA

Ineffective management of **Therapeutic** regimen r/t complexity of therapeutic regimen, decisional conflicts, economic difficulties, nonsupportive family, insufficient cues to action, deficient knowledge, mistrust, lack of acknowledgment of seriousness of condition

*See Diabetes Mellitus*

## HYPERKALEMIA

Risk for **Activity** intolerance r/t muscle weakness

Risk for decreased **Cardiac** output r/t possible dysrhythmia

Risk for excess **Fluid** volume r/t untreated renal failure

## HYPERNATREMIA

Risk for deficient **Fluid** volume r/t abnormal water loss, inadequate water intake

## HYPEROSMOLAR HYPERGLYCEMIC NONKETOTIC COMA (HHNC)

Deficient **Fluid** volume r/t polyuria, inadequate fluid intake

Disturbed **Thought** processes r/t dehydration, electrolyte imbalance

Risk for **Injury**: seizures r/t hyperosmolar state, electrolyte imbalance

*See Diabetes Mellitus; Diabetes Mellitus, Juvenile*

## HYPERPHOSPHATEMIA

Deficient **Knowledge** r/t dietary changes needed to control phosphate levels

*See Renal Failure*

## HYPERSENSITIVITY TO SLIGHT CRITICISM

Defensive **Coping** r/t situational crisis, psychological impairment, substance abuse

## HYPERTENSION

Imbalanced **Nutrition**: more than body requirements r/t lack of knowledge of relationship between diet and disease process

Ineffective **Health** maintenance r/t deficient knowledge regarding treatment and control of disease process

**Noncompliance** r/t side effects of treatment

## HYPERTHERMIA

**Hyperthermia** r/t exposure to hot environment, vigorous activity, medications, anesthesia, inappropriate clothing, increased metabolic rate, illness, trauma, dehydration, inability or decreased ability to perspire

## HYPERTHYROIDISM

**Activity** intolerance r/t increased oxygen demands from increased metabolic rate

**Anxiety** r/t increased stimulation, loss of control

**Diarrhea** r/t increased gastric motility

Disturbed **Sleep** pattern r/t anxiety, excessive sympathetic discharge

Imbalanced **Nutrition**: less than body requirements r/t increased metabolic rate, increased gastrointestinal activity

Ineffective **Health** maintenance r/t deficient knowledge regarding medications, methods of coping with stress

Risk for **Injury**: eye damage r/t exophthalmos

## HYPERVENTILATION

Ineffective **Breathing** pattern r/t anxiety, acid-base imbalance

## HYPOCALCEMIA

**Activity** intolerance r/t neuromuscular irritability

Imbalanced **Nutrition**: less than body requirements r/t effects of vitamin D deficiency, renal failure, malabsorption, laxative use

Ineffective **Breathing** pattern r/t laryngospasm

## HYPOGLYCEMIA

Disturbed **Thought** processes r/t insufficient blood glucose to brain

Imbalanced **Nutrition**: less than body requirements r/t imbalance of glucose and insulin level

Ineffective **Health** maintenance r/t deficient knowledge regarding disease process, self-care

*See Diabetes Mellitus; Diabetes Mellitus, Juvenile*

## HYPOKALEMIA

**Activity** intolerance r/t muscle weakness

Decreased **Cardiac** output r/t possible dysrhythmia from electrolyte imbalance

## HYPOMAGNESEMIA

**Imbalanced Nutrition**: less than body requirements r/t deficient knowledge of nutrition, alcoholism

*See Alcoholism*

## HYPOMANIA

Disturbed **Sleep** pattern r/t psychological stimulus

*See Manic Disorder, Bipolar I*

## HYPONATREMIA

Disturbed **Thought** processes r/t electrolyte imbalance

Excess **Fluid** volume r/t excessive intake of hypotonic fluids

H

Risk for **Injury** r/t seizures, new onset of confusion

## HYPOPLASTIC LEFT LUNG

*See Congenital Heart Disease/Cardiac Anomalies*

## HYPOTENSION

Decreased **Cardiac** output r/t decreased preload, decreased contractility

Disturbed **Thought** processes r/t decreased oxygen supply to brain

Ineffective **Tissue** perfusion: cardiopulmonary/peripheral r/t hypovolemia, decreased contractility, decreased afterload

Risk for deficient **Fluid** volume r/t excessive fluid loss

*See cause of Hypotension*

## HYPOTHERMIA

**Hypothermia** r/t exposure to cold environment, illness, trauma, damage to hypothalamus, malnutrition, aging

## HYPOTHYROIDISM

**Activity** intolerance r/t muscular stiffness, shortness of breath on exertion

**Constipation** r/t decreased gastric motility

Disturbed **Thought** processes r/t altered metabolic process

Imbalanced **Nutrition**: more than body requirements r/t decreased metabolic process

Impaired **Gas** exchange r/t possible respiratory depression

Impaired **Skin** integrity r/t edema, dry or scaly skin

Ineffective **Health** maintenance r/t deficient knowledge regarding disease process and self-care

## HYPOVOLEMIC SHOCK

Deficient **Fluid** volume r/t trauma, third spacing, loss of fluid from body

*See Shock*

## HYPOXIA

Acute **Confusion** r/t decreased oxygen supply to brain

Disturbed **Thought** processes r/t decreased oxygen supply to brain

**Fear** r/t breathlessness

Impaired **Gas** exchange r/t altered oxygen supply, inability to transport oxygen

## HYSTERECTOMY

Acute **Pain** r/t surgical injury

Anticipatory **Grieving** r/t change in body image, loss of reproductive status

**Constipation** r/t opioids, anesthesia, bowel manipulation during surgery

Ineffective **Coping** r/t situational crisis of surgery

Ineffective **Health** maintenance r/t deficient knowledge regarding precautions and self-care following surgery

Risk for **Constipation** r/t narcotics, anesthesia, bowel manipulation during surgery

Risk for deficient **Fluid** volume r/t abnormal blood loss, hemorrhage

Risk for ineffective **Tissue** perfusion r/t thromboembolism

Risk for urge urinary **Incontinence** r/t edema in area, anesthesia, narcotics, pain

Risk for **Urinary** retention r/t edema in area, anesthesia, opioids, pain

**Sexual** dysfunction r/t disturbance in self-concept

*See Surgery, Perioperative; Surgery, Preoperative; Surgery, Postoperative*

# I

## IBS (IRRITABLE BOWEL SYNDROME)

Chronic **Pain** r/t spasms, increased motility of bowel

**Constipation** r/t low-residue diet, stress

**Diarrhea** r/t increased motility of intestines associated with stress

Ineffective **Health** maintenance r/t deficient knowledge regarding self-care with IBS

Ineffective **Therapeutic** regimen management r/t deficient knowledge, powerlessness

Readiness for enhanced **Therapeutic** regimen management r/t an expressed desire to manage illness and prevent onset of symptoms

## ICD (IMPLANTABLE CARDIOVERTER/ DEFIBRILLATOR)

Ineffective **Health** maintenance r/t deficient knowledge regarding self-care, action of internal cardiac defibrillator

Decreased **Cardiac** output r/t possible dysrhythmia

## IDDM (INSULIN-DEPENDENT DIABETES)

*See Diabetes Mellitus*

## IDENTITY DISTURBANCE

Disturbed personal **Identity** r/t situational crisis, psychological impairment, chronic illness, pain

Readiness for enhanced **Coping** r/t seeking social support

**Spiritual** distress r/t expression of alienation from others

## IDIOPATHIC THROMBOCYTOPENIC PURPURA

*See ITP (Idiopathic Thrombocytopenic Purpura)*

## ILEAL CONDUIT

Deficient **Knowledge** r/t care of stoma

Disturbed **Body** image r/t presence of stoma

Ineffective **Sexuality** patterns r/t altered body function and structure

Ineffective **Therapeutic** regimen management r/t new skills required to care for appliance and self

Readiness for enhanced **Therapeutic** regimen management r/t expressed desire to care for stoma

Risk for impaired **Skin** integrity r/t difficulty obtaining tight seal of appliance

Risk for latex **Allergy** response r/t repeated exposures to latex associated with treatment and management of disease

**Social** isolation r/t alteration in physical appearance, fear of accidental spill of ostomy contents

## ILEOSTOMY

Chronic **Sorrow** r/t physical changes associated with presence of stoma

**Constipation/Diarrhea** r/t dietary changes, change in intestinal motility

Deficient **Knowledge** r/t limited practice of stoma care, dietary modifications

Disturbed **Body** image r/t presence of stoma

Ineffective **Sexuality** patterns r/t altered body function and structure

Ineffective **Therapeutic** regimen management r/t new skills required to care for appliance and self

Risk for impaired **Skin** integrity r/t difficulty obtaining tight seal of appliance, caustic drainage

**Social** isolation r/t alteration in physical appearance, fear of accidental spill of ostomy contents

## ILEUS

Acute **Pain** r/t pressure, abdominal distention

**Constipation** r/t decreased gastric motility

Deficient **Fluid** volume r/t loss of fluids from vomiting, fluids trapped in bowel

**Nausea** r/t gastrointestinal irritation

## IMMOBILITY

Adult **Failure** to thrive r/t limited physical mobility

**Constipation** r/t immobility

Disturbed **Thought** processes r/t sensory deprivation from immobility

Impaired physical **Mobility** r/t medically imposed bedrest

Impaired **Transfer** ability r/t limited physical mobility

Impaired **Walking** r/t limited physical mobility

Ineffective **Breathing** pattern r/t inability to deep breathe in supine position

Ineffective **Tissue** perfusion: peripheral r/t interruption of venous flow

**Powerlessness** r/t forced immobility from health care environment

Risk for **Disuse** syndrome r/t immobilization

Risk for impaired **Skin** integrity r/t pressure on immobile parts, shearing forces when moved

## IMMUNOSUPPRESSION

Ineffective **Protection** r/t medications, treatments or pathology suppressing immune system function

Risk for **Infection** r/t immunosuppression

## IMPACTION OF STOOL

**Constipation** r/t decreased fluid intake, less than adequate amounts of fiber and bulk-forming foods in diet, medication effect, or immobility

Readiness for enhanced **Therapeutic** regimen management r/t to appropriate nutritional choices to prevent constipation

## IMPERFORATE ANUS

**Anxiety** r/t ability to care for newborn

Deficient **Knowledge** r/t home care for newborn

Impaired **Skin** integrity r/t pruritus

Risk for impaired **Skin** integrity r/t presence of stool at surgical repair site

## IMPETIGO

Ineffective **Health** maintenance r/t parental deficient knowledge regarding care of impetigo

*See Communicable Diseases, Childhood*

## IMPLANTABLE CARDIOVERTER/ DEFIBRILLATOR

*See ICD (Implantable Cardioverter/ Defibrillator)*

## IMPOTENCE

Readiness for enhanced **Knowledge** of treatment information for erectile dysfunction

**Self-esteem** disturbance r/t physiological crisis, inability to practice usual sexual activity

**Sexual** dysfunction r/t altered body function

## INACTIVITY

**Activity** intolerance r/t imbalance between oxygen supply and demand, sedentary lifestyle, weakness, immobility

Impaired physical **Mobility** r/t intolerance to activity, decreased strength and endurance, depression, severe anxiety, musculoskeletal impairment, perceptual or cognitive impairment, neuromuscular impairment, pain, discomfort

Risk for **Constipation** r/t insufficient physical activity

## INCOMPETENT CERVIX
*See Premature Dilation of the Cervix*

## INCONTINENCE OF STOOL

**Bowel** incontinence r/t decreased awareness of need to defecate, loss of sphincter control

Deficient **Knowledge** r/t lack of information on normal bowel elimination

Disturbed **Body** image r/t inability to control elimination of stool

Risk for impaired **Skin** integrity r/t presence of stool

Situational low **Self-esteem** r/t inability to control elimination of stool

Toileting **Self-care** deficit r/t toileting needs

## INCONTINENCE OF URINE

Functional **Incontinence** r/t altered environment; sensory, cognitive, or mobility deficits

Reflex **Incontinence** r/t neurological impairment

Risk for impaired **Skin** integrity r/t presence of urine

Risk for urge urinary **Incontinence** r/t effects of alcohol, caffeine, decreased bladder capacity, irritation of bladder stretch receptors causing spasm, increased urine concentration, overdistention of bladder

Toileting **Self-care** deficit r/t toileting needs

Situational low **Self-esteem** r/t inability to control passage of urine

Stress urinary **Incontinence** r/t degen-erative change in pelvic muscles and structural supports associated with increased age, high intraabdominal pressure (e.g., from obesity, gravid uterus), incompetent bladder outlet, overdistention between voidings, weak pelvic muscles and structural supports

Total urinary **Incontinence** r/t neuropathy preventing transmission of reflex indicating bladder fullness, neurological dysfunction causing triggering of micturition at unpredictable times, independent contraction of detrusor reflex resulting from surgery, trauma or disease affecting spinal cord nerves, anatomical fistula

Urge urinary **Incontinence** r/t decreased bladder capacity (i.e., history of pelvic inflammatory disease, abdominal surgeries, indwelling urinary catheter), irritation of bladder stretch receptors causing spasm (e.g., bladder infection), alcohol, caffeine, increased fluids, increased urine concentration, overdistention of bladder

## INDIGESTION

Imbalanced **Nutrition**: less than body requirements r/t discomfort when eating

Impaired **Comfort** r/t burning, bloating, heaviness, unpleasant sensations experienced when eating

**Nausea** r/t gastrointestinal irritation

## INDUCTION OF LABOR

**Anxiety** r/t medical interventions

Decisional **Conflict** r/t perceived threat to idealized birth

Ineffective **Coping** r/t situational crisis of medical intervention in birthing process

Readiness for enhanced **Family** processes r/t family support during induction of labor

I

Risk for imbalanced **Fluid** volume r/t intravenous fluid therapy

Risk for **Injury**: maternal and fetal r/t hypertonic uterus, potential prematurity of newborn

**Self-esteem** disturbance r/t inability to carry out normal labor

## INFANT APNEA

*See Premature Infant; Respiratory Conditions of the Neonate; SIDS (Sudden Infant Death Syndrome)*

## INFANT BEHAVIOR

Disorganized **Infant** behavior r/t pain, oral/motor problems, feeding intolerance, environmental overstimulation, lack of containment/boundaries, prematurity, invasive/painful procedures

Readiness for enhanced organized **Infant** behavior r/t prematurity, pain

Risk for disorganized **Infant** behavior r/t pain, oral/motor problems, environmental overstimulation, lack of containment/boundaries

## INFANT FEEDING PATTERN, INEFFECTIVE

Disorganized **Infant** behavior r/t prematurity, immature neurological system

Impaired **Swallowing** r/t prematurity

Ineffective **Infant** feeding pattern r/t prematurity, neurological impairment or delay, oral hypersensitivity, prolonged NPO

Risk for imbalanced **Fluid** volume r/t intravenous fluid therapy, inadequate intake or absorption of fluids, regurgitation

## INFANT OF DIABETIC MOTHER

Deficient **Fluid** volume r/t increased urinary excretion and osmotic diuresis

Delayed **Growth** and development r/t prolonged and severe postnatal hypoglycemia

Imbalanced **Nutrition**: less than body requirements r/t hypotonia, lethargy, poor sucking, postnatal metabolic changes from hyperglycemia to hypoglycemia and hyperinsulinism

Risk for decreased **Cardiac** output r/t increased incidence of cardiomegaly

Risk for delayed **Development** r/t prolonged and severe postnatal hypoglycemia

Risk for disproportionate **Growth** r/t prolonged and severe postnatal hypoglycemia

Risk for impaired **Gas** exchange r/t increased incidence of cardiomegaly, prematurity

*See Premature Infant; Respiratory Conditions of the Neonate*

## INFANT OF SUBSTANCE-ABUSING MOTHER (FETAL ALCOHOL SYNDROME, CRACK BABY, OTHER DRUG WITHDRAWAL INFANTS)

Delayed **Growth** and development r/t effects of maternal use of drugs, effects of neurological impairment, decreased attentiveness to environmental stimuli or inadequate stimuli

**Diarrhea** r/t effects of withdrawal, increased peristalsis secondary to hyperirritability

Disturbed **Sensory** perception r/t hypersensitivity to environmental stimuli

Disturbed **Sleep** pattern r/t hyperirritability/hypersensitivity to environmental stimuli

Imbalanced **Nutrition**: less than body requirements r/t feeding problems; uncoordinated or ineffective suck and swallow; effects of diarrhea, vomiting, or colic associated with maternal substance abuse

Impaired **Parenting** r/t impaired or absent attachment behaviors, inadequate support systems

Ineffective **Airway** clearance r/t pooling of secretions secondary to lack of adequate cough reflex, effects of viral or bacterial lower airway infection secondary to altered protective state

Ineffective **Infant** feeding pattern r/t uncoordinated or ineffective sucking reflex

Ineffective **Protection** r/t effects of maternal substance abuse

Interrupted **Breastfeeding** r/t use of drugs or alcohol by mother

Risk for delayed **Development** r/t substance abuse

Risk for disproportionate **Growth** r/t substance abuse

Risk for **Infection**: skin, meningeal, respiratory r/t effects of withdrawal

*See Cerebral Palsy; Failure to Thrive, Nonorganic; Hospitalized Child; Hyperactive Syndrome; SIDS (Sudden Infant Death Syndrome)*

### INFANTILE POLYARTERITIS

*See Kawasaki Syndrome*

### INFANTILE SPASMS

*See Seizure Disorders, Childhood*

### INFECTION

**Hyperthermia** r/t increased metabolic rate

Ineffective **Protection** r/t inadequate nutrition, abnormal blood profiles, drug therapies, treatments

### INFECTION, POTENTIAL FOR

Risk for **Infection** r/t inadequate primary defenses (e.g., broken skin, traumatized tissue, decrease in ciliary action, stasis of body fluids, change in pH secretions, altered peristalsis), inadequate secondary defenses

(e.g., decreased hemoglobin, leukopenia suppressed inflammatory response), immunosuppression, inadequate acquired immunity, tissue destruction and increased environmental exposure, chronic disease, invasive procedures, malnutrition, pharmaceutical agents, trauma, rupture of amniotic membranes, insufficient knowledge to avoid exposure to pathogens

### INFERTILITY

Chronic **Sorrow** r/t inability to conceive a child

Ineffective **Therapeutic** regimen management r/t deficient knowledge about infertility

**Powerlessness** r/t infertility

Risk for **Powerlessness** r/t inability to conceive a child

**Spiritual** distress r/t inability to conceive a child

### INFLAMMATORY BOWEL DISEASE (CHILD AND ADULT)

Acute **Pain** r/t abdominal cramping and anal irritation

Deficient **Fluid** volume r/t frequent and loose stools

**Diarrhea** r/t effects of inflammatory changes of the bowel

Imbalanced **Nutrition**: less than body requirements r/t anorexia, decreased absorption of nutrients from gastrointestinal tract

Impaired **Skin** integrity r/t frequent stools, development of anal fissures

Ineffective **Coping** r/t repeated episodes of diarrhea

**Social** isolation r/t diarrhea

*See Child with Chronic Condition; Crohn's Disease; Hospitalized Child; Maturational Issues, Adolescent*

## INFLUENZA

Acute **Pain** r/t inflammatory changes in joints

Deficient **Fluid** volume r/t inadequate fluid intake

**Hyperthermia** r/t infectious process

Ineffective **Health** maintenance r/t deficient knowledge regarding self-care

Ineffective **Therapeutic** regimen management r/t lack of knowledge regarding preventive immunizations

Readiness for enhanced **Knowledge** of information to prevent influenza

## INGUINAL HERNIA REPAIR

Acute **Pain** r/t surgical procedure

Impaired physical **Mobility** r/t pain at surgical site and fear of causing hernia to "break open"

Risk for **Infection** r/t surgical procedure

**Urinary** retention r/t possible edema at surgical site

## INJURY

Risk for **Falls** r/t orthostatic hypertension, impaired physical mobility, diminished mental status

Risk for **Injury** r/t environmental conditions interacting with client's adaptive and defensive resources

## INSOMNIA

**Anxiety** r/t actual or perceived loss of sleep

Disturbed **Sleep** pattern r/t sensory alterations, internal factors, external factors

**Sleep** deprivation r/t sustained inadequate sleep hygiene, prolonged use of pharmacological agents, aging-related sleep stage shifts

## INSULIN SHOCK

*See Hypoglycemia*

## INTERMITTENT CLAUDICATION

Acute **Pain** r/t decreased circulation to extremities with activity

Deficient **Knowledge** r/t lack of knowledge of cause and treatment of peripheral vascular diseases

Ineffective **Tissue** perfusion: peripheral r/t interruption of arterial flow

Readiness for enhanced **Knowledge** of prevention of pain and impaired circulation

Risk for **Injury** r/t tissue hypoxia

Risk for **Peripheral** neurovascular dysfunction r/t disruption in arterial flow

*See Peripheral Vascular Disease*

## INTERNAL CARDIOVERTER DEFIBRILLATOR

*See ICD (Internal Cardioverter Defibrillator)*

## INTERNAL FIXATION

Impaired **Walking** r/t repair of fracture

Risk for **Infection** r/t traumatized tissue, broken skin

*See Fracture*

## INTERSTITIAL CYSTITIS

Acute **Pain** r/t inflammatory process

Impaired **Urinary** elimination r/t inflammation of bladder

Risk for **Infection** r/t suppressed inflammatory response

Risk for urge urinary **Incontinence** r/t effects of alcohol, caffeine, decreased bladder capacity, irritation of bladder stretch receptors causing spasm, increased urine concentration, overdistention of bladder

## INTERVERTEBRAL DISK EXCISION

*See Laminectomy*

## INTESTINAL OBSTRUCTION

*See Ileus*

## INTOXICATION

Acute **Confusion** r/t alcohol abuse

**Anxiety** r/t loss of control of actions

Disturbed **Sensory** perception r/t neurochemical imbalance in brain

Disturbed **Thought** processes r/t effect of substance on central nervous system

Impaired **Memory** r/t effects of alcohol on mind

Ineffective **Coping** r/t use of mind-altering substances as a means of coping

Risk for **Falls** r/t diminished mental status

Risk for other-directed **Violence** r/t inability to control thoughts and actions

## INTRAAORTIC BALLOON COUNTERPULSATION

**Anxiety** r/t device providing cardiovascular assistance

Compromised family **Coping** r/t seriousness of significant other's medical condition

Decreased **Cardiac** output r/t failing heart needing counterpulsation

Impaired physical **Mobility** r/t restriction of movement because of mechanical device

Risk for **Peripheral** neurovascular dysfunction r/t vascular obstruction of balloon catheter, thrombus formation, emboli, edema

## INTRACRANIAL PRESSURE, INCREASED

Acute **Confusion** r/t increased intracranial pressure

Adult **Failure** to thrive r/t undetected changes from increased intracranial pressure

Decreased **Intracranial** adaptive capacity r/t sustained increase in intracranial pressure

Disturbed **Sensory** perception r/t pressure damage to sensory centers in brain

Disturbed **Thought** processes r/t pressure damage to brain

Impaired **Memory** r/t neurological disturbance

Ineffective **Breathing** pattern r/t pressure damage to breathing center in brain stem

Ineffective **Tissue** perfusion: cerebral r/t effects of increased intracranial pressure

*See cause of Increased Intracranial Pressure*

## INTRAUTERINE GROWTH RETARDATION

**Anxiety**: maternal r/t threat to fetus

Delayed **Growth** and development r/t insufficient supply of oxygen and nutrients

Imbalanced **Nutrition**: less than body requirements r/t insufficient placenta

Impaired **Gas** exchange r/t insufficient placental perfusion

Ineffective **Coping**: maternal r/t situational crisis, threat to fetus

Risk for delayed **Development** r/t insufficient supply of oxygen and nutrients

Risk for disproportionate **Growth** r/t insufficient supply of oxygen and nutrients

Risk for **Injury** r/t insufficient supply of oxygen and nutrients

Risk for **Powerlessness** r/t unknown outcome of fetus

Situational low **Self-esteem**: maternal r/t guilt about threat to fetus

**Spiritual** distress r/t unknown outcome of fetus

I

## INTUBATION, ENDOTRACHEAL OR NASOGASTRIC

Acute **Pain** r/t presence of tube

Disturbed **Body** image r/t altered appearance with mechanical devices

Imbalanced **Nutrition**: less than body requirements r/t inability to ingest food resulting from presence of tubes

Impaired **Oral** mucous membrane r/t presence of tubes

Impaired verbal **Communication** r/t endotracheal tube

## IRREGULAR PULSE

*See Dysrhythmia*

## IRRITABLE BOWEL SYNDROME

*See IBS (Irritable Bowel Syndrome)*

## ISOLATION

Adult **Failure** to thrive r/t depression

Risk for **Loneliness** r/t lack of affection, physical isolation, cathectic deprivation, social isolation

Risk for situational low **Self-esteem** r/t decreased power, control over environment

**Social** isolation r/t factors contributing to absence of satisfying personal relationships, such as delay in accomplishing developmental tasks, immature interests, alterations in mental status, unacceptable social behavior, unacceptable social values, altered state of wellness, inadequate personal resources, inability to engage in satisfying personal relationships

## ITCHING

Impaired **Comfort** r/t irritation of the skin

Risk for **Infection** r/t potential break in skin

## ITP (IDIOPATHIC THROMBOCYTOPENIC PURPURA)

Deficient **Diversional** activity r/t activity restrictions, safety precautions

Impaired **Home** health maintenance r/t parental lack of ability to follow through with safety precautions secondary to child's developmental stage (active toddler)

Ineffective **Protection** r/t decreased platelet count

Risk for **Injury** r/t decreased platelet count, developmental level, age-appropriate play

*See Hospitalized Child*

## JAUNDICE

Disturbed **Thought** processes r/t toxic blood metabolites

Impaired **Comfort**: pruritus r/t toxic metabolites excreted in the skin

Risk for impaired **Skin** integrity r/t pruritus, itching

*See Cirrhosis and Hepatitis*

## JAUNDICE, NEONATAL

Readiness for enhanced **Knowledge** of information on assessing jaundice when infant is discharged from the hospital, when to call the physician and possible preventive measures such as frequent breastfeeding

*See Hyperbilirubinemia*

## JAW PAIN AND HEART ATTACKS

*See Chest Pain; MI (Myocardial Infarction)*

## JAW SURGERY

Acute **Pain** r/t surgical procedure

Deficient **Knowledge** r/t emergency care for wired jaws (e.g., cutting bands and wires), oral care

Imbalanced **Nutrition**: less than body requirements r/t jaws wired closed

Impaired **Swallowing** r/t edema from surgery

Risk for **Aspiration** r/t wired jaws

## JET LAG PREVENTION

Readiness for enhanced **Knowledge** of getting adequate sleep prior to travel, drinking extra water and avoiding caffeine and alcohol, engaging in regular exercise but not at bedtime

## JITTERY

**Anxiety** r/t unconscious conflict about essential values and goals, threat to or change in health status

Death **Anxiety** r/t unresolved issues relating to end of life

Risk for **Post-trauma** syndrome r/t occupation, survivor's role in event, inadequate social support

## JOCK ITCH

Impaired **Skin** integrity r/t moisture and irritating or tight-fitting clothing

Ineffective **Therapeutic** regimen management r/t prevention and treatment

*See Itching*

## JOINT INFLAMMATION

*See Arthritis*

## JOINT PAIN

*See Arthritis; Bursitis; JRA (Juvenile Rheumatoid Arthritis); Osteoarthritis; Rheumatoid Arthritis*

## JOINT REPLACEMENT

Risk for **Peripheral** neurovascular dysfunction r/t orthopedic surgery

*See Total Joint Replacement*

## JRA (JUVENILE RHEUMATOID ARTHRITIS)

Acute **Pain** r/t swollen or inflamed joints, restricted movement, physical therapy

Delayed **Growth** and development r/t effects of physical disability, chronic illness

**Fatigue** r/t chronic inflammatory disease

Impaired physical **Mobility** r/t pain, restricted joint movement

Risk for impaired **Skin** integrity r/t splints, adaptive devices

Risk for **Injury** r/t impaired physical mobility, splints, adaptive devices, increased bleeding potential secondary to antiinflammatory medications

Risk for situational low **Self-esteem** r/t disturbed body image

**Self-care** deficits: feeding, bathing/hygiene, dressing/grooming, toileting r/t restricted joint movement, pain

*See Child with Chronic Condition; Hospitalized Child*

## JUVENILE ONSET DIABETES

*See Diabetes Mellitus, Juvenile*

# K

## KAPOSI'S SARCOMA

Risk for dysfunctional **Grieving** r/t preloss psychological symptoms associated with unknown prognosis and outcome of disease

Risk for impaired **Religiosity** r/t illness/hospitalization

*See AIDS (Acquired Immunodeficiency Syndrome)*

## KAWASAKI SYNDROME (FORMERLY MUCOCUTANEOUS LYMPH NODE SYNDROME)

Acute **Pain** r/t enlarged lymph nodes; erythematous skin rash that progresses to desquamation, peeling, denuding of skin

**Anxiety**: parental r/t progression of disease, complications of arthritis and cardiac involvement

**Hyperthermia** r/t inflammatory disease process

Imbalanced **Nutrition**: less than body requirements r/t impaired oral mucous membrane

Impaired **Oral** mucous membrane r/t inflamed mouth and pharynx; swollen lips that become dry, cracked, fissured

Impaired **Skin** integrity r/t inflammatory skin changes

*See Hospitalized Child*

## KEGEL EXERCISE

**Health**-seeking behavior r/t desire for information to relieve incontinence

Risk for urge urinary **Incontinence** r/t effects of alcohol, caffeine, decreased bladder capacity, irritation of bladder stretch receptors causing spasm, increased urine concentration, overdistention of bladder

Stress urinary **Incontinence** r/t degenerative change in pelvic muscles

Urge urinary **Incontinence** r/t decreased bladder capacity

## KELOIDS

Disturbed **Body** image r/t presence of scar tissue at site of a healed skin injury

Readiness for enhanced **Therapeutic** regimen management r/t desire to have information to decrease discoloration of skin from sun exposure: covering the area and using sunblock

at least 6 months after the injury or surgery for an adult and 18 months for a child

## KERATOCONJUNCTIVITIS SICCA

Risk for **Infection** r/t dry eyes

*See Conjunctivitis*

## KERATOPLASTY

*See Corneal Transplant*

## KETOACIDOSIS, DIABETIC

Deficient **Fluid** volume r/t excess excretion of urine, nausea, vomiting, increased respiration

Imbalanced **Nutrition**: less than body requirements r/t body's inability to use nutrients

Impaired **Memory** r/t fluid and electrolyte imbalance

Ineffective **Therapeutic** regimen management r/t denial of illness, lack of understanding of preventive measures and adequate blood sugar control

**Noncompliance**: diabetic regimen r/t ineffective coping with chronic disease

Risk for **Powerlessness** r/t illness-related regimen

*See Diabetes Mellitus*

## KETOACIDOSIS, ALCOHOLIC

*See Alcohol Withdrawal; Alcoholism*

## KEYHOLE HEART SURGERY

*See MIDCAB (Minimally Invasive Direct Coronary Bypass)*

## KIDNEY FAILURE

*See Renal Failure*

## KIDNEY STONE

Acute **Pain** r/t obstruction from renal calculi

Deficient **Knowledge** r/t fluid requirements and dietary restrictions

Impaired **Urinary** elimination: urgency

and frequency r/t anatomical obstruction, irritation caused by stone

Risk for deficient **Fluid** volume r/t nausea, vomiting

Risk for **Infection** r/t obstruction of urinary tract with stasis of urine

## KIDNEY TRANSPLANT

Decisional **Conflict** r/t acceptance of donor kidney

Ineffective **Protection** r/t immunosuppressive therapy

Readiness for enhanced **Family** processes r/t adapting to life without dialysis

Readiness for enhanced **Spiritual** well-being r/t heightened coping, living without dialysis

Readiness for enhanced **Therapeutic** regimen management r/t desire to manage the treatment and prevention of complications post transplant

*See Surgery, Perioperative Care; Surgery, Postoperative Care; Surgery, Preoperative Care*

## KIDNEY TUMOR

*See Wilms' Tumor*

## KISSING DISEASE

*See Mononucleosis*

## KNEE REPLACEMENT

*See Total Joint Replacement*

## KNOWLEDGE

Readiness for enhanced **Knowledge** of (specify) r/t the following: expresses an interest in learning, explains knowledge of the topic, displays behaviors congruent with expressed knowledge, describes previous experiences pertaining to the topic

## KNOWLEDGE, DEFICIENT

Deficient **Knowledge** r/t lack of exposure, lack of recall, information misinterpretation, cognitive limitation, lack

of interest in learning, unfamiliarity with information resources

Ineffective **Health** maintenance r/t lack of or significant alteration in communication skills (written, verbal, and/or gestural)

Ineffective **Therapeutic** regimen management r/t complexity of therapeutic regimen

## KOCK POUCH

*See Continent Ileostomy*

## KORSAKOFF'S SYNDROME

Acute **Confusion** r/t alcohol abuse

Dysfunctional **Family** processes: alcoholism r/t possible cause of syndrome

Impaired **Memory** r/t neurological changes

Risk for **Falls** r/t cognitive impairment

Risk for imbalanced **Nutrition**: less than body requirements r/t lack of adequate balanced intake

Risk for **Injury** r/t sensory dysfunction, lack of coordination when ambulating

# L

## LABOR, INDUCTION OF

*See Induction of Labor*

## LABOR, NORMAL

Acute **Pain** r/t uterine contractions, stretching of cervix and birth canal

**Anxiety** r/t fear of the unknown, situational crisis

Death **Anxiety** r/t threat of maternal mortality

Deficient **Knowledge** r/t lack of preparation for labor

**Fatigue** r/t childbirth

**Health**-seeking behaviors r/t healthy outcome of pregnancy, prenatal care, and childbirth education

Impaired **Tissue** integrity r/t passage of infant through birth canal, episiotomy

Readiness for enhanced family **Coping** r/t significant other providing support during labor

Risk for deficient **Fluid** volume r/t excessive loss of blood

Risk for **Infection** r/t multiple vaginal examinations, tissue trauma, prolonged rupture of membranes

Risk for **Injury**: fetal r/t hypoxia

Risk for **Post-trauma** syndrome r/t trauma or violence associated with labor pains, birth process, medical/surgical interventions, history of sexual abuse

Risk for **Powerlessness** r/t labor process

## LABYRINTHITIS

Risk for **Injury** r/t dizziness

Ineffective **Therapeutic** regimen management r/t delay in seeking treatment for respiratory and ear infections

Readiness for enhanced **Therapeutic** regimen management r/t management of episodes: keep still and rest during attacks, gradually resume activity, avoid sudden position changes, do not try to read during attacks, avoid bright lights.

## LACTATION

*See Breastfeeding, Effective; Breastfeeding, Ineffective; Breastfeeding, Interrupted.*

## LACTOSE INTOLERANCE

Readiness for enhanced **Knowledge** r/t interest in identifying lactose intolerance, treatment, and substitutes for mild products

*See Abdominal Distention; Diarrhea*

## LAMINECTOMY

Acute **Pain** r/t localized inflammation and edema

**Anxiety** r/t change in health status, surgical procedure

Deficient **Knowledge** r/t appropriate postoperative and postdischarge activities

Disturbed **Sensory** perception: tactile r/t possible edema or nerve injury

Impaired physical **Mobility** r/t neuromuscular impairment

Risk for impaired **Tissue** perfusion r/t edema, hemorrhage, or embolism

Risk for perioperative positioning **Injury** r/t prone position

**Urinary** retention r/t competing sensory impulses, effects of narcotics/anesthesia

*See Scoliosis; Surgery, Perioperative; Surgery, Postoperative; Surgery, Preoperative*

## LAPAROSCOPIC LASER CHOLECYSTECTOMY

*See Cholecystectomy; Laser Surgery*

## LAPAROSCOPY

Acute **Pain**: shoulder r/t gas irritating the diaphragm

Urge urinary **Incontinence** r/t pressure on the bladder from gas

## LAPAROTOMY

*See Abdominal Surgery*

## LARYNGECTOMY

Anticipatory **Grieving** r/t loss of voice, fear of death

Chronic **Sorrow** r/t change in body image

Death **Anxiety** r/t unknown results of surgery

Disturbed **Body** image r/t change in body structure and function

Imbalanced **Nutrition**: less than body requirements r/t absence of oral feeding, difficulty swallowing, increased need for fluids

Impaired **Oral** mucous membrane r/t absence of oral feeding

Impaired **Swallowing** r/t edema, laryngectomy tube

Impaired verbal **Communication** r/t removal of larynx

Ineffective **Airway** clearance r/t surgical removal of glottis, decreased humidification of air

Ineffective **Health** maintenance r/t deficient knowledge regarding self-care with laryngectomy

Interrupted **Family** processes r/t surgery, serious condition of family member, difficulty communicating

Risk for dysfunctional **Grieving** r/t loss and major life event

Risk for **Infection** r/t invasive procedure, surgery

Risk for **Powerlessness** r/t chronic illness, change in communication

Risk for situational low **Self-esteem** r/t disturbed body image

## LASER SURGERY

Acute **Pain** r/t heat from laser

**Constipation** r/t laser intervention in vulval and perianal areas

Deficient **Knowledge** r/t preoperative and postoperative care associated with laser procedure

Risk for **Infection** r/t delayed heating reaction of tissue exposed to laser

Risk for **Injury** r/t accidental exposure to laser beam

## LASIK EYE SURGERY (LASER-ASSISTED *IN SITU* KERATOMILEUSIS)

Decisional **Conflict** r/t decision to have the surgery

Readiness for enhanced **Therapeutic** regimen management r/t preexamination preparation, contact lens wearing, surgical procedure pre- and postoperative teaching and expectations

## LATEX ALLERGY

Latex **Allergy** r/t hypersensitivity to natural latex rubber

Readiness for enhanced **Knowledge** of prevention and treatment of exposure to latex products

Risk for latex **Allergy** response r/t multiple surgical procedures, especially from infancy (e.g., spina bifida); allergies to bananas, avocados, tropical fruits, kiwi fruit, chestnuts; professions with daily exposure to latex (e.g., medicine, nursing, dentistry); conditions needing continuous or intermittent catheterization; history of reactions to latex (e.g., balloons, condoms, gloves); allergies to poinsettia plants; history of allergies and asthma

## LAXATIVE ABUSE

Perceived **Constipation** r/t health belief, faulty appraisal, impaired thought processes

## LEAD POISONING

Impaired **Home** maintenance r/t presence of lead paint

Risk for delayed **Development** r/t lead poisoning

## LEGIONNAIRES' DISEASE

Ineffective community **Therapeutic** regimen management r/t contaminated air systems in large buildings

Risk for **Infection** r/t increased environmental exposure to pathogens (contaminated water in air-conditioning systems and sometimes showers)

*See Pneumonia*

## LENS IMPLANT

*See Cataract Extraction; Vision Impairment*

L

## LETHARGY/LISTLESSNESS

Adult **Failure** to thrive r/t apathy

Disturbed **Sleep** pattern r/t internal or external stressors

**Fatigue** r/t decreased metabolic energy production

Ineffective **Tissue** perfusion: cerebral r/t lack of oxygen supply to brain

*See cause of Lethargy/Listlessness*

## LEUKEMIA

Ineffective **Protection** r/t abnormal blood profile

Risk for deficient **Fluid** volume r/t nausea, vomiting, bleeding, side effects of treatment

Risk for **Infection** r/t ineffective immune system

*See Cancer; Chemotherapy*

## LEUKOPENIA

Ineffective **Protection** r/t leukopenia

Risk for **Infection** r/t low white blood cell count

## LEVEL OF CONSCIOUSNESS, DECREASED

*See Confusion, Acute; Confusion, Chronic*

## LICE

Impaired **Comfort** r/t pruritus secondary to infestation

Impaired **Home** maintenance r/t close overcrowded conditions

Readiness for enhanced **Therapeutic** regimen management to prevent and treat infestation

*See Communicable Diseases, Childhood*

## LIGHTHEADEDNESS

*See Dizziness*

## LIMB REATTACHMENT PROCEDURES

Anticipatory **Grieving** r/t unknown outcome of reattachment procedure

**Anxiety** r/t unknown outcome of reattachment procedure, use and appearance of limb

Disturbed **Body** image r/t unpredictability of function and appearance of reattached body part

Risk for deficient **Fluid** volume: hemorrhage r/t severed vessels

Risk for impaired **Religiosity** r/t pain, suffering, hospitalization

Risk for perioperative positioning **Injury** r/t immobilization

Risk for **Peripheral** neurovascular dysfunction r/t trauma, orthopedic and neurovascular surgery, compression of nerves and blood vessels

Risk for **Powerlessness** r/t unknown outcome of procedure

**Spiritual** distress r/t anxiety about condition

*See Surgery, Postoperative Care*

## LIPOSUCTION

Disturbed **Body** image r/t dissatisfaction with unwanted fat deposits in body

Readiness for enhanced **Self-concept** r/t satisfaction with new body image

*See Surgery, Perioperative Care; Surgery, Postoperative Care; Surgery, Preoperative Care*

## LITHOTRIPSY

Readiness for enhanced **Therapeutic** regimen management r/t desire for information related to procedure and after care and prevention of stones

*See Kidney Stone*

## LIVER BIOPSY

**Anxiety** r/t procedure and results

Risk for deficient **Fluid** volume r/t hemorrhage from biopsy site

Risk for **Powerlessness** r/t inability to control outcome of procedure

## LIVER DISEASE

*See Cirrhosis; Hepatitis*

## LIVER TRANSPLANT

Decisional **Conflict** r/t acceptance of donor liver

Readiness for enhanced **Family** processes r/t change in physical needs of family member

Ineffective **Protection** r/t immunosuppressive therapy

Readiness for enhanced **Spiritual** well-being r/t heightened coping

Readiness for enhanced **Therapeutic** regimen management r/t desire to manage the treatment and prevention of complications posttransplant

*See Surgery, Perioperative Care; Surgery, Postoperative Care; Surgery, Preoperative Care*

## LIVING WILL

Readiness for enhanced **Religiosity** r/t request to meet with religious leaders/facilitators

Readiness for enhanced **Spiritual** well-being r/t acceptance of and preparation for end of life

*See Advance Directives*

## LOBECTOMY

*See Thoracotomy*

## LONELINESS

Risk for impaired **Religiosity** r/t lack of social interaction

Risk for **Loneliness** r/t lack of affection, physical isolation, cathectic deprivation, social isolation

Risk for situational low **Self-esteem** r/t failure, rejection

**Spiritual** distress r/t loneliness/social alienation

## LOOSE STOOLS

**Diarrhea** r/t increased gastric motility

*See cause of Loose Stools*

## LOU GEHRIG'S DISEASE

*See ALS (Amyotrophic Lateral Sclerosis)*

## LOW BACK PAIN

Chronic **Pain** r/t degenerative processes, musculotendinous strain, injury, inflammation, congenital deformities

Impaired physical **Mobility** r/t back pain

Ineffective **Health** maintenance r/t deficient knowledge regarding self-care with back pain

Readiness for enhanced **Therapeutic** regimen management r/t expressed desire for information to manage pain

Risk for **Powerlessness** r/t living with chronic pain

**Urinary** retention r/t possible spinal cord compression

## LUMBAR PUNCTURE

Acute **Pain**: headache r/t possible loss of cerebrospinal fluid

**Anxiety** r/t invasive procedure and unknown results

Deficient **Knowledge** r/t information about procedure

Risk for **Infection** r/t invasive procedure

## LUMPECTOMY

Decisional **Conflict** r/t treatment choices

Readiness for enhanced **Knowledge**: pre- and post-operative care

L

Readiness for enhanced **Spiritual** well-being r/t hope of benign diagnosis

*See Cancer*

## LUNG CANCER

*See Cancer; Chemotherapy; Radiation Therapy; Thoracotomy*

## LUPUS ERYTHEMATOSUS

Acute **Pain** r/t inflammatory process

Chronic **Sorrow** r/t presence of chronic illness

Disturbed **Body** image r/t change in skin, rash, lesions, ulcers, mottled erythema

**Fatigue** r/t increased metabolic requirements

Impaired **Religiosity** r/t ineffective coping with disease

Ineffective **Health** maintenance r/t deficient knowledge regarding medication, diet, and activity

**Powerlessness** r/t unpredictability of course of disease

Risk for impaired **Skin** integrity r/t chronic inflammation, edema, altered circulation

**Spiritual** distress r/t chronicity of disease, unknown etiology

## LYME DISEASE

Acute **Pain** r/t inflammation of joints, urticaria, rash

Deficient **Knowledge** r/t lack of information concerning disease, prevention, treatment

**Fatigue** r/t increased energy requirements

Risk for decreased **Cardiac** output r/t dysrhythmia

Risk for **Powerlessness** r/t possible chronic condition

## LYMPHEDEMA

Deficient **Knowledge** r/t management of condition

Disturbed **Body** image r/t change in appearance of body part with edema

Excess **Fluid** volume r/t compromised regulatory system; inflammation, obstruction, or removal of lymph glands

Risk for situational low **Self-esteem** r/t disturbed body image

## LYMPHOMA

*See Cancer*

# M

## MACULAR DEGENERATION

Impaired **Adjustment** r/t deteriorating vision

Compromised **Family** coping r/t deteriorating vision of family member

Disturbed **Sensory** perception: visual r/t blurred, distorted, dim, or absent central vision

Effective management of **Therapeutic** regimen r/t practicing good nutrition, vitamin use; zinc, and abstaining from tobacco use

**Hopelessness** r/t deteriorating vision

Ineffective **Coping** r/t visual loss

Risk for **Falls** r/t visual difficulties

Risk for impaired **Religiosity** r/t possible lack of transportation

Risk for **Injury** r/t inability to distinguish traffic lights

Risk for **Powerlessness** r/t deteriorating vision

Sedentary **Lifestyle** r/t visual loss

**Social** isolation r/t inability to drive associated with visual changes

## MAD COW DISEASE

Risk for dysfunctional **Grieving** r/t possible rapid fatal outcome of disease

*See CJD (Creutzfeldt-Jakob Disease)*

## MAGNETIC RESONANCE IMAGING

*See MRI (Magnetic Resonance Imaging)*

## MAJOR DEPRESSIVE DISORDER

Interrupted **Family** processes r/t change in health status of family member

Risk for **Loneliness** r/t social isolation associated with feelings of sadness, hopelessness

*See Depression*

## MALABSORPTION SYNDROME

Deficient **Knowledge** r/t lack of information about diet and nutrition

**Diarrhea** r/t lactose intolerance, gluten sensitivity, resection of small bowel

Imbalanced **Nutrition**: less than body requirements r/t inability of body to absorb nutrients because of biological factors

Risk for deficient **Fluid** volume r/t diarrhea

Risk for disproportionate **Growth** r/t malnutrition from malabsorption

*See Abdominal Distention*

## MALADAPTIVE BEHAVIOR

*See Crisis; Post-Trauma Syndrome; Suicide Attempt*

## MALAISE

*See Fatigue*

## MALARIA

**Health seeking** behaviors r/t countries requiring malaria prophylaxis, appropriate malaria regimen, use of protective clothing and insecticides

Readiness for enhanced **Knowledge** r/t countries requiring malaria prophylaxis, appropriate malaria regi-

men, use of protective clothing and insecticides

Risk for **Infection** r/t increased environmental exposure (not wearing protective clothing, not using insecticide or repellant on skin and in room in areas where infected mosquitoes are present); inadequate defense mechanisms (inappropriate use of prophylactic regimen)

*See Anemia*

## MALIGNANCY

*See Cancer*

## MALIGNANT HYPERTHERMIA

Effective **Therapeutic** regimen management r/t use of a general anesthetic: pretreatment with dantrolene sodium is recommended; if there is a family history of anesthesia-induced problems, it is imperative to alert the surgeon and anesthesiologist

**Hyperthermia** r/t anesthesia reaction associated with inherited condition

M

## MALNUTRITION

Adult **Failure** to thrive r/t undetected malnutrition

Deficient **Knowledge** r/t misinformation about normal nutrition, social isolation, lack of food-preparation facilities

Imbalanced **Nutrition**: less than body requirements r/t inability to ingest food, digest food, or absorb nutrients because of biological, psychological, or economic factors; institutionalization (i.e., lack of menu choices)

Ineffective **Protection** r/t inadequate nutrition

Ineffective **Therapeutic** regimen management r/t economic difficulties

Risk for disproportionate **Growth** r/t malnutrition

Risk for **Powerlessness** r/t possible inability to provide adequate nutrition

## MAMMOGRAPHY

Effective **Therapeutic** regimen management r/t women schedule mammograms 1 to 2 years after age 40 or at earlier age based on family history of breast cancer or to evaluate a woman who has symptoms of a breast disease, such as a lump, nipple discharge, breast pain, dimpling of the skin on the breast, or retraction of the nipple

**Health-seeking** behavior r/t information regarding mammograms: frequency and age recommendations; preparation; no deodorant, perfume, powders, or ointments under the arms or on the breasts on the day of the mammogram

## MANIC DISORDER, BIPOLAR I

**Anxiety** r/t change in role function

Deficient **Fluid** volume r/t decreased intake

Disturbed **Sleep** pattern r/t constant anxious thoughts

Disturbed **Thought** processes r/t mania

Imbalanced **Nutrition**: less than body requirements r/t lack of time and motivation to eat, constant movement

Impaired **Home** maintenance r/t altered psychological state, inability to concentrate

Ineffective **Coping** r/t situational crisis

Ineffective **Denial** r/t fear of inability to control behavior

Ineffective **Role** performance r/t impaired social interactions

Interrupted **Family** processes r/t family member's illness

Ineffective **Therapeutic** regimen management r/t lack of social supports

Ineffective **Therapeutic** regimen management: families r/t unpredictability of client, excessive demands on family, chronicity of condition

**Noncompliance** r/t denial of illness

Risk for **Caregiver** role strain r/t unpredictability of condition, mood swings

Risk for impaired **Religiosity** r/t depression

Risk for **Powerlessness** r/t inability to control changes in mood

Risk for self- or other-directed **Violence** r/t hallucinations, delusions

Risk for **Spiritual** distress r/t depression

Risk for **Suicide** r/t bipolar disorder

**Sleep** deprivation r/t hyperagitated state

## MANIPULATION OF ORGANS, SURGICAL INCISION

Deficient **Knowledge** r/t lack of exposure to information regarding care after surgery and at home

Risk for **Infection** r/t presence of urinary catheter

**Urinary** retention r/t swelling of urinary meatus

## MANIPULATIVE BEHAVIOR

Defensive **Coping** r/t superior attitude toward others

Impaired **Social** interaction r/t self-concept disturbance

Ineffective **Coping** r/t inappropriate use of defense mechanisms

Risk for **Loneliness** r/t inability to interact appropriately with others

Risk for **Self-mutilation** r/t inability to cope with increased psychological or physiological tension in healthy manner

Risk for situational low **Self-esteem** r/t history of learned helplessness

**Self-mutilation** r/t use of manipulation to obtain nurturing relationship with others

## MARASMUS

*See Failure to Thrive, Nonorganic*

## MARFAN SYNDROME

Decreased **Cardiac** output r/t dilation of the aortic root, dissection or rupture of the aorta

Effective **Therapeutic** regimen management r/t medication to slow the heart rate (beta blockers) to help prevent stress on the aorta; not participating in competitive athletics and contact sports; yearly echocardiogram to assess the aortic root; surgical replacement of the aortic root and valve if needed

Disturbed **Sensory** perception; visual r/t myopia associated with Marfan syndrome

Readiness for enhanced **Therapeutic** regimen management r/t good oral health and routine dental evaluation; antibiotics before dental work or other procedures expected to contaminate the bloodstream with bacteria for all clients who have valvular heart disease, including a composite graft repair or placement of an artificial valve

*See Mitral Valve Prolapse; Scoliosis*

## MARSHALL-MARCHETTI-KRANTZ OPERATION

### PREOPERATIVE

Stress urinary **Incontinence** r/t weak pelvic muscles and pelvic supports

### POSTOPERATIVE

Acute **Pain** r/t manipulation of organs, surgical incision

Deficient **Knowledge** r/t lack of exposure to information regarding care after surgery and at home

Risk for **Infection** r/t presence of urinary catheter

**Urinary** retention r/t swelling of urinary meatus

## MASTECTOMY

Acute **Pain** r/t surgical procedure

Chronic **Sorrow** r/t disturbed body image, unknown long-term health status

Death **Anxiety** r/t threat of mortality associated with breast cancer

Deficient **Knowledge** r/t self-care activities

Disturbed **Body** image r/t loss of sexually significant body part

**Fear** r/t change in body image, prognosis

**Nausea** r/t chemotherapy

Risk for impaired physical **Mobility** r/t nerve or muscle damage, pain

Risk for **Post-trauma** syndrome r/t loss of body part, surgical wounds

Risk for **Powerlessness** r/t fear of unknown outcome of procedure

**Sexual** dysfunction r/t change in body image, fear of loss of femininity

**Spiritual** distress r/t change in body image

*See Cancer; Modified Radical Mastectomy; Surgery, Perioperative; Surgery, Postoperative; Surgery, Preoperative*

## MASTITIS

Acute **Pain** r/t infectious disease process, swelling of breast tissue

**Anxiety** r/t threat to self, concern over safety of milk for infant

Deficient **Knowledge** r/t antibiotic regimen, comfort measures

Ineffective **Breastfeeding** r/t breast pain, conflicting advice from health care providers

Ineffective **Role** performance r/t change in capacity to function in expected role

M

## MATERNAL INFECTION

Ineffective **Protection** r/t invasive procedures, traumatized tissue, stress of recent childbirth

*See Postpartum, Normal Care*

## MATURATIONAL ISSUES, ADOLESCENT

Deficient **Knowledge**: potential for enhanced health maintenance r/t information misinterpretation, lack of education regarding age-related factors

Impaired **Social** interaction r/t ineffective, unsuccessful, or dysfunctional interaction with peers

Ineffective **Coping** r/t maturational crises

Interrupted **Family** processes r/t developmental crises of adolescence secondary to challenge of parental authority and values, situational crises secondary to change in parental marital status

Readiness for enhanced **Communication** r/t expressing willingness to communicate with parental figures

Risk for **Injury/Trauma** r/t thrill-seeking behaviors

Risk for situational low **Self-esteem** r/t developmental changes

**Social** isolation r/t perceived alteration in physical appearance, social values not accepted by dominant peer group

*See Sexuality, Adolescent; Substance Abuse (If relevant)*

## MAZE III PROCEDURE

*See Open Heart Surgery; Dysrhythmia*

## MEASLES (RUBEOLA)

*See Communicable Diseases, Childhood*

## MECONIUM ASPIRATION

*See Respiratory Conditions of the Neonate*

## MELANOMA

Acute **Pain** r/t surgical incision

Disturbed **Body** image r/t altered pigmentation, surgical incision

**Fear** r/t threat to well-being

Ineffective **Health** maintenance r/t deficient knowledge regarding self-care and treatment of melanoma

*See Cancer*

## MELENA

**Fear** r/t presence of blood in feces

Risk for deficient **Fluid** volume r/t hemorrhage

*See GI Bleed (Gastrointestinal Bleeding)*

## MEMORY DEFICIT

Impaired **Memory** r/t acute or chronic hypoxia, anemia, decreased cardiac output, fluid and electrolyte imbalance, neurological disturbance, excessive environmental disturbances

Impaired environmental **Interpretation** syndrome r/t dementia

## MENIERE'S DISEASE

Effective **Therapeutic** regimen management r/t prompt treatment of ear infection

Readiness for enhanced **Therapeutic** regimen management r/t avoiding sudden movements that may aggravate symptoms; help with walking due to loss of balance during attacks; rest during severe episodes, and gradually increase activity; during episodes, avoiding bright lights, television, and reading, which may make symptoms worse

Risk for **Injury** r/t symptoms from disease; avoiding hazardous activities

M

such as driving, operating heavy machinery, climbing, and similar activities until one week after symptoms disappear.

*See Dizziness*

## MENINGITIS/ENCEPHALITIS

Acute **Pain** r/t neck (nuchal) rigidity, inflammation of meninges, headache

Decreased **Intracranial** adaptive capacity r/t sustained increase in intracranial pressure

Delayed **Growth** and development r/t brain damage secondary to infectious process, increased intracranial pressure

Disturbed **Sensory** perception: hearing r/t central nervous system infection, ear infection

Disturbed **Sensory** perception: kinesthetic r/t central nervous system infection

Disturbed **Sensory** perception: visual r/t photophobia secondary to central nervous system infection

Disturbed **Thought** processes r/t inflammation of brain, fever

Excess **Fluid** volume r/t increased intracranial pressure, syndrome of inappropriate secretion of antidiuretic hormone (SIADH)

Impaired **Comfort** r/t central nervous system inflammation

Impaired **Comfort**: photophobia r/t increased sensitivity to external stimuli secondary to central nervous system inflammation

Impaired **Mobility** r/t neuromuscular or central nervous system insult

Ineffective **Airway** clearance r/t seizure activity

Ineffective **Tissue** perfusion: cerebral r/t inflamed cerebral tissues and meninges, increased intracranial pressure

Risk for **Aspiration** r/t seizure activity

Risk for **Falls** r/t neuromuscular dysfunction

Risk for **Injury** r/t seizure activity

*See Hospitalized Child*

## MENINGOCELE

*See Neurotube Defects*

## MENOPAUSE

**Health**-seeking behavior r/t menopause, therapies associated with change in hormonal levels

Impaired **Memory** r/t change in hormonal levels

Ineffective **Sexuality** patterns r/t altered body structure, lack of physiological lubrication, lack of knowledge of artificial lubrication

Ineffective **Thermoregulation** r/t changes in hormonal levels

Readiness for enhanced **Spiritual** well-being r/t desire for harmony of mind, body, and spirit

Readiness for enhanced **Therapeutic** regimen management r/t verbalized desire to manage menopause

Risk for imbalanced **Nutrition**: more than body requirements r/t change in metabolic rate caused by fluctuating hormone levels

Risk for **Powerlessness** r/t changes associated with menopause

Risk for situational low **Self-esteem** r/t developmental changes: menopause

Risk for urge urinary **Incontinence** r/t changes in hormonal levels affecting bladder function

## MENORRHAGIA

**Fear** r/t loss of large amounts of blood

Risk for deficient **Fluid** volume r/t excessive loss of menstrual blood

M

## MENTAL ILLNESS

Chronic **Sorrow** r/t presence of mental illness

Compromised family **Coping** r/t lack of available support from client

Defensive **Coping** r/t psychological impairment, substance abuse

Disabled family **Coping** r/t chronically unexpressed feelings of guilt, anxiety, hostility, or despair

Disturbed **Thought** processes r/t head injury, mental disorder, personality disorder, organic mental disorder, substance abuse, severe interpersonal conflict, sleep deprivation, sensory deprivation or overload, impaired cerebral perfusion

Ineffective community **Therapeutic** regimen management r/t inadequate services to care for mentally ill clients, lack of information regarding how to access services

Ineffective **Coping** r/t situational crisis, coping with mental illness

Ineffective **Denial** r/t refusal to acknowledge abuse problem, fear of the social stigma of disease

Ineffective **Therapeutic** regimen management: families r/t chronicity of condition, unpredictability of client, unknown prognosis

Risk for **Loneliness** r/t social isolation

Risk for **Powerlessness** r/t lifestyle of helplessness

## MENTAL RETARDATION

Chronic low **Self-esteem** r/t perceived differences

Delayed **Growth** and development r/t cognitive or perceptual impairment, developmental delay

**Grieving** r/t loss of perfect child, birth of child with congenital defect or subsequent head injury

Impaired **Home** maintenance r/t insufficient support systems

Impaired **Social** interaction r/t developmental lag or delay, perceived differences

Impaired **Swallowing** r/t neuromuscular impairment

Impaired verbal **Communication** r/t developmental delay

Interrupted **Family** processes r/t crisis of diagnosis and situational transition

Parental role **Conflict** r/t home care of child with special needs

Readiness for enhanced family **Coping** r/t adaptation and acceptance of child's condition and needs

Risk for delayed **Development** r/t cognitive or perceptual impairment

Risk for disproportionate **Growth** r/t mental retardation

Risk for impaired **Religiosity** r/t social isolation

Risk for **Self-mutilation** r/t separation anxiety, depersonalization

**Self-care** deficit: bathing/hygiene, dressing/grooming, feeding, toileting r/t perceptual or cognitive impairment

**Self-mutilation** r/t inability to express tension verbally

**Spiritual** distress r/t chronic condition of child with special needs

*See Child with Chronic Condition; Safety, Childhood*

## METABOLIC ACIDOSIS

*See Ketoacidosis, Diabetic; Ketoacidosis, Alcoholic*

## METABOLIC ALKALOSIS

Deficient **Fluid** volume r/t fluid volume loss, vomiting, gastric suctioning, failure of regulatory mechanisms

## METASTASIS

*See Cancer*

## MI (MYOCARDIAL INFARCTION)

Acute **Pain** r/t myocardial tissue damage from inadequate blood supply

**Anxiety** r/t threat of death, possible change in role status

**Constipation** r/t decreased peristalsis from decreased physical activity, medication effect, change in diet

Death **Anxiety** r/t seriousness of medical condition

Decreased **Cardiac** output r/t ventricular damage, ischemia, dysrhythmias

**Fear** r/t threat to well-being

Ineffective **Denial** r/t fear, deficient knowledge about heart disease

Ineffective family **Coping** r/t spouse or significant other's fear of partner loss

Ineffective **Health** maintenance r/t deficient knowledge regarding self-care and treatment

Ineffective **Sexuality** patterns r/t fear of chest pain, possibility of heart damage

Ineffective **Therapeutic** regimen management r/t knowledge deficit

Interrupted **Family** processes r/t crisis, role change

Readiness for enhanced **Knowledge** of heart problems and rehabilitation and prevention

Risk for **Powerlessness** r/t acute illness

Risk for **Spiritual** distress r/t physical illness: MI

Situational low **Self-esteem** r/t crisis of MI

## MIDCAB (MINIMALLY INVASIVE DIRECT CORONARY BYPASS)

Readiness for enhanced **Therapeutic** regimen management r/t pre- and postoperative care associated with the surgery

Risk for **Infection** r/t large breasts on incision line

*See Angioplasty, Coronary; Coronary Artery Bypass Grafting*

## MIDLIFE CRISIS

Ineffective **Coping** r/t inability to deal with changes associated with aging

**Powerlessness** r/t lack of control over life situation

Readiness for enhanced **Spiritual** well-being r/t desire to find purpose and meaning to life

**Spiritual** distress r/t questioning belief/value system

## MIGRAINE HEADACHE

Acute **Pain**: headache r/t vasodilation of cerebral and extracerebral vessels

Disturbed **Energy** field r/t pain, disruption of normal flow of energy

Ineffective **Health** maintenance r/t deficient knowledge regarding prevention and treatment of headaches

Readiness for enhanced **Therapeutic** regimen management r/t expressed desire to obtain information to prevent and treat pain associated with migraines

## MILK INTOLERANCE

*See Lactose Intolerance*

## MINIMALLY INVASIVE HEART SURGERY

*See MIDCAB (Minimally Invasive Direct Coronary Bypass); OPCAB (Off-Pump Coronary Artery Bypass)*

## MISCARRIAGE

*See Pregnancy Loss*

## MITRAL STENOSIS

**Activity** intolerance r/t imbalance between oxygen supply and demand

M

**Anxiety** r/t possible worsening of symptoms, activity intolerance, fatigue

Decreased **Cardiac** output r/t incompetent heart valves, abnormal forward or backward blood flow, flow into a dilated chamber, flow through an abnormal passage between chambers

**Fatigue** r/t reduced cardiac output

Ineffective **Health** maintenance r/t deficient knowledge regarding self-care with disorder

## MITRAL VALVE PROLAPSE

Acute **Pain** r/t mitral valve regurgitation

**Anxiety** r/t symptoms of condition: palpitations, chest pain

Effective management of **Therapeutic** regimen r/t prophylactic antibiotic therapy prior to invasive procedure such as dental work

**Fatigue** r/t abnormal catecholamine regulation, decreased intravascular volume

**Fear** r/t lack of knowledge about mitral valve prolapse, feelings of having a heart attack

Ineffective **Health** maintenance r/t deficient knowledge regarding methods to relieve pain and treat dysrhythmia and shortness of breath, need for prophylactic antibiotics before invasive procedures

Ineffective **Tissue** perfusion: cerebral r/t postural hypotension

Readiness for enhanced **Knowledge** of methods to treat and prevent symptoms associated with condition

Risk for **Infection** r/t invasive procedures

Risk for **Powerlessness** r/t unpredictability of onset of symptoms

## MOBILITY, IMPAIRED BED

Impaired bed **Mobility** r/t impaired ability to turn side to side; move from supine to sitting or sitting to supine; "scoot" or reposition self in bed; move from supine to prone or prone to supine; move from supine to long sitting or long sitting to supine

## MOBILITY, IMPAIRED PHYSICAL

Impaired physical **Mobility** r/t intolerance to activity, decreased strength and endurance, pain, discomfort, perceptual or cognitive impairment, neuromuscular impairment, musculoskeletal impairment, depression, severe anxiety

Risk for **Falls** r/t impaired physical mobility

## MOBILITY, IMPAIRED WHEELCHAIR

Impaired wheelchair **Mobility** r/t impaired ability to operate manual or power wheelchair on even or uneven surface; impaired ability to operate manual or power wheelchair on an incline or decline; impaired ability to operate wheelchair on curbs

## MODIFIED RADICAL MASTECTOMY

Decisional **Conflict** r/t treatment of choice

Readiness for enhanced **Communication** r/t willingness to discuss options for treatment

*See Mastectomy*

## MONONUCLEOSIS

**Activity** intolerance r/t generalized weakness

Acute **Pain** r/t enlargement of lymph nodes, irritation of oropharyngeal cavity

**Fatigue** r/t disease state, stress

Hyperthermia r/t infectious process

Impaired **Swallowing** r/t irritation of oropharyngeal cavity

Ineffective **Health** maintenance r/t deficient knowledge concerning transmission and treatment of disease

Risk for **Injury** r/t possible rupture of spleen

## MOOD DISORDERS

**Caregiver** role strain r/t symptoms associated with disorder of care receiver

Impaired **Adjustment** r/t hopelessness, altered locus of control

Readiness for enhanced **Communication** r/t willingness to communicate with others regarding problems associated with mood disorder

Risk for situational low **Self-esteem** r/t unpredictable changes in mood

**Social** isolation r/t alterations in mental status

*See specific disorder: Depression; Dysthymic Disorder; Hypomania; Manic Disorder, Bipolar I*

## MOON FACE

Disturbed **Body** image r/t change in appearance from disease and medication

Risk for situational low **Self-esteem** r/t change in body image

*See Cushing's Syndrome*

## MORAL/ETHICAL DILEMMAS

Decisional **Conflict** r/t questioning personal values and belief, which alter decision

Readiness for enhanced **Religiosity** r/t requests assistance in expanding religious options

Readiness for enhanced **Spiritual** well-being r/t request for interaction with others regarding difficult decisions

Risk for **Powerlessness** r/t lack of knowledge to make a decision

Risk for **Spiritual** distress r/t moral or ethical crisis

## MOTTLING OF PERIPHERAL SKIN

Ineffective **Tissue** perfusion: peripheral r/t interruption of arterial flow, decreased circulating blood volume

## MOURNING

*See Grieving*

## MOUTH LESIONS

*See Mucous Membranes, Impaired Oral*

## MRI (MAGNETIC RESONANCE IMAGING)

**Anxiety** r/t fear of being in closed spaces

Deficient **Knowledge** r/t preparation for examination, contraindications to test, especially presence of any metal in body

Readiness for enhanced **Knowledge** r/t appropriate preparation for exam

Readiness for enhanced **Therapeutic** regimen management r/t removing any metallic objects prior to the examination

## MUCOCUTANEOUS LYMPH NODE SYNDROME

*See Kawasaki Syndrome*

## MUCOUS MEMBRANES, IMPAIRED ORAL

Impaired **Oral** mucous membrane r/t chemotherapy, chemical irritants (e.g., alcohol, tobacco, acidic foods, drugs, regular use of inhalers or other noxious agents), depression, immunosuppression, aging related loss of connective, adipose, or bone tissue, barriers to professional care, cleft lip or palate, medication side effects, lack of or decreased salivation, trauma, pathological conditions; oral cavity (radiation to head or neck), NPO for more than 24 hours, mouth

**M**

breathing, malnutrition or vitamin deficiency, dehydration, infection, ineffective oral hygiene, mechanical (e.g., ill-fitting dentures, braces, tubes [endotracheal/nasogastric], surgery in oral cavity), decreased platelets, immunocompromised, radiation therapy, barriers to oral self-care, diminished hormone levels (women), stress, loss of supportive structures

## MULTIINFARCT DEMENTIA

*See Dementia*

## MULTIPLE GESTATION

**Anxiety** r/t uncertain outcome of pregnancy

Death **Anxiety** r/t maternal complications associated with multiple gestation

Deficient **Knowledge** r/t caring for more than one infant

Disturbed **Sleep** pattern r/t discomforts of multiple gestation or care of infants

**Fatigue** r/t physiological demands of a multi-fetal pregnancy and/or care of more than one infant

Imbalanced **Nutrition**: less than body requirements r/t physiological demands of a multi-fetal pregnancy

Impaired **Home** maintenance r/t fatigue

Impaired physical **Mobility** r/t increased uterine size

Impaired **Transfer** ability r/t enlarged uterus

Readiness for enhanced **Family** processes r/t family adapting to change with more than one infant

Risk for **Constipation** r/t enlarged uterus

Risk for delayed **Development**: fetus r/t multiple gestation

Risk for disproportionate **Growth**: fetus r/t multiple gestation

Risk for ineffective **Breastfeeding** r/t

lack of support, physical demands of feeding more than one infant

Stress urinary **Incontinence** r/t increased pelvic pressure

## MULTIPLE PERSONALITY DISORDER (DISSOCIATIVE IDENTITY DISORDER)

**Anxiety** r/t loss of control of behavior and feelings

Chronic low **Self-esteem** r/t inability to deal with life events, history of abuse

Defensive **Coping** r/t unresolved past traumatic events, severe anxiety

Disturbed **Body** image r/t feelings of powerlessness with personality changes

Disturbed personal **Identity** r/t severe child abuse

**Hopelessness** r/t long-term stress

Ineffective **Coping** r/t history of abuse

Readiness for enhanced **Communication** r/t willingness to discuss problems associated with condition

Risk for **Self-mutilation** r/t need to act out to relieve stress

*See Dissociative Identity Disorder*

## MULTIPLE SCLEROSIS (MS)

Chronic **Sorrow** r/t loss of physical ability

Disturbed **Energy** field r/t disruption in energy flow resulting from disharmony between mind and body

Disturbed **Sensory** perception: specify r/t pathology in sensory tracts

Impaired physical **Mobility** r/t neuromuscular impairment

Ineffective **Airway** clearance r/t decreased energy/fatigue

**Powerlessness** r/t progressive nature of disease

Readiness for enhanced **Spiritual** well-being r/t struggling with chronic debilitating condition

Readiness for enhanced **Therapeutic** regimen management r/t expressing a desire to manage condition

Risk for **Disuse** syndrome r/t physical immobility

Risk for imbalanced **Nutrition**: less than body requirements r/t impaired swallowing, depression

Risk for impaired **Religiosity** r/t illness

Risk for **Injury** r/t altered mobility, sensory dysfunction

Risk for latex **Allergy** response r/t possible repeated exposures to latex associated with intermittent catheterizations

Risk for **Powerlessness** r/t chronic illness

**Self-care** deficit: specify r/t neuromuscular impairment

**Sexual** dysfunction r/t biopsychosocial alteration of sexuality

**Spiritual** distress r/t perceived hopelessness of diagnosis

**Urinary** retention r/t inhibition of the reflex arc

*See Neurological Disorders*

## MUMPS

*See Communicable Diseases, Childhood*

## MURMURS

Decreased **Cardiac** output r/t incompetent heart valves, abnormal forward or backward blood flow, flow into a dilated chamber, flow through an abnormal passage between chambers

## MUSCULAR ATROPHY/WEAKNESS

Risk for **Disuse** syndrome r/t impaired physical mobility

Risk for **Falls** r/t impaired physical mobility

## MUSCULAR DYSTROPHY (MD)

**Activity** intolerance r/t fatigue

**Constipation** r/t immobility

Decreased **Cardiac** output r/t effects of CHF

Disturbed **Energy** field r/t illness

**Fatigue** r/t increased energy requirements to perform activities of daily living

Imbalanced **Nutrition**: less than body requirements r/t impaired swallowing or chewing

Imbalanced **Nutrition**: more than body requirements r/t inactivity

Impaired **Mobility** r/t muscle weakness and development of contractures

Impaired **Transfer** ability r/t muscle weakness

M

Impaired **Walking** r/t muscle weakness

Ineffective **Airway** clearance r/t muscle weakness and decreased ability to cough

Readiness for enhanced **Self-concept** r/t acceptance of strength and abilities

Risk for **Aspiration** r/t impaired swallowing

Risk for **Disuse** syndrome r/t complications of immobility

Risk for **Falls** r/t muscle weakness

Risk for impaired **Gas** exchange r/t ineffective airway clearance and ineffective breathing pattern secondary to muscle weakness

Risk for impaired **Religiosity** r/t illness

Risk for impaired **Skin** integrity r/t immobility, braces, or adaptive devices

Risk for ineffective **Breathing** pattern r/t muscle weakness

Risk for **Infection** r/t pooling of pulmonary secretions secondary to immobility and muscle weakness

Risk for **Injury** r/t muscle weakness and unsteady gait

Risk for **Powerlessness** r/t chronic condition

Risk for situational low **Self-esteem** r/t presence of chronic condition

**Self-care** deficits: feeding, bathing, dressing, toileting r/t muscle weakness and fatigue

*See Child with Chronic Condition; Hospitalized Child*

## MVA (MOTOR VEHICLE ACCIDENT)

*See Fracture; Head Injury; Injury; Pneumothorax*

## MYASTHENIA GRAVIS

**Fatigue** r/t paresthesia, aching muscles

Imbalanced **Nutrition**: less than body requirements r/t difficulty eating and swallowing

Impaired physical **Mobility** r/t defective transmission of nerve impulses at the neuromuscular junction

Impaired **Swallowing** r/t neuromuscular impairment

Ineffective **Airway** clearance r/t decreased ability to cough and swallow

Ineffective **Therapeutic** regimen management r/t lack of knowledge of treatment, uncertainty of outcome

Interrupted **Family** processes r/t crisis of dealing with diagnosis

Readiness for enhanced **Spiritual** well being r/t heightened coping with serious illness

Risk for **Caregiver** role strain r/t severity of illness of client

Risk for impaired **Religiosity** r/t illness

*See Neurological Disorders*

## MYCOPLASMA PNEUMONIA

*See Pneumonia*

## MYELOCELE

*See Neurotube Defects*

## MYELOGRAM, CONTRAST

Acute **Pain** r/t irritation of nerve roots

Risk for deficient **Fluid** volume r/t possible dehydration, loss of cerebrospinal fluid

Risk for ineffective **Tissue** perfusion: cerebral r/t hypotension, loss of cerebrospinal fluid

**Urinary** retention r/t pressure on spinal nerve roots

## MYELOMENINGOCELE

*See Neurotube Defects*

## MYOCARDIAL INFARCTION

*See MI (Myocardial Infarction)*

## MYOCARDITIS

**Activity** intolerance r/t reduced cardiac reserve and prescribed bedrest

Decreased **Cardiac** output r/t impaired contractility of ventricles

Deficient **Knowledge** r/t treatment of disease

Readiness for enhanced **Knowledge** r/t serious life changing disease

*See CHF (Congestive Heart Failure), if appropriate*

## MYRINGOTOMY

Acute **Pain** r/t surgical procedure

Disturbed **Sensory** perception r/t possible hearing impairment

**Fear** r/t hospitalization, surgical procedure

Ineffective **Health** maintenance r/t deficient knowledge regarding self-care following surgery

Risk for **Infection** r/t invasive procedure

## MYXEDEMA

*See Hypothyroidism*

**N**

## NARCISSISTIC PERSONALITY DISORDER

Decisional **Conflict** r/t lack of realistic problem-solving skills

Defensive **Coping** r/t grandiose sense of self

Disturbed **Personal** identity r/t psychological impairment

Impaired **Social** interaction r/t self-concept disturbance

Interrupted **Family** processes r/t taking advantage of others to achieve own goals

Risk for **Loneliness** r/t inability to interact appropriately with others

Risk for **Self-mutilation** r/t inadequate coping

## NARCOLEPSY

**Anxiety** r/t fear of lack of control over falling asleep disturbed

Disturbed **Sleep** pattern r/t uncontrollable desire to sleep

Readiness for enhanced **Sleep** r/t expression of willingness to enhance sleep

Risk for **Trauma** r/t falling asleep during potentially dangerous activity

## NARCOTIC USE

Risk for **Constipation** r/t effects of opioids on peristalsis

*See Substance Abuse (if relevant)*

## NASOGASTRIC SUCTION

Impaired **Comfort** r/t presence of nasogastric tube

Impaired **Oral** mucous membrane r/t presence of nasogastric tube

Risk for deficient **Fluid** volume r/t loss of gastrointestinal fluids without adequate replacement

## NAUSEA

### TREATMENT RELATED

**Nausea** r/t gastric irritation: pharmaceuticals (e.g., aspirin, nonsteroidal antiinflammatory drugs, steroids, antibiotics), alcohol, iron, blood; gastric distention: delayed gastric emptying caused by pharmacological interventions (e.g., narcotics administration, anesthesia agents); pharmaceuticals (e.g., analgesics, antiviral agents for HIV, aspirin, opioids, chemotherapeutic agents); toxins (e.g., radiotherapy)

### BIOPHYSICAL

**Nausea** r/t biochemical disorders (e.g., uremia, diabetic ketoacidosis, pregnancy), cardiac pain, cancer of the stomach or intraabdominal tumors (e.g., pelvic or colorectal cancers), esophageal or pancreatic disease, gastric distention due to delayed gastric emptying, pyloric intestinal obstruction, genitourinary and biliary distension, upper bowel stasis, external compression of the stomach (liver, spleen, or other organ), enlargement that slows the stomach functioning (squashed stomach syndrome), excess food intake, gastric irritation due to pharyngeal and/or peritoneal inflammation, liver or splenetic capsule stretch, local tumors (e.g., acoustic neuroma, primary or secondary brain tumors, bone metastases at base of skull), motion sickness, Meniere's disease or labyrinthitis, physical factors (e.g., increased intracranial pressure, meningitis), toxins (e.g., tumor-produced peptides, abnormal metabolites due to cancer)

**N**

## SITUATIONAL

**Nausea** r/t psychological factors (e.g., pain, fear, anxiety, noxious odors, taste, unpleasant visual stimulation)

### NEAR-DROWNING

Anticipatory **Grieving** r/t potential death of child, unknown sequelae, guilt about accident

**Aspiration** r/t aspiration of fluid into the lungs

**Fear**: parental r/t possible death of child, possible permanent and debilitating sequelae

**Hypothermia** r/t central nervous system injury, prolonged submersion in cold water

Impaired **Gas** exchange r/t laryngospasm, holding breath, aspiration

Ineffective **Airway** clearance r/t aspiration, impaired gas exchange

Ineffective **Health** maintenance r/t parental deficient knowledge regarding safety measures appropriate for age

Readiness for enhanced **Spiritual** well-being r/t struggle with survival of life-threatening situation

Risk for delayed **Development** and disproportionate growth r/t hypoxemia, cerebral anoxia

Risk for **Infection** r/t aspiration, invasive monitoring

*See Child with Chronic Condition; Hospitalized Child; Safety, Childhood; Terminally Ill Child/ Death of Child*

### NEARSIGHTEDNESS

Effective management of **Therapeutic** regimen r/t early diagnosis and appropriate referral for eyeglasses or contact lenses when nearsightedness is suspected; signs, which may indicate a vision problem: sitting close to television, holding books very close when reading, or having difficulty reading the blackboard in school or signs on a wall

### NEAR-SIGHTEDNESS; CORNEAL SURGERY

*See LASIK Eye Surgery (Laser-Assisted In Situ Keratomileusis)*

### NECK VEIN DISTENTION

Decreased **Cardiac** output r/t decreased contractility of heart and resulting increased preload

Excess **Fluid** volume r/t excess fluid intake, compromised regulatory mechanisms

*See CHF (Congestive Heart Failure)*

### NECROSIS—RENAL TUBULAR; ATN (ACUTE TUBULAR NECROSIS); NECROSIS—ACUTE TUBULAR

*See Renal Failure*

### NECROTIZING ENTEROCOLITIS (NEC)

Deficient **Fluid** volume r/t vomiting, gastrointestinal bleeding

Disturbed **Energy** field r/t illness

Imbalanced **Nutrition**: less than body requirements r/t decreased ability to absorb nutrients, decreased perfusion to gastrointestinal tract

Ineffective **Breathing** pattern r/t abdominal distention, hypoxia

Ineffective **Tissue** perfusion: gastrointestinal r/t shunting of blood away from mesenteric circulation and toward vital organs secondary to perinatal stress, hypoxia

Risk for **Infection** r/t bacterial invasion of gastrointestinal tract, invasive procedures

*See Hospitalized Child; Premature Infant (Child)*

## NECROTIZING FASCIITIS (FLESH-EATING BACTERIA)

Acute **Pain** r/t toxins interfering with blood flow

Anticipatory **Grieving** r/t poor prognosis associated with disease

Decreased **Cardiac** output r/t tachycardia and hypotension

**Fear** r/t possible fatal outcome of disease

**Hyperthermia** r/t presence of infection

Ineffective **Protection** r/t cellulitis resistant to treatment

Ineffective **Tissue** perfusion: peripheral r/t thrombosis of the subcutaneous blood vessels, leading to necrosis of nerve fibers

*See Renal Failure; Septicemia*

## NEGATIVE FEELINGS ABOUT SELF

Chronic low **Self-esteem** r/t longstanding negative self-evaluation

Readiness for enhanced **Self-concept** r/t expressed willingness to enhance self-concept

**Self-esteem** disturbance r/t inappropriate learned negative feelings about self

## NEGLECT, UNILATERAL

*See Unilateral Neglect of One Side of Body*

## NEGLECTFUL CARE OF FAMILY MEMBER

**Caregiver** role strain r/t care demands of family member, lack of social or financial support

Deficient **Knowledge** r/t care needs

Disabled family **Coping** r/t highly ambivalent family relationships, lack of respite care

Ineffective community **Therapeutic** regimen management r/t deficits in community for support of caregivers, detection of client neglect

Interrupted **Family** processes r/t situational transition or crisis

## NEONATE

*See Newborn, Normal; Newborn, Postmature; Newborn, Small for Gestational Age*

## NEOPLASM

**Fear** r/t possible malignancy

*See Cancer*

## NEPHRECTOMY

Acute **Pain** r/t incisional discomfort

**Anxiety** r/t surgical recovery, prognosis

**Constipation** r/t lack of return of peristalsis

Impaired **Urinary** elimination r/t loss of kidney

Ineffective **Breathing** pattern r/t location of surgical incision

Risk for deficient **Fluid** volume r/t vascular losses, decreased intake

Risk for **Infection** r/t invasive procedure, lack of deep breathing because of location of surgical incision

**Spiritual** distress r/t chronic illness

## NEPHROSTOMY, PERCUTANEOUS

Acute **Pain** r/t invasive procedure

Impaired **Urinary** elimination r/t nephrostomy tube

Risk for **Infection** r/t invasive procedure

## NEPHROTIC SYNDROME

**Activity** intolerance r/t generalized edema

Disturbed **Body** image r/t edematous appearance and side effects of steroid therapy

Excess **Fluid** volume r/t edema secondary to oncotic fluid shift resulting from serum protein loss and renal retention of salt and water

Imbalanced **Nutrition**: less than body requirements r/t anorexia, protein loss

Imbalanced **Nutrition**: more than body requirements r/t increased appetite secondary to steroid therapy

Impaired **Comfort** r/t edema

Risk for impaired **Skin** integrity r/t edema

Risk for **Infection** r/t altered immune mechanisms secondary to disease and effects of steroids

Risk for **Noncompliance** r/t side effects of home steroid therapy

**Social** isolation r/t edematous appearance

*See Child with Chronic Condition; Hospitalized Child*

## NERVE ENTRAPMENT

*See Carpal Tunnel Syndrome*

## NEURITIS

**Activity** intolerance r/t pain with movement

Acute **Pain** r/t stimulation of affected nerve endings, inflammation of sensory nerves

Ineffective **Health** maintenance r/t deficient knowledge regarding self-care with neuritis

## NEUROFIBROMATOSIS

Compromised **Family** coping r/t cost and emotional needs of disease

Disturbed **Energy** field r/t disease

Disturbed **Sensory** perception r/t optic nerve gliomas associated with disease

Effective **Therapeutic** regimen management r/t evaluate visual disturbances, associated with optic pathway tumors: dimness of vision, headache, visual field defects, nystagmus and distortion of binocular fixation, decreased

visual acuity, proptosis or a droopy eyelid

Impaired **Skin** integrity r/t café-au-lait spots

Readiness for enhanced **Therapeutic** regimen management r/t seek cancer screening, education, and genetic counseling

Risk for delayed **Development**: learning disorders including attention deficit/ hyperactivity disorder (ADHD), low intelligent quotient (IQ) scores, and developmental delay r/t genetic disorder

Risk for decreased **Cardiac** output r/t hypertension associated with condition

Risk for **Constipation** r/t intestinal neurofibromas

Risk for disproportionate **Growth**: short stature, precocious puberty, delayed maturation, thyroid disorders r/t genetic disorder

Risk for **Injury** r/t possible problems with balance

Risk for **Spiritual** distress r/t possible severity of disease

*See Abdominal Distension; Surgery, Perioperative; Surgery, Postoperative; Surgery, Preoperative*

## NEUROGENIC BLADDER

Reflex **Incontinence** r/t neurological impairment

Risk for latex **Allergy** response r/t repeated exposures to latex associated with possible repeated catheterizations

**Urinary** retention r/t interruption in the lateral spinal tracts

## NEUROLOGICAL DISORDERS

Acute **Confusion** r/t dementia, alcohol abuse, drug abuse, delirium

Anticipatory **Grieving** r/t loss of usual body functioning

Disturbed **Energy** field r/t illness

Imbalanced **Nutrition**: less than body requirements r/t impaired swallowing, depression, difficulty feeding self

Impaired **Home** maintenance r/t client's or family member's disease

Impaired **Memory** r/t neurological disturbance

Impaired physical **Mobility** r/t neuromuscular impairment

Impaired **Swallowing** r/t neuromuscular dysfunction

Ineffective **Airway** clearance r/t perceptual or cognitive impairment, decreased energy, fatigue

Ineffective **Coping** r/t disability requiring change in lifestyle

Interrupted **Family** processes r/t situational crisis, illness, or disability of family member

**Powerlessness** r/t progressive nature of disease

Risk for **Disuse** syndrome r/t physical immobility, neuromuscular dysfunction

Risk for impaired **Religiosity** r/t life transition

Risk for impaired **Skin** integrity r/t altered sensation, altered mental status, paralysis

Risk for **Injury** r/t altered mobility, sensory dysfunction, cognitive impairment

**Self-care** deficit: specify r/t neuromuscular dysfunction

**Sexual** dysfunction r/t biopsychosocial alteration of sexuality

**Social** isolation r/t altered state of wellness

**Wandering** r/t cognitive impairment

## NEUROPATHY, PERIPHERAL

Chronic **Pain** r/t damage to nerves in the peripheral nervous system secondary to medication side effects, vitamin deficiency, or diabetes

Ineffective **Thermoregulation** r/t decreased ability to regulate body temperature

Risk for **Injury** r/t lack of muscle control and decreased sensation

Risk for **Peripheral** neurovascular dysfunction r/t compression, entrapment

*See Peripheral Vascular Disease*

## NEUROSURGERY

*See Crainiectomy/Craniotomy*

## NEUROTUBE DEFECTS (MENINGOCELE, MYELOMENINGOCELE, SPINA BIFIDA, ANENCEPHALY)

Chronic low **Self-esteem** r/t perceived differences, decreased ability to participate in physical and social activities at school

**Constipation** r/t immobility or less than adequate mobility

Delayed **Growth** and development r/t physical impairments, possible cognitive impairment

Disturbed **Sensory** perception: visual r/t altered reception secondary to strabismus

**Grieving** r/t loss of perfect child, birth of child with congenital defect

Impaired **Mobility** r/t neuromuscular impairment

Impaired **Skin** integrity r/t incontinence

Readiness for enhanced family **Coping** r/t effective adaptive response by family members

Readiness for enhanced **Family** processes r/t family supporting each other

Reflex **Incontinence** r/t neurogenic impairment

Risk for delayed **Development** r/t chronic illness

N

Risk for disproportionate **Growth** r/t chronic illness

Risk for imbalanced **Nutrition**: more than body requirements r/t diminished, limited, or impaired physical activity

Risk for impaired **Skin** integrity: lower extremities r/t decreased sensory perception

Risk for latex **Allergy** response r/t multiple exposures to latex products

Risk for **Powerlessness** r/t debilitating disease

Total urinary **Incontinence** r/t neurogenic impairment

Urge urinary **Incontinence** r/t neurogenic impairment

*See Child with Chronic Condition; Premature Infant (Child)*

## NEWBORN, NORMAL

Effective **Breastfeeding** r/t normal oral structure and gestational age >34 weeks

Ineffective **Protection** r/t immature immune system

Ineffective **Thermoregulation** r/t immaturity of neuroendocrine system

Readiness for enhanced organized **Infant** behavior r/t appropriate environmental stimuli

Readiness for enhanced **Parenting** r/t providing emotional and physical needs of infant

Risk for **Infection** r/t open umbilical stump

Risk for **Injury** r/t immaturity, need for caretaking

Risk for sudden infant **Death** syndrome r/t lack of knowledge regarding infant sleeping in prone or sidelying position, prenatal or postnatal infant smoke exposure, infant overheating/overwrapping, soft underlayment/loose articles in the sleep environment

## NEWBORN, POSTMATURE

**Hypothermia** r/t depleted stores of subcutaneous fat

Impaired **Skin** integrity r/t cracked and peeling skin secondary to decreased vernix

Risk for ineffective **Airway** clearance r/t meconium aspiration

Risk for **Injury** r/t hypoglycemia secondary to depleted glycogen stores

## NEWBORN, SMALL FOR GESTATIONAL AGE (SGA)

Imbalanced **Nutrition**: less than body requirements r/t history of placental insufficiency

Ineffective **Thermoregulation** r/t decreased brown fat, subcutaneous fat

Risk for delayed **Development** r/t history of placental insufficiency

Risk for disproportionate **Growth** r/t history of placental insufficiency

Risk for **Injury** r/t hypoglycemia, perinatal asphyxia, meconium aspiration

Risk for sudden infant **Death** syndrome r/t low birth weight

## NICOTINE ADDICTION

Ineffective **Health** maintenance r/t lack of ability to make a judgment about smoking cessation

**Powerlessness** r/t perceived lack of control over ability to give up nicotine

Readiness for enhanced **Therapeutic** regimen management r/t expresses desire to learn measures to stop smoking

## NIDDM (NON–INSULIN-DEPENDENT DIABETES MELLITUS)

**Health**-seeking behaviors r/t desiring information on exercise and diet to manage diabetes

*See Diabetes Mellitus*

## NIGHTMARES

Disturbed **Energy** field r/t disharmony of body and mind

**Post-trauma** response r/t disaster, war, epidemic, rape, assault, torture, catastrophic illness, or accident

**Rape-trauma** syndrome: compound reaction/silent reaction r/t forced violent sexual penetration against the victim's will and consent

## NIPPLE SORENESS

Acute **Pain** r/t injury to nipples

*See Painful Breasts, Sore Nipples*

## NOCTURIA

Impaired **Urinary** elimination r/t sensory motor impairment, urinary tract infection

Risk for **Powerlessness** r/t inability to control nighttime voidings

Total **Urinary** incontinence r/t neuropathy preventing transmission of reflex indicating bladder fullness, neurological dysfunction causing triggering of micturition at unpredictable times, independent contraction of detrusor reflex as a result of surgery, trauma, or disease affecting spinal cord nerves, anatomical fistula

Urge urinary **Incontinence** r/t decreased bladder capacity, irritation of bladder stretch receptors causing spasm, alcohol, caffeine, increased fluids, increased urine concentration, overdistention of bladder

## NOCTURNAL MYOCLONUS

*See Restless Leg Syndrome; Stress*

## NOCTURNAL PAROXYSMAL DYSPNEA

*See PND (Paroxysmal Nocturnal Dyspnea)*

## NONCOMPLIANCE

**Noncompliance** r/t *Healthcare Plan:* duration, significant others, cost, intensity, complexity; *Individual Factors:* personal and developmental abilities, health beliefs, cultural influences, spiritual values, knowledge and skill relevant to the regimen behavior, motivational forces; *Health System:* satisfaction with care, credibility of provider, access and convenience of care, financial flexibility of plan, client-provider relationships, provider reimbursement of teaching and follow-up, provider continuity and regular follow-up, individual health coverage, communication and teaching skills of the provider; *Network:* involvement of members in health plan, social value regarding plan, perceived belief of significant others

## NON–INSULIN-DEPENDENT DIABETES MELLITUS (NIDDM)

*See Diabetes Mellitus*

## NORMAL PRESSURE HYDROCEPHALUS (NPH)

Acute **Confusion** r/t dementia secondary to obstruction to flow of cerebrospinal fluid (CSF)

Impaired **Memory** r/t neurological disturbance

Impaired verbal **Communication** r/t obstruction of flow of cerebrospinal fluid

Ineffective **Tissue** perfusion: cerebral r/t obstruction to flow of CSF secondary to closed head injury, craniotomy, meningitis, or subarachnoid hemorrhage

Risk for **Falls** r/t unsteady gait secondary to obstruction of CSF

## NORWALK VIRUS

*See Viral Gastroenteritis*

## NURSING

*See Breastfeeding, Effective; Breastfeeding, Ineffective; Breastfeeding, Interrupted*

**N**

## NUTRITION

Readiness for enhanced **Nutrition** r/t expresses willingness to enhance nutrition, eats regularly, consumes adequate food and fluid, expresses knowledge of healthy food and fluid choices, follows an appropriate standard for intake (e.g., the food guide pyramid or America Diabetic Association guidelines), safe preparation and storage for food and fluids, attitude toward eating and drinking is congruent with health goals

## NUTRITION, IMBALANCED

Imbalanced **Nutrition**: less than body requirements r/t inability to ingest or digest food or absorb nutrients because of biological, psychological, economic factors

Imbalanced **Nutrition**: more than body requirements r/t excessive intake in relation to metabolic need

Risk for imbalanced **Nutrition**: more than body requirements r/t reported use of solid food as major food source before 5 months of age; concentrating food intake at end of day; reported or observed obesity in one or both parents; rapid transition across growth percentiles in infants or children; pairing food with other activities; observed use of food as reward or comfort measure; eating in response to external cues (e.g., time of day, social situation); dysfunctional eating patterns

## OBESITY

Chronic low **Self-esteem** r/t ineffective coping, overeating

Disturbed **Body** image r/t eating disorder, excess weight

Imbalanced **Nutrition**: more than body requirements r/t caloric intake exceeding energy expenditure

Readiness for enhanced **Nutrition** r/t expressing willingness to enhance nutrition

## OBS (ORGANIC BRAIN SYNDROME)

*See Organic Mental Disorders*

## OBSESSIVE-COMPULSIVE DISORDER

**Anxiety** r/t threat to self-concept, unmet needs

Decisional **Conflict** r/t inability to make a decision for fear of reprisal

Disabled family **Coping** r/t family process being disrupted by client's ritualistic activities

Disturbed **Thought** processes r/t persistent thoughts, ideas, impulses that seem irrelevant and will not relent

Ineffective **Coping** r/t expression of feelings in an unacceptable way, ritualistic behavior

**Powerlessness** r/t unrelenting repetitive thoughts to perform irrational activities

Risk for situational low **Self-esteem** r/t inability to control repetitive thoughts and actions

## OBSTRUCTION, BOWEL

*See Bowel Obstruction*

## OBSTRUCTIVE SLEEP APNEA

Disturbed **Sleep** pattern r/t blocked airway

**Health-seeking** behaviors r/t seeking nutritional information to control weight that may be contributing to sleep apnea

Imbalanced **Nutrition**: more than body requirements r/t excessive intake related to metabolic need

*See PND (Paroxysmal Nocturnal Dyspnea)*

## ODD

*See Oppositional Defiant Disorder (ODD)*

## OLDER ADULT

*See Aging*

## OLIGOHYDRAMNIOS

**Anxiety**: maternal r/t fear of unknown, threat to fetus

Risk for **Injury**: fetal r/t decreased umbilical cord blood flow secondary to compression

## OLIGURIA

Deficient **Fluid** volume r/t active fluid loss, failure of regulatory mechanism

*See Cardiac Output Decrease; Renal Failure; Shock*

## OMPHALOCELE

*See Gastroschisis/Omphalocele*

## ONYCHOMYCOSIS

*See Ringworm of Nails*

## OOPHORECTOMY

Risk for ineffective **Sexuality** patterns r/t altered body function

*See Surgery, Perioperative; Surgery, Postoperative; Surgery, Preoperative*

## OPCAB (OFF-PUMP CORONARY ARTERY BYPASS)

Acute **Confusion** r/t possible decreased cerebral tissue perfusion

Acute **Pain** r/t possible gastrointestinal dysfunction

Decreased **Cardiac** output r/t increased vasodilation

Impaired **Gas** exchange r/t alveolar-capillary membrane changes

Impaired **Memory** r/t possible decreased cerebral tissue perfusion

Readiness for enhanced **Therapeutic** regimen management r/t pre- and postoperative care associated with the surgery

Risk for deficient **Fluid** volume r/t bleeding associated with anticoagulant therapy

*See Angioplasty, Coronary; Coronary Artery Bypass Grafting*

## OPEN HEART SURGERY

Decreased **Cardiac** output r/t altered preload or afterload

Impaired **Gas** exchange r/t cardiac surgery

*See Coronary Artery Bypass Grafting; Dysrhythmia*

## OPEN REDUCTION OF FRACTURE WITH INTERNAL FIXATION (FEMUR)

**Anxiety** r/t outcome of corrective procedure

Impaired physical **Mobility** r/t postoperative position, abduction of leg, avoidance of acute flexion

**Powerlessness** r/t loss of control, unanticipated change in lifestyle

Risk for perioperative positioning **Injury** r/t immobilization

Risk for **Peripheral** neurovascular dysfunction r/t mechanical compression, orthopedic surgery, immobilization

*See Surgery, Postoperative Care*

## OPIATE USE

Risk for **Constipation** r/t effects of opiates on peristalsis

*See Drug Abuse; Drug Withdrawal*

## OPPORTUNISTIC INFECTION

Delayed **Surgical** recovery r/t abnormal blood profiles, impaired healing

Risk for **Infection** r/t abnormal blood profiles

O

*See AIDS (Acquired Immunodeficiency Syndrome); HIV (Human Immunodeficiency Virus)*

## OPPOSITIONAL DEFIANT DISORDER (ODD)

**Anxiety** r/t feelings of anger and hostility towards authority figures

Chronic or situational low **Self-esteem** r/t poor self-control and disruptive behaviors

Disabled **Family** coping r/t feelings of anger, hostility; defiant behavior toward authority figures

Disturbed **Thought** processes r/t difficulty thinking, making appropriate decisions

Impaired **Adjustment** r/t multiple stressors associated with condition

Impaired **Social** interaction r/t being touchy or easily annoyed, blaming others for own mistakes, constant trouble in school

Ineffective **Coping** r/t lack of self-control or perceived lack of self-control

Ineffective family **Therapeutic** regimen management r/t difficulty in limit setting and managing oppositional behaviors

Risk for impaired **Parenting** r/t childrens' difficult behaviors and inability to set limits

Risk for other-directed **Violence** r/t history of violence, threats of violence against others; history of antisocial behavior; history of indirect violence

Risk for **Powerlessness** r/t inability to deal with difficulty behaviors

Risk for **Spiritual** distress r/t anxiety and stress in dealing with difficulty behaviors

**Social** isolation r/t unaccepted social behavior

## ORAL MUCOUS MEMBRANE, IMPAIRED

Impaired **Oral** mucous membrane r/t pathological conditions—oral cavity (radiation to head or neck), dehydration, chemical trauma (e.g., acidic foods, drugs, noxious agents, alcohol), mechanical trauma (e.g., ill-fitting dentures, braces, endotracheal and nasogastric tubes, surgery in oral cavity), NPO for more than 24 hours, ineffective oral hygiene, mouth breathing, malnutrition, infection, lack of or decreased salivation, medication

## ORAL THRUSH

*See Candidiasis, Oral*

## ORCHITIS

Readiness for enhanced **Therapeutic** regimen management r/t follows recommendations for mumps vaccination

*See Epididymitis*

## ORGANIC MENTAL DISORDERS

Adult **Failure** to thrive r/t undetected organic mental disorder

Impaired **Social** interaction r/t disturbed thought processes

Risk for **Injury** r/t disorientation to time, place, person

*See Dementia*

## ORTHOPEDIC TRACTION

Impaired **Social** interaction r/t limited physical mobility

Impaired **Transfer** ability r/t limited physical mobility

Ineffective **Role** performance r/t limited physical mobility

Risk for impaired **Religiosity** r/t immobility

*See Traction and Casts*

## ORTHOPNEA

Decreased **Cardiac** output r/t inability of heart to meet demands of body

Ineffective **Breathing** pattern r/t inability to breathe with head of bed flat

## ORTHOSTATIC HYPOTENSION

*See Dizziness*

## OSTEOARTHRITIS

**Activity** intolerance r/t pain after exercise or use of joint

Acute **Pain** r/t movement

Impaired **Transfer** ability r/t pain

*See Arthritis*

## OSTEOMYELITIS

Acute **Pain** r/t inflammation in affected extremity

Deficient **Diversional** activity r/t prolonged immobilization, hospitalization

**Fear**: parental r/t concern regarding possible growth plate damage secondary to infection, concern that infection may become chronic

**Hyperthermia** r/t infectious process

Impaired physical **Mobility** r/t imposed immobility secondary to infected area

Ineffective **Health** maintenance r/t continued immobility at home, possible extensive casts, continued antibiotics

Risk for **Constipation** r/t immobility

Risk for impaired **Skin** integrity r/t irritation from splint/cast

Risk for **Infection** r/t inadequate primary and secondary defenses

*See Hospitalized Child*

## OSTEOPOROSIS

Acute **Pain** r/t fracture, muscle spasms

Deficient **Knowledge** r/t diet, exercise, need to abstain from alcohol and nicotine

Effective **Therapeutic** regimen management: individual r/t appropriate choices for diet and exercise to prevent and manage condition

Imbalanced **Nutrition**: less than body requirements r/t inadequate intake of calcium and vitamin D

Impaired physical **Mobility** r/t pain, skeletal changes

Readiness for enhanced **Therapeutic** regimen management r/t expressing desire to manage the treatment of illness and prevention of complications

Risk for **Injury**: fracture r/t lack of activity, risk of falling resulting from environmental hazards, neuromuscular disorders, diminished senses, cardiovascular responses, responses to drugs

Risk for **Powerlessness** r/t debilitating disease

## OSTOMY

*See Child with Chronic Condition; Colostomy; Ileal Conduit; Ileostomy*

## OTITIS MEDIA

Acute **Pain** r/t inflammation, infectious process

Disturbed **Sensory** perception: auditory r/t incomplete resolution of otitis media, presence of excess drainage in middle ear

Readiness for enhanced **Knowledge** of information relating to treatment and prevention of disease

Risk for delayed **Development** r/t frequent otitis media

Risk for **Infection** r/t eustachian tube obstruction, traumatic eardrum perforation, infectious disease process

## OVARIAN CARCINOMA

Death **Anxiety** r/t unknown outcome, possible poor prognosis

O

**Fear** r/t unknown outcome, possible poor prognosis

Ineffective **Health** maintenance r/t deficient knowledge regarding self-care, treatment of condition

*See Chemotherapy; Hysterectomy; Radiation Therapy*

## OXYURIASIS

*See Pinworms*

# P

## PACEMAKER

Acute **Pain** r/t surgical procedure

**Anxiety** r/t change in health status, presence of pacemaker

Death **Anxiety** r/t worry over possible malfunction of pacemaker

Deficient **Knowledge** r/t self-care program, when to seek medical attention

Readiness for enhanced **Therapeutic** regimen management r/t appropriate health care management of pacemaker

Risk for decreased **Cardiac** output r/t malfunction of pacemaker

Risk for **Infection** r/t invasive procedure, presence of foreign body (catheter and generator)

Risk for **Powerlessness** r/t presence of electronic device to stimulate heart

## PAGET'S DISEASE

Chronic **Sorrow** r/t chronic condition with altered body image

Deficient **Knowledge** r/t appropriate diet high in protein and calcium, mild exercise

Disturbed **Body** image r/t possible enlarged head, bowed tibias, kyphosis

Risk for **Trauma**: fracture r/t excessive bone destruction

## PAIN, ACUTE

Acute **Pain** r/t injury agents (biological, chemical, physical, psychological)

Disturbed **Energy** field r/t unbalanced energy field

## PAIN, CHRONIC

Chronic **Pain** r/t chronic physical or psychosocial disability

Disturbed **Energy** field r/t unbalanced energy field

## PAINFUL BREASTS, ENGORGEMENT

Acute **Pain** r/t distention of breast tissue

Impaired **Tissue** integrity r/t excessive fluid in breast tissues

Ineffective **Role** performance r/t change in physical capacity to assume role of breastfeeding mother

Risk for ineffective **Breastfeeding** r/t pain, infant's inability to latch on to engorged breast

Risk for **Infection** r/t milk stasis

## PAINFUL BREASTS, SORE NIPPLES

Acute **Pain** r/t cracked nipples

Impaired **Skin** integrity r/t mechanical factors involved in suckling, breastfeeding management

Ineffective **Breastfeeding** r/t pain

Ineffective **Role** performance r/t change in physical capacity to assume role of breastfeeding mother

Risk for **Infection** r/t break in skin

## PALLOR OF EXTREMITIES

Ineffective **Tissue** perfusion: peripheral r/t interruption of vascular flow

## PALPITATIONS (HEART PALPITATIONS)

*See Dysrhythmia*

## PANCREATIC CANCER

Anticipatory **Grieving** r/t shortened life span

Death **Anxiety** r/t possible poor prognosis of disease process

Deficient **Knowledge** r/t disease-induced diabetes, home management

**Fear** r/t poor prognosis of the disease

Ineffective family **Coping** r/t poor prognosis

**Spiritual** distress r/t poor prognosis

*See Cancer; Chemotherapy; Radiation Therapy; Surgery, Perioperative; Surgery, Postoperative; Surgery, Preoperative*

## PANCREATITIS

Acute **Pain** r/t irritation and edema of the inflamed pancreas

Chronic **Sorrow** r/t chronic illness

**Diarrhea** r/t decrease in pancreatic secretions resulting in steatorrhea

Deficient **Fluid** volume r/t vomiting, decreased fluid intake, fever, diaphoresis, fluid shifts

Imbalanced **Nutrition**: less than body requirements r/t inadequate dietary intake, increased nutritional needs secondary to acute illness, increased metabolic needs caused by increased body temperature

Ineffective **Breathing** pattern r/t splinting from severe pain

Ineffective **Denial** r/t ineffective coping, alcohol use

Ineffective **Health** maintenance r/t deficient knowledge concerning diet, alcohol use, medication

**Nausea** r/t irritation of gastrointestinal system

## PANIC DISORDER

**Anxiety** r/t situational crisis

Ineffective **Coping** r/t personal vulnerability

**Post-trauma** syndrome r/t previous catastrophic event

Readiness for enhanced **Coping** r/t seeking problem-oriented and emotion-oriented strategies to manage condition

Risk for **Loneliness** r/t inability to socially interact because of fear of losing control

Risk for **Post-trauma** syndrome r/t perception of the event, diminished ego strength

Risk for **Powerlessness** r/t ineffective coping skills

**Social** isolation r/t fear of lack of control

*See Anxiety; Anxiety Disorder*

## PARALYSIS

Acute **Pain** r/t prolonged immobility

Chronic **Sorrow** r/t loss of physical mobility

**Constipation** r/t effects of spinal cord disruption, inadequate fiber in diet

Disturbed **Body** image r/t biophysical changes, loss of movement, immobility

Impaired **Home** maintenance r/t physical disability

Impaired physical **Mobility** r/t neuromuscular impairment

Impaired **Transfer** ability r/t paralysis

Ineffective **Health** maintenance r/t deficient knowledge regarding self-care with paralysis

**Powerlessness** r/t illness-related regimen

Reflex **Incontinence** r/t neurological impairment

Risk for **Disuse** syndrome r/t paralysis

Risk for **Falls** r/t to paralysis

P

Risk for impaired **Religiosity** r/t immobility, possible lack of transportation

Risk for impaired **Skin** integrity r/t altered circulation, altered sensation, immobility

Risk for **Injury** r/t altered mobility, sensory dysfunction

Risk for latex **Allergy** response r/t possible repeated urinary catheterizations

Risk for **Post-trauma** syndrome r/t event causing paralysis

Risk for situational low **Self-esteem** r/t change in body image and function

**Self-care** deficit: specify r/t neuromuscular impairment

**Sexual** dysfunction r/t loss of sensation, biopsychosocial alteration

*See Child with Chronic Condition; Hemiplegia; Hospitalized Child; Neurotube Defects; Spinal Cord Injury*

## PARALYTIC ILEUS

Acute **Pain** r/t pressure, abdominal distention

**Constipation** r/t decreased gastric motility

Deficient **Fluid** volume r/t loss of fluids from vomiting, retention of fluid in bowel

Impaired **Oral** mucous membrane r/t presence of nasogastric tube

**Nausea** r/t gastrointestinal irritation

## PARANOID PERSONALITY DISORDER

**Anxiety** r/t uncontrollable intrusive, suspicious thoughts

Chronic low **Self-esteem** r/t inability to trust others

Disturbed personal **Identity** r/t difficulty with reality testing

Disturbed **Sensory** perception: specify r/t psychological dysfunction, suspicious thoughts

Disturbed **Thought** processes r/t psychological conflicts

Impaired **Adjustment** r/t intense emotional state

Risk for **Loneliness** r/t social isolation

Risk for other-directed **Violence** r/t being suspicious of others and others' actions

Risk for **Post-trauma** syndrome r/t exaggerated sense of responsibility

Risk for **Suicide** r/t psychiatric illness

**Social** isolation r/t inappropriate social skills

## PARAPLEGIA

*See Spinal Cord Injury*

## PARATHYROIDECTOMY

**Anxiety** r/t surgery

Risk for impaired verbal **Communication** r/t possible laryngeal damage, edema

Risk for ineffective **Airway** clearance r/t edema or hematoma formation, airway obstruction

Risk for **Infection** r/t surgical procedure

*See Hypocalcemia*

## PARENT ATTACHMENT

Chronic **Sorrow** r/t difficult parent-child relationship

Risk for impaired parent/infant/child **Attachment** r/t physical barriers; anxiety associated with parental role; substance abuse; premature infant; ill infant/child who is unable to effectively initiate parental contact as a result of altered behavioral organization; lack of privacy; inability of parents to meet personal needs; separation

Risk for **Spiritual** distress r/t altered relationships

## PARENTAL ROLE CONFLICT

Chronic **Sorrow** r/t difficult parent-child relationship

Parental role **Conflict** r/t change in marital status; home care of a child with special needs (e.g., apnea monitoring, postural drainage, hyperalimentation); interruptions of family life because of home care regimen (e.g., treatments, caregivers, lack of respite); specialized care center policies; separation from child because of chronic illness; intimidation with invasive or restrictive modalities (e.g., isolation, intubation)

Readiness for enhanced **Parenting** r/t willingness to enhance parenting

Risk for **Spiritual** distress r/t altered relationships

## PARENTING

Readiness for enhanced **Parenting** r/t expresses willingness to enhance parenting; children or other dependent person(s) express satisfaction with home, environment; emotional and tacit support of children or dependent person(s) evident; bonding or attachment evident; physical and emotional needs of children/dependent person(s) are met; realistic expectations of children/dependent person(s) exhibited

## PARENTING, IMPAIRED

Chronic **Sorrow** r/t difficult parent-child relationship

Impaired **Parenting** r/t *Social:* Lack of access to resources; social isolation; lack of resources; poor home environment; lack of family cohesiveness; inadequate child care arrangements; lack of transportation; unemployment or job problems; role strain or overload; marital conflict, declining satisfaction; lack of value of parenthood; change in family unit; low socioeconomic class; unplanned or unwanted pregnancy; presence of stress (e.g., financial, legal, recent crisis, cultural move); lack of, or poor, parental role model; single parent; lack of social support networks; father of child not involved; history of being abusive; history of being abused; financial difficulties; maladaptive coping strategies; poverty; poor problem-solving skills; inability to put child's needs before own; low self-esteem; relocations; legal difficulties. *Knowledge:* Lack of knowledge about child health maintenance; lack of knowledge about parenting skills; unrealistic expectation for self, infant, partner; limited cognitive functioning; lack of knowledge about child development; inability to recognize and act on infant cues; low educational level or attainment; poor communication skills; lack of cognitive readiness for parenthood; preference for physical punishment. *Physiological:* Physical illness. *Infant or Child:* Premature birth; illness; prolonged separation from parent; not desired gender; attention deficit/hyperactivity disorder; difficult temperament; separation from parent at birth; lack of goodness of fit (temperament) with parental expectations; unplanned or unwanted child; handicapping condition or developmental delay; multiple births; altered perceptual abilities. *Psychological:* History of substance abuse or dependencies; disability; depression; difficult labor and/or delivery; young age, especially adolescent; history of mental illness; high number or closely spaced pregnancies; sleep deprivation or disruption; lack of, or late, prenatal care; separation from infant/child

Risk for **Spiritual** distress r/t altered relationships

P

## PARENTING, RISK FOR IMPAIRED

Chronic **Sorrow** r/t difficult parent-child relationship

Risk for impaired **Parenting** r/t *Social:* Marital conflict, declining satisfaction; history of being abused; poor problem-solving skills; role strain/overload; social isolation; legal difficulties; lack of access to resources; lack of value of parenthood; relocation; poverty; poor home environment; lack of family cohesiveness; lack of or poor parental role model; father of child not involved; history of being abusive; financial difficulties; low self-esteem; lack of resources; unplanned or unwanted pregnancy; inadequate child care arrangements; maladaptive coping strategies; low socioeconomic class; lack of transportation; change in family unit; unemployment or job problems; single parent; lack of social support network; inability to put child's needs before own; stress. *Knowledge:* Low educational level or attainment; unrealistic expectations of child; lack of knowledge about parenting skills; poor communication skills; preference for physical punishment; inability to recognize and act on infant cues functioning; lack of knowledge about child health maintenance; lack of knowledge about child development; lack of cognitive readiness for parenthood. *Physiological:* Physical illness. *Infant or Child:* Multiple births; handicapping condition or developmental delay; illness; altered perceptual abilities; lack of goodness of fit (temperament) with parental expectations; unplanned or unwanted child; premature birth; not gender desired; difficult temperament; attention deficit/hyperactivity disorder; prolonged separation from parent; separation from parent at birth. *Psycholog-*

*ical:* Separation from infant/child; high number or closely spaced children; disability; sleep deprivation or disruption; difficult labor and/or delivery; young age, especially adolescent; depression; history of mental illness; lack of, or late, prenatal care; history of substance abuse or dependence

Risk for **Spiritual** distress r/t altered relationships

## PARESTHESIA

Disturbed **Sensory** perception: tactile r/t altered sensory reception, transmission, integration

Risk for **Injury** r/t inability to feel temperature changes, pain

## PARKINSON'S DISEASE

Chronic **Sorrow** r/t loss of physical capacity

**Constipation** r/t weakness of defecation muscles, lack of exercise, inadequate fluid intake, decreased autonomic nervous system activity

Imbalanced **Nutrition**: less than body requirements r/t tremor, slowness in eating, difficulty in chewing and swallowing

Impaired verbal **Communication** r/t decreased speech volume, slowness of speech, impaired facial muscles

Risk for **Injury** r/t tremors, slow reactions, altered gait

*See Neurological Disorders*

## PAROXYSMAL NOCTURNAL DYSPNEA

*See PND (Paroxysmal Nocturnal Dyspnea)*

## PATENT DUCTUS ARTERIOSUS (PDA)

*See Congenital Heart Disease/Cardiac Anomalies*

## PATIENT-CONTROLLED ANALGESIA

*See PCA (Patient-Controlled Analgesia)*

## PATIENT EDUCATION

Deficient **Knowledge** r/t lack of exposure to information, information misinterpretation, unfamiliarity with information resources

Effective **Therapeutic** regimen management r/t verbalized desire to manage illness, prevent complications

**Health-seeking** behaviors r/t expressed or observed desire to seek a higher level of wellness, control of health practices

Readiness for enhanced **Knowledge** of (specify) r/t interest in learning, knowledge of the topic, behaviors congruent with expressed knowledge, previous experiences pertaining to the topic

Readiness for enhanced **Spiritual** well-being r/t desire to reach harmony with self, others, higher power/God

Readiness for enhanced **Therapeutic** regimen management r/t the following: expresses a desire to manage the treatment of illness and prevent sequelae, makes choices of daily living that are appropriate for meeting the goals of treatment or prevention, expresses little to no difficulty with regulation/integration of one or more prescribed regimens for treatment of illness or prevention of complications, describes reduction of risk factors for progression of illness and sequelae, shows no unexpected acceleration of illness symptoms

## PCA (PATIENT-CONTROLLED ANALGESIA)

Deficient **Knowledge** r/t self-care of pain control

Effective **Therapeutic** regimen management r/t ability to manage pain with appropriate use of PCA

Impaired **Comfort**: pruritus, nausea, vomiting r/t side effects of medication

Readiness for enhanced **Knowledge** of appropriate management of PCA

Risk for **Injury** r/t possible complications associated with PCA

## PEDICULOSIS

*See Lice*

## PELVIC INFLAMMATORY DISEASE

*See PID (Pelvic Inflammatory Disease)*

## PENILE PROSTHESIS

**Health-seeking** behaviors r/t information regarding use and care of prosthesis

Ineffective **Sexuality** pattern r/t use of penile prosthesis

Risk for **Infection** r/t invasive surgical procedure

Risk for situational low **Self-esteem** r/t ineffective Sexuality patterns

*See Impotence*

## PEPTIC ULCER

*See Ulcer, Peptic*

## PERCUTANEOUS TRANSLUMINAL CORONARY ANGIOPLASTY (PTCA)

*See Angioplasty, Coronary*

## PERICARDIAL FRICTION RUB

Acute **Pain** r/t inflammation, effusion

Decreased **Cardiac** output r/t inflammation in pericardial sac, fluid accumulation compressing heart

Delayed **Surgical** recovery r/t complications associated with cardiac problems

P

P

## PERICARDITIS

**Activity** intolerance r/t reduced cardiac reserve, prescribed bed rest

Acute **Pain** r/t biological injury, inflammation

Delayed **Surgical** recovery r/t complications associated with cardiac problems

Deficient **Knowledge** r/t unfamiliarity with information sources

Ineffective **Tissue** perfusion: cardiopulmonary/peripheral r/t risk for development of emboli

Risk for decreased **Cardiac** output r/t inflammation in pericardial sac, fluid accumulation compressing heart function

Risk for imbalanced **Nutrition**: less than body requirements r/t fever, hypermetabolic state associated with fever

## PERIOPERATIVE POSITIONING

Risk for perioperative positioning **Injury** r/t disorientation, edema, emaciation, immobilization, muscle weakness, obesity, sensory/perceptual disturbances resulting from anesthesia

## PERIPHERAL NEUROPATHY

*See Neuropathy, Peripheral*

## PERIPHERAL NEUROVASCULAR DYSFUNCTION

Risk for **Peripheral** neurovascular dysfunction r/t trauma, vascular obstruction; orthopedic surgery; fractures; burns; mechanical compression (e.g., tourniquet, cane, cast, brace, dressing, restraint); immobilization

*See Neuropathy, Peripheral; Peripheral Vascular Disease*

## PERIPHERAL VASCULAR DISEASE

**Activity** intolerance r/t imbalance between peripheral oxygen supply and demand

Chronic **Pain**: intermittent claudication r/t ischemia

Ineffective **Health** maintenance r/t deficient knowledge regarding self-care and treatment of disease

Ineffective **Tissue** perfusion: peripheral r/t interruption of vascular flow

Readiness for enhanced **Therapeutic** regimen management r/t self-care and treatment of disease

Risk for **Falls** r/t altered mobility

Risk for impaired **Skin** integrity r/t altered circulation or sensation

Risk for **Injury** r/t tissue hypoxia, altered mobility, altered sensation

Risk for **Peripheral** neurovascular dysfunction r/t possible vascular obstruction

*See Neuropathy, Peripheral; Peripheral Neurovascular Dysfunction*

## PERITONEAL DIALYSIS

Acute **Pain** r/t instillation of dialysate, temperature of dialysate

Chronic **Sorrow** r/t chronic disability

Deficient **Knowledge** r/t treatment procedure, self-care with peritoneal dialysis

Impaired **Home** maintenance r/t complex home treatment of client

Risk for **Fluid** Volume excess r/t retention of dialysate

Risk for ineffective **Breathing** pattern r/t pressure from dialysate

Risk for ineffective **Coping** r/t disability requiring change in lifestyle

Risk for **Infection**: peritoneal r/t invasive procedure, presence of catheter, dialysate

Risk for **Powerlessness** r/t chronic condition and care involved

*See Child with Chronic Condition; Hospitalized Child; Renal Failure; Renal Failure, Acute/Chronic—Child*

## PERITONITIS

Acute **Pain** r/t inflammation, stimulation of somatic nerves

**Constipation** r/t decreased oral intake, decrease of peristalsis

Deficient **Fluid** volume r/t retention of fluid in bowel with loss of circulating blood volume

Imbalanced **Nutrition**: less than body requirements r/t nausea, vomiting

Ineffective **Breathing** pattern r/t pain, increased abdominal pressure

**Nausea** r/t gastrointestinal irritation

## PERNICIOUS ANEMIA

**Diarrhea** r/t malabsorption of nutrients

Effective **Therapeutic** regimen management r/t follows treatment plan; lifelong replacement of vitamin $B_{12}$

**Fatigue** r/t imbalanced Nutrition; less than body requirements

Imbalanced **Nutrition**: less than body requirements r/t lack of appetite associated with nausea and altered oral mucous membrane

Impaired **Memory** r/t anemia; lack of adequate red blood cells

Impaired **Oral** mucous membranes r/t vitamin deficiency; inability to absorb vitamin $B_{12}$ associated with lack of intrinsic factor

**Nausea** r/t altered oral mucous membrane; sore tongue, bleeding gums

Risk for **Peripheral** neurovascular dysfunction r/t anemia

Risk for **Falls** r/t dizziness, lightheadedness

## PERSISTENT FETAL CIRCULATION

*See Congenital Heart Disease/Cardiac Anomalies*

## PERSONAL IDENTITY PROBLEMS

Disturbed personal **Identity** r/t situational crisis, psychological impairment, chronic illness, pain

## PERSONALITY DISORDER

Chronic low **Self-esteem** r/t inability to set and achieve goals

Compromised family **Coping** r/t inability of client to provide positive feedback to family, chronicity exhausting family

Decisional **Conflict** r/t low self-esteem, feelings that choices will always be wrong

Disturbed personal **Identity** r/t lack of consistent positive self-image

Impaired **Adjustment** r/t ambivalent behavior toward others, testing of others' loyalty

Impaired **Social** interaction r/t knowledge or skill deficit regarding ways to interact effectively with others, self-concept disturbances

Readiness for enhanced **Self-concept** r/t expressing willingness to enhance self-concept

Risk for **Loneliness** r/t inability to interact appropriately with others

Risk for **Self-mutilation** r/t disturbed interpersonal relationships, borderline personality disorders

Risk for situational low **Self-esteem** r/t history of learned helplessness

**Spiritual** distress r/t lack of identifiable values, lack of meaning to life

*See Antisocial Personality Disorder; Borderline Personality Disorder;*

P

*Obsessive-Compulsive Disorder; Paranoid Personality Disorder*

## PERTUSSIS (WHOOPING COUGH)

*See Respiratory Infections, Acute Childhood*

## PESTICIDE CONTAMINATION

**Effective Therapeutic** regimen management r/t verbalizes intent to reduce risk factors associated with environmental toxins; meticulous hand hygiene

**Health-seeking** behaviors r/t expression of concern about environmental conditions

Risk for disproportionate **Growth** r/t environmental contamination

## PETECHIAE

*See Clotting Disorder; Anticoagulant Therapy; DIC (Disseminated Intravascular Coagulation); Hemophilia*

## PETIT MAL SEIZURE

**Effective Therapeutic** regimen management r/t follows prescribed medication regimen

Readiness for enhanced **Therapeutic** regimen management r/t wears medical alert bracelet; limits hazardous activities such as driving, swimming, skiing, working at heights, operating equipment

*See Epilepsy*

## PHARYNGITIS

*See Sore Throat*

## PHENYLKETONURIA

*See PKU (Phenylketonuria)*

## PHEOCHROMOCYTOMA

**Anxiety** r/t symptoms from increased catecholamines—headache, palpitations, sweating, nervousness, nausea, vomiting, syncope

Disturbed **Sleep** pattern r/t high levels of catecholamines

Ineffective **Health** maintenance r/t deficient knowledge regarding treatment and self-care

**Nausea** r/t increased catecholamines

Risk for ineffective **Tissue** perfusion: cardiopulmonary and renal r/t episodes of hypertension

*See Surgery, Perioperative; Surgery, Postoperative; Surgery, Preoperative*

## PHLEBITIS

*See Thrombophlebitis*

## PHOBIA (SPECIFIC)

**Anxiety** r/t inability to control emotions when dreaded object or situation is encountered

**Fear** r/t presence or anticipation of specific object or situation

Ineffective **Coping** r/t transfer of fears from self to dreaded object situation

**Powerlessness** r/t anxiety about encountering unknown or known entity

Readiness for enhanced **Communication** r/t willingness to discuss situation

Risk for **Post-trauma** syndrome r/t exposure to dreaded object or situation

Risk for **Powerlessness** r/t inadequate coping patterns

Risk for situational low **Self-esteem** r/t decreased power/control over fears

*See Anxiety; Anxiety Disorder; Panic Disorder*

## PHOTOSENSITIVITY

Ineffective **Health** maintenance r/t deficient knowledge regarding medications inducing photosensitivity

Risk for impaired **Skin** integrity r/t exposure to sun

## PHYSICAL ABUSE

*See Abuse, Child; Abuse, Spouse, Parent, or Significant Other*

## PICA

**Anxiety** r/t stress from urge to eat nonnutritive substances

Imbalanced **Nutrition**: less than body requirements r/t eating nonnutritive substances

Impaired **Parenting** r/t lack of supervision, food deprivation

Risk for **Constipation** r/t presence of undigestible materials in gastrointestinal tract

Risk for **Infection** r/t ingestion of infectious agents via contaminated substances

Risk for **Poisoning** r/t ingestion of substances containing lead

## PID (PELVIC INFLAMMATORY DISEASE)

Acute **Pain** r/t biological injury; inflammation, edema, congestion of pelvic tissues

Ineffective **Health** maintenance r/t deficient knowledge regarding self-care, treatment of disease

Ineffective **Sexuality** patterns r/t medically imposed abstinence from sexual activities until acute infection subsides, change in reproductive potential

Risk for **Infection** r/t insufficient knowledge to avoid exposure to pathogens; proper hygiene, nutrition, other health habits

Risk for urge urinary **Incontinence** r/t inflammation, edema, congestion of pelvic tissues

*See Maturational Issues, Adolescent*

## PIH (PREGNANCY-INDUCED HYPERTENSION/ PREECLAMPSIA)

**Anxiety** r/t fear of the unknown, threat to self and infant, change in role functioning

Death **Anxiety** r/t seriousness of condition

Deficient **Diversional** activity r/t bed rest

Deficient **Knowledge** r/t lack of experience with situation

Excess **Fluid** volume r/t decreased renal function

Impaired **Home** maintenance r/t bed rest

Impaired **Parenting** r/t bed rest

Impaired physical **Mobility** r/t medically prescribed limitations

Impaired **Social** interaction r/t imposed bed rest

Ineffective **Role** performance r/t change in physical capacity to assume role of pregnant woman or resume other roles

Interrupted **Family** processes r/t situational crisis

**Powerlessness** r/t complication threatening pregnancy, medically prescribed limitations

Readiness for enhanced **Knowledge** r/t desire for information on managing condition

Risk for imbalanced **Fluid** volume r/t hypertension, altered renal function

Risk for **Injury**: fetal r/t decreased uteroplacental perfusion, seizures

Risk for **Injury**: maternal r/t vasospasm, high blood pressure

Situational low **Self-esteem** r/t loss of idealized pregnancy

P

## PILOERECTION

**Hypothermia** r/t exposure to cold environment

## PIMPLES

*See Acne*

## PINWORMS

Impaired **Comfort**: itching r/t worms and eggs in the anal area

Disturbed **Sleep** pattern r/t discomfort

Effective **Therapeutic** regimen management r/t adheres to guidelines for antiparasitic medication for infected person and members of household; check for pinworms with flashlight; check for eggs; place tape over anal area in the morning (tape is placed on slide and taken to health care provider to look for eggs)

Impaired **Home** maintenance r/t inadequate cleaning of bed linen and toilet seats

Readiness for enhanced **Therapeutic** regimen r/t proper hand washing; short clean fingernails; avoiding hand, mouth, nose contact with unwashed hands; appropriate cleaning of bed linen and toilet seats

## PITUITARY, CUSHING'S

*See Cushing's Syndrome*

## PKU (PHENYLKETONURIA)

Effective **Therapeutic** regimen management r/t testing of newborn for PKU and following prescribed dietary regimen if test is positive

Risk for delayed **Development** r/t not following strict dietary program; eating foods extremely low in phenylalanine; avoiding eggs, milk, any foods containing aspartame (Nutrasweet)

## PLACENTA ABRUPTIO

Acute **Pain**: abdominal/back r/t premature separation of placenta before delivery

Death **Anxiety** r/t threat of mortality associated with bleeding

**Fear** r/t threat to self and fetus

Ineffective **Health** maintenance r/t deficient knowledge regarding treatment and control of hypertension associated with placenta abruptio

Risk for deficient **Fluid** volume r/t maternal blood loss

Risk for **Powerlessness** r/t complications of pregnancy and unknown outcome

Risk for **Spiritual** distress r/t fear from unknown outcome of pregnancy

## PLACENTA PREVIA

Death **Anxiety** r/t threat of mortality associated with bleeding

Deficient **Diversional** activity r/t long-term hospitalization

Disturbed **Body** image r/t negative feelings about body and reproductive ability, feelings of helplessness

**Fear** r/t threat to self and fetus, unknown future

Impaired **Home** maintenance r/t maternal bed rest, hospitalization

Impaired physical **Mobility** r/t medical protocol, maternal bed rest

Ineffective **Coping** r/t threat to self and fetus

Ineffective **Role** performance r/t maternal bed rest, hospitalization

Ineffective **Tissue** perfusion: placental r/t dilation of cervix, loss of placental implantation site

Interrupted **Family** processes r/t maternal bed rest, hospitalization

Risk for **Constipation** r/t bed rest, pregnancy

Risk for deficient **Fluid** volume r/t maternal blood loss

Risk for imbalanced **Fluid** volume r/t maternal blood loss

Risk for impaired **Parenting** r/t maternal bed rest, hospitalization

Risk for **Injury**: fetal and maternal r/t threat to uteroplacental perfusion, hemorrhage

Risk for **Powerlessness** r/t complications of pregnancy and unknown outcome

Situational low **Self-esteem** r/t situational crisis

**Spiritual** distress r/t inability to participate in usual religious rituals, situational crisis

### PLEURAL EFFUSION

Acute **Pain** r/t inflammation, fluid accumulation

Excess **Fluid** volume r/t compromised regulatory mechanisms; heart, liver, or kidney failure

**Hyperthermia** r/t increased metabolic rate secondary to infection

Ineffective **Breathing** pattern r/t pain

### PLEURAL FRICTION RUB

Acute **Pain** r/t inflammation, fluid accumulation

Ineffective **Breathing** pattern r/t pain

*See cause of Pleural Friction Rub*

### PLEURAL TAP

*See Pleural Effusion*

### PLEURISY

Acute **Pain** r/t pressure on pleural nerve endings associated with fluid accumulation or inflammation

Ineffective **Breathing** pattern r/t pain

Risk for impaired **Gas** exchange r/t ventilation perfusion imbalance

Risk for impaired physical **Mobility** r/t activity intolerance, inability to "catch breath"

Risk for ineffective **Airway** clearance r/t increased secretions, ineffective cough because of pain

### PMS (PREMENSTRUAL TENSION SYNDROME)

Acute **Pain** r/t hormonal stimulation of gastrointestinal structures

Deficient **Knowledge** r/t methods to deal with and prevent syndrome

Excess **Fluid** volume r/t alterations of hormonal levels inducing fluid retention

**Fatigue** r/t hormonal changes

Readiness for enhanced **Communication** r/t willingness to express thoughts and feelings about PMS

Readiness for enhanced **Therapeutic** regimen management r/t desire for information to manage and prevent symptoms

Risk for **Powerlessness** r/t lack of knowledge and ability to deal with symptoms

### PND (PAROXYSMAL NOCTURNAL DYSPNEA)

**Anxiety** r/t inability to breathe during sleep

Decreased **Cardiac** output r/t failure of the left ventricle

Disturbed **Sleep** pattern r/t suffocating feeling from fluid in lungs on awakening from sleep

Ineffective **Breathing** pattern r/t increase in carbon dioxide levels, decrease in oxygen levels

Readiness for enhanced **Sleep** r/t expressing willingness to learn measures to enhance sleep

Risk for **Powerlessness** r/t inability to control nocturnal dyspnea

**Sleep** deprivation r/t inability to breathe during sleep

### PNEUMONIA

**Activity** intolerance r/t imbalance between oxygen supply and demand

Deficient **Knowledge** r/t risk factors

P

predisposing person to pneumonia, treatment

**Hyperthermia** r/t dehydration, increased metabolic rate, illness

Imbalanced **Nutrition**: less than body requirements r/t loss of appetite

Impaired **Gas** exchange r/t decreased functional lung tissue

Impaired **Oral** mucous membrane r/t dry mouth from mouth breathing, decreased fluid intake

Ineffective **Airway** clearance r/t inflammation and presence of secretions

Ineffective **Health** maintenance r/t deficient knowledge regarding self-care and treatment of disease

Risk for deficient **Fluid** volume r/t inadequate intake of fluids

*See Respiratory Infections, Acute Childhood*

## PNEUMOTHORAX

Acute **Pain** r/t recent injury, coughing, deep breathing

**Fear** r/t threat to own well-being, difficulty breathing

Impaired **Gas** exchange r/t ventilation-perfusion imbalance

Risk for **Injury** r/t possible complications associated with closed chest drainage system

## POISONING, RISK FOR

### EXTERNAL

Risk for **Poisoning** r/t unprotected contact with heavy metals or chemicals; medicine stored in unlocked cabinets accessible to children or confused people; presence of poisonous vegetation; presence of atmospheric pollutants; paint or lacquer used in poorly ventilated areas or without effective protection; flaking or peeling paint or plaster in presence of young children; chemical contamination of food and water; availability

of illicit drugs potentially contaminated by poisonous additives; large supplies of drugs in house, dangerous products placed or stored within the reach of children or confused persons

### INTERNAL

Risk for **Poisoning** r/t reduced vision, verbalization of occupational settings without adequate safeguards; reduced vision; lack of safety or drug education, lack of proper precaution; insufficient finances; cognitive or emotional difficulties

## POLYDIPSIA

Readiness for enhanced **Fluid** balance r/t no excessive thirst when diabetes is controlled

*See Diabetes Mellitus*

## POLYPHAGIA

Readiness for enhanced **Nutrition** r/t knowledge of appropriate diet for diabetes

*See Diabetes Mellitus*

## POLYURIA

Readiness for enhanced **Urinary** elimination r/t willingness to learn measures to enhance urinary elimination

*See Diabetes Mellitus*

## POSTOPERATIVE CARE

*See Surgery, Postoperative*

## POSTPARTUM BLUES

**Anxiety** r/t new responsibilities of parenting

Chronic **Sorrow** r/t loss of ideal postpartum experience or ideal parent-infant relationship

Deficient **Knowledge** r/t lifestyle changes

Disturbed **Body** image r/t normal postpartum recovery

Disturbed **Sleep** pattern r/t new responsibilities of parenting

**Fatigue** r/t childbirth, postpartum state

Impaired **Adjustment** r/t lack of support systems

Impaired **Home** maintenance r/t fatigue, care of newborn

Impaired **Parenting** r/t hormone-induced depression

Impaired **Social** interaction r/t change in role functioning

Ineffective **Coping** r/t hormonal changes, maturational crisis

Ineffective **Role** performance r/t new responsibilities of parenting

Risk for **Post-trauma** syndrome r/t trauma or violence associated with labor and birth process, medical/surgical interventions, history of sexual abuse

Risk for situational low **Self-esteem** r/t decreased power over feelings of sadness

Risk for **Spiritual** distress r/t altered relationships, social isolation

**Sexual** dysfunction r/t fear of another pregnancy, postpartum pain, lochia flow

## POSTPARTUM HEMORRHAGE

**Activity** intolerance r/t anemia from loss of blood

**Acute Pain** r/t nursing and medical interventions to control bleeding

Death **Anxiety** r/t threat of mortality associated with bleeding

Decreased **Cardiac** output r/t hypovolemia

Deficient **Fluid** volume r/t uterine atony, loss of blood

Deficient **Knowledge** r/t lack of exposure to situation

Disturbed **Body** image r/t loss of ideal childbirth

**Fear** r/t threat to self, unknown future

Impaired **Home** maintenance r/t lack of stamina

Ineffective **Tissue** perfusion r/t hypovolemia

Interrupted **Breastfeeding** r/t separation from infant for medical treatment

Risk for imbalanced **Fluid** volume r/t maternal blood loss

Risk for **Infection** r/t loss of blood, depressed immunity

Risk for impaired **Parenting** r/t weakened maternal condition

Risk for **Powerlessness** r/t acute illness

## POSTPARTUM, NORMAL CARE

Acute **Pain** r/t episiotomy, lacerations, bruising, breast engorgement, headache, sore nipples, epidural or intravenous (IV) site, hemorrhoids

**Anxiety** r/t change in role functioning, parenting

**Constipation** r/t hormonal effects on smooth muscles, fear of straining with defecation, effects of anesthesia

Deficient **Knowledge**: infant care r/t lack of preparation for parenting

Disturbed **Sleep** pattern r/t care of infant

Effective **Breastfeeding** r/t basic breastfeeding knowledge, support of partner and health care provider

**Fatigue** r/t childbirth, new responsibilities of parenting, body changes

**Health-seeking** behaviors r/t postpartum recovery and adaptation

Impaired **Skin** integrity r/t episiotomy, lacerations

Impaired **Urinary** elimination r/t effects of anesthesia, tissue trauma

Ineffective **Breastfeeding** r/t lack of knowledge, lack of support, lack of motivation

P

Ineffective **Role** performance r/t new responsibilities of parenting

Readiness for enhanced family **Coping** r/t adaptation to new family member

Readiness for enhanced **Parenting** r/t expressing willingness to enhance parenting skills

Risk for **Constipation** r/t hormonal effects on smooth muscles, fear of straining with defecation, effects of anesthesia

Risk for imbalanced **Fluid** volume r/t shift in blood volume, edema

Risk for impaired **Parenting** r/t lack of role models, deficient knowledge

Risk for **Infection** r/t tissue trauma, blood loss

Risk for **Post-trauma** syndrome r/t trauma or violence associated with labor and birth process, medical/surgical interventions, history of sexual abuse

Risk for urge urinary **Incontinence** r/t effects of anesthesia or tissue trauma

**Sexual** dysfunction r/t fear of pain or pregnancy

## P POST-TRAUMA SYNDROME

**Post-trauma** syndrome r/t events outside the range of the usual human experience; physical and psychosocial abuse; tragic occurrence involving multiple deaths; epidemics; sudden destruction of one's home or community; being held as a prisoner of war or enduring criminal victimization (torture), wars; rape; natural or produced disasters; serious accidents; assault; witnessing mutilation, violent death, other horrors; serious threat or injury to self or loved ones; industrial and motor vehicle accidents; military combat

## POST-TRAUMA SYNDROME, RISK FOR

Risk for **Post-trauma** syndrome r/t exaggerated sense of responsibility; perception of event; survivor's role in the event; occupation (e.g., police, fire, rescue, corrections, emergency room staff, mental health worker); displacement from home; inadequate social support, nonsupportive environment; diminished ego strength; duration of the event

## POST-TRAUMATIC STRESS DISORDER

**Anxiety** r/t exposure to internal or external cues that symbolize or resemble an aspect of the traumatic event

Death **Anxiety** r/t psychological stress associated with traumatic event

Disturbed **Energy** field r/t disharmony of mind, body, spirit

Disturbed **Sensory** perception r/t psychological stress

Disturbed **Sleep** pattern r/t recurring nightmares

Disturbed **Thought** processes r/t sense of reliving the experience (flashbacks)

Ineffective **Breathing** pattern r/t hyperventilation associated with anxiety

Ineffective **Coping** r/t extreme anxiety

**Post-trauma** syndrome r/t exposure to a traumatic event

Readiness for enhanced **Communication** r/t willingness to express feelings and thoughts

Readiness for enhanced **Spiritual** wellbeing r/t desire for harmony after stressful event

Risk for **Powerlessness** r/t flashbacks, reliving event

Risk for self- or other-directed **Violence** r/t fear of self or others

**Sleep** deprivation r/t nightmares associated with traumatic event

**Spiritual** distress r/t feelings of detachment or estrangement from others

## POTASSIUM, INCREASE/DECREASE

*See Hyperkalemia; Hypokalemia*

## POWERLESSNESS

**Powerlessness** r/t health care environment, illness-related regimen, interpersonal interaction, lifestyle of helplessness

Risk for **Powerlessness** r/t *Physiological:* Chronic or acute illness (hospitalization, intubation, ventilator, suctioning); acute injury or progressive debilitating disease process (e.g., spinal cord injury, multiple sclerosis); aging (decreased physical strength, decreased mobility); dying. *Psychological:* Lack of knowledge of illness or health care style, lifestyle of dependency with inadequate coping patterns, absence of integrality, decreased self-esteem, low or unstable body image

## PREECLAMPSIA

*See PIH (Pregnancy-Induced Hypertension/Preeclampsia)*

## PREGNANCY LOSS

Acute **Pain** r/t surgical intervention

**Anxiety** r/t threat to role functioning, health status, situational crisis

Chronic **Sorrow** r/t loss of a fetus or child

Compromised family **Coping** r/t lack of support by significant other because of personal suffering

Ineffective **Coping** r/t situational crisis

Ineffective **Role** performance r/t inability to assume parenting role

Ineffective **Sexuality** patterns r/t self-esteem disturbance resulting from

pregnancy loss and anxiety about future pregnancies

Readiness for enhanced **Communication** r/t willingness to express feelings and thoughts about loss

Readiness for enhanced **Spiritual** well-being r/t desire for acceptance of loss

Risk for deficient **Fluid** volume r/t blood loss

Risk for dysfunctional **Grieving** r/t loss of pregnancy

Risk for ineffective **Sexuality** patterns r/t self-esteem disturbance, anxiety, grief

Risk for **Infection** r/t retained products of conception

Risk for **Powerlessness** r/t situational crisis

Risk for **Spiritual** distress r/t intense suffering

**Spiritual** distress r/t intense suffering

## PREGNANCY, CARDIAC DISORDERS

*See Cardiac Disorders in Pregnancy*

## PREGNANCY, NORMAL

P

Deficient **Knowledge** r/t primiparity

Disturbed **Body** image r/t altered body function and appearance

Disturbed **Sleep** pattern r/t sleep deprivation secondary to uncomfortable pregnancy state

**Fear** r/t labor and delivery

**Health-seeking** behaviors r/t desire to promote optimal fetal and maternal health

Imbalanced **Nutrition**: less than body requirements r/t growing fetus, nausea

Imbalanced **Nutrition**: more than body requirements r/t deficient knowledge regarding nutritional needs of pregnancy

Ineffective **Coping** r/t personal vulnerability, situational crisis

Interrupted **Family** processes r/t developmental transition of pregnancy

**Nausea** r/t hormonal changes of pregnancy

Readiness for enhanced family **Coping** r/t satisfying partner relationship, attention to gratification of needs, effective adaptation to developmental tasks of pregnancy

Readiness for enhanced **Parenting** r/t expressing willingness to enhance parenting skills

**Sexual** dysfunction r/t altered body function, self-concept, body image with pregnancy

*See Discomforts of Pregnancy*

## PREGNANCY-INDUCED HYPERTENSION/ PREECLAMPSIA

*See PIH (Pregnancy Induced Hypertension/Preeclampsia)*

## PREMATURE DILATION OF THE CERVIX (INCOMPETENT CERVIX)

Anticipatory **Grieving** r/t potential loss of infant

Deficient **Diversional** activity r/t bed rest

Deficient **Knowledge** r/t treatment regimen, prognosis for pregnancy

**Fear** r/t potential loss of infant

Ineffective **Coping** r/t bed rest, threat to fetus

Ineffective **Role** performance r/t inability to continue usual patterns of responsibility

Impaired physical **Mobility** r/t imposed bed rest to prevent preterm birth

Impaired **Social** interaction r/t bed rest

**Powerlessness** r/t inability to control outcome of pregnancy

Risk for **Infection** r/t invasive procedures to prevent preterm birth

Risk for **Injury**: fetal r/t preterm birth, use of anesthetics

Risk for **Injury**: maternal r/t surgical procedures to prevent preterm birth (e.g., cerclage)

Risk for **Spiritual** distress r/t physical/ psychological stress

**Sexual** dysfunction r/t fear of harm to fetus

Situational low **Self-esteem** r/t inability to complete normal pregnancy

## PREMATURE INFANT, CHILD

Delayed **Growth** and development: developmental lag r/t prematurity, environmental and stimulation deficiencies, multiple caretakers

Disorganized **Infant** behavior r/t prematurity

Disturbed **Sensory** perception r/t noxious stimuli, noisy environment

Disturbed **Sleep** pattern r/t noisy and noxious intensive care environment

Imbalanced **Nutrition**: less than body requirements r/t delayed or understimulated rooting reflex, easy fatigue during feeding, diminished endurance

Impaired **Gas** exchange r/t effects of cardiopulmonary insufficiency

Impaired **Swallowing** r/t decreased or absent gag reflex, fatigue

Ineffective **Thermoregulation** r/t large body surface/weight ratio, immaturity of thermal regulation, state of prematurity

Readiness for enhanced organized **Infant** behavior r/t prematurity

Risk for delayed **Development** r/t prematurity

Risk for disproportionate **Growth** r/t prematurity

Risk for **Infection** r/t inadequate, immature, or undeveloped acquired immune response

Risk for **Injury** r/t prolonged mechanical ventilation, retinopathy of prematurely (ROP) secondary to 100% oxygen environment

## PREMATURE INFANT (PARENT)

Anticipatory **Grieving** r/t loss of perfect child possibly leading to dysfunctional grieving

Chronic **Sorrow** r/t threat of loss of a child, prolonged hospitalization

Compromised family **Coping** r/t disrupted family roles and disorganization, prolonged condition exhausting supportive capacity of significant persons

Decisional **Conflict** r/t support system deficit, multiple sources of information

Dysfunctional **Grieving** (prolonged) r/t unresolved conflicts

Ineffective **Breastfeeding** r/t disrupted establishment of effective pattern secondary to prematurity or insufficient opportunities

Parental role **Conflict** r/t expressed concerns, expressed inability to care for child's physical, emotional, or developmental needs

Readiness for enhanced **Family** process r/t adaptation to change associated with premature infant

Risk for impaired parent/infant/child **Attachment** r/t separation, physical barriers, lack of privacy

Risk for **Powerlessness** r/t inability to control situation

Risk for **Spiritual** distress r/t challenged belief or value systems regarding moral or ethical implications of treatment plans

**Spiritual** distress r/t challenged belief or value systems regarding moral or ethical implications of treatment plans

*See Child with Chronic Condition; Hospitalized Child*

## PREMATURE RUPTURE OF MEMBRANES

Anticipatory **Grieving** r/t potential loss of infant

**Anxiety** r/t threat to infant's health status

Disturbed **Body** image r/t inability to carry pregnancy to term

Ineffective **Coping** r/t situational crisis

Risk for **Infection** r/t rupture of membranes

Risk for **Injury**: fetal r/t risk of premature birth

Situational low **Self-esteem** r/t inability to carry pregnancy to term

## PREMENSTRUAL TENSION SYNDROME

*See PMS (Premenstrual Tension Syndrome)*

## PRENATAL CARE, NORMAL

**Anxiety** r/t unknown future, threat to self secondary to pain of labor

**Constipation** r/t decreased gastrointestinal motility secondary to hormonal stimulation

Deficient **Knowledge** r/t lack of experience with pregnancy and care

Disturbed **Sleep** pattern r/t discomforts of pregnancy and fetal activity

**Fatigue** r/t increased energy demands

**Health-seeking** behaviors r/t consistent prenatal care and education

Imbalanced **Nutrition**: less than body requirements r/t nausea from normal hormonal changes

Impaired **Urinary** elimination r/t frequency caused by increased pelvic pressure and hormonal stimulation

P

Ineffective **Breathing** pattern r/t increased intrathoracic pressure and decreased energy secondary to enlarged uterus

Interrupted **Family** processes r/t developmental transition

Readiness for enhanced **Knowledge** of appropriate prenatal care

Readiness for enhanced **Nutrition** r/t desire for knowledge of appropriate nutrition during pregnancy

Readiness for enhanced **Parenting** r/t realistic expectations of new role as parent

Readiness for enhanced **Spiritual** well-being r/t oncoming new role as parent

Risk for **Activity** intolerance r/t enlarged abdomen, increased cardiac workload

Risk for **Constipation** r/t decreased gastrointestinal motility secondary to hormonal stimulation

Risk for **Injury**: maternal r/t change in balance and center of gravity secondary to enlarged abdomen

Risk for **Sexual** dysfunction r/t enlarged abdomen, fear of harm to infant

## PRENATAL TESTING

Acute **Pain** r/t invasive procedures

**Anxiety** r/t unknown outcome, delayed test results

**Health-seeking** behaviors r/t desire to have information regarding prenatal testing

Risk for **Infection** r/t invasive procedures during amniocentesis or chorionic villi sampling

Risk for **Injury**: fetal r/t invasive procedures

## PREOPERATIVE TEACHING

**Health-seeking** behaviors r/t preoperative regimens, postoperative precautions, expectations of role of client during preoperative or postoperative time

*See Surgery, Preoperative Care*

## PRESSURE ULCER

Acute **Pain** r/t tissue destruction, exposure of nerves

Imbalanced **Nutrition**: less than body requirements r/t limited access to food, inability to absorb nutrients because of biological factors, anorexia

Impaired bed **Mobility** r/t intolerance to activity, pain, cognitive impairment, depression, severe anxiety

Impaired **Skin** integrity: stage I or II pressure ulcer r/t physical immobility, mechanical factors, altered circulation, skin irritants

Impaired **Tissue** integrity: stage III or IV pressure ulcer r/t altered circulation, impaired physical mobility

Risk for **Infection** r/t physical immobility, mechanical factors (shearing forces, pressure, restraint, altered circulation, skin irritants)

Total urinary **Incontinence** r/t neurological dysfunction

## PRETERM LABOR

Anticipatory **Grieving** r/t loss of idealized pregnancy, potential loss of fetus

**Anxiety** r/t threat to fetus, change in role functioning, change in environment and interaction patterns, use of tocolytic drugs

Deficient **Diversional** activity r/t long-term hospitalization

Disturbed **Sleep** pattern r/t change in usual pattern secondary to contractions, hospitalization, treatment regimen

Impaired **Home** maintenance r/t medical restrictions

Impaired physical **Mobility** r/t medically imposed restrictions

Impaired **Social** interaction r/t prolonged bed rest or hospitalization

Ineffective **Coping** r/t situational crisis, preterm labor

Ineffective **Role** performance r/t inability to carry out normal roles secondary to bedrest or hospitalization, change in expected course of pregnancy

Readiness for enhanced **Communication** r/t willingness to discuss thoughts and feelings about situation

Risk for **Injury**: fetal r/t premature birth, immature body systems

Risk for **Injury**: maternal r/t use of tocolytic drugs

Risk for **Powerlessness** r/t lack of control over preterm labor

**Sexual** dysfunction r/t actual or perceived limitation imposed by preterm labor and/or prescribed treatment, separation from partner because of hospitalization

Situational low **Self-esteem** r/t threatened ability to carry pregnancy to term

## PROBLEM-SOLVING ABILITY

Defensive **Coping** r/t situational crisis

Impaired **Adjustment** r/t altered locus of control

Ineffective **Coping** r/t situational crisis

Readiness for enhanced **Communication** r/t willingness to share ideas with others

Readiness for enhanced **Spiritual** well-being r/t desire to draw on inner strength and find meaning and purpose to life

## PROJECTION

**Anxiety** r/t threat to self-concept

Chronic low **Self-esteem** r/t failure

Defensive **Coping** r/t inability to acknowledge that own behavior may be a problem, blaming others

Impaired **Social** interaction r/t self-concept disturbance, confrontational communication style

Risk for **Loneliness** r/t blaming others for problems

Risk for **Post-trauma** syndrome r/t diminished ego strength

## PROLAPSED UMBILICAL CORD

**Fear** r/t threat to fetus, impending surgery

Ineffective **Tissue** perfusion: fetal r/t interruption in umbilical blood flow

Risk for **Injury**: fetal r/t cord compression, ineffective tissue perfusion

Risk for **Injury**: maternal r/t emergency surgery

## PROLONGED GESTATION

**Anxiety** r/t potential change in birthing plans, need for increased medical intervention, unknown outcome for fetus

Defensive **Coping** r/t underlying feeling of inadequacy regarding ability to give birth normally

Imbalanced **Nutrition**: less than body requirements (fetal) r/t aging of placenta

**Powerlessness** r/t perceived lack of control over outcome of pregnancy

Situational low **Self-esteem** r/t perceived inadequacy of body functioning

## PROSTATECTOMY

*See TURP (Transurethral Resection of the Prostate)*

## PROSTATIC HYPERTROPHY

Disturbed **Sleep** pattern r/t nocturia

Ineffective **Health** maintenance r/t deficient knowledge regarding self-care and prevention of complications

Risk for **Infection** r/t urinary residual

P

after voiding, bacterial invasion of bladder

Risk for urge urinary **Incontinence** r/t small bladder capacity

**Urinary** retention r/t obstruction

*See BPH (Benign Prostatic Hypertrophy)*

## PROSTATITIS

Ineffective **Health** maintenance r/t deficient knowledge regarding treatment

Ineffective **Protection** r/t depressed immune system

Risk for urge **Incontinence** r/t irritation of bladder

## PROTECTION, ALTERED

Ineffective **Protection** r/t abnormal blood profiles (e.g., leukopenia, thrombocytopenia, anemia, coagulation), inadequate nutrition, extremes of age; drug therapies (e.g., antineoplastic, corticosteroid, immune, anticoagulant, thrombolytic); alcohol abuse; treatments (e.g., surgery, radiation); diseases such as cancer, immune disorders

## PRURITUS

Deficient **Knowledge** r/t methods to treat and prevent itching

Impaired **Comfort**: pruritus r/t inflammation in tissues

Risk for impaired **Skin** integrity r/t scratching from pruritus

## PSORIASIS

Disturbed **Body** image r/t lesions on body

Impaired **Skin** integrity r/t lesions on body

Ineffective **Health** maintenance r/t deficient knowledge regarding treatment modalities

**Powerlessness** r/t lack of control over

condition with frequent exacerbations and remissions

## PSYCHOSIS

**Anxiety** r/t unconscious conflict with reality

Chronic **Sorrow** r/t chronic mental illness

Disturbed **Sleep** pattern r/t sensory alterations contributing to fear and anxiety

Disturbed **Thought** processes r/t inaccurate interpretations of environment

**Fear** r/t altered contact with reality

Imbalanced **Nutrition**: less than body requirements r/t lack of awareness of hunger, disinterest toward food

Impaired **Home** maintenance r/t impaired cognitive or emotional functioning, inadequate support systems

Impaired **Social** interaction r/t impaired communication patterns, self-concept disturbance, disturbed thought processes

Impaired verbal **Communication** r/t psychosis, inaccurate perceptions, hallucinations, delusions

Ineffective **Coping** r/t inadequate support systems, unrealistic perceptions, disturbed thought processes, impaired communication

Ineffective **Health** maintenance r/t cognitive impairment, ineffective individual and family coping

Interrupted **Family** processes r/t inability to express feelings, impaired communication

Risk for **Post-trauma** syndrome r/t diminished ego strength

Risk for self- or other-directed **Violence** r/t lack of trust, panic, hallucinations, delusional thinking

Risk for **Suicide** r/t psychiatric illness/disorder

**Self-care** deficit r/t loss of contact with reality, impairment of perception

**Self-esteem** disturbance r/t excessive use of defense mechanisms (e.g., projection, denial, rationalization)

**Social** isolation r/t lack of trust, regression, delusional thinking, repressed fears

*See Schizophrenia*

## PTCA (PERCUTANEOUS TRANSLUMINAL CORONARY ANGIOPLASTY)

*See Angioplasty, Coronary*

## PULMONARY EDEMA

**Anxiety** r/t fear of suffocation

Impaired **Gas** exchange r/t extravasation of extravascular fluid in lung tissues and alveoli

Ineffective **Breathing** pattern r/t presence of tracheobronchial secretions

Ineffective **Health** maintenance r/t deficient knowledge regarding treatment regimen

**Sleep** deprivation r/t inability to breathe

*See CHF (Congestive Heart Failure)*

## PULMONARY EMBOLISM

Acute **Pain** r/t biological injury, lack of oxygen to cells

Deficient **Knowledge** r/t activities to prevent embolism, self-care after diagnosis of embolism

Delayed **Surgical** recovery r/t complications associated with respiratory difficulty

**Fear** r/t severe pain, possible death

Impaired **Gas** exchange r/t altered blood flow to alveoli secondary to lodged embolus

Ineffective **Tissue** perfusion: pulmonary r/t interruption of pulmonary blood flow secondary to lodged embolus

Risk for decreased **Cardiac** output r/t right ventricular failure secondary to obstructed pulmonary artery

*See Anticoagulant Therapy*

## PULMONARY STENOSIS

*See Congenital Heart Disease/ Cardiac Anomalies*

## PULSE DEFICIT

Decreased **Cardiac** output r/t dysrhythmia

*See Dysrhythmia*

## PULSE OXIMETRY

Readiness for enhanced **Knowledge** r/t treatment regimen

*See Hypoxia*

## PULSE PRESSURE, INCREASED

*See Intracranial Pressure, Increased*

## PULSE PRESSURE, NARROWED

*See Shock*

## PULSES, ABSENT OR DIMINISHED PERIPHERAL

Ineffective **Tissue** perfusion: peripheral r/t interruption of arterial flow

Risk for **Peripheral** neurovascular dysfunction r/t fractures, mechanical compression, orthopedic surgery trauma, immobilization, burns, vascular obstruction

*See cause of Absent or Diminished Peripheral Pulses*

## PURPURA

*See Clotting Disorder*

## PYELONEPHRITIS

Acute **Pain** r/t inflammation and irritation of urinary tract

Disturbed **Sleep** pattern r/t urinary frequency

Impaired **Comfort** r/t chills and fever

P

Impaired **Urinary** elimination r/t irritation of urinary tract

Ineffective **Health** maintenance r/t deficient knowledge regarding self-care, treatment of disease, prevention of further urinary tract infections

Risk for urge urinary **Incontinence** r/t irritation of urinary tract

## PYLORIC STENOSIS

Acute **Pain** r/t surgical incision

Deficient **Fluid** volume r/t vomiting, dehydration

Imbalanced **Nutrition**: less than body requirements r/t vomiting secondary to pyloric sphincter obstruction

Ineffective **Health** maintenance r/t parental deficient knowledge regarding home care feeding regimen, wound care

*See Hospitalized Child*

# Q

## QUADRIPLEGIA

Disturbed **Energy** field r/t illness, grieving of loss of normal function

**Grieving** r/t loss of normal lifestyle, severity of disability

Impaired **Transfer** ability r/t quadriplegia

Impaired wheelchair **Mobility** r/t quadriplegia

Ineffective **Breathing** pattern r/t inability to use intercostal muscles

Readiness for enhanced **Spiritual** well being r/t heightened coping associated with disability

Risk for **Autonomic** dysreflexia r/t bladder distention, bowel distention, skin irritation, lack of client and caregiver knowledge

Risk for impaired **Religiosity** r/t immobility and possible lack of transportation

*See Spinal Cord Injury*

# R

## RA

*See Rheumatoid Arthritis*

## RABIES

Acute **Pain** r/t multiple immunization injections

**Health**-seeking behaviors r/t prophylactic immunization of domestic animals, avoidance of contact with wild animals

**Hopelessness** r/t poor prognosis

Ineffective **Health** maintenance r/t deficient knowledge regarding care of wound, isolation, and observation of infected animal

## RADIAL NERVE DYSFUNCTION

Acute **Pain** r/t trauma to hand/arm

*See Neuropathy, Peripheral*

## RADIATION THERAPY

**Activity** intolerance r/t fatigue from possible anemia

Deficient **Knowledge** r/t what to expect with radiation therapy

**Diarrhea** r/t irradiation effects

Disturbed **Body** image r/t change in appearance, hair loss

Imbalanced **Nutrition**: less than body requirements r/t anorexia, nausea, vomiting, irradiation of areas of pharynx and esophagus

Impaired **Oral** mucous membrane r/t irradiation effects

Ineffective **Protection** r/t suppression of bone marrow

**Nausea** r/t side effects of radiation

Risk for impaired **Skin** integrity r/t irradiation effects

Risk for **Powerlessness** r/t medical treatment and possible side effects

Risk for **Spiritual** distress r/t radiation treatment, prognosis

## RADICAL NECK DISSECTION

*See Laryngectomy*

## RAGE

Risk for other-directed **Violence** r/t panic state, manic excitement, organic brain syndrome

Risk for **Self-mutilation** r/t command hallucinations

Risk for **Suicide** r/t desire to kill oneself

## RAPE-TRAUMA SYNDROME

Chronic **Sorrow** r/t forced loss of virginity

**Rape-trauma** syndrome r/t forced, violent sexual penetration against victim's will and consent

**Rape-trauma** syndrome: compound reaction r/t forced and violent sexual penetration against victim's will and consent, activation of previous health disruptions (e.g., physical illness, psychiatric illness, substance abuse)

**Rape-trauma** syndrome: silent reaction r/t forced and violent sexual penetration against victim's will and consent, demonstration of repression of incident

Risk for **Post-trauma** syndrome r/t trauma or violence associated with rape

Risk for **Powerlessness** r/t inability to control thoughts about incident

Risk for **Spiritual** distress r/t forced loss of virginity

## RASH

Impaired **Comfort**: pruritus r/t inflammation in skin

Impaired **Skin** integrity r/t mechanical trauma

Risk for **Infection** r/t traumatized tissue, broken skin

Risk for latex **Allergy** r/t multiple surgical procedures, allergies to products associated with latex allergy, professions with daily associations with latex, history of reactions to latex

## RATIONALIZATION

Defensive **Coping** r/t situational crisis, inability to accept blame for consequences of own behavior

Ineffective **Denial** r/t fear of consequences, actual or perceived loss

Readiness for enhanced **Communication** r/t expressing desire to share thoughts and feelings

Readiness for enhanced **Spiritual** well-being r/t possibility of seeking harmony with self, others, higher power/God

Risk for **Post-trauma** syndrome r/t survivor's role in event

## RATS, RODENTS IN THE HOME

Impaired **Home** maintenance r/t lack of knowledge, insufficient finances

*See Filthy Home Environment*

## RAYNAUD'S DISEASE

Deficient **Knowledge** r/t lack of information about disease process, possible complications, self-care needs regarding disease process and medication

Ineffective **Tissue** perfusion: peripheral r/t transient reduction of blood flow

## RDS (RESPIRATORY DISTRESS SYNDROME)

*See Respiratory Conditions of the Neonate*

R

## RECTAL FULLNESS

**Constipation** r/t decreased activity level, decreased fluid intake, inadequate fiber in diet, decreased peristalsis, side effects from antidepressant or antipsychotic therapy

Risk for **Constipation** r/t habitual denial/ignoring of urge to defecate

## RECTAL PAIN/BLEEDING

Acute **Pain** r/t pressure of defecation

**Constipation** r/t pain on defecation

Deficient **Knowledge** r/t possible causes of rectal bleeding, pain, treatment modalities

Risk for deficient **Fluid** volume: bleeding r/t untreated rectal bleeding

## RECTAL LUMP

*See Hemorrhoids*

## RECTAL SURGERY

*See Hemorrhoidectomy*

## RECTOCELE REPAIR

Acute **Pain** r/t surgical procedure

**Constipation** r/t painful defecation

Ineffective **Health** maintenance r/t deficient knowledge of postoperative care of surgical site, dietary measures, exercise to prevent constipation

Risk for **Infection** r/t surgical procedure, possible contamination of site with feces

Risk for urge urinary **Incontinence** r/t edema from surgery

**Urinary** retention r/t edema from surgery

## REFLEX INCONTINENCE

Reflex **Incontinence** r/t neurological impairment

## REGRESSION

**Anxiety** r/t threat to or change in health status

Defensive **Coping** r/t denial of obvious problems, weaknesses

Ineffective **Role** performance r/t powerlessness over health status

**Powerlessness** r/t health care environment

*See Hospitalized Child; Separation Anxiety*

## REGRETFUL

**Anxiety** r/t situational or maturational crises

Death **Anxiety** r/t feelings of not having accomplished goals in life

Risk for **Spiritual** distress r/t inability to forgive

## REHABILITATION

Impaired **Comfort** r/t difficulty in performing rehabilitation tasks

Impaired physical **Mobility** r/t injury, surgery, psychosocial condition warranting rehabilitation

Ineffective **Coping** r/t loss of normal function

Readiness for enhanced **Self-concept** r/t accepts strengths and limitations

Readiness for enhanced **Therapeutic** regimen management r/t expression of desire to manage rehabilitation

**Self-care** deficit r/t impaired physical mobility

## RELAXATION TECHNIQUES

**Anxiety** r/t disturbed energy field

**Health-seeking** behaviors r/t requesting information about ways to relieve stress

Readiness for enhanced **Religiosity** r/t requests religious materials and/or experiences

Readiness for enhanced **Self-concept** r/t willingness to enhance self-concept

Readiness for enhanced **Spiritual**

well-being r/t seeking comfort from higher power

## RELIGIOSITY

Impaired **Religiosity** r/t *Physical*: Sickness/illness, pain. *Psychological*: Ineffective support/coping, personal disaster/crisis, lack of security, anxiety, fear of death, ineffective coping with disease, use of religion to manipulate. *Sociocultural*: Barriers to practicing religion (cultural and environmental), lack of social integration, lack of social/cultural interaction. *Spiritual*: Spiritual crises, suffering. *Developmental and Situational*: End-stage life crises, life transitions, aging

Readiness for enhanced **Religiosity** r/t expresses desire to strengthen religious belief patterns and customs that had provided comfort/religion in the past; request for assistance to increase participation in prescribed religious beliefs through: religious ceremonies, dietary regulations/rituals, clothing, prayer, worship/religious services, private religious behaviors/reading religious materials/media, holiday observances; requests assistance expanding religious options; requests meeting with religious leaders/facilitators; requests forgiveness, reconciliation; requests religious material and/or experiences; questions or rejects belief patterns and customs that are harmful

Risk for impaired **Religiosity** r/t *Physical*: Illness/hospitalization, pain. *Psychological*: Ineffective support/coping/caregiving, depression; lack of security. *Sociocultural*: Lack of social interaction, cultural barrier to practicing religion, social isolation. *Spiritual*: Suffering. *Environmental*: Lack of transportation, environmental barriers to practicing religion. *Developmental*: Life transitions

## RELIGIOUS CONCERNS

Readiness for enhanced **Spiritual** well-being r/t desire for increased spirituality

Risk for impaired **Religiosity** r/t ineffective support/coping/caregiving

Risk for **Spiritual** distress r/t physical or psychological stress

**Spiritual** distress r/t separation from religious or cultural ties

## RELOCATION STRESS SYNDROME

**Relocation** stress syndrome r/t unpredictability of experience; isolation from family/friends; past, concurrent, recent losses; feeling of powerlessness; lack of adequate support system; lack of predeparture counseling; passive coping; impaired psychosocial health; language barrier; decreased health status

## RENAL FAILURE

**Activity** intolerance r/t effects of anemia, CHF

Chronic **Sorrow** r/t chronic illness

Death **Anxiety** r/t unknown outcome of disease

Decreased **Cardiac** output r/t effects of congestive heart failure, elevated potassium levels interfering with conduction system

Excess **Fluid** volume r/t decreased urine output, sodium retention, inappropriate fluid intake

Fatigue r/t effects of chronic uremia and anemia

Imbalanced **Nutrition**: less than body requirements r/t anorexia, nausea, vomiting, altered taste sensation, dietary restrictions

Impaired **Comfort**: pruritus r/t effects of uremia

Impaired **Oral** mucous membrane r/t ir-

R

ritation from nitrogenous waste products

Impaired **Urinary** elimination r/t effects of disease, need for dialysis

Ineffective **Coping** r/t depression secondary to chronic disease

Risk for impaired **Oral** mucous membrane r/t dehydration, effects of uremia

Risk for **Infection** r/t altered immune functioning

Risk for **Injury** r/t bone changes, neuropathy, muscle weakness

Risk for **Noncompliance** r/t complex medical therapy

Risk for **Powerlessness** r/t chronic illness

**Spiritual** distress r/t dealing with chronic illness

### RENAL FAILURE, ACUTE/CHRONIC, CHILD

Deficient **Diversional** activity r/t immobility during dialysis

Disturbed **Body** image r/t growth retardation, bone changes, visibility of dialysis access devices (shunt, fistula), edema

*See Child with Chronic Condition; Hospitalized Child; Renal Failure*

### RENAL FAILURE, NONOLIGURIC

**Anxiety** r/t change in health status

Risk for deficient **Fluid** volume r/t loss of large volumes of urine

*See Renal Failure*

### RENAL TRANSPLANTATION, DONOR

Decisional **Conflict** r/t harvesting of kidney from traumatized donor

Readiness for enhanced **Communication** r/t expressing thoughts and feelings about situation

Readiness for enhanced family **Coping** r/t decision to allow organ donation

Readiness for enhanced **Spirituality** r/t inner peace resulting from allowance of organ donation

**Spiritual** distress r/t anticipatory grieving from loss of significant person

*See Nephrectomy*

### RENAL TRANSPLANTATION, RECIPIENT

**Anxiety** r/t possible rejection, procedure

Deficient **Knowledge** r/t specific nutritional needs, possible paralytic ileus, fluid or sodium restrictions

Impaired **Health** maintenance r/t long-term home treatment after transplantation, diet, signs of rejection, use of medications

Impaired **Urinary** elimination r/t possible impaired renal function

Ineffective **Protection** r/t immunosuppression therapy

Readiness for enhanced **Spiritual** well-being r/t acceptance of situation

Risk for **Infection** r/t use of immunosuppressive therapy to control rejection

Risk for **Spiritual** distress r/t obtaining transplanted kidney from someone's traumatic loss

### RESPIRATORY ACIDOSIS

*See Acidosis, Respiratory*

### RESPIRATORY CONDITIONS OF THE NEONATE (RESPIRATORY DISTRESS SYNDROME [RDS], MECONIUM ASPIRATION, DIAPHRAGMATIC HERNIA)

**Fatigue** r/t increased energy requirements and metabolic demands

Impaired **Gas** exchange r/t decreased surfactant, immature lung tissue

Ineffective **Airway** clearance r/t sequelae of attempts to breathe in utero resulting in meconium aspiration

Ineffective **Breathing** pattern r/t prolonged ventilator dependence

Risk for **Infection** r/t tissue destruction or irritation secondary to aspiration of meconium fluid

*See Bronchopulmonary Dysplasia; Hospitalized Child; Premature Infant, Child*

## RESPIRATORY DISTRESS

*See Dyspnea*

## RESPIRATORY DISTRESS SYNDROME (RDS)

*See Respiratory Conditions of the Neonate*

## RESPIRATORY INFECTIONS, ACUTE CHILDHOOD (CROUP, EPIGLOTTITIS, PERTUSSIS, PNEUMONIA, RESPIRATORY SYNCYTIAL VIRUS)

**Activity** intolerance r/t generalized weakness, dyspnea, fatigue, poor oxygenation

**Anxiety**/fear r/t oxygen deprivation, difficulty breathing

Deficient **Fluid** volume r/t insensible losses (fever, diaphoresis), inadequate oral fluid intake

**Hyperthermia** r/t infectious process

Imbalanced **Nutrition**: less than body requirements r/t anorexia, fatigue, generalized weakness, poor sucking and breathing coordination, dyspnea

Impaired **Gas** exchange r/t insufficient oxygenation secondary to inflammation or edema of epiglottis, larynx, bronchial passages

Ineffective **Airway** clearance r/t excess tracheobronchial secretions

Ineffective **Breathing** pattern r/t inflamed bronchial passages, coughing

Risk for **Aspiration** r/t inability to coordinate breathing, coughing, sucking

Risk for **Infection**: transmission to others r/t virulent infectious organisms

Risk for **Injury** (to pregnant others) r/t exposure to aerosolized medications (e.g., ribavirin, pentamidine), resultant potential fetal toxicity

Risk for **Suffocation** r/t inflammation of larynx, epiglottis

*See Hospitalized Child*

## RESPIRATORY SYNCYTIAL VIRUS

*See Respiratory Infections, Acute Childhood*

## RESTLESS LEG SYNDROME

Disturbed **Sleep** pattern r/t leg discomfort during sleep relieved by frequent leg movement

**Sleep** deprivation r/t frequent leg movements

*See Stress*

## RETARDED GROWTH AND DEVELOPMENT

*See Growth and Development Lag*

## RETCHING

Imbalanced **Nutrition**: less than body requirements r/t inability to ingest food

**Nausea** r/t chemotherapy, postsurgical anesthesia, irritation to gastrointestinal system, stimulation of neuropharmacological mechanisms

## RETINAL DETACHMENT

**Anxiety** r/t change in vision, threat of loss of vision

Deficient **Knowledge** r/t symptoms, need for early intervention to prevent permanent damage

Disturbed **Sensory** perception: visual r/t changes in vision, sudden flashes of light, floating spots, blurring of vision

Risk for impaired **Home** mainte-

R

nance r/t postoperative care, activity limitations, care of affected eye

*See Vision Impairment*

## RETINOPATHY, DIABETIC

*See Diabetic Retinopathy*

## RETINOPATHY OF PREMATURITY (ROP)

Effective **Therapeutic** regimen management r/t at least two eye examinations, by a qualified ophthalmologist, for very low birth weight or premature babies (less than 28 weeks gestational age), as well as other premature or low birth weight babies who have unstable conditions; follow-up exams at appropriate times

Risk for **Injury** r/t prolonged mechanical ventilation, retinopathy of prematurely (ROP) secondary to 100% oxygen environment

*See Retinal Detachment*

## REYE'S SYNDROME

Anticipatory **Grieving** r/t uncertain prognosis and sequelae

Compromised family **Coping** r/t acute situational crisis

Deficient **Fluid** volume r/t vomiting, hyperventilation

Disturbed **Sensory** perception r/t cerebral edema

Disturbed **Thought** processes r/t degenerative changes in fatty brain tissue

Excess **Fluid** volume: cerebral r/t cerebral edema

Imbalanced **Nutrition**: less than body requirements r/t effects of liver dysfunction, vomiting

Impaired **Gas** exchange r/t hyperventilation, sequelae of increased intracranial pressure

Impaired **Skin** integrity r/t effects of decorticate or decerebrate posturing, seizure activity

Ineffective **Breathing** pattern r/t neuromuscular impairment

Ineffective **Health** maintenance r/t deficient knowledge regarding use of salicylates during viral illness of child

Risk for **Injury** r/t combative behavior, seizure activity

Situational low **Self-esteem**: family r/t negative perceptions of self, perceived inability to manage family situation, expressions of guilt

*See Hospitalized Child*

## RH FACTOR INCOMPATIBILITY

**Anxiety** r/t unknown outcome of pregnancy

Deficient **Knowledge** r/t treatment regimen from lack of experience with situation

Effective **Therapeutic** regimen management r/t following recommended protocol; if the father of the infant is Rh-positive, and the mother Rh-negative, the mother is given a mid-term injection of RhoGAM and a second injection within a few days of delivery

**Health-seeking** behaviors r/t prenatal care, compliance with diagnostic and treatment regimen

**Powerlessness** r/t perceived lack of control over outcome of pregnancy

Risk for fetal **Injury** r/t intrauterine destruction of red blood cells, transfusions

## RHABDOMYOLYIS

Impaired physical **Mobility** r/t myalgia and muscle weakness

Impaired **Urinary** elimination r/t presence of myoglobin in the kidneys

Ineffective **Coping** r/t seriousness of condition

Readiness for enhanced **Therapeutic**

regimen management r/t seeks information to avoid condition

Risk for deficient **Fluid** volume r/t reduced blood flow to kidneys

*See Renal Failure*

## RHEUMATIC FEVER

*See Endocarditis*

## RHEUMATOID ARTHRITIS

Chronic **Pain** r/t swollen or inflamed joints, restricted movement, physical therapy

Effective **Therapeutic** regimen management r/t following prescribed medication and adhering to exercise program; physical therapy

**Fatigue** r/t chronic inflammatory disease

Impaired physical **Mobility** r/t pain, limited range of motion

Imbalanced **Nutrition**: less than body requirements r/t loss of appetite

Risk for impaired **Skin** integrity r/t splints, adaptive devices

Risk for **Injury** r/t impaired physical mobility, splints, adaptive devices, increased bleeding potential secondary to antiinflammatory medications

Risk for situational low **Self-esteem** r/t disturbed body image

**Self-care** deficits: feeding, bathing/hygiene, dressing/grooming, toileting r/t restricted joint movement, pain

*See Arthritis; JRA (Juvenile Rheumatoid Arthritis)*

## RIB FRACTURE

Acute **Pain** r/t movement, deep breathing

Ineffective **Breathing** pattern r/t fractured ribs

*See Ventilator Client (if relevant)*

## RIDICULE OF OTHERS

Defensive **Coping** r/t situational crisis, psychological impairment, substance abuse

Risk for **Post-trauma** syndrome r/t perception of the event

## RINGWORM OF BODY

Impaired **Skin** integrity r/t presence of macules associated with fungus

Ineffective **Therapeutic** regimen management r/t deficient knowledge of prevention, treatment

*See Itching*

## RINGWORM OF NAILS

Disturbed **Body** image r/t appearance of nails, removed nails

Ineffective **Therapeutic** regimen management r/t deficient knowledge of prevention, treatment

## RINGWORM OF SCALP

Disturbed **Body** image r/t possible hair loss (alopecia)

Ineffective **Therapeutic** regimen management r/t deficient knowledge of prevention, treatment

*See Itching*

## RISK FOR RELOCATION STRESS SYNDROME

*See Relocation Stress Syndrome*

## ROACHES, INVASION OF HOME WITH

Impaired **Home** maintenance r/t lack of knowledge, insufficient finances

*See Filthy Home Environment*

## ROLE PERFORMANCE, ALTERED

Ineffective **Role** performance r/t *Social:* inadequate or inappropriate linkage with the healthcare system; job schedule demands; young age; developmental level; lack of rewards;

R

poverty; family conflict; inadequate support system; inadequate role socialization (e.g., role model, expectations, responsibilities); *Knowledge:* inadequate role preparation (e.g., role transition, skill rehearsal, validation); lack of knowledge about role, role skills, role transition, lack of opportunity for role rehearsal; developmental transitions; unrealistic role expectations education attainment level; lack of or inadequate role model; *Physiological:* inadequate/inappropriate linkage with health care system; substance abuse; mental illness; body image alteration' physical illness; cognitive deficits; health alterations (e.g., physical health, body image, self-esteem, mental health, psychosocial health, cognition, learning style, neurological health); depression; low self-esteem; pain; fatigue

## ROP

*See Retinopathy of Prematurity (ROP)*

## RSV (RESPIRATORY SYNCYTIAL VIRUS)

*See Respiratory Infection, Acute Childhood*

## RUBELLA

*See Communicable Diseases, Childhood*

## RUBOR OF EXTREMITIES

Ineffective **Tissue** perfusion: peripheral r/t interruption of arterial flow

*See Peripheral Vascular Disease*

## RUPTURED DISK

*See Low Back Pain*

# S

## SAD (SEASONAL AFFECTIVE DISORDER)

Effective **Therapeutic** regimen management r/t uses SAD lights during winter months

*See Depression*

## SADNESS

Adult **Failure** to thrive r/t depression, apathy

Dysfunctional **Grieving** r/t actual or perceived loss

Readiness for enhanced **Communication** r/t willingness to share feelings and thoughts

Readiness for enhanced **Spiritual** well-being r/t desire for harmony following actual or perceived loss

Risk for **Powerlessness** r/t actual or perceived loss

Risk for **Spiritual** distress r/t loss of loved one

**Spiritual** distress r/t intense suffering

*See Depression*

## SAFE SEX

Effective **Therapeutic** regimen management r/t taking appropriate precautions sexual activity to keep from contacting a sexually transmitted disease

*See Sexuality, Adolescent; STD (Sexually Transmitted Disease)*

## SAFETY, CHILDHOOD

Deficient **Knowledge**: potential for enhanced health maintenance r/t parental knowledge and skill acquisition regarding appropriate safety measures

**Health-seeking** behaviors: enhanced parenting r/t adequate support systems, appropriate requests for help, desire and request for safety information, requests for information or assistance regarding parenting skills

Risk for altered **Health** maintenance r/t parental deficient knowledge regarding appropriate safety needs per developmental stage, childproofing house, infant and child car restraints, water safety, teaching child ways to avoid molestation

Risk for **Aspiration** and/or **Suffocation** r/t pillow or propped bottle placed in infant's crib; sides of playpen/crib being wide enough for child to get head through; child left in car with engine running; enclosed areas; plastic bags or small objects used as toys; toys with small, breakaway parts; refrigerators or freezers with doors accessible as play areas; child left unattended in or near bathtub, pool, spa; low clotheslines; electric garage doors without automatic stop/reopen; pacifier hung around infant's neck; food not cut into small, bite-size, age-appropriate pieces; balloons, hot dogs, nuts, or popcorn given to infant or young child, especially <1 year of age; use of baby powder

Risk for impaired **Parenting** r/t lack of available and effective role model, lack of knowledge; misinformation from other family members (old wives' tales)

Risk for **Injury/Trauma** r/t developmental age, altered home maintenance management (house not childproofed); impaired parenting; hot liquids within child's reach, no infant or child car restraints, no gate at top of stairs, lack of immunization; no fences or pool or spa covers; child left unattended in car with closed windows in hot weather; firearms loaded and within child's reach

Risk for **Poisoning** r/t use of lead-based paint; presence of asbestos or radon gas; drugs not locked in cabinet; household products left in accessible area (bleach, detergent, drain cleaners, household cleaners); alcohol and perfume within reach of child; presence of poisonous plants; atmospheric pollutants

## SALMONELLA

Readiness for enhanced **Therapeutic** regimen management r/t avoiding improperly prepared or stored food, wearing gloves when handling pet reptiles or its feces

Impaired **Home** maintenance r/t improper preparation or storage of food, lack of safety measures when caring for pet reptile

*See Gastroenteritis; Gastroenteritis, Child*

## SALPINGECTOMY

Anticipatory **Grieving** r/t possible loss due to tubal pregnancy

Decisional **Conflict** r/t sterilization procedure

Risk for impaired **Urinary** elimination r/t trauma to ureter during surgery

*See Hysterectomy; Surgery, Perioperative Care; Surgery, Postoperative Care; Surgery, Preoperative Care*

## SARCOIDOSIS

Acute **Pain** r/t possible disease affecting joints

**Anxiety** r/t change in health status

Impaired **Gas** exchange r/t ventilation-perfusion imbalance

Ineffective **Health** maintenance r/t deficient knowledge regarding home care and medication regimen

Risk for decreased **Cardiac** output r/t dysrhythmias

## SARS (SEVERE ACUTE RESPIRATORY SYNDROME)

Risk for **Infection** r/t increased environmental exposure (travelers in close proximity to infected persons, traveling when a fever is present)

Readiness for enhanced **Knowledge** of information regarding travel and precautions to avoid exposure to SARS

Effective **Therapeutic** regimen management r/t uses appropriate hand hygiene

*See Pneumonia*

## SBE (SELF-BREAST EXAMINATION)

Effective **Therapeutic** regimen management r/t practices self-breast examination per recommended protocol

**Health-seeking** behaviors r/t desire to have information about self-breast examination

Readiness for enhanced **Knowledge** of self-breast examination

## SCABIES

*See Communicable Diseases, Childhood*

## SCARED

**Anxiety** r/t threat of death, threat to or change in health status

Death **Anxiety** r/t unresolved issues surrounding end-of-life decisions

**Fear** r/t hospitalization, real or imagined threat to own well-being

Readiness for enhanced **Communication** r/t willingness to share thoughts and feelings

## SCHIZOPHRENIA

**Anxiety** r/t unconscious conflict with reality

Chronic **Sorrow** r/t chronic mental illness

Deficient **Diversional** activity r/t social isolation, possible regression

Disturbed **Sleep** pattern r/t sensory alterations contributing to fear and anxiety

Disturbed **Sensory** perception r/t biochemical imbalances for sensory distortion (illusions, hallucinations)

Disturbed **Thought** processes r/t inaccurate interpretations of environment

**Fear** r/t altered contact with reality

Imbalanced **Nutrition**: less than body requirements r/t fear of eating, lack of awareness of hunger, disinterest toward food

Impaired **Home** maintenance r/t impaired cognitive or emotional functioning, insufficient finances, inadequate support systems

Impaired **Social** interaction r/t impaired communication patterns, self-concept disturbance, disturbed thought processes

Impaired verbal **Communication** r/t psychosis, disorientation, inaccurate perception, hallucinations, delusions

Ineffective **Coping** r/t inadequate support systems, unrealistic perceptions, inadequate coping skills, disturbed thought processes, impaired communication

Ineffective **Health** maintenance r/t cognitive impairment, ineffective individual and family coping, lack of material resources

Ineffective family **Therapeutic** regimen management r/t chronicity and unpredictability of condition

Interrupted **Family** processes r/t inability to express feelings, impaired communication

Risk for **Caregiver** role strain r/t bizarre behavior of client, chronicity of condition

Risk for impaired **Religiosity** r/t ineffective coping; lack of security

Risk for **Loneliness** r/t inability to interact socially

Risk for **Post-trauma** syndrome r/t diminished ego strength

Risk for **Powerlessness** r/t intrusive, distorted thinking

Risk for self- and other-directed **Violence** r/t lack of trust, panic, hallucinations, delusional thinking

Risk for **Suicide** r/t psychiatric illness

**Self-care** deficit r/t loss of contact with reality, impairment of perception

**Self-esteem** disturbance r/t excessive use of defense mechanisms (e.g., projection, denial, rationalization)

**Sleep** deprivation r/t intrusive thoughts, nightmares

**Social** isolation r/t lack of trust, regression, delusional thinking, repressed fears

**Spiritual** distress r/t loneliness/social alienation

## SCIATICA

*See Neuropathy, Peripheral*

## SCOLIOSIS

Acute **Pain** r/t musculoskeletal restrictions, surgery, reambulation with cast or spinal rod

Chronic **Sorrow** r/t chronic disability

Disturbed **Body** image r/t use of therapeutic braces, postsurgery scars, restricted physical activity

Impaired **Adjustment** r/t lack of developmental maturity to comprehend long-term consequences of noncompliance with treatment procedures

Impaired **Gas** exchange r/t restricted lung expansion secondary to severe presurgery curvature of spine, immobilization

Impaired physical **Mobility** r/t restricted movement, dyspnea secondary to severe curvature of spine

Impaired **Skin** integrity r/t braces, casts, surgical correction

Ineffective **Breathing** pattern r/t restricted lung expansion secondary to severe curvature of spine

Ineffective **Health** maintenance r/t deficient knowledge regarding treatment modalities, restrictions, home care, postoperative activities

Readiness for enhanced **Therapeutic** regimen management r/t desire for knowledge regarding treatment for condition

Risk for **Infection** r/t surgical incision

Risk for perioperative positioning **Injury** r/t prone position

*See Hospitalized Child; Maturational Issues, Adolescent*

## SEDENTARY LIFESTYLE

**Activity** intolerance r/t sedentary lifestyle

Readiness for enhanced **Coping** r/t seeking knowledge of new strategies to adjust to sedentary lifestyle

**Sedentary** lifestyle r/t deficient knowledge of health benefits of physical exercise; lack of motivation, interest, training for accomplishment of physical exercise; lack of resources: time, money, companionship, facilities

## SEIZURE DISORDERS, ADULT

Acute **Confusion** r/t postseizure state

Impaired **Memory** r/t seizure activity

Ineffective **Health** maintenance r/t lack of knowledge regarding anticonvulsive therapy

Readiness for enhanced **Knowledge** of anticonvulsive therapy

Risk for disturbed **Thought** processes r/t effects of anticonvulsant medications

Risk for **Falls** r/t uncontrolled seizure activity

Risk for ineffective **Airway** clearance r/t accumulation of secretions during seizure

S

Risk for **Injury** r/t uncontrolled movements during seizure, falls, drowsiness secondary to anticonvulsants

Risk for **Powerlessness** r/t possible seizure

**Social** isolation r/t unpredictability of seizures, community-imposed stigma

*See Epilepsy*

## SEIZURE DISORDERS, CHILDHOOD (EPILEPSY, FEBRILE SEIZURES, INFANTILE SPASMS)

Ineffective **Health** maintenance r/t lack of knowledge regarding anticonvulsive therapy, fever reduction (febrile seizures)

Risk for delayed **Development** and disproportionate growth r/t effects of seizure disorder, parental overprotection

Risk for disturbed **Thought** processes r/t effects of anticonvulsant medications

Risk for **Falls** r/t possible seizure

Risk for ineffective **Airway** clearance r/t accumulation of secretions during seizure

Risk for **Injury** r/t uncontrolled movements during seizure, falls, drowsiness secondary to anticonvulsants

**Social** isolation r/t unpredictability of seizures, community-imposed stigma

*See Epilepsy*

## SELF-BREAST EXAMINATION

*See SBE (Self-Breast Examination)*

## SELF-CARE DEFICIT, BATHING/HYGIENE

Bathing/hygiene **Self-care** deficit r/t decreased or lack of motivation; weakness and tiredness; severe anxiety; inability to perceive body part or spatial relationship; perceptual or cognitive impairment; pain; neuromuscular, musculoskeletal impairment; environmental barriers

## SELF-CARE DEFICIT, DRESSING/GROOMING

Dressing/grooming **Self-care** deficit r/t decreased or lack of motivation; pain; severe anxiety; perceptual or cognitive impairment; weakness or tiredness; neuromuscular, musculoskeletal impairment; discomfort; environmental barriers

## SELF-CARE DEFICIT, FEEDING DISCOMFORT

Feeding **Self-care** deficit: r/t weakness or tiredness, severe anxiety, neuromuscular impairment, pain, perceptual or cognitive impairment, discomfort, environmental barriers, decreased or lack of motivation, musculoskeletal impairment

## SELF-CARE DEFICIT, TOILETING

Toileting **Self-care** deficit r/t environmental barriers, weakness or tiredness, decreased or lack of motivation, severe anxiety, impaired mobility status, impaired transfer ability, musculoskeletal impairment, neuromuscular impairment, pain, perceptual or cognitive impairment

## SELF-CONCEPT

Readiness for enhanced **Self-concept** r/t expresses willingness to enhance self-concept; expresses satisfaction with thoughts about self, sense of worthiness, role performance, body image, personal identity; actions are congruent with expressed feelings and thoughts; expresses confidence in abilities; accepts strengths and limitations

## SELF-DESTRUCTIVE BEHAVIOR

**Post-trauma** response r/t unresolved feelings from traumatic event

Risk for self-directed **Violence** r/t panic state, history of child abuse, toxic reaction to medication

Risk for **Self-mutilation** r/t feelings of depression, rejection, self-hatred, depersonalization; command hallucinations

Risk for **Suicide** r/t history of self-destructive behavior

## SELF-ESTEEM, CHRONIC LOW

Chronic low **Self-esteem** r/t long-standing negative self-evaluation

## SELF-ESTEEM, SITUATIONAL LOW

Risk for situational low **Self-esteem** r/t developmental changes (specify); disturbed body image; functional impairment (specify); loss (specify); social role changes (specify); history of learned helplessness; history of abuse, neglect, or abandonment; unrealistic self-expectations; behavior inconsistent with values; lack of recognition/rewards; failures/rejections; decreased power; control over environment; physical illness (specify)

**Self-esteem** disturbance r/t inappropriate and learned negative feelings about self

Situational low **Self-esteem** r/t developmental changes (specify); disturbed body image; functional impairment (specify); loss (specify); social role changes (specify); lack of recognition/rewards; behavior inconsistent with values; failures/rejections

## SELF-MUTILATION, RISK FOR

Risk for **Self-mutilation**: psychotic state (command hallucinations) r/t inability to express tension verbally; child-

hood sexual abuse; violence between parental figures; family divorce, alcoholism; family history of self-destructive behaviors; adolescence; peers who self-mutilate; isolation from peers; perfectionism; substance abuse; eating disorders; sexual identity crisis; low or unstable self-esteem; low or unstable body image; labile behavior (mood swings); history of inability to plan solutions or see long-term consequences; use of manipulation to obtain nurturing relationship with others; chaotic/disturbed interpersonal relationships; emotionally disturbed and/or battered children; feels threatened with actual or potential loss of significant relationship; loss of parent/parental relationships; experiences dissociation or depersonalization; experiences mounting tension that is intolerable; impulsivity; inadequate coping; experiences irresistible urge to cut/damage self; needs quick reduction of stress; childhood illness or surgery; foster, group, or institutional care; incarceration; character disorders; borderline personality disorders; loss of control over problem-solving situations; developmentally delayed or autistic individuals; history of self-injurious behavior; feelings of depression, rejection, self-hatred, separation anxiety, guilt, depersonalization

**Self-mutilation** r/t psychotic state (command hallucinations); inability to express tension verbally; childhood sexual abuse; violence between parental figures; family divorce; family alcoholism; family history of self-destructive behaviors; adolescence; peers who self-mutilate; isolation from peers; perfectionism; substance abuse; eating disorders; sexual identity crisis; low or unstable self-esteem; low or unstable body image; labile behavior (mood swings); history of inability to plan solutions or see long-term

S

consequences; use of manipulation to obtain nurturing relationship with others; chaotic/disturbed interpersonal relationships; emotionally disturbed; battered child; feels threatened with actual or potential loss of significant relationship (e.g., loss of parent, parental relationship); experiences dissociation or depersonalization; mounting tension that is intolerable; impulsivity; inadequate coping; irresistible urge to cut/damage self; needs quick reduction of stress; childhood illness or surgery; foster, group, or institutional care; incarceration; character disorders; borderline personality disorders; developmentally delayed or autistic individual; history of self-injurious behavior; feelings of depression, rejection, self-hatred, separation anxiety, guilt, depersonalization; poor parent adolescent communication; lack of family confidant

## SENILE DEMENTIA

**Sedentary** lifestyle r/t lack of interest

*See Dementia*

## SENSORY/PERCEPTUAL ALTERATIONS

Disturbed **Sensory** perception: visual, auditory, kinesthetic, gustatory, tactile, olfactory r/t altered sensory perception; excessive environmental stimuli; psychological stress; altered sensory reception, transmission, and/or integration; insufficient environmental stimuli; biochemical imbalances for sensory distortion (e.g., illusions, hallucinations); electrolyte imbalance; biochemical imbalance

## SEPARATION ANXIETY

Disturbed **Sleep** patterns r/t separation for significant others

Ineffective **Coping** r/t maturational and situational crises, vulnerability secondary to developmental age, hospital-ization, separation from family and familiar surroundings, multiple caregivers

Risk for impaired parent/infant/child **Attachment** r/t separation

*See Hospitalized Child*

## SEPSIS, CHILD

Delayed **Surgical** recovery r/t presence of infection

Imbalanced **Nutrition**: less than body requirements r/t anorexia, generalized weakness, poor sucking reflex

Impaired **Comfort**: increased sensitivity to environmental stimuli r/t disturbed sensory perceptions: visual, auditory, kinesthetic

Ineffective **Thermoregulation** r/t infectious process, septic shock

Ineffective **Tissue** perfusion: cardiopulmonary, peripheral r/t arterial or venous blood flow exchange problems, septic shock

Risk for impaired **Skin** integrity r/t desquamation secondary to disseminated intravascular coagulation (DIC)

*See Hospitalized Child; Premature Infant, Child*

## SEPTICEMIA

Deficient **Fluid** volume r/t vasodilation of peripheral vessels, leaking of capillaries

Imbalanced **Nutrition**: less than body requirements r/t anorexia, generalized weakness

Ineffective **Tissue** perfusion r/t decreased systemic vascular resistance

*See Sepsis, Child; Shock; Shock, Septic*

## SEVERE ACUTE RESPIRATORY SYNDROME

*See SARS (Severe Acute Respiratory Syndrome); Pneumonia*

## SEXUAL DYSFUNCTION

Chronic **Sorrow** r/t loss of ideal sexual experience, altered relationships

**Sexual** dysfunction r/t misinformation or lack of knowledge; vulnerability; values conflict; psychosocial abuse (e.g., harmful relationships); physical abuse; lack of privacy; ineffectual or absent role models; altered body structure or function (e.g., pregnancy, recent childbirth, drugs, surgery, anomalies, disease process, trauma, radiation); lack of significant other; biopsychosocial alteration of sexuality

*See Erectile Dysfunction*

## SEXUALITY, ADOLESCENT

Decisional **Conflict**: sexual activity r/t undefined personal values or beliefs, multiple or divergent sources of information, lack of relevant information

Deficient **Knowledge**: potential for enhanced health maintenance r/t multiple or divergent sources of information or lack of relevant information regarding sexual transmission of disease, contraception, prevention of toxic shock syndrome

Disturbed **Body** image r/t anxiety secondary to unachieved developmental milestone (puberty) or deficient knowledge regarding reproductive maturation as manifested by amenorrhea or expressed concerns regarding lack of growth of secondary sex characteristics

Risk for **Rape-trauma** syndrome r/t date rape, campus rape, insufficient knowledge regarding self-protection mechanisms

*See Maturational Issues, Adolescent*

## SEXUALITY PATTERNS, INEFFECTIVE

Ineffective **Sexuality** patterns r/t lack of significant other; conflicts with sexual orientation or variant preferences; fear of pregnancy or acquiring a sexually transmitted disease; impaired relationship with a significant other; ineffective or absent role models; knowledge skill deficit regarding alternative responses to health-related transitions, altered body function or structure, illness or medical treatment; lack of privacy

## SEXUALLY TRANSMITTED DISEASE

*See STD (Sexually Transmitted Disease)*

## SHAKEN BABY SYNDROME

Decreased **Intracranial** adaptive capacity r/t brain injury

Impaired **Parenting** r/t stress, history of being abusive

Risk for other-directed **Violence** r/t history of violence against others; perinatal complications

*See Child Abuse; Suspected Child Abuse and Neglect (SCAN), Child; Suspected Child Abuse and Neglect (SCAN), Parent*

## SHAKINESS

**Anxiety** r/t situational or maturational crisis, threat of death

## SHAME

**Self-esteem** disturbance r/t inability to deal with past traumatic events, blaming of self for events not under one's control

S

## SHINGLES

Acute **Pain** r/t vesicular eruption along the nerves

Ineffective **Protection** r/t abnormal blood profiles

Risk for **Infection** r/t tissue destruction

**Social** isolation r/t altered state of wellness, contagiousness of disease

*See Itching*

## SHIVERING

Hypothermia r/t exposure to cool environment

## SHOCK

**Fear** r/t serious threat to health status

Ineffective **Tissue** perfusion: cardio-pulmonary; peripheral r/t arterial/venous blood flow exchange problems

Risk for **Injury** r/t prolonged shock resulting in multiple organ failure, death

*See Shock, Cardiogenic; Shock, Hypovolemic; Shock, Septic*

## SHOCK, CARDIOGENIC

Decreased **Cardiac** output r/t decreased myocardial contractility, dysrhythmia

*See Shock*

## SHOCK, HYPOVOLEMIC

Deficient **Fluid** volume r/t abnormal loss of fluid

*See Shock*

## SHOCK, SEPTIC

Deficient **Fluid** volume r/t abnormal loss of fluid through capillaries, pooling of blood in peripheral circulation

Ineffective **Protection** r/t inadequately functioning immune system

*See Sepsis, Child; Septicemia; Shock*

## SHOULDER REPAIR

Risk for perioperative positioning **Injury** r/t immobility

**Self-care** deficit: bathing/hygiene, dressing/grooming, feeding r/t immobilization of affected shoulder

*See Surgery, Preoperative; Surgery, Perioperative; Surgery, Postoperative; Total Joint Replacement*

## SICKLE CELL ANEMIA/CRISIS

**Activity** intolerance r/t fatigue, effects of chronic anemia

Acute **Pain** r/t viscous blood, tissue hypoxia

Deficient **Fluid** volume r/t decreased intake, increased fluid requirements during sickle cell crisis, decreased ability of kidneys to concentrate urine

Impaired physical **Mobility** r/t pain, fatigue

Risk for ineffective **Tissue** perfusion: renal, cerebral, cardiac, gastrointestinal, peripheral r/t effects of red cell sickling; infarction of tissues

Risk for **Infection** r/t alterations in splenic function

*See Child with Chronic Condition; Hospitalized Child*

## SIDS (SUDDEN INFANT DEATH SYNDROME)

Anticipatory **Grieving** r/t potential loss of infant

**Anxiety/Fear**: parental r/t life-threatening event

Deficient **Knowledge**: potential for enhanced health maintenance r/t knowledge or skill acquisition of cardiopulmonary resuscitation (CPR) and home apnea monitoring

Disturbed **Sleep** pattern: parental/infant r/t home apnea monitoring

Interrupted **Family** processes r/t stress secondary to special care needs of infant with apnea

Risk for **Powerlessness** r/t unanticipated life-threatening event

Risk for sudden infant **Death** syndrome r/t modifiable risk factors such as infants placed to sleep in the prone or side-lying position, prenatal and/or postnatal infant smoke exposure, infant overheating/overwrapping, soft underlayment/loose articles in the sleep environment, delayed or nonattendance of prenatal care; potentially modifiable risk factors such as

S

low birth weight, prematurity, young maternal age; nonmodifiable risk factors such as male gender, ethnicity (e.g., African American, Native American race of mother), seasonality of SIDS deaths (higher in winter and fall months); peaking of SIDS mortality between infant ages of 2 and 4 months

*See Terminally Ill Child/Death of Child, Parent*

## SITUATIONAL CRISIS

Ineffective **Coping** r/t situational crisis

Interrupted **Family** processes r/t situational crisis

Readiness for enhanced **Communication** r/t willingness to share feelings and thoughts

Readiness for enhanced **Religiosity** r/t requests religious material and/ or experiences

Readiness for enhanced **Spiritual** well-being r/t desire for harmony following crisis

## SKIN CANCER

Impaired **Skin** integrity r/t abnormal cell growth in skin, treatment of skin cancer

Ineffective **Health** maintenance r/t deficient knowledge regarding self-care with skin cancer

Readiness for enhanced **Knowledge** of self-care to prevent and treat skin cancer

## SKIN DISORDERS

### INTERNAL

Impaired **Skin** integrity r/t altered metabolic state, skeletal prominence; immunological deficit; developmental factors; altered sensation; altered nutritional state (e.g., obesity, emaciation); altered pigmentation; altered circulation; alterations in turgor (change in elasticity); altered fluid status

### EXTERNAL

Impaired **Skin** integrity r/t hyperthermia; hypothermia; chemical substances; humidity mechanical factors (e.g., shearing forces, pressure, restraint); physical immobilization; radiation; extremes in age, moisture, medication

## SKIN INTEGRITY, RISK FOR IMPAIRED

### INTERNAL

Risk for impaired **Skin** integrity r/t medication; skeletal prominence; immunologic factors; developmental factors; altered sensation; altered pigmentation; altered metabolic state; altered circulation; alterations to skin turgor (changes in elasticity); alterations in nutritional state (e.g., obesity, emaciation); psychogenetic

### EXTERNAL

Risk for impaired **Skin** integrity r/t radiation, physical immobilization, mechanical factors (e.g., shearing forces, pressure, restraint); hypothermia or hyperthermia; humidity; chemical substance; excretions and/or secretions; moisture; extremes of age

## SKIN TURGOR, CHANGE IN ELASTICITY

Deficient **Fluid** volume r/t active fluid loss (decreased skin turgor can be a normal finding in the elderly)

S

## SLEEP

Readiness for enhanced **Sleep** r/t expresses willingness to enhance sleep, amount of sleep and rapid eye movement (REM) sleep is congruent with developmental needs, expressed feeling of being rested after sleep, following sleep routines that promote sleep habits, occasional or infrequent use of medications to induce sleep

## SLEEP APNEA

*See PND (Paroxysmal Nocturnal Dyspnea)*

## SLEEP DEPRIVATION

Disturbed **Sensory** perception r/t lack of sleep

**Fatigue** r/t lack of sleep

**Sleep** deprivation r/t prolonged physical discomfort; prolonged psychological discomfort; sustained inadequate sleep hygiene; prolonged use of pharmacological or dietary antisoporifics; aging-related sleep stage shifts; sustained circadian asynchrony; inadequate daytime activity; sustained environmental stimulation; sustained unfamiliar or uncomfortable sleep environment; non–sleep-inducing parenting practices; sleep apnea; periodic limb movement (e.g., restless leg syndrome, nocturnal myoclonus); sundown syndrome; narcolepsy; idiopathic central nervous system hypersomnolence; sleep walking; sleep terror; sleep-related enuresis; nightmares; familial sleep paralysis; sleep-related painful erections; dementia

## SLEEP PATTERN DISORDERS

Disturbed **Sleep** pattern r/t *Psychological:* Ruminative presleep thought; daytime activity pattern; thinking about home; body temperature; temperament; dietary; childhood onset; inadequate sleep hygiene; sustained use of antisleep agents; circadian asynchrony; frequently changing sleep-wake schedule; depression; loneliness; frequent travel across time zones; daylight/darkness exposure; grief; anticipation; shift work; delayed or advance sleep phase syndrome; loss of sleep partner; life change; preoccupation with trying to sleep; periodic gender related hormonal shifts; biochemical agents; fear; separation from significant others; social schedule inconsistent with chronotype; aging-related sleep shifts; anxiety; medications; fear of insomnia; maladaptive conditioned wakefulness; fatigue; boredom; *Environmental:* Noise; lighting; unfamiliar sleep furnishings; ambient temperature, humidity; other-generated awakening; excessive stimulation; physical restraint; lack of sleep privacy/control; interruptions for therapeutics, monitoring, lab tests; sleep partner; noxious odors; *Parental:* Mother's sleep-wake pattern; parent-infant interaction; mother's emotional support; *Physiological:* Urinary urgency, incontinence; fever; nausea; stasis of secretions; shortness of breath; position; gastroesophageal reflux

## SLEEP PATTERN, DISTURBED, PARENT/CHILD

Disturbed **Sleep** pattern: child r/t anxiety or apprehension secondary to parental deprivation, fear, night terrors, enuresis, inconsistent parental responses to child's requests to alter bedtime rules, frequent nighttime awakening, inability to wean from parents' bed, hypervigilance

Disturbed **Sleep** pattern: parent r/t time-intensive home treatments, increased caretaker demands

*See Suspected Child Abuse and Neglect*

## SLURRING OF SPEECH

Impaired verbal **Communication** r/t decrease in circulation to brain, brain tumor, anatomical defect, cleft palate

Situational low **Self-esteem** r/t speech impairment

*See Communication Problems*

## SMALL BOWEL RESECTION

*See Abdominal Surgery*

S

## SMELL, LOSS OF ABILITY TO

Risk for **Injury** r/t inability to detect gas fumes, smoke smells

*See Anosmia*

## SMOKING BEHAVIOR

Altered **Health** maintenance r/t denial of effects of smoking, lack of effective support for smoking withdrawal

Readiness for enhanced **Knowledge** of smoking cessation

## SOCIAL INTERACTION, IMPAIRED

Impaired **Social** interaction r/t knowledge/skill deficit regarding ways to enhance mutuality; therapeutic isolation; sociocultural dissonance; limited physical mobility; environmental barriers; communication barriers; altered thought processes; absence of available significant others or peers; self-concept disturbance

## SOCIAL ISOLATION

**Social** isolation r/t alterations in mental status; inability to engage in satisfying personal relationships; unacceptable social values; unacceptable social behavior; inadequate personal resources; immature interests; factors contributing to absence of satisfying personal relationships (e.g., delay in accomplishing developmental tasks); alterations in physical appearance; altered state of wellness

## SOCIOPATHIC PERSONALITY

*See Antisocial Personality Disorder*

## SODIUM, DECREASE/INCREASE

*See Hyponatremia/Hypernatremia*

## SOMATIZATION DISORDER

**Anxiety** r/t unresolved conflicts channeled into physical complaints or conditions

Chronic **Pain** r/t unexpressed anger, multiple physical disorders, depression

Ineffective **Coping** r/t lack of insight into underlying conflicts

Ineffective **Denial** r/t displaces psychological stress to physical symptoms

## SORE NIPPLES, BREASTFEEDING

Ineffective **Breastfeeding** r/t deficient knowledge regarding correct feeding procedure

*See Painful Breasts, Sore Nipples*

## SORE THROAT

Acute **Pain** r/t inflammation, irritation, dryness

Deficient **Knowledge** r/t treatment, relief of discomfort

Impaired **Oral** mucous membrane r/t inflammation or infection of oral cavity

Impaired **Swallowing** r/t irritation of oropharyngeal cavity

## SORROW

Anticipatory **Grieving** r/t impending loss of significant person or object

Chronic **Sorrow** r/t unresolved grief

**Grieving** r/t loss of significant person, object, or role

Readiness for enhanced **Communication** r/t expresses thoughts and feelings

Readiness for enhanced **Spiritual** well-being r/t desire to find purpose and meaning of loss

## SPASTIC COLON

*See IBS (Irritable Bowel Syndrome)*

## SPEECH DISORDERS

**Anxiety** r/t difficulty with communication

Delayed **Growth** and development r/t effects of physical/mental disability

Disturbed **Sensory** perception (audi-

S

tory) r/t altered sensory reception, transmission, and/or integration

Impaired verbal **Communication** r/t anatomical defect, cleft palate, psychological barriers, decrease in circulation to brain

## SPINA BIFIDA

Risk for latex **Allergy** response r/t multiple exposures to latex products

*See Neurotube Defects*

## SPINAL CORD INJURY

Chronic **Sorrow** r/t immobility, change in body function

**Constipation** r/t immobility, loss of sensation

Deficient **Diversional** activity r/t long-term hospitalization, frequent lengthy treatments

Disturbed **Body** image r/t change in body function

Dysfunctional **Grieving** r/t loss of usual body function

**Fear** r/t powerlessness over loss of body function

Impaired **Home** maintenance r/t change in health status, insufficient family planning or finances, deficient knowledge, inadequate support systems

Impaired physical **Mobility** r/t neuromuscular impairment

Ineffective **Health** maintenance r/t deficient knowledge regarding self-care with spinal cord injury

Reflex **Incontinence** r/t spinal cord lesion interfering with conduction of cerebral messages

Risk for **Autonomic** dysreflexia r/t bladder or bowel distention, skin irritation, deficient knowledge of client and caregiver

Risk for **Disuse** syndrome r/t paralysis

Risk for impaired **Skin** integrity r/t immobility, paralysis

Risk for ineffective **Breathing** pattern r/t neuromuscular impairment

Risk for **Infection** r/t chronic disease, stasis of body fluids

Risk for latex **Allergy** response r/t continuous or intermittent catherization

Risk for **Loneliness** r/t physical immobility

Risk for **Powerlessness** r/t loss of function

**Self-care** deficit r/t neuromuscular impairment

**Sedentary** lifestyle r/t lack of resources/interest

**Sexual** dysfunction r/t altered body function

**Urinary** retention r/t inhibition of reflex arc

*See Child with Chronic Condition; Hospitalized Child; Neurotube Defects*

## SPINAL FUSION

Impaired bed **Mobility** r/t impaired ability to turn side-to-side keeping spine in proper alignment

Impaired physical **Mobility** r/t musculoskeletal impairment associated with surgery, possible back brace

Readiness for enhanced **Knowledge** r/t expresses interest in information associated with surgery

*See Acute Back; Back Pain; Scoliosis; Surgery, Preoperative Care; Surgery, Perioperative Care; Surgery, Postoperative Care*

## SPIRITUAL DISTRESS

Risk for **Spiritual** distress r/t *Physical:* Physical illness, substance abuse/ excessive drinking, chronic illness; *Psychosocial:* Low self-esteem, depression, anxiety, stress, poor relationships, separate from support systems, blocks to experiencing love, inability to forgive, loss; *Sociocultural:* Racial/cultural conflict, change in religious rituals; *Spiritual:* change in spiritual practices; *Developmental:* Life transitions; *Environmental:* Environmental changes, natural disasters

**Spiritual** distress r/t self-alienation, loneliness/social isolation, anxiety, sociocultural deprivation, death and dying of self or others, pain, life change, chronic illness of self or others

## SPIRITUAL WELL-BEING

Readiness for enhanced **Spiritual** well-being r/t health-seeking behaviors, empathy, self-care, self-awareness, desire for harmonious interconnectedness, desire to find meaning and purpose in life

## SPLENECTOMY

*See Abdominal Surgery*

## SPRAINS

Acute **Pain** r/t physical injury

Effective **Therapeutic** regimen management r/t not exercising when tired or in pain; maintaining healthy weight; wearing properly fitting shoes; appropriate warm up, stretching and cool down exercises; wearing protective equipment; running on even surfaces; staying physically fit

Impaired physical **Mobility** r/t injury

## STAPEDECTOMY

Acute **Pain** r/t headache

Disturbed **Sensory** perception: auditory r/t hearing loss caused by edema from surgery

Risk for **Falls** r/t dizziness

Risk for **Infection** r/t invasive procedure

Risk for **Injury**: falls r/t dizziness

## STASIS ULCER

Impaired **Tissue** integrity r/t chronic venous congestion

*See CHF (Congestive Heart Failure); Varicose Veins*

## STD (SEXUALLY TRANSMITTED DISEASE)

Acute **Pain** r/t biological or psychological injury

Ineffective **Health** maintenance r/t deficient knowledge regarding transmission, symptoms, treatment of STD

Ineffective **Sexuality** patterns r/t illness, altered body function

**Fear** r/t altered body function, risk for social isolation, fear of incurable illness

Readiness for enhanced **Knowledge** of prevention and treatment of STDs

Risk for **Infection**/spread of infection r/t lack of knowledge concerning transmission of disease

**Social** isolation r/t fear of contracting or spreading disease

*See Maturational Issues, Adolescent*

## STERILIZATION SURGERY

Decisional **Conflict** r/t multiple or divergent sources of information; unclear personal values/beliefs

*See Surgery, Preoperative Care; Surgery, Perioperative Care; Surgery, Postoperative Care; Tubal Ligation; Vasectomy*

## STERTOROUS RESPIRATIONS

Ineffective **Airway** clearance r/t pharyngeal obstruction

## STILLBIRTH

*See Pregnancy Loss*

## STOMA

*See Colostomy; Ileostomy*

S

## STOMATITIS

Impaired **Oral** mucous membrane r/t pathological conditions of oral cavity

## STONE, KIDNEY

*See Kidney Stone*

## STOOL, HARD/DRY

**Constipation** r/t inadequate fluid intake, inadequate fiber intake, decreased activity level, decreased gastric motility

## STRAINING WITH DEFECATION

**Constipation** r/t less than adequate fluid intake, less than adequate dietary intake

Risk for decreased **Cardiac** output r/t vagal stimulation with dysrhythmia secondary to Valsalva maneuver

## STRESS

**Anxiety** r/t feelings of helplessness, feelings of being threatened

Disturbed **Energy** field r/t low energy level, feelings of hopelessness

**Fear** r/t powerlessness over feelings

Ineffective **Coping** r/t ineffective use of problem-solving process, feelings of apprehension or helplessness

Readiness for enhanced **Communication** r/t willingness to share thoughts and feelings

Readiness for enhanced **Spiritual** well-being r/t desire for harmony and peace in stressful situation

Risk for **Post-trauma** syndrome r/t perception of event, survivor's role in event

**Self-esteem** disturbance r/t inability to deal with life events

## STRESS URINARY INCONTINENCE

Risk for urge urinary **Incontinence** r/t involuntary sphincter relaxation

Stress urinary **Incontinence** r/t degenerative change in pelvic muscles

*See Incontinence of Urine*

## STRIDOR

Ineffective **Airway** clearance r/t obstruction, tracheobronchial infection, trauma

## STROKE

*See CVA (Cerebrovascular Accident)*

## STUTTERING

**Anxiety** r/t impaired verbal communication

Impaired verbal **Communication** r/t anxiety, psychological problems

## SUBARACHNOID HEMORRHAGE

Acute **Pain**: headache r/t irritation of meninges from blood, increased intracranial pressure

Ineffective **Tissue** perfusion: cerebral r/t bleeding from cerebral vessel

*See Intracranial Pressure, Increased*

## SUBSTANCE ABUSE

**Anxiety** r/t loss of control

Compromised/disabled family **Coping** r/t codependency issues

Defensive **Coping** r/t substance abuse

Disturbed **Sleep** pattern r/t irritability, nightmares, tremors

Dysfunctional **Family** processes: alcohol r/t inadequate coping skills

Imbalanced **Nutrition**: less than body requirements r/t anorexia

Ineffective **Coping** r/t use of substances to cope with life events

Ineffective **Denial** r/t refusal to acknowledge substance abuse problem

Ineffective **Protection** r/t malnutrition, sleep deprivation

**Powerlessness** r/t substance addiction

Readiness for enhanced **Coping** r/t seeking social support and seeking knowledge of new strategies

Readiness for enhanced **Self-concept** r/t accepting strengths and limitations

Risk for impaired parent/infant/child **Attachment** r/t substance abuse

Risk for **Injury** r/t alteration in sensory perception

Risk for self- or other-directed **Violence** r/t reactions to substances used, impulsive behavior, disorientation, impaired judgment

Risk for **Suicide** r/t substance abuse

**Self-esteem** disturbance r/t failure at life events

**Social** isolation r/t unacceptable social behavior or values

*See Maturational Issues, Adolescent*

## SUBSTANCE ABUSE, ADOLESCENT

*See Alcohol Withdrawal; Maturational Issues, Adolescent; Substance Abuse*

## SUBSTANCE ABUSE IN PREGNANCY

Altered **Health** maintenance r/t addiction

Defensive **Coping** r/t denial of situation, differing value system

Deficient **Knowledge** r/t lack of exposure to information regarding effects of substance abuse in pregnancy

**Health-seeking** behaviors (substance abuse counseling) r/t desire to provide child with substance-free perinatal period

**Noncompliance** r/t differing value system, cultural influences, addiction

Risk for fetal **Injury** r/t effects of drugs on fetal growth and development

Risk for impaired parent-infant **Attachment** r/t substance abuse, inability

of parent to meet infant's/own personal needs

Risk for impaired **Parenting** r/t lack of ability to meet infant's needs

Risk for **Infection** r/t intravenous drug use, lifestyle

Risk for maternal **Injury** r/t drug use

*See Substance Abuse*

## SUCKING REFLEX

Effective **Breastfeeding** r/t regular and sustained suckling and swallowing at breast

## SUDDEN INFANT DEATH SYNDROME

*See SIDS (Sudden Infant Death Syndrome)*

## SUFFOCATION, RISK FOR

### INTERNAL

Risk for **Suffocation** r/t reduced olfactory sensation, reduced motor abilities; cognitive or emotional difficulties, disease or injury process, lack of safety education, lack of safety precautions

### EXTERNAL

Risk for **Suffocation** r/t vehicle running in closed garage, use of fuel-burning heaters not vented to outside, smoking in bed, children playing with plastic bags or inserting small objects into mouth or nose, propped bottle placed in infant's crib, pillow placed in an infant's crib, person who eats large mouthfuls of food, discarded or unused refrigerators or freezers without removed doors, children left unattended in bathtubs or pools, household gas leaks, low-strung clothesline, pacifier hung around infant's neck

## SUICIDE ATTEMPT

**Hopelessness** r/t perceived or actual loss, substance abuse, low self-concept, inadequate support systems

S

Ineffective **Coping** r/t anger, dysfunctional grieving

**Post-trauma** response r/t history of traumatic events, abuse, rape, incest, war, torture

Readiness for enhanced **Communication** r/t willingness to share thoughts and feelings

Readiness for enhanced **Spiritual** well-being r/t desire for harmony and inner strength to help redefine purpose for life

Risk for **Post-trauma** syndrome r/t survivor's role in suicide attempt

Risk for **Suicide** r/t *Behavioral:* History of prior suicide attempt; impulsiveness; buying a gun; stockpiling medicines; making or changing a will; giving away possessions; sudden euphoric recovery from major depression; marked changes in behavior, attitude, or school performance; *Verbal:* Threats of killing oneself; states desire to die/end it all; *Situational:* Living alone; retirement; relocation, institutionalization; economic instability; loss of autonomy/independence; presence of gun in home; adolescents living in nontraditional setting (e.g., juvenile detention center, prison, half-way house, group home); *Psychological:* Family history of suicide; alcohol and substance use/abuse; psychiatric illness/disorder (e.g., depression, schizophrenia, bipolar disorder); abuse in childhood; guilt; gay or lesbian orientation in youth; *Demographic:* Age: elderly, young adult male, adolescents; Race: Caucasian, Native American; Gender: male; Marital status: divorced, widowed; *Physical:* Physical illness; terminal illness; chronic pain; *Social:* Loss of important relationship; disrupted family life; grief, bereavement; poor support systems; loneliness; hopelessness; helplessness; social isolation; legal or disciplinary problems; cluster suicides

**Self-esteem** disturbance r/t guilt, inability to trust, feelings of worthlessness or rejection

**Social** isolation r/t inability to engage in satisfying personal relationships

**Spiritual** distress r/t hopelessness, despair

*See Violent Behavior*

## SUPPORT SYSTEM

Readiness for enhanced family **Coping** r/t ability to adapt to tasks associated with care, support of significant other during health crisis

Readiness for enhanced **Family** processes r/t activities support the growth of family members

Readiness for enhanced **Parenting** r/t children or other dependent person(s) expressing satisfaction with home environment

## SUPPRESSION OF LABOR

*See Preterm Labor; Tocolytic Therapy*

## SURGERY, PERIOPERATIVE CARE

Risk for imbalanced **Fluid** volume r/t surgery

Risk for perioperative positioning **Injury** r/t predisposing condition, prolonged surgery

## SURGERY, POSTOPERATIVE CARE

**Activity** intolerance r/t pain, surgical procedure

Acute **Pain** r/t inflammation or injury in surgical area

**Anxiety** r/t change in health status, hospital environment

Deficient **Knowledge** r/t postoperative expectations, lifestyle changes

Imbalanced **Nutrition**: less than body

requirements r/t anorexia, nausea, vomiting, decreased peristalsis

**Nausea** r/t manipulation of gastrointestinal tract, postsurgical anesthesia

Risk for **Constipation** r/t decreased activity, decreased food or fluid intake, anesthesia, pain medication

Risk for deficient **Fluid** volume r/t hypermetabolic state, fluid loss during surgery, presence of indwelling tubes

Risk for ineffective **Breathing** pattern r/t pain, location of incision, effects of anesthesia/narcotics

Risk for ineffective **Tissue** perfusion: peripheral r/t hypovolemia, circulatory stasis, obesity, prolonged immobility, decreased coughing, decreased deep breathing

Risk for **Infection** r/t invasive procedure, pain, anesthesia, location of incision, weakened cough as a result of aging

**Urinary** retention r/t anesthesia, pain, fear, unfamiliar surroundings, client's position

## SURGERY, PREOPERATIVE CARE

**Anxiety** r/t threat to or change in health status, situational crisis, fear of the unknown

Deficient **Knowledge** r/t preoperative procedures, postoperative expectations

Disturbed **Sleep** pattern r/t anxiety about upcoming surgery

Readiness for enhanced **Knowledge** of preoperative and postoperative expectations for self-care

## SUSPECTED CHILD ABUSE AND NEGLECT (SCAN), CHILD

Acute **Pain** r/t physical injuries

**Anxiety/Fear**: child r/t threat of punishment for perceived wrongdoing

Chronic low **Self-esteem** r/t lack of positive feedback, excessive negative feedback

Deficient **Diversional** activity r/t diminished or absent environmental or personal stimuli

Delayed **Growth** and development: regression vs. delayed r/t diminished or absent environmental stimuli, inadequate caretaking, inconsistent responsiveness by caretaker

Disturbed **Sleep** pattern r/t hypervigilance, anxiety

Imbalanced **Nutrition**: less than body requirements r/t inadequate caretaking

Impaired **Skin** integrity r/t altered nutritional state, physical abuse

**Post-trauma** response r/t physical abuse, incest, rape, molestation

**Rape-trauma** syndrome: compound/silent reaction r/t altered lifestyle secondary to abuse, changes in residence

Readiness for enhanced community **Coping** r/t obtaining resources to prevent child abuse, neglect

Risk for **Poisoning** r/t inadequate safeguards, lack of proper safety precautions, accessibility of illicit substances secondary to impaired home maintenance

Risk for **Suffocation**: secondary to aspiration r/t propped bottle, unattended child

Risk for **Trauma** r/t inadequate precautions, cognitive or emotional difficulties

**Social** isolation: family-imposed r/t fear of disclosure of family dysfunction and abuse

*See Hospitalized Child; Maturational Issues, Adolescent*

S

## SUSPECTED CHILD ABUSE AND NEGLECT (SCAN), PARENT

Chronic low **Self-esteem** r/t lack of successful parenting experiences

Disabled family **Coping** r/t dysfunctional family, underdeveloped nurturing parental role, lack of parental support systems or role models

Dysfunctional **Family** processes: alcoholism r/t inadequate coping skills

Impaired **Home** maintenance r/t disorganization, parental dysfunction, neglect of safe and nurturing environment

Impaired **Parenting** r/t unrealistic expectations of child; lack of effective role model; unmet social, emotional, or maturational needs of parents; interruption in bonding process

Ineffective **Health** maintenance r/t deficient knowledge of parenting skills secondary to unachieved developmental tasks

**Powerlessness** r/t inability to perform parental role responsibilities

Risk for **Violence** toward child r/t inadequate coping mechanisms, unresolved stressors, unachieved maturational level by parent

## SUSPICION

Impaired **Social** interaction r/t disturbed thought processes, paranoid delusions, hallucinations

**Powerlessness** r/t repetitive paranoid thinking

Risk for self- or other-directed **Violence** r/t inability to trust

## SWALLOWING DIFFICULTIES

Impaired **Swallowing** r/t *Congenital Defects*: upper airway anomalies; failure to thrive or protein energy malnutrition; conditions with severe hyptonia; respiratory disorders; history of tube feeding; behavioral problems; self-injurious behavior; neuromuscular impairment (e.g., decreased or absent gag reflex, decreased strength or excursion of muscles involved in mastication, perceptual impairment, facial paralysis); mechanical obstruction (e.g., edema, tracheostomy tube, tumor); congenital heart disease; cranial nerve involvement; *Neurological:* upper airway anomalies; laryngeal abnormalities; achalasia; gastrointestinal reflux disease; acquired anatomic defects; cerebral palsy; internal or external traumas; tracheal, laryngeal, esophageal defects; traumatic head injury; developmental delay; nasal or nasopharyngeal cavity defects; oral cavity or oropharynx abnormalities; premature infants

## SYNCOPE

**Anxiety** r/t fear of falling

Decreased **Cardiac** output r/t dysrhythmia

Impaired physical **Mobility** r/t fear of falling

Ineffective **Tissue** perfusion: cerebral r/t interruption of blood flow

Risk for **Falls** r/t syncope

Risk for **Injury** r/t altered sensory perception, transient loss of consciousness, risk for falls

**Social** isolation r/t fear of falling

## SYPHILIS

*See STD (Sexually Transmitted Disease)*

## SYSTEMIC LUPUS ERYTHEMATOSUS

*See Lupus Erythematosus*

# T

## T & A (TONSILLECTOMY AND ADENOIDECTOMY)

Acute **Pain** r/t surgical incision

Deficient **Knowledge**: potential for enhanced health maintenance r/t insufficient knowledge regarding postoperative nutritional and rest requirements, signs and symptoms of complications, positioning

Impaired **Comfort** r/t effects of anesthesia (nausea and vomiting)

Ineffective **Airway** clearance r/t hesitation or reluctance to cough secondary to pain

Risk for **Aspiration/Suffocation** r/t postoperative drainage and impaired swallowing

Risk for deficient **Fluid** volume r/t decreased intake secondary to painful swallowing, effects of anesthesia (nausea, vomiting), hemorrhage

Risk for imbalanced **Nutrition**: less than body requirements r/t hesitation or reluctance to swallow

## TACHYCARDIA

*See Dysrhythmia*

## TACHYPNEA

Ineffective **Breathing** pattern r/t pain, anxiety

*See cause of Tachypnea*

## TARDIVE DYSKINESIA

Deficient **Knowledge** r/t cognitive limitation in assimilating information relating to side effects associated with neuroleptic medications

Disturbed sensory **Perception** r/t tardive dyskinesia

Risk for **Injury** r/t drug induced abnormal body movements

## TASTE ABNORMALITY

Adult **Failure** to thrive r/t imbalanced nutrition: less than body requirements associated with taste abnormality

Disturbed **Sensory** perception: gustatory r/t medication side effects; altered sensory reception, transmission, integration; aging changes

## TB (PULMONARY TUBERCULOSIS)

**Fatigue** r/t disease state (TB)

**Hyperthermia** r/t infection

Impaired **Gas** exchange r/t disease process

Impaired **Home** maintenance management r/t client/family member with disease

Ineffective **Airway** clearance r/t increased secretions, excessive mucus

Ineffective **Breathing** pattern r/t decreased energy/ fatigue

Ineffective **Therapeutic** regimen management r/t deficient knowledge of prevention and treatment regimen

Readiness for enhanced **Therapeutic** regimen management r/t taking medications according to prescribed protocol for prevention and treatment

Risk for **Infection** r/t insufficient knowledge regarding avoidance of exposure to pathogens

## TBI (TRAUMATIC BRAIN INJURY)

Acute **Confusion** r/t brain injury

Chronic **Sorrow** r/t change in person's health status and functional ability

Decreased **Intracranial** adaptive capacity r/t brain injury

Disturbed **Sensory** perception: specify r/t pressure damage to sensory centers in brain

T

Disturbed **Thought** processes r/t pressure damage to brain

Impaired **Memory** r/t neurological disturbances

Ineffective **Tissue** perfusion: cerebral r/t effects of increased intracranial pressure

Ineffective **Breathing** pattern r/t pressure damage to breathing center in brain stem

Interrupted **Family** processes r/t traumatic injury to family member

Risk for **Post-trauma** syndrome r/t perception of event causing traumatic brain injury

Risk for impaired **Religiosity** r/t impaired physical mobility

## TD (TRAVELER'S DIARRHEA)

Risk for deficient **Fluid** volume r/t excessive loss of fluids; diarrhea

Risk for **Infection** r/t insufficient knowledge regarding avoidance of exposure to pathogens (water supply, iced drinks, local cheeses, ice cream, undercooked meat, fish and shellfish, uncooked vegetables, unclean eating utensils, improper hand washing)

## TEMPERATURE, DECREASED

**Hypothermia** r/t exposure to cold environment

## TEMPERATURE, INCREASED

**Hyperthermia** r/t dehydration, illness, trauma

## TEMPERATURE REGULATION, IMPAIRED

Ineffective **Thermoregulation** r/t trauma, illness

## TENSION

**Anxiety** r/t threat to or change in health status, situational crisis

Disturbed **Energy** field r/t change in health status, discouragement, pain

Readiness for enhanced **Communication** r/t willingness to share feelings and thoughts

*See Stress*

## TERMINALLY ILL ADULT

Anticipatory **Grieving** r/t loss of self or significant other

Compromised family **Coping** r/t inability to discuss impending death

Death **Anxiety** r/t unresolved issues relating to death and dying

Decisional **Conflict** r/t planning for advance directives

Disturbed **Energy** field r/t impending disharmony of mind, body, spirit

Readiness for enhanced **Religiosity** r/t requests religious material and or/experiences

Readiness for enhanced **Spiritual** well-being r/t desire to achieve harmony of mind, body, spirit

Risk for **Spiritual** distress r/t impending death

**Spiritual** distress r/t suffering while dying

## TERMINALLY ILL CHILD, ADOLESCENT

Disturbed **Body** image r/t effects of terminal disease, already critical feelings of group identity and self-image

Impaired **Social** interaction/social isolation r/t forced separation from peers

Ineffective **Coping** r/t inability to establish personal and peer identity secondary to threat of being different or not being, inability to achieve maturational tasks

*See Child with Chronic Condition; Hospitalized Child*

## TERMINALLY ILL CHILD, INFANT/TODDLER

Ineffective **Coping** r/t separation from parents and familiar environment

T

secondary to inability to grasp external meaning of death

*See Child with Chronic Condition*

### TERMINALLY ILL CHILD, PRESCHOOL CHILD

**Fear** r/t perceived punishment, bodily harm, feelings of guilt secondary to magical thinking (i.e., believing that thoughts cause events)

*See Child with Chronic Condition*

### TERMINALLY ILL CHILD, SCHOOL-AGE CHILD/ PREADOLESCENT

**Fear** r/t perceived punishment, body mutilation, feelings of guilt

*See Child with Chronic Condition*

### TERMINALLY ILL CHILD/DEATH OF CHILD, PARENT

Anticipatory **Grieving** r/t possible, expected, or imminent death of child

Compromised family **Coping** r/t inability or unwillingness to discuss impending death and feelings with child or to support child through terminal stages of illness

Decisional **Conflict** r/t continuation or discontinuation of treatment, do not resuscitate decision, ethical issues regarding organ donation

Disturbed **Sleep** pattern r/t grieving process

**Grieving** r/t death of child

**Hopelessness** r/t overwhelming stresses secondary to terminal illness

Impaired **Parenting** r/t risk for overprotection of surviving siblings

Impaired **Social** interaction r/t dysfunctional grieving

Ineffective **Denial** r/t dysfunctional grieving

Interrupted **Family** processes r/t situational crisis

**Powerlessness** r/t inability to alter course of events

Readiness for enhanced family **Coping** r/t impact of crisis on family values, priorities, goals, or relationships; expressed interest or desire to attach meaning to child's life and death

Risk for dysfunctional **Grieving** r/t prolonged, unresolved, obstructed progression through stages of grief and mourning

**Social** isolation: imposed by others r/t feelings of inadequacy in providing support to grieving parents

**Social** isolation: self-imposed r/t unresolved grief, perceived inadequate parenting skills

**Spiritual** distress r/t sudden and unexpected death, prolonged suffering before death, questioning the death of youth, questioning the meaning of one's own existence

### TETRALOGY OF FALLOT

*See Congenital Heart Disease/ Cardiac Anomalies*

### THERAPEUTIC REGIMEN, EFFECTIVE MANAGEMENT

Effective **Therapeutic** regimen management r/t appropriate choices of daily activities for meeting goals of a treatment or prevention program, illness symptoms within normal range of expectation, verbalization of desire to manage treatment of illness and prevention of sequelae, verbalization of intent to reduce risk factors for progression of illness and sequelae

### THERAPEUTIC REGIMEN, INEFFECTIVE MANAGEMENT

Ineffective **Therapeutic** regimen management r/t perceived barriers, social support deficits, powerlessness; perceived susceptibility, perceived benefits; mistrust of regimen and/or health care personnel, knowl-

T

edge deficit, family patterns of health care, family conflict, excessive demands made on individual or family, economic difficulties; decisional conflicts, complexity of therapeutic regimen, complexity of health care system, faulty perception of illness seriousness, inadequate number and types of cues to action

## THERAPEUTIC REGIMEN, INEFFECTIVE MANAGEMENT: COMMUNITY

Ineffective community **Therapeutic** regimen management r/t illness symptoms above the norm expected for the number and type of population, unexpected acceleration of illness(es), number of health care resources insufficient for the incidence or prevalence of illness(es), deficits in advocates for aggregates, deficits in people and programs to be accountable for illness care of aggregates, deficits in community activities for secondary and tertiary prevention, unavailable health care resources for illness care

## THERAPEUTIC REGIMEN, INEFFECTIVE MANAGEMENT: FAMILY

Ineffective family **Therapeutic** regimen management r/t complexity of health care system, complexity of therapeutic regimen, decisional conflicts, economic difficulties, excessive demands on individual or family, family conflict

## THERAPEUTIC REGIMEN MANAGEMENT, READINESS FOR ENHANCED

Readiness for enhanced **Therapeutic** regimen management r/t the following: expresses desire to manage the treatment of illness and prevention of sequelae, makes choices of daily living that are appropriate for meeting the goals of treatment or prevention, expresses little to no difficulty with

regulation/integration of one or more prescribed regimens for treatment of illness or prevention of complications, describes reduction of risk factors for progression of illness and sequelae, shows no unexpected acceleration of illness symptoms

## THERAPEUTIC TOUCH

Disturbed **Energy** field r/t low energy levels, disturbance in energy fields, pain, depression, fatigue

## THERMOREGULATION, INEFFECTIVE

Ineffective **Thermoregulation** r/t aging, fluctuating environmental temperature, immaturity trauma or illness

## THORACENTESIS

*See Pleural Effusion*

## THORACOTOMY

**Activity** intolerance r/t pain, imbalance between oxygen supply and demand, presence of chest tubes

Acute **Pain** r/t surgical procedure, coughing, deep breathing

Deficient **Knowledge** r/t self-care, effective breathing exercises, pain relief

Ineffective **Airway** clearance r/t drowsiness, pain with breathing and coughing

Ineffective **Breathing** pattern r/t decreased energy, fatigue, pain

Risk for **Infection** r/t invasive procedure

Risk for **Injury** r/t disruption of closed-chest drainage system

Risk for perioperative positioning **Injury** r/t lateral positioning, immobility

## THOUGHT DISORDERS

Disturbed **Thought** processes r/t disruption in cognitive thinking, processing

*See Schizophrenia*

## THOUGHT PROCESSES, DISTURBED

Disturbed **Thought** processes r/t head injury, mental disorder, personality disorder, organic mental disorder, substance abuse, severe interpersonal conflict, sleep deprivation, sensory deprivation or overload, impaired cerebral perfusion

## THROMBOCYTOPENIC PURPURA

*See ITP (Idiopathic Thrombocytopenic Purpura)*

## THROMBOPHLEBITIS

Acute **Pain** r/t vascular inflammation, edema

**Constipation** r/t inactivity, bed rest

Deficient **Diversional** activity r/t bed rest

Deficient **Knowledge** r/t pathophysiology of condition, self-care needs, treatment regimen and outcome

Delayed **Surgical** recovery r/t complication associated with inactivity

Impaired physical **Mobility** r/t pain in extremity, forced bed rest

Ineffective **Tissue** perfusion: peripheral r/t interruption of venous blood flow

Risk for **Injury** r/t possible embolus

Sedentary lifestyle r/t deficient knowledge of benefits of physical exercise

*See Anticoagulant Therapy*

## THYROIDECTOMY

Risk for altered verbal **Communication** r/t edema, pain, vocal cord of laryngeal nerve damage

Risk for ineffective **Airway** clearance r/t edema or hematoma formation, airway obstruction

Risk for **Injury** r/t possible parathyroid damage or removal

*See Surgery, Preoperative Care; Surgery, Perioperative Care; Surgery, Postoperative Care*

## TIA (TRANSIENT ISCHEMIC ATTACK)

Acute **Confusion** r/t hypoxia

**Health-seeking** behaviors r/t obtaining knowledge regarding treatment, prevention of inadequate oxygenation

Ineffective **Tissue** perfusion: cerebral r/t lack of adequate oxygen supply to brain

Risk for decreased **Cardiac** output r/t dysrhythmia contributing to inadequate oxygen supply to brain

Risk for **Falls** r/t hypoxia

Risk for **Injury** r/t possible syncope

*See Syncope*

## TIC DISORDER

*See Tourette's Syndrome (TS)*

## TINEA CAPITIS

*See Ringworm of Scalp*

## TINEA CORPORIS

*See Ringworm of Body*

## TINEA CRURIS

*See Jock Itch; Itching*

## TINEA PEDIS

*See Athlete's Foot; Itching*

## TINEA UNGUIUM (ONYCHOMYCOSIS)

*See Ringworm of Nails*

T

## TINNITUS

Disturbed **Sensory** perception: auditory r/t altered sensory reception, transmission, integration

Ineffective **Health** maintenance r/t deficient knowledge regarding self-care with tinnitus

## TISSUE DAMAGE, CORNEAL, INTEGUMENTARY, OR SUBCUTANEOUS

Impaired **Tissue** integrity r/t mechanical irritants (pressure, shear, friction); radiation (including therapeutic radiation); nutritional deficit or excess; thermal irritants (temperature extremes); knowledge deficit; irritants; chemical (including body excretions; secretions, medications); impaired physical mobility; altered circulation; fluid deficit or excess

## TISSUE PERFUSION, DECREASED

Ineffective **Tissue** perfusion r/t hypovolemia, hypervolemia; interruption of flow, arterial; exchange problems; interruption of flow, venous; mechanical reduction of venous and/or arterial blood flow; hypoventilation; impaired transport of oxygen across alveolar and/or capillary membrane; mismatch of ventilation with blood flow; decreased hemoglobin concentration in blood; enzyme poisoning; altered affinity of hemoglobin for oxygen

## TOCOLYTIC THERAPY

Ineffective **Health** maintenance r/t deficient knowledge regarding management of preterm labor, treatment regimen

Risk for **Fluid** volume excess r/t effects of tocolytic drugs

*See Preterm Labor*

## TOILET TRAINING

**Health-seeking** behaviors: bladder/bowel training r/t achievement of developmental milestone secondary to enhanced parenting skills

## TOILETING PROBLEMS

Impaired **Transfer** ability r/t neuromuscular deficits

**Self-care** deficit: toileting r/t impaired transfer ability, impaired mobility status, intolerance of activity, neuromuscular impairment, cognitive impairment

## TONSILLECTOMY AND ADENOIDECTOMY

*See T & A (Tonsillectomy and Adenoidectomy)*

## TOOTHACHE

Acute **Pain** r/t inflammation/infection

Impaired **Dentition** r/t ineffective oral hygiene, barriers to self-care, economic barriers to professional care, nutritional deficits, lack of knowledge regarding dental health

## TOTAL ANOMALOUS PULMONARY VENOUS RETURN

*See Congenital Heart Disease/Cardiac Anomalies*

## TOTAL JOINT REPLACEMENT (TOTAL HIP/TOTAL KNEE/SHOULDER)

Acute **Pain** r/t possible edema, physical injury, surgery

Deficient **Knowledge** r/t self-care, treatment regimen, outcomes

Disturbed **Body** image r/t large scar, presence of prosthesis

Impaired physical **Mobility** r/t musculoskeletal impairment, surgery, prosthesis

Risk for **Infection** r/t invasive procedure, anesthesia, immobility

Risk for **Injury**: neurovascular r/t altered peripheral tissue perfusion, altered mobility, prosthesis

*See Surgery, Perioperative Care; Surgery, Postoperative Care; Surgery, Preoperative Care*

## TOTAL PARENTERAL NUTRITION

*See TPN (Total Parenteral Nutrition)*

## TOTAL URINARY INCONTINENCE

Total urinary **Incontinence** r/t neuropathy preventing transmission of reflex indication bladder fullness; trauma or disease affecting spinal cord nerves; anatomic (fistula); independent contraction of detrusor reflex due to surgery; neurological dysfunction causing triggering of micturition at unpredictable times

## TOURETTE'S SYNDROME (TS)

**Hopelessness** r/t inability to control behavior

Risk for situational low **Self-esteem** r/t uncontrollable behavior, motor/phonic tics

*See Attention Deficit Disorder*

## TOXEMIA

*See PIH (Pregnancy-Induced Hypertension/Preeclampsia)*

## TPN (TOTAL PARENTERAL NUTRITION)

Imbalanced **Nutrition**: less than body requirements r/t inability to ingest or digest food or absorb nutrients as a result of biological or psychological factors

Risk for **Fluid** volume excess r/t rapid administration of TPN

Risk for **Infection** r/t concentrated glucose solution, invasive administration of fluids

## TRACHEOESOPHAGEAL FISTULA

Imbalanced **Nutrition**: less than body requirements r/t difficulties in swallowing

Ineffective **Airway** clearance r/t aspiration of feeding secondary to inability to swallow

Risk for **Aspiration** r/t common passage of air and food

*See Respiratory Conditions of the Neonate; Hospitalized Child*

## TRACHEOSTOMY

Acute **Pain** r/t edema, surgical procedure

**Anxiety** r/t impaired verbal communication, ineffective airway clearance

Deficient **Knowledge** r/t self-care, home maintenance management

Disturbed **Body** image r/t abnormal opening in neck

Impaired verbal **Communication** r/t presence of mechanical airway

Risk for **Aspiration** r/t presence of tracheostomy

Risk for ineffective **Airway** clearance r/t increased secretions, mucous plugs

Risk for **Infection** r/t invasive procedure, pooling of secretions

## TRACTION AND CASTS

Acute **Pain** r/t immobility, injury, or disease

**Constipation** r/t immobility

Deficient **Diversional** activity r/t immobility

Impaired physical **Mobility** r/t imposed restrictions on activity secondary to bone or joint disease injury

Impaired **Transfer** ability r/t presence of traction, casts

Risk for **Disuse** syndrome r/t mechanical immobilization

Risk for impaired **Skin** integrity r/t contact of traction or cast with skin

Risk for **Peripheral** neurovascular dysfunction r/t mechanical compression

**Self-care** deficit: feeding, dressing/grooming, bathing/hygiene, toileting r/t degree of impaired physical mobility, body area affected by traction or cast

T

## TRANSFER ABILITY

Impaired **Transfer** ability r/t intolerance of activity, decreased strength and endurance, pain or discomfort, perceptual or cognitive impairment, neuromuscular impairment, musculoskeletal impairment, depression, severe anxiety

## TRANSIENT ISCHEMIC ATTACK

*See TIA (Transient Ischemic Attack)*

## TRANSPOSITION OF GREAT VESSELS

*See Congenital Heart Disease/Cardiac Anomalies*

## TRANSURETHRAL RESECTION OF THE PROSTATE

*See TURP (Transurethral Resection of the Prostate)*

## TRAUMA IN PREGNANCY

Acute **Pain** r/t trauma

**Anxiety** r/t threat to self or fetus, unknown outcome

Deficient **Knowledge** r/t lack of exposure to situation

Impaired **Skin** integrity r/t trauma

Risk for deficient **Fluid** volume r/t blood loss

Risk for fetal **Injury** r/t premature separation of placenta

Risk for **Infection** r/t traumatized tissue

## TRAUMA, RISK FOR

### INTERNAL

Risk for **Trauma** r/t lack of safety education, insufficient finances to purchase safety equipment or effect repairs, history of previous trauma, lack of safety precautions, poor vision, reduced temperature and/or tactile sensation, balancing difficulties, cognitive or emotional difficulties, reduced large or small muscle coordination, weakness, reduced hand-eye coordination

### EXTERNAL

Risk for **Trauma** r/t high-crime neighborhood and vulnerable clients; pot handles facing toward front of stove; knives stored uncovered; inappropriate call-for-aid mechanisms for bed-resting client; inadequately stored combustibles or corrosives (e.g., matches, oily rags, lye); highly flammable children's toys or clothing; obstructed passageways; high beds; large icicles hanging from the roof; nonuse or misuse of seat restraints; overexposure to sun, sun lamps, radiotherapy; overloaded electrical outlets; overloaded fuse boxes; play or work near vehicle pathways (e.g., driveways, lanes, railroad tracks); playing with fireworks of gunpowder; guns or ammunition stored unlocked; contact with rapidly moving machinery, industrial belts, or pulleys; litter of liquid spills on floor or stairways; defective appliances; bathing in very hot water (e.g., unsupervised bathing of young children); bathtub without hand grip or antislip equipment; children playing with matches, candles, cigarettes, sharp-edged toys; children playing without gates at top of stairs; children riding in the front seat in car; delayed lighting of gas burner or oven; contact with intense cold; grease waste collected on stoves; driving a mechanically unsafe vehicle; driving after partaking of alcoholic beverages or drugs; driving at excessive speeds; entering unlighted rooms; experimenting with chemical or gasoline; exposure to dangerous machinery; faulty electrical plugs; frayed wires; contact with acids or alkalis; unsturdy or absent stair rails; use of unsteady ladders or chairs; use of cracked dishware or glasses; wearing plastic apron or flowing clothes around open flame; unscreened fires or heaters; unsafe window protection in homes with young children; sliding on coarse bed linen or struggling within bed restraints; use of thin or worn potholders; unanchored electric wires; misuse of necessary headgear for motorized cyclists or young children carried on adult bicycles; potential igniting of gas leaks; unsafe road or road crossing conditions; slippery floors (e.g., wet or highly waxed); smoking in bed or near oxygen; snow or ice collected on stairs, walkways; unanchored rugs; driving without necessary visual aids

## TRAUMATIC BRAIN INJURY (TBI)

*See TBI (Traumatic Brain Injury); Intracranial Pressure, Increased*

## TRAUMATIC EVENT

**Post-trauma** syndrome r/t previously experienced trauma

## TRAVELER'S DIARRHEA

*See TD (Traveler's Diarrhea)*

## TREMBLING OF HANDS

**Anxiety/Fear** r/t threat to or change in health status, threat of death, situational crisis

## TRICUSPID ATRESIA

*See Congenital Heart Disease/Cardiac Anomalies*

## TRIGEMINAL NEURALGIA

Acute **Pain** r/t irritation of trigeminal nerve

Imbalanced **Nutrition**: less than body requirements r/t pain when chewing

Ineffective **Therapeutic** regimen management r/t deficient knowledge regarding prevention of stimuli that trigger pain

Risk for **Injury** (eye) r/t possible decreased corneal sensation

## TRUNCUS ARTERIOSUS

*See Congenital Heart Disease/Cardiac Anomalies*

## TS (TOURETTE'S SYNDROME)

*See Tourette's Syndrome (TS)*

## TSE (TESTICULAR SELF-EXAMINATION)

**Health-seeking** behavior r/t procedure for doing testicular self-examinations

## TUBAL LIGATION

Decisional **Conflict** r/t tubal sterilization

*See Laparoscopy*

## TUBE FEEDING

Risk for **Aspiration** r/t improperly administered feeding, improper placement of tube, improper positioning of client during and after feeding, excessive residual feeding or lack of digestion, altered gag reflex

Risk for deficient **Fluid** volume r/t inadequate water administration with concentrated feeding

Risk for imbalanced **Nutrition**: less than body requirements r/t intolerance to tube feeding, inadequate calorie replacement to meet metabolic needs

## TUBERCULOSIS

*See TB (Pulmonary Tuberculosis)*

## TURP (TRANSURETHRAL RESECTION OF THE PROSTATE)

Acute **Pain** r/t incision, irritation from catheter, bladder spasms, kidney infection

Deficient **Knowledge** r/t postoperative self-care, home maintenance management

Risk for deficient **Fluid** volume r/t fluid loss, possible bleeding

Risk for **Infection** r/t invasive procedure, route for bacteria entry

T

Risk for urge urinary **Incontinence** r/t edema from surgical procedure

Risk for **Urinary** retention r/t obstruction of urethra or catheter with clots

## ULCER, PEPTIC (DUODENAL OR GASTRIC)

Acute **Pain** r/t irritated mucosa from acid secretion

**Fatigue** r/t loss of blood, chronic illness

Ineffective **Health** maintenance r/t lack of knowledge regarding health practices to prevent ulcer formation

**Nausea** r/t gastrointestinal irritation

*See GI Bleed (Gastrointestinal Bleeding)*

## ULCERATIVE COLITIS

*See Inflammatory Bowel Disease (Child and Adult)*

## ULCERS, STASIS

*See Stasis Ulcer*

## UNILATERAL NEGLECT OF ONE SIDE OF BODY

Unilateral **Neglect** r/t effects of disturbed perceptual abilities (e.g., hemianopia); neurological illness or trauma; one-sided blindness

## UNSANITARY LIVING CONDITIONS

Impaired **Home** maintenance r/t impaired cognitive or emotional functioning, lack of knowledge, insufficient finances

## URGENCY TO URINATE

Risk for urge urinary **Incontinence** r/t effects of alcohol, caffeine, decreased bladder capacity, irritation of bladder stretch receptors causing

spasm, increased urine concentration, overdistention of bladder

Urge urinary **Incontinence** r/t decreased bladder capacity, irritation of bladder stretch receptors causing spasm, alcohol, caffeine, increased fluids, increased urine concentration, overdistention of bladder

## URINARY DIVERSION

*See Ileal Conduit*

## URINARY ELIMINATION, ALTERED

Impaired **Urinary** elimination r/t anatomical obstruction, sensory motor impairment, urinary tract infection

## URINARY INCONTINENCE

*See Incontinence of Urine*

## URINARY READINESS

Readiness for enhanced **Urinary** elimination

## URINARY RETENTION

**Urinary** retention r/t high urethral pressure caused by weak detrusor, inhibition of reflex arc, strong sphincter, blockage

## URINARY TRACT INFECTION (UTI)

*See UTI (Urinary Tract Infection)*

## UROLITHIASIS

*See Kidney Stone*

## UTERINE ATONY IN LABOR

*See Dystocia*

## UTERINE ATONY IN POSTPARTUM

*See Postpartum Hemorrhage*

## UTERINE BLEEDING

*See Hemorrhage; Postpartum Hemorrhage; Shock*

## UTI (URINARY TRACT INFECTION)

Acute **Pain**: dysuria r/t inflammatory process in bladder

Impaired **Urinary** elimination: frequency r/t urinary tract infection

Ineffective **Health** maintenance r/t deficient knowledge regarding methods to treat and prevent UTIs

Risk for urge urinary **Incontinence** r/t hyperreflexia from cystitis

## VAGINAL HYSTERECTOMY

Risk for **Infection** r/t surgical site

Risk for **Perioperative** positioning injury r/t lithotomy position

Risk for urge urinary **Incontinence** r/t edema, congestion of pelvic tissues

**Urinary** retention r/t edema at surgical site

*See Postpartum Hemorrhage*

## VAGINITIS

Acute **Pain**: pruritus r/t inflamed tissues, edema

Ineffective **Health** maintenance r/t deficient knowledge regarding self-care with vaginitis

Ineffective **Sexuality** patterns r/t abstinence during acute stage, pain

Risk for **Infection** r/t spread of infection, risk of reinfection

## VAGOTOMY

*See Abdominal Surgery*

## VALUE SYSTEM CONFLICT

Decisional **Conflict** r/t unclear personal values/beliefs

Readiness for enhanced **Spiritual** well-being r/t desire for harmony with self, others, higher power/God

**Spiritual** distress r/t challenged value system

## VARICOSE VEINS

Chronic **Pain** r/t impaired circulation

Ineffective **Health** maintenance r/t deficient knowledge regarding health care practices, prevention, treatment regimen

Ineffective **Tissue** perfusion: peripheral r/t venous stasis

Risk for impaired **Skin** integrity r/t altered peripheral tissue perfusion

## VASCULAR DEMENTIA (FORMERLY CALLED *MULTIINFARCT DEMENTIA*)

*See Dementia*

## VASCULAR OBSTRUCTION—PERIPHERAL

Acute **Pain** r/t vascular obstruction

**Anxiety** r/t lack of circulation to body part

Ineffective **Tissue** perfusion: peripheral r/t interruption of circulatory flow

Risk for **Peripheral** neurovascular dysfunction r/t vascular obstruction

## VASECTOMY

Decisional **Conflict** r/t surgery as method of permanent sterilization

Effective **Therapeutic** regimen management r/t practices alternate forms of contraception until two to three sperm counts are negative

## VASOCOGNOPATHY

*See Alzheimer's Type Dementia*

## VENEREAL DISEASE

*See STD (Sexually Transmitted Disease)*

## VENTILATION, INABILITY TO SUSTAIN SPONTANEOUS

Impaired spontaneous **Ventilation** r/t respiratory muscle fatigue, metabolic factors

### VENTILATOR CLIENT

Dysfunctional **Ventilatory** weaning response r/t psychological, situational, physiological factors

**Fear** r/t inability to breathe on own, difficulty communicating

Impaired **Gas** exchange r/t ventilation-perfusion imbalance

Impaired spontaneous **Ventilation** r/t metabolic factors, respiratory muscle fatigue

Impaired verbal **Communication** r/t presence of endotracheal tube, decreased mentation

Ineffective **Airway** clearance r/t increased secretions, decreased cough and gag reflex

Ineffective **Breathing** pattern r/t decreased energy and fatigue secondary to possible altered nutrition: less than body requirements

**Powerlessness** r/t health treatment regimen

Risk for **Infection** r/t presence of endotracheal tube, pooled secretions

Risk for latex **Allergy** r/t repeated exposure to latex products

**Social** isolation r/t impaired mobility, ventilator dependence

*See Child with Chronic Condition; Hospitalized Child; Respiratory Conditions of the Neonate*

## VENTILATORY, DYSFUNCTIONAL WEANING RESPONSE (DVWR)

Dysfunctional **Ventilatory** weaning response r/t *Psychological:* Patient perceived inefficacy about the ability to wean; powerlessness; anxiety: moderate, severe; knowledge deficit of the weaning process, patient role; hopelessness; fear; decreased motivation; decreased self-esteem; insufficient trust in the nurse. *Situational:* Uncontrolled episodic energy demands or problems; history of multiple unsuccessful weaning attempts; adverse environment (e.g., noisy, active environment, negative events in the room, low nurse-patient ratio, extended nurse absence from bedside, unfamiliar nursing staff); history of ventilator dependence >4 days to 1 week; inappropriate pacing of diminished ventilator support; inadequate social support. *Physiological:* Inadequate nutrition, sleep pattern disturbance, uncontrolled pain or discomfort, ineffective airway clearance

## VENTRICULAR FIBRILLATION

*See Dysrhythmia*

## VERTIGO

Disturbed **Sensory** perception: kinesthetic r/t altered sensory reception, transmission, integration; medications

Ineffective **Tissue** perfusion: cerebral r/t decreased blood supply to brain

Risk for **Falls** r/t vertigo

Risk for **Injury** r/t disturbed sensory perception

## VIOLENT BEHAVIOR

Risk for other-directed **Violence** r/t body language; rigid posture, clenching of fists and jaw, hyperactivity, pacing, breathlessness, threatening stances; history of violence against others (e.g., hitting someone, kicking someone, spitting at someone, scratching someone, throwing objects at someone, biting someone, attempted rape, rape, sexual molestation, urinating/defecating on a person); history of threats of violence (e.g., verbal threats against property, verbal threats against person, social threats, cursing, threatening notes/letters, threatening gestures, sexual threats); history of violent antisocial behavior (e.g., stealing, insistent borrowing, insistent demands for privileges, insistent interruption of meetings, refusal to eat, refusal to take medication, ignoring instructions); history of violence, indirect (e.g., tearing of clothes, ripping objects off walls, writing on walls, urinating on floor, defecating on floor, stamping feet, temper tantrum, running in corridors, yelling, throwing objects, breaking a window, slamming doors, sexual advances); neurological impairment (e.g., positive EEG, CAT, MRI, neurological findings; head trauma; seizure disorders); cognitive impairment (e.g., learning disabilities, attention deficit/hyperactivity disorder, decreased intellectual functioning); history of childhood abuse; history of witnessing family violence; cruelty to animals, fire setting; pre/perinatal complications/abnormalities; history of drug/alcohol abuse/pathological intoxication; psychotic symptomatology (e.g., auditory, visual, command hallucinations; paranoid delusions; loose, rambling, or illogical thought processes); motor vehicle offenses (e.g., frequent traffic violations, use of a motor vehicle to release anger); suicidal behavior; impulsivity; availability/possession of weapon(s)

Risk for self-directed **Violence** r/t suicidal ideation (frequent, intense prolonged); suicidal plan (clear and specific lethality; method and availability of destructive means); history of multiple suicide attempts; behavioral clues (e.g., writing forlorn love notes, directing angry messages at a significant other who has rejected the person, giving away personal items,

taking out a large life insurance policy); verbal clues (e.g., talking about death, "better off without me," asking questions about lethal dosages of drugs); emotional status (hopelessness, despair, increased anxiety, panic, anger, hostility); mental health (severe depression, psychosis, severe personality disorder, alcoholism or drug abuse); physical health (hypochondriasis, chronic or terminal illness); employment (unemployed, recent job loss/failure; age 15 to 19; age over 45; marital status (single, widowed, divorced); occupation (executive, administrator/owner of business, professional, semiskilled worker); conflicting interpersonal relationships; family background (chaotic or conflicting, history of suicide); sexual orientation (bisexual [active], homosexual [inactive]); personal resources (poor insight, affect unavailable and poorly controlled); social resources (poor rapport, social isolated, unresponsive family); people who engage in autoerotic sexual acts

## VIRAL GASTROENTERITIS

**Diarrhea** r/t infectious process, rotavirus and Norwalk virus

Ineffective **Therapeutic** regimen management r/t inadequate handwashing

Ineffective community **Therapeutic** regimen management r/t contaminated food and/or water

*See Gastroenteritis, Child*

## VISION IMPAIRMENT

Disturbed **Sensory** perception r/t altered sensory reception associated with impaired vision

**Fear** r/t loss of sight

Risk for **Injury** r/t disturbed sensory perception

**Self-care** deficit: specify r/t perceptual impairment

V

**Social** isolation r/t altered state of wellness, inability to see

*See Blindness*

## VOMITING

**Nausea** r/t chemotherapy, postsurgical anesthesia, irritation to the gastrointestinal system, stimulation of neuropharmacological mechanisms

Risk for deficient **Fluid** volume r/t decreased intake, loss of fluids with vomiting

Risk for imbalanced **Nutrition**: less than body requirements r/t inability to ingest food

## VON RECKLINGHAUSE'S DISEASE

*See Neurofibromatosis*

## WALKING IMPAIRMENT

Impaired **Walking** r/t intolerance to activity, decreased strength and endurance, pain or discomfort, perceptual or cognitive impairment, neuromuscular impairment, musculoskeletal impairment, depression, severe anxiety, lower extremity amputation

## WANDERING

**Wandering** r/t cognitive impairment, specifically memory and recall deficits, disorientation, poor visuoconstructive (or visuospatial) ability, language (primarily expressive) defects; cortical atrophy; premorbid behavior (e.g., outgoing, sociable personality; premorbid dementia); separation from familiar people and places; sedation; emotional state, especially frustration, anxiety, boredom, or depression (agitation); overstimulating/understimulating social or physical environment; physiological state or need

(e.g., hunger/thirst, pain, urination, constipation); time of day

## WEAKNESS

**Fatigue** r/t decreased or increased metabolic energy production

Risk for **Falls** r/t weakness

## WEIGHT GAIN

Imbalanced **Nutrition**: more than body requirements r/t excessive intake in relation to metabolic need

## WEIGHT LOSS

Imbalanced **Nutrition**: less than body requirements r/t inability to ingest food because of biological, psychological, economic factors

## WELLNESS-SEEKING BEHAVIOR

**Health-seeking** behaviors r/t expressed desire for increased control of health practice

## WERNICKE KORSAKOFF SYNDROME

*See Korsakoff's Syndrome*

## WEST NILE VIRUS

Effective **Therapeutic** regimen management r/t avoid mosquito bites, use mosquito-repellant products containing DEET and wear long sleeves and pants, mosquito-proof the home, community spraying for mosquitos

*See Meningitis/Encephalitis*

## WHEELCHAIR USE PROBLEMS

Impaired wheelchair **Mobility** r/t intolerance to activity, decreased strength and endurance, pain or discomfort, perceptual or cognitive impairment, neuromuscular impairment, musculoskeletal impairment, depression, severe anxiety, amputation

W

## WHEEZING

Ineffective **Airway** clearance r/t tracheobronchial obstructions, secretions

## WILMS' TUMOR

Acute **Pain** r/t pressure from tumor

**Constipation** r/t obstruction associated with presence of tumor

*See Chemotherapy; Hospitalized Child; Radiation Therapy; Surgery, Preoperative Care; Surgery, Perioperative Care; Surgery, Postoperative Care*

## WITHDRAWAL FROM ALCOHOL

*See Alcohol Withdrawal*

## WITHDRAWAL FROM DRUGS

*See Drug Withdrawal*

## WOUND DEBRIDEMENT

Acute **Pain** r/t debridement of wound

Impaired **Tissue** integrity r/t debridement, open wound

Risk for **Infection** r/t open wound, presence of bacteria

## WOUND DEHISCENCE, EVISCERATION

**Fear** r/t client fear of body parts falling out, surgical procedure not going as planned

Imbalanced **Nutrition**: less than body requirements r/t inability to digest nutrients, need for increased protein for healing

Risk for deficient **Fluid** volume r/t inability to ingest nutrients, obstruction, fluid loss

Risk for delayed **Surgical** recovery r/t separation of wound, exposure of abdominal contents

Risk for **Injury** r/t exposed abdominal contents

## WOUND INFECTION

Disturbed **Body** image r/t dysfunctional open wound

**Hyperthermia** r/t increased metabolic rate, illness, infection

Imbalanced **Nutrition**: less than body requirements r/t biological factors, infection, hyperthermia

Impaired **Tissue** integrity r/t wound, presence of infection

Risk for deficient **Fluid** volume r/t increased metabolic rate

Risk for delayed **Surgical** recovery r/t presence of infection

Risk for **Infection**: spread of r/t imbalanced nutrition: less than body requirements

W

# Guide to Planning Care

# Activity intolerance

## NANDA Definition

Insufficient physiological or psychological energy to endure or complete required or desired daily activities

## Defining Characteristics

Verbal report of fatigue or weakness; abnormal heart rate or blood pressure response to activity; exertional discomfort or dyspnea; electrocardiographic changes reflecting dysrhythmias or ischemia

## Related Factors (r/t)

Bed rest or immobility; generalized weakness; sedentary lifestyle; imbalance between oxygen supply and demand

## Client Outcomes

### Client Will (Specify Time Frame):

- Participate in prescribed physical activity with appropriate increases in heart rate, blood pressure, and breathing rate; maintain monitor patterns (rhythm and ST segment) within normal limits.
- State symptoms of adverse effects of exercise and report on-set of symptoms immediately.
- Maintain normal skin color and keep skin warm and dry with activity.
- Verbalize an understanding of the need to gradually increase activity based on testing, tolerance, and symptoms.
- Express an understanding of the need to balance rest and activity.
- Demonstrate increased activity tolerance.

## Nursing Interventions

- Determine cause of activity intolerance (see Related Factors) and decide whether cause is physical, psychological, or motivational.

• = Independent          ▲ = Collaborative

- Assess client daily for appropriateness of activity and bed rest orders.
- If client is mainly on bed rest, minimize cardiovascular deconditioning by positioning the client in an upright position several times daily.
- If client is mostly immobile, consider use of a transfer chair—a chair that becomes a stretcher.
- When appropriate, gradually increase activity, allowing the client to assist with positioning, transferring, and self-care as possible. Progress from sitting in bed to dangling, to standing, to ambulation.
- When getting a client up, observe for symptoms of intolerance such as nausea, pallor, dizziness, visual dimming, and impaired consciousness, as well as changes in vital signs.
▲ If a client experiences syncope with activity, refer for evaluation by a physician.
- Perform range-of-motion exercises if the client is unable to tolerate activity or is mostly immobile.
- Monitor and record the client's ability to tolerate activity: note pulse rate, blood pressure, monitor pattern, dyspnea, use of accessory muscles, and skin color before and after activity. If the following signs and symptoms of cardiac decompensation develop, activity should be stopped immediately:
  - Onset of chest discomfort
  - Dyspnea
  - Palpitations
  - Excessive fatigue
  - Lightheadedness, confusion, ataxia, pallor, cyanosis, nausea, or any peripheral circulatory insufficiency
  - Dysrhythmia (symptomatic supraventricular tachycardia, ventricular tachycardia, exercise-induced intraventricular conduction defect, second- or third-degree atrioventricular block, frequent premature ventricular contractions)
  - Exercise hypotension (drop in systolic blood pressure

• = Independent          ▲ = Collaborative

A

of 10 mm Hg from baseline blood pressure despite an increase in workload)

- Excessive rise in blood pressure (systolic >180 mm Hg or diastolic >110 mm Hg) (NOTE: These are upper limits; activity may be stopped before these values are reached.)
- Inappropriate bradycardia (drop in heart rate >10 beats/min or <50 beats/min)
- Increased heart rate above 100 beats/min

▲ Instruct the client to stop the activity immediately and report to the physician if the following symptoms are experienced: new or worsened intensity or increased frequency of discomfort; tightness or pressure in chest, back, neck, jaw, shoulders, and/or arms; palpitations; dizziness; weakness; unusual and extreme fatigue; excessive air hunger.

• Observe and document skin integrity several times a day.

• Assess for constipation. If present, refer to care plan for **Constipation.**

▲ Refer the client to physical therapy to help increase activity levels and strength.

▲ Consider dietitian referral to assess nutritional needs related to activity intolerance. Recognize that undernutrition causes significant morbidity due to the loss of lean body mass.

• Identify the factors that contribute to undernutrition in hospital patients.

• Provide emotional support and encouragement to the client to gradually increase activity.

• Observe for pain before activity. If possible, treat pain before activity, and ensure that the client is not heavily sedated.

• Obtain any necessary assistive devices or equipment needed before ambulating the client (e.g., walkers, canes, crutches, portable oxygen).

• Use a gait walking belt when ambulating the client.

• Work with the client to set mutual goals that increase activity levels.

▲ If the client is scheduled for a surgical intervention that

• = Independent          ▲ = Collaborative

A

will result in bed rest in intensive care, consider referring to physical therapy for a prehabilitation program including warm-up, aerobic conditioning, strength building, and flexibility enhancement.

## Activity Intolerance Due to Respiratory Disease

- • If the client is able to walk and has chronic obstructive pulmonary disease (COPD), consider the use of an accelerometer to assess walking ability or use the traditional 6-minute walk distance.
- ▲ Ensure that the chronic pulmonary client has oxygen saturation testing with exercise. Use supplemental oxygen to keep oxygen saturation 90% or above or as prescribed with activity.
- • Monitor a COPD client's response to activity by observing for symptoms of respiratory intolerance such as increased dyspnea, loss of ability to control breathing rhythmically, use of accessory muscles, and skin tone changes such as pallor and cyanosis.
- • Instruct and assist a COPD client in using conscious controlled breathing techniques including pursing their lips and diaphragmatic breathing.
- ▲ Refer the COPD client to a pulmonary rehabilitation program.

## Activity Intolerance Due to Cardiovascular Disease

- • If the client is able to walk and has heart failure, consider use of the 6-minute walk test to determine physical ability.
- • Allow for periods of rest before and after planned exertion periods such as meals, baths, treatments, and physical activity.
- ▲ Refer to heart failure program or cardiac rehabilitation program for education, evaluation, and guided support to increase activity and rebuild life.

## Geriatric

- • Slow the pace of care. Allow the client extra time to carry out activities. Encourage families to help/allow an

• = Independent          ▲ = Collaborative

**A**

elderly client to be independent in whatever activities possible.

▲ If the client has heart disease causing activity intolerance, refer for cardiac rehabilitation.

▲ Refer the client to physical therapy for resistance exercise training as able, including exercises such as abdominal crunch, leg press, leg extension, leg curl, and calf press.

• When mobilizing the elderly client, watch for orthostatic hypotension accompanied by dizziness and fainting.

• Once the client is able to walk independently and needs an exercise program, suggest the client enter an exercise program with a friend.

## Home Care

▲ Begin discharge planning as soon as possible with case manager or social worker to assess the need for home support systems and the need for community or home health services.

▲ Assess the home environment for factors that precipitate or contribute to decreased activity tolerance: stairs; lack of assistive bed or bathroom devices; distance to bathroom; presence of allergens such as dust, smoke, and those associated with pets; home temperature; energy-intensive activity patterns; and furniture placement. Refer to occupational therapy if needed to assist the client in restructuring the home and the patterns of activities of daily living (ADL).

▲ Refer to physical therapy for strength training and possible weight training.

▲ Support strength training program prescribed by physical therapist.

• Normalize the client's activity intolerance; encourage progress with positive feedback. The client's experience should be validated within expected norms. Recognition of progress enhances motivation.

• Teach the client/family the importance of and methods for setting priorities for activities, especially those having a high energy demand (e.g., home/family events). In-

• = Independent          ▲ = Collaborative

struct in realistic expectations. The client and/or family may assume a more rapid rate of energy recovery than actually occurs. Assistance may be needed to ensure accuracy of expectations for the client.

- Provide the client/family with resources such as senior centers, exercise classes, educational and recreational programs, and volunteer opportunities that can aid in promoting socialization and appropriate activity.
- Discuss the importance of sexual activity as part of daily living. Instruct the client in adaptive techniques to conserve energy during sexual interactions.
- Instruct the client and family in the importance of maintaining proper nutrition, rest, and behavioral pacing for energy conservation and rehabilitation. Instruct in use of dietary supplements as indicated.
▲ Refer to medical social services as necessary to assist the family in adjusting to major changes in patterns of living.
- Assess the need for long-term support for optimal activity tolerance of priority activities (e.g., assistive devices, oxygen, medication, catheters, massage), especially for a hospice client. Evaluate intermittently.
▲ Refer to home health aide services to support the client and family through changing levels of activity tolerance. Introduce aide support early. Instruct the aide to promote independence in activity as tolerated.
- Be aware of increased risk of bone fracture even after muscle strength is normalized, especially in osteoporosis-prone individuals such as estrogen-deficient women and the elderly.
- Allow terminally ill clients and their families to guide care.
- Provide increased attention to comfort and dignity for the terminally ill client in care planning.
- Institute case management of frail elderly to support continued independent living.
▲ In the presence of psychiatric illness, refer to psychiatric home health care services for client reassurance and implementation of a therapeutic regimen.

• = Independent          ▲ = Collaborative

A

## Client/Family Teaching

- Instruct the client on the reasons and techniques for avoiding inactivity.
- Teach the client to use controlled breathing techniques with activity.
- Teach the client the importance and proper technique for coughing and clearing secretions.
- Instruct the client in the use of relaxation techniques during activity.
- Help the client with energy conservation and work simplification techniques in ADLs.
- Teach the client the importance of proper nutrition.
- Describe to the client the symptoms of activity intolerance, including which symptoms to report to the physician.
- Explain to the client how to use assistive devices or medications before or during activity.
- Help the client develop an activity log to record exercise and exercise tolerance.

# Risk for Activity intolerance

## NANDA Definition

At risk for experiencing insufficient physiological or psychological energy to endure or complete required or desired daily activities

## Risk Factors

History of intolerance to activity; deconditioned status; presence of circulatory or respiratory problems; inexperience with activity

## Related Factors (r/t)

See Risk Factors.

## Client Outcomes, Nursing Interventions, and Client/Family Teaching

See care plan for **Activity intolerance.**

• = Independent        ▲ = Collaborative

# Impaired Adjustment

A

## NANDA Definition

Inability to modify lifestyle/behavior in a manner consistent with a change in health status

## Defining Characteristics

Denial of health status change; failure to take actions that would prevent further health problems; failure to achieve optimal sense of control; demonstration of nonacceptance of health status change

## Related Factors (r/t)

Low state of optimism; intense emotional state; negative attitudes toward health behavior; absence of intent to change behavior; multiple stressors; absence of social support for changed beliefs and practices; disability or health status change requiring change in lifestyle; lack of motivation to change behaviors

## Client Outcomes

### Client Will (Specify Time Frame):

- State acceptance of change in health status.
- Request assistance in altering behaviors to adapt to change.
- State personal goals for dealing with change in health status and means to prevent further health problems.
- State experience of a period of grief that is proportional to the actual or perceived effect of the loss.
- Report and/or demonstrate behavioral changes mutually agreed upon with nurse as evidence of positive adaptation.

## Nursing Interventions

- Assess the client's perception about the illness/event. Ask the client to state feelings related to the change in health status.
- Assess the client and family for the presence of addi-

• = Independent          ▲ = Collaborative

**A**

tional stressors (e.g., financial difficulty, health of other family members, occupational changes).

- Assess the client's feelings about whether change in health status is personally being dealt with effectively.
- Assess for negative affect and internalization of problems.
- Assess the socioeconomic status of all clients.
- Allow the client adequate time to express feelings about the change in health status.
- Help the client work through the stages of grief. Denial is usually the initial response. Acknowledge that grief takes time, and give the client permission to grieve; accept crying.
- Recognize that denial may be adaptive at certain stages of a threatening encounter.
- Discuss resources (e.g., the client's support system) that have worked previously when dealing with changes in lifestyle or health status.
▲ Refer to community resources. Provide general and contact information for ease of use.
- Use open-ended questions to allow the client free expression (e.g., "Tell me about your last hospitalization" or "How does this time compare?").
- Discuss the client's current goals. If appropriate, have the client list goals so that they can be referred to and steps can be taken to accomplish them.
- List the client activities that may require assistance and those that can be performed independently.
- Allow the client choices in daily care, particularly choices that result from the change in health status.
- Allow the client time to adjust to new situations. Introduce new material gradually to prevent overload. Ask for frequent feedback.
- Give the client positive feedback for accomplishments, no matter how small.
- Manipulate the environment to decrease stress; allow the client to display personal items that have meaning.
- Maintain consistency and continuity in daily schedule. When possible, provide the same caregiver.

● = Independent          ▲ = Collaborative

- Foster communication between the client/family and medical staff.
- Promote use of positive spiritual influences.

### Geriatric

- ▲ Assess for signs of depression resulting from illness-associated changes and make appropriate referral.
- Monitor the client for agitation.
- Increase and mobilize support available to the elderly client. Encourage interaction with family and friends.

### Multicultural

- Assess for the influence of cultural beliefs, norms, and values on the client's ability to modify health behavior.
- Encourage spirituality as a source of support for coping.
- Discuss with the client those aspects of his or her health behavior/lifestyle that will remain unchanged by his or her health status.
- Negotiate with the client regarding the aspects of health behavior that will need to be modified.
- Assess the role of fatalism in the client's ability to modify health behavior.
- Identify which family members the client can rely on for support.
- Validate the client's feelings regarding the impact of health status on current lifestyle.
- ▲ Assess for signs of depression and level of social support and make appropriate referrals.

### Home Care

- Include a spiritual assessment in the overall assessment of client and family resources.
- ▲ Refer to medical social services to facilitate the listed interventions and support client care goals.
- Assess affective climate within family and family support system.
- ▲ Observe for signs of caregiver stress on an ongoing basis. Refer to necessary support services.
- ▲ Refer the client to counselor or therapist for follow-up

• = Independent          ▲ = Collaborative

**A**

care. Initiate community referrals as needed (e.g., grief counseling, self-help groups).
- Assist client to recognize and exercise power in using self-care management to adjust to health change. Refer to care plan for **Powerlessness.**
- Take the client's perspective into consideration, and use a holistic approach in assessing and responding to client planning for the future.

## Client/Family Teaching

- Assess family/caregivers for coping and teaching/learning styles.
- Teach the client to maintain a positive outlook by listing current strengths.
- Teach the client and his or her family relaxation techniques (controlled breathing, guided imagery) and help them practice.
- Allow the client to proceed at own pace in learning; provide time for return demonstrations (e.g., self-injection of insulin).
- Involve significant others in planning and teaching.
- If long-term deficits are expected, inform the family as soon as possible.
- Teach family members intervention techniques such as setting limits, communicating acceptable behavior, and having time-outs.
- Educate and prepare families regarding the appearance of the client and the environment before initial exposure.

# Ineffective Airway clearance

## NANDA Definition

Inability to clear secretions or obstructions from the respiratory tract to maintain a clear airway

● = Independent          ▲ = Collaborative

## Defining Characteristics

Dyspnea; diminished breath sounds; orthopnea; adventitious breath sounds (crackles, wheezes); cough, ineffective or absent; sputum production; cyanosis; difficulty vocalizing; wide-eyed; changes in respiratory rate and rhythm; restlessness

## Related Factors (r/t)

### Environmental

Smoking; smoke inhalation; second-hand smoke; obstructed airway; airway spasm; retained secretions; excessive mucus; presence of artificial airway; foreign body in airway; secretions in bronchi; exudate in alveoli

### Physiological

Neuromuscular dysfunction; hyperplasia of bronchial walls; COPD; infection; asthma; allergic airways

## Client Outcomes

### Client Will (Specify Time Frame):

- Demonstrate effective coughing and clear breath sounds; be free of cyanosis and dyspnea.
- Maintain a patent airway at all times.
- Relate methods to enhance secretion removal.
- Relate the significance of changes in sputum to include color, character, amount, and odor.
- Identify and avoid specific factors that inhibit effective airway clearance.

## Nursing Interventions

- Auscultate breath sounds every 1 to 4 hours. Breath sounds are normally clear or scattered fine crackles at bases, which clear with deep breathing.
- Monitor respiratory patterns, including rate, depth, and effort. A normal respiratory rate for an adult without dyspnea is 12 to 16 respirations/min.
- Monitor blood gas values and pulse oxygen saturation levels as available. An oxygen saturation less than 90%

• = Independent          ▲ = Collaborative

A

(normal: 95% to 100%) or a partial pressure of oxygen less than 80 (normal: 80 to 100) indicates significant oxygenation problems.

- Position the client to optimize respiration (e.g., head of bed elevated 45 degrees and patient repositioned at least every 2 hours).
- If the client has unilateral lung disease, alternate a semi-Fowler's position with a lateral position (with a 10- to 15-degree elevation and "good lung down") for 60 to 90 minutes. This method is contraindicated for a client with a pulmonary abscess or hemorrhage or with interstitial emphysema.
- Help the client to deep breathe and perform controlled coughing. Have the client inhale deeply, hold breath for several seconds, and cough two or three times with mouth open while tightening the upper abdominal muscles.
- If the client has COPD, cystic fibrosis, or bronchiectasis, consider helping the client use the forced expiratory technique—the "huff cough." The client performs a series of coughs while saying the word "huff."
- Encourage the client to use an incentive spirometer.
- Assist with clearing secretions from pharynx by offering tissues and gentle suction of the oropharynx if necessary.
- Observe sputum, noting color, odor, and volume.
- When suctioning an endotracheal tube or tracheostomy tube for a client on a ventilator, do the following:
  - Explain the process of suctioning before the procedure and ensure the client is not in pain or overly anxious.
  - Hyperoxygenate before and between endotracheal suction sessions.
  - Use a closed, in-line suction system.
  - Avoid saline instillation during suctioning.
  - Document results of coughing and suctioning, particularly client tolerance and secretion characteristics such as color, odor, and volume.
- Provide oral care every 4 hours using a toothbrush.

• = Independent        ▲ = Collaborative

A

- Encourage activity and ambulation as tolerated. If unable to ambulate the client, turn the client from side to side at least every 2 hours.
- If client is intubated, consider use of kinetic therapy, using a kinetic bed that slowly moves the client with 40-degree turns.
- Encourage fluid intake of up to 2500 ml/day within cardiac or renal reserve.
▲ Administer oxygen as ordered.
▲ Administer medications such as bronchodilators or inhaled steroids as ordered.
▲ Provide postural drainage, percussion, and vibration only as ordered.
▲ Refer for physical therapy or respiratory therapy for further treatment.

## Geriatric

- Encourage ambulation as tolerated without causing exhaustion.
- Actively encourage the elderly to deep breathe and cough.
- Ensure adequate hydration within cardiac and renal reserves.

## Home Care

- Some of the above interventions may be adapted for home care use.
▲ Begin discharge planning with case manager or social worker as soon as possible to assess need for home support systems, assistive devices, and community or home health services.
- Assess home environment for factors that exacerbate airway clearance problems (e.g., presence of allergens, lack of adequate humidity in air, poor air flow, stressful family relationships).
- Assess affective climate within family and family support system. Refer to care plan for **Caregiver role strain.**
- Refer to GOLD and ACP-ASIM/ACCP guidelines for

A

COPD for management of home care and indications of hospital admission criteria.

- Provide the client with emotional support in dealing with symptoms of respiratory distress.
- When respiratory procedures (e.g., apneic monitoring for an infant) are being implemented, explain equipment and procedures to family members, and provide needed emotional support.
- When electrically based equipment for respiratory support is being implemented, evaluate the home environment for electrical safety or proper grounding, for example. Ensure that notification is sent to the local utility company, the emergency medical team, and the police and fire departments.
- Support clients' efforts at self-care. Ensure they have all the information they need to participate in care.
- Provide family with support for care of a client with chronic or terminal illness.
- Instruct the client to avoid exposure to persons with upper respiratory tract infections.
▲ Provide/teach percussion and postural drainage per physician orders. Teach adaptive breathing techniques.
- Determine client adherence to medical regimen. Instruct the client and family in importance of reporting effectiveness of current medications to physician.
- Teach the client when and how to use inhalant or nebulizer treatments at home.
- Teach the client/family importance of maintaining regimen and having necessary drugs easily accessible at all times.
- Teach the client/family the importance of and methods for setting priorities for activities, especially those having a high energy demand (e.g., home/family events). Instruct in realistic expectations.
- Instruct the client and family in the importance of maintaining proper nutrition, adequate fluids, rest, and be-

havioral pacing for energy conservation and rehabilitation.
- Instruct in use of dietary supplements as indicated.
- Identify an emergency plan, including criteria for use.
▲ Refer for home health aide services for assistance with ADLs.
▲ Assess family for role changes and coping skills. Refer to medical social services as necessary.
▲ Institute case management of frail elderly to support continued independent living.

## Client/Family Teaching

▲ Teach importance of not smoking. Be aggressive in approach, setting a date for smoking cessation and recommending nicotine replacement therapy (nicotine patch or gum). Refer to smoking cessation programs, and encourage clients who relapse to try again.
- Teach the client how to use a flutter clearance device if ordered, which vibrates to loosen mucus and gives positive pressure to keep airways open.
▲ Teach the client how to use a peak expiratory flow rate (PEFR) meter if ordered and when to seek medical attention if the PEFR reading drops. Also teach how to use metered dose inhalers and self-administer inhaled corticosteroids following precautions to decrease side effects.
- Teach the client how to deep breathe and cough effectively.
- Teach the client/family to identify and avoid specific factors that exacerbate ineffective airway clearance, including known allergens and especially smoking (if relevant) or exposure to second-hand smoke.
- Educate the client and family about the significance of changes in sputum characteristics, including color, character, amount, and odor.
- Teach the client/family the necessity of finishing entire prescription of antibiotics.

• = Independent          ▲ = Collaborative

**A**

# Latex Allergy Response

## NANDA Definition

An immunological reaction to natural latex rubber (NLR) products

## Defining Characteristics

**Type I reactions:** Immediate reactions (<1 hour) to latex proteins (can be life-threatening); contact urticaria progressing to generalized symptoms; edema of the lips, tongue, uvula, and/or throat; shortness of breath, tightness in chest, wheezing, bronchospasm leading to respiratory arrest; hypotension, syncope, cardiac arrest

**May also include:** Orofacial characteristics: edema of sclera or eyelids, erythema and/or itching of the eyes, tearing of the eyes, nasal congestion, itching and/or erythema, rhinorrhea, facial erythema, facial itching, oral itching; gastrointestinal characteristics: abdominal pain, nausea; generalized characteristics: flushing, general discomfort, generalized edema, increasing complaint of total body warmth, restlessness

**Type IV reactions:** Delayed onset (hours); eczema; irritation; reaction to additives (e.g., thiurams, carbamates) causes discomfort; redness

**Irritant reactions:** Erythema; chapped or cracked skin; blisters

## Related Factors (r/t)

No immune mechanism response

## Client Outcomes

### Client Will (Specify Time Frame):

- Identify presence of NRL allergy.
- List history of risk factors.
- Identify type of reaction.
- State reasons to avoid latex and to have a latex-safe environment.
- Experience a latex-safe environment for all health care procedures.

● = Independent          ▲ = Collaborative

A

- Avoid areas where there is powder from NRL gloves.
- Wear a Medic Alert bracelet and state the importance of wearing one.
- Carry an emergency kit with a supply of nonlatex gloves, antihistamines, and an autoinjectable epinephrine syringe (EpiPen), and state the importance of the kit.

## Nursing Interventions

- Identify clients at risk: those persons who are most likely to exhibit a sensitivity to NRL that may result in varying degrees of reactivity. Consider the following client groups:
  - Persons with neural tube defects, including spina bifida, myelomeningocele/meningocele
  - Children who have experienced three or more surgeries, particularly as a neonate
  - Children with chronic renal failure
  - Atopic individuals (persons with a tendency to have multiple allergic conditions), especially those with allergies to food products, such as bananas, avocados, celery, figs, chestnuts, papayas, potatoes, tomatoes, melons, and passion fruit
  - Persons who possess a known or suspected NRL allergy by having exhibited an allergic or anaphylactic reaction, positive skin testing, or positive immunoglobulin E (IgE) antibodies against latex
  - Persons who have had an ongoing occupational exposure to NRL, including health care workers, rubber industry workers, bakers, laboratory personnel, food handlers, hairdressers, janitors, policemen, and firefighters
- Take a thorough history of the client at risk.
- Question the client about associated symptoms of itching, swelling, and redness after contact with rubber products such as rubber gloves, balloons, and barrier contraceptives, or swelling of the tongue and lips after dental examinations.
- Consider a skin prick test with NRL extracts to identify IgE-mediated immunity.

• = Independent          ▲ = Collaborative

- All latex-sensitive clients are treated as if they have NRL allergy.
- Patients with spina bifida and others with a positive history of NRL sensitivity or NRL allergy should have all medical/surgical/dental procedures performed in a latex-controlled environment.
- The most effective approach to preventing NRL anaphylaxis is complete latex avoidance. Medications may reduce certain symptoms.
- Materials and items that contain NRL must be identified, and latex-free alternatives must be found.
- In health care settings, general use of latex gloves having negligible allergen content, powder-free latex gloves, and nonlatex gloves and medical articles should be considered in an effort to minimize exposure to latex allergen.
- ▲ If latex gloves are chosen for protection from blood or body fluids, a reduced-protein, powder-free glove should be selected.
- See Box II-1 for examples of products that may contain NRL and safe alternatives that are available.

## Home Care
- Assess the home environment for presence of NRL products (e.g., balloons, condoms, gloves, and products of related allergies, such as bananas, avocados, and poinsettia plants).
- At onset of care, assess client history and current status of NRL allergy response.
- ▲ Seek medical care as necessary.
- Do not use NRL products in caregiving.
- Assist the client in identifying and obtaining alternatives to NRL products.

## Client/Family Teaching
- Provide written information about NRL allergy and sensitivity.
- Instruct the client to inform health care professionals if

●  = Independent          ▲ = Collaborative

| BOX    II-I | Products That May Contain Latex and Latex-Free Alternatives Used in Healthcare Settings |
|---|---|

| Frequently Contain Latex | Latex-Free Alternative |
|---|---|
| Ace wraps | Ted hose, pneumatic boots |
| Airways | Hudson airways, oxygen masks |
| Ambu (bag-valve) masks (black or blue reusable) | Clear, disposable ambu bags |
| Band-Aids | Sterile dressing with plastic tape or Tegaderm |
| Blood pressure cuffs | Dura-Cuf Critikon Vital Answers or use over gown or stockinette |
| Catheter, indwelling | Silocone Foley (Kendall, Argyle, Baxter) |
| Catheter, straight | Plastic (Mentor, Bard) Double, triple lumen (Bard, Rusch) |
| Chux | Disposable underpads |
| Disposable gloves, latex, non-sterile | Sensicare gloves |
| Dressings—Moleskin, Micropore, Coban (3M) | Tegaderm (3M), Steri-strips |
| Electrode pads | 3M, Baxter electrocardiogram pads Dantec surface electrocardiogram pads |
| Endotracheal tubes | Mallinckrodt, Sheridan, Portex tube stylets Laryngeal mask airway |
| Gloves, sterile and exam, surgical and medical | Vinyl, neoprene gloves (Neolon, Tachylon, Tru-touch, Elastryn) |
| Heplock-PRN adapter | Use stopcock to inject medications |
| IV solutions and tubing systems | Baxter, Abbott, Walrus tubing Walrus anesthesia sets are latex-free Abbott IV fluid |

*Continued*

• = Independent       ▲ = Collaborative

A

| BOX II-I | Products That May Contain Latex and Latex-Free Alternatives Used in Healthcare Settings—cont'd |
|---|---|

| Frequently Contain Latex | Latex-Free Alternative |
|---|---|
| Medication syringes | Becton Dickinson angiocaths and syringes<br>Concord Portex, Bard syringes |
| Medication vial | Remove latex stopper |
| Oral and nasal airways | Hudson airways, oxygen masks |
| OR caps with elastic (bouffant) | Caps with ties |
| Oxygen tubing | Nasal, face mask |
| Stethoscope tubing | Do not let tubing touch patient, cover with web roll |
| Suction tubing | Mallinckrodt, Yankauer, Davol suction catheters |
| Tape—cloth, adhesive, paper | Plastic, silk, 3M Microfoam, Blenderm, Durapore |
| Tourniquets | Latex-free tourniquet (blue) |

Adapted from American Association of Nurse Anesthetists: *AANA latex protocol,* pp 1-9, Park Ridge, Ill, 1998, The Association; National Institute for Occupational Safety and Health: *Preventing allergic reactions to natural rubber latex in the workplace,* Cincinnati, July 1998, The Institute; Hepner DL, Castells MC: Latex allergy: an update, *Anesth Analg* 96(4):1219-1229, 2003.

he or she has an NRL allergy, particularly if scheduled for surgery.
- Teach the client what products contain NRL and to avoid direct contact with all latex products and foods that trigger allergic reactions.
- See Box II-2 for examples of products found in the community that may contain NRL and safe alternatives that are available.
- Teach the client to avoid areas where powdered latex gloves are used, and where latex balloons are inflated or deflated.

• = Independent          ▲ = Collaborative

| BOX II-2 | Latex Products and Safe Alternatives Outside of the Health Care Setting | A |
|---|---|---|

| Containing Latex | Latex-Free Alternative |
|---|---|
| Balloons | Mylar balloons |
| Balls, Koosh ball | Vinyl, Thornton sport ball |
| Belt for clothing | Leather or cloth belts |
| Beach shoes | Cotton socks |
| Bungee cords | Rope or twine |
| Cleaning/kitchen gloves | Vinyl gloves |
| Condoms | Polyurethane Avanti for males Polyurethane Reality for females |
| Crib mattress pads | Heavy cotton pads |
| Elastic bands | Paper clips, staples, twine |
| Elastic on legs, waist of clothing, disposable diapers, rubber pants | Velcro closures Cloth diapers |
| Halloween rubber masks | Plastic mask or water-based paints |
| Pacifiers | Plastic pacifier "The First Years" Silicone—Pur, Gerber, Soft-Flex |
| Racquet handles | Leather handles |
| Raincoats/slickers | Nylon or synthetic waterproof coats |
| Swim fins | Clear plastic fins |
| Telephone cords | Clear cords |

Adapted from American Association of Nurse Anesthetists: *AANA latex protocol*, pp 1-9, Park Ridge, Ill, 1998, The Association; National Institute for Occupational Safety and Health: *Preventing allergic reactions to natural rubber latex in the workplace*, Cincinnati, July 1998, The Institute; Hepner DL, Castells MC: Latex allergy: an update, *Anesth Analg* 96(4):1219-1229, 2003.

• = Independent        ▲ = Collaborative

**A**

- Instruct the client with NRL allergy to wear a medical identification bracelet and/or carry a medical identification card.
- Instruct the client to carry an emergency kit with a supply of nonlatex gloves, antihistamines, and an autoinjectable epinephrine syringe (EpiPen).

## Risk for Latex Allergy Response

### NANDA Definition

At risk for allergic response to natural rubber latex (NRL) products

### Risk Factors

Multiple surgical procedures, especially from infancy (e.g., spina bifida); allergies to bananas, avocados, tropical fruits, kiwis, chestnuts; professions with daily exposure to latex (e.g., medicine, nursing, dentistry); conditions associated with continuous or intermittent catheterization; history of reactions to latex (e.g., balloons, condoms, gloves); allergies to poinsettia plants; history of allergies and asthma

### Client Outcomes

**Client Will (Specify Time Frame):**

- State risk factors for NRL allergy.
- Request latex-free environment.
- Demonstrate knowledge of plan to treat NRL allergic reaction.

### Nursing Interventions

- Clients at high risk need to be identified, such as those with frequent bladder catheterizations, occupational exposure to latex, past history of atopy (hay fever, asthma, dermatitis, or food allergy to fruits such as ba-

● = Independent        ▲ = Collaborative

nanas, avocados, papayas, chestnuts, or kiwis); those with a history of anaphylaxis of uncertain etiology, especially if associated with surgery; health care workers; and females exposed to barrier contraceptives and routine examinations during gynecological and obstetric procedures.

- Clients with spina bifida are a high-risk group for NRL allergy and should remain latex-free from the first day of life.
- Children who are on home ventilation should be assessed for NRL allergy.
- Children with chronic renal failure should be assessed for NRL allergy.
- Assess for NRL allergy in clients who are exposed to "hidden" latex.
- See care plan for **Latex Allergy response.**

## Home Care

▲ Ensure that the client has a medical plan if a response develops. Prompt treatment decreases potential severity of response.
- See care plan for **Latex Allergy response.** Note client history and environmental assessment.

## Client/Family Teaching

▲ A client who has had symptoms of NRL allergy or who suspects he or she is allergic to latex should tell his or her employer and contact his or her institution's occupational health services.
- Provide written information about latex allergy and sensitivity.
- Health care workers should avoid the use of latex gloves and seek alternatives such as gloves made from nitrile.
- Health care institutions should develop prevention programs for the use of latex-free gloves and the absence of powdered gloves; they should also establish latex-safe areas in their facilities.

• = Independent        ▲ = Collaborative

# A Anxiety

## NANDA Definition

Anxiety is a vague, uneasy feeling of discomfort or dread accompanied by an autonomic response, with the source often nonspecific or unknown to the individual; it is a feeling of apprehension caused by anticipation of danger. Anxiety is an alerting signal that warns of impending danger and enables the individual to take measures to deal with a threat.

## Defining Characteristics

### Behavioral

Diminished productivity; scanning and vigilance; poor eye contact; restlessness; glancing about; extraneous movement (e.g., foot shuffling, hand/arm movements); expressed concerns due to change in life events; insomnia; fidgeting

### Affective

Regretful; irritability; anguish; scared; jittery; overexcited; painful and persistent increased helplessness; rattled; uncertainty; increased wariness; focus on self; feelings of inadequacy; fearful; distressed; worried or apprehensive; anxious

### Physiological

Voice quivering; trembling/hand tremors; shakiness; increased respiration (sympathetic); urinary urgency (parasympathetic); increased pulse (sympathetic); pupil dilation (sympathetic); increased reflexes (sympathetic); abdominal pain (parasympathetic); sleep disturbance (parasympathetic); tingling in extremities (parasympathetic); cardiovascular excitation (sympathetic); increased perspiration; facial tension; anorexia (sympathetic); heart pounding (sympathetic); diarrhea (parasympathetic); urinary hesitancy (parasympathetic); fatigue (parasympathetic); dry mouth (sympathetic); weakness (sympathetic); decreased pulse (parasympathetic); facial flushing (sympathetic); superficial vasoconstriction (sympathetic); twitching (sympathetic); decreased

• = Independent          ▲ = Collaborative

blood pressure (parasympathetic); nausea (parasympathetic); urinary frequency (parasympathetic); faintness (parasympathetic); respiratory difficulties (sympathetic); increased blood pressure (sympathetic)

## Cognitive
Blocking of thought; confusion; preoccupation; forgetfulness; rumination; impaired attention; decreased perceptual field; fear of unspecified consequences; tendency to blame others; difficulty concentrating; diminished ability to problem-solve and/or learn; awareness of physiological symptoms

## Related Factors (r/t)

Exposure to toxins; unconscious conflict about essential values/goals of life; familial association/heredity; unmet needs; interpersonal transmission/contagion; situational/maturational crises; threat of death; threat to self-concept; stress; substance abuse; threat to or change in role status, health status, interaction patterns, role function, environment, and/or economic status

## Client Outcomes

### Client Will (Specify Time Frame):

- Identify and verbalize symptoms of anxiety.
- Identify, verbalize, and demonstrate techniques to control anxiety.
- Verbalize absence of or decrease in subjective distress.
- Have vital signs that reflect baseline or decreased sympathetic stimulation.
- Have posture, facial expressions, gestures, and activity levels that reflect decreased distress.
- Demonstrate improved concentration and accuracy of thoughts.
- Identify and verbalize anxiety precipitants, conflicts, and threats.
- Demonstrate return of basic problem-solving skills.
- Demonstrate increased external focus.
- Demonstrate some ability to reassure self.

• = Independent        ▲ = Collaborative

## Nursing Interventions

A

- Assess the client's level of anxiety and physical reactions to anxiety (e.g., tachycardia, tachypnea, nonverbal expressions of anxiety). Use the Sheehan Patient-Rated Anxiety Scale (SPRAS). Validate observations by asking the client, "Are you feeling anxious now?" Consider the use of a "faces scale" to assess anxiety in critically ill clients.
- If the situational response is rational, use empathy to encourage the client to interpret the anxiety symptoms as normal.
- If irrational thoughts or fears are present, offer the client accurate information and encourage the client to talk about the meaning of the events contributing to the anxiety.
- Encourage the client to use positive self-talk such as the following: "Anxiety won't kill me," "I can do this one step at a time," "Right now I need to breathe and stretch," "I don't have to be perfect."
- Intervene when possible to remove sources of anxiety.
- Explain all activities, procedures, and issues that involve the client; use nonmedical terms and calm, slow speech. Do this in advance of procedures when possible, and validate the client's understanding.
- Ascertain client preferences about the desire to be distracted before and during noxious medical procedures.
- Explore coping skills previously used by client to relieve anxiety; reinforce these skills and explore other outlets.
- Provide back rubs/massage for the client to decrease anxiety.
- Use therapeutic touch and healing touch techniques.
- Use guided imagery to decrease anxiety.
- Provide clients with a means to listen to music or audiotapes of their choice. Provide a quiet place and encourage clients to listen for 20 minutes.
- Incorporate animal-assisted therapy (AAT) into the care of perioperative clients.
- Rule out withdrawal from alcohol, sedatives, or smoking as the cause of anxiety.

• = Independent          ▲ = Collaborative

▲ Identify and limit, discontinue, or be aware of the use of any stimulants such as caffeine, nicotine, theophylline, terbutaline sulfate, amphetamines, and cocaine.

## Geriatric

▲ Monitor the client for depression. Use appropriate interventions and referrals.
- Provide a protective and safe environment. Use consistent caregivers and maintain the accustomed environmental structure.
- Observe for adverse changes if antianxiety drugs are taken.
- Provide a quiet environment with diversion.

## Multicultural

- Assess for the presence of culture-bound anxiety states.
- Assess for the influence of cultural beliefs, norms, and values on the client's perspective of a stressful situation.
- Identify how anxiety is manifested in the culturally diverse client.
- Acknowledge that value conflicts from acculturation stresses may contribute to increased anxiety.
- Acknowledge that socioeconomic factors may contribute to increased stress and anxiety.
- For the diverse client experiencing preoperative anxiety, provide music of their choice. Music intervention was found to have cross-cultural validity in the reduction of preoperative anxiety in Chinese male clients.

## Home Care

- Above interventions may be adapted for home care use.
- Approach the client's anxiety in nonjudgmental fashion.
- Assist family to be supportive of the client in the face of anxiety symptoms.
- Adapt treatment needs to specific anxiety type.
- Assess for influence of anxiety on medical regimen.
- Assess for presence of depression.
- ▲ Consider referral for the prescription of antianxiety or antidepressant medications for clients who have panic

• = Independent          ▲ = Collaborative

A

disorder (PD) or other anxiety-related psychiatric disorders.

▲ Assist the client/family to institute medication regimen appropriately. Instruct in side effects, importance of taking medications as ordered, and side effects that should be reported immediately to nurse or physician.

▲ Assess for suicidal ideation. Implement emergency plan as indicated. Refer to care plan for **Risk of Suicide.**

▲ Encourage use of appropriate community resources: family, friends, neighbors, self-help and support groups, volunteer agencies, churches, clubs and centers for recreation, and other persons with similar interests.

▲ Refer for psychiatric home health care services for client reassurance and implementation of a therapeutic regimen.

## Client/Family Teaching

- Teach the client/family the symptoms of anxiety.
- Help client to define anxiety levels (from "easily tolerated" to "intolerable") and select appropriate interventions.
- Teach the client techniques to self-manage anxiety.
- Teach progressive muscle relaxation techniques.
- Teach relaxation breathing for occasional use: client should breathe in through nose, fill slowly from abdomen upward while thinking "re," and then breathe out through mouth, from chest downward, and think "lax."
- Teach the client to visualize or fantasize about the absence of anxiety or pain, successful experience of the situation, resolution of conflict, or outcome of procedure.
- Teach relationship between a healthy physical and emotional lifestyle and a realistic mental attitude. Health and well-being are influenced by how well-defined and well-met needs are in areas of safety, diet, exercise, sleep, work, pleasure, and social belonging.

▲ Teach use of appropriate community resources in emergency situations (e.g., suicidal thoughts), such as hotlines, emergency departments, law enforcement, and judicial systems.

• = Independent          ▲ = Collaborative

▲ Provide family members with information to help them
distinguish between a panic attack and serious physical illness symptoms. Instruct family members to
consult a health care professional if they have
questions.

A

# Death Anxiety

## NANDA Definition

Apprehension, worry, or fear related to death or dying

## Defining Characteristics

Worrying about impact of one's own death on significant others;
feeling powerless over issues related to dying; fear of loss of
physical and/or mental abilities when dying; anticipated pain
related to dying; deep sadness; fear of dying process; concerns of
overworking caregiver as terminal illness incapacitates self; concern about meeting one's creator or feeling doubtful about
existence of God or Higher Being; total loss of control over any
aspect of one's own death; negative death images or unpleasant
thoughts about any event related to death or dying; fear of
delayed demise; fear of premature death because it prevents
accomplishment of important life goals; worrying about being the
cause of others' grief and suffering; fear of leaving family alone
after death; fear of developing a terminal illness; denial of one's
own mortality or impending death

## Related Factors (r/t)

To be developed—see Defining Characteristics

## Client Outcomes

### Client Will (Specify Time Frame):
- State concerns about impact of death on others.
- Express feelings associated with dying.
- Seek help in dealing with feelings.
- Discuss concerns about God or Higher Being.

• = Independent      ▲ = Collaborative

A

- Discuss realistic goals.
- Use prayer or other religious practice for comfort.

## Nursing Interventions

- Assess psychosocial maturity of the individual. Erikson's scale of task accomplishment may be used.
- Assist clients to identify with their culture and its values.
- Assess clients for pain and provide pain relief measures.
- Assess client for fears related to death.
- Assist clients with life planning: consider and redefine main life goals, focus on areas of strength and/or goals that will provide satisfaction, adopt realistic goals, and recognize goals that are impossible to achieve.
- Assist clients with life review and reminiscence.
- Provide requested music to a client.
- Provide social support for families receiving CPR training to save the life of a family member at risk for sudden death.
- Encourage clients to pray.

## Geriatric

- Carefully assess older adults for issues regarding death anxiety.
- Provide back massage for clients who have anxiety regarding issues such as death.
- Refer to care plan for **Anticipatory Grieving.**

## Multicultural

Refer to care plans for **Anxiety** and **Anticipatory Grieving.**

## Home Care

- Above interventions may be adapted for home care.
- Identify times and places where anxiety is greatest. Provide for psychological support at those times, using such strategies as personal contact, telephone contact, diversionary activities, or therapeutic self.
- Support religious beliefs; encourage client to participate in services and activities of choice.

● = Independent          ▲ = Collaborative

▲ Refer to medical social services or mental health services, including support groups as appropriate (e.g., anticipatory grieving groups from hospice, visiting volunteers of hospice).

• Encourage the client to verbalize feelings to family/caregivers, counselors, and self.

• Identify client's preferences for end-of-life care; provide assistance in honoring preferences as much as practicable.

• Assist the client in making contact with death-related planning organizations, if appropriate, such as the Cremation Society and funeral homes.

• Assist the client in creating a memento book reflecting life achievements. Leave in the home for regular review by client. If family will be the recipient, a memento book serves as both an opportunity for life review and a means of proactively leaving something behind for survivors. Refer to care plan for **Powerlessness.**

• With client/caregivers, establish realistic life goals for anticipated life span of self or others. Create manageable, tangible steps that client can refer to and use to measure activity. Memento books and written life goals are tangible milestones related to life and death.

▲ Refer for psychiatric home health care services for client reassurance and implementation of a therapeutic regimen. Psychiatric home care nurses can address issues relating to client's death anxiety, including family relationships.

## Client/Family Teaching

• Promote more effective communication to family members engaged in the caregiving role. Encourage them to talk to their loved one about areas of concern.

• Allow family members to be physically close to their dying loved one, giving them permission, instruction, and opportunities to touch. Keep family members informed.

• To increase clients' knowledge about end-of-life issues, teach them and their family members about options for care, such as advance directives.

• = Independent        ▲ = Collaborative

# Risk for Aspiration

## NANDA Definition

At risk for entry of gastrointestinal secretions, oropharyngeal secretions, solids, or fluids into the tracheobronchial passages

## Risk Factors

Increased intragastric pressure; tube feedings; situations hindering elevation of upper body; reduced level of consciousness; presence of tracheostomy or endotracheal tube; medication administration; wired jaws; increased gastric residual; incomplete lower esophageal sphincter; impaired swallowing; gastrointestinal tubes; facial, oral, or neck surgery or trauma; depressed cough and gag reflexes; decreased gastrointestinal motility; delayed gastric emptying

## Client Outcomes

### Client Will (Specify Time Frame):
- Swallow and digest oral, nasogastric, or gastric feeding without aspiration.
- Maintain patent airway and clear lung sounds.

## Nursing Interventions

- Monitor respiratory rate, depth, and effort. Note any signs of aspiration such as dyspnea, cough, cyanosis, wheezing, or fever.
- Auscultate lung sounds frequently and before and after feedings; note any new onset of crackles or wheezing.
- Take vital signs frequently, noting onset of a fever.
- Before initiating oral feeding, check client's gag reflex and ability to swallow by feeling the laryngeal prominence as the client attempts to swallow.
- When feeding client, watch for signs of impaired swallowing or aspiration, including coughing, choking, spitting food, or excessive drooling. If client is having

• = Independent          ▲ = Collaborative

problems swallowing, see Nursing Interventions for **Impaired Swallowing.**

- Have suction machine available when feeding high-risk clients. If aspiration does occur, suction immediately.
- Keep head of bed elevated when feeding and for at least an hour afterward.
▲ Note presence of any nausea, vomiting, or diarrhea. Treat nausea promptly with antiemetics.
- Listen to bowel sounds frequently, noting if they are decreased, absent, or hyperactive.
- Note new onset of abdominal distention or increased rigidity of abdomen.
▲ If client has a tracheostomy, ask for referral to speech pathologist for swallowing studies before attempting to feed. After evaluation, decision should be made to have cuff either inflated or deflated when client eats.
- If client shows symptoms of nausea and vomiting, position on side.
- If client needs to be fed, feed slowly and allow adequate time for chewing and swallowing. Position upright during and after feedings.

## Enteral Feedings

- Insert nasogastric feeding tube using the internal nares to introduce the tube distal to the esophageal sphincter.
▲ Ensure nasogastric tube is inserted a sufficient distance into the stomach, to the "distallower esophageal distance."
- Keep nasogastric tube securely taped. Use pink tape to secure the tube.
- Determine placement of feeding tube before each feeding or every 4 hours if client is on continuous feeding. Check pH of aspirate and note characteristic appearance of aspirate; do not rely on air insufflation method.
- Check for gastric residual during continuous feedings or before feedings; if residual is greater than 400 ml, hold feedings following institutional protocol.
- Test for the presence of glucose in tracheobronchial se-

A

cretions or the presence of pepsin to detect aspiration of enteral feedings. Recognize that the glucose test may not be accurate if there is blood in the aspirate or if a low-glucose feeding is being used.
- Do not use blue dye to tint enteral feedings.
- During enteral feedings, position client with head of bed elevated 30 to 40 degrees; maintain for 30 to 45 minutes after feeding.
- Use a closed versus an open enteral delivery system of tube feeding if possible.
- Stop continual feeding temporarily when turning or moving client.

## Geriatric

- Carefully check elderly client's gag reflex and ability to swallow before feeding.
- Watch for signs of aspiration pneumonia in the elderly with cerebrovascular accidents, even if there are no apparent signs of difficulty swallowing or of aspiration.
- ▲ Use central nervous system depressants cautiously; elderly clients may have an increased incidence of aspiration with altered levels of consciousness.
- Keep the elderly, mostly bedridden client sitting upright for 2 hours following meals.
- ▲ Recommend to families that tube feedings not be used for clients with dementia; instead use increased feeding assistance, modified food consistency as needed, or environmental alterations.

## Home Care

- Above interventions may be adapted for home care use.
- ▲ For clients at high risk for aspiration, obtain complete information from the discharging institution regarding institutional management.
- Assess the client and family for willingness and cognitive ability to learn and cope with swallowing, feeding, and related disorders.
- Assess caregiver understanding and reinforce teaching re-

• = Independent          ▲ = Collaborative

garding positioning and assessment of the client for possible aspiration.

**A**

- Provide the client with emotional support in dealing with
  fears of aspiration. Refer to care plan for **Anxiety.**
- Establish emergency and contingency plans for care of
  client.
- ▲ Have both speech and occupational therapists assess client's swallowing ability and other physiological factors
  and recommend strategies for working with client in the
  home (e.g., pureeing foods served to client, providing
  adaptive equipment for independence in eating).
- Obtain suction equipment for the home as necessary.
- Teach caregivers safe, effective use of suctioning devices.
  Inform client and family that only individuals instructed in suctioning should perform the procedure.
- ▲ Institute case management of frail elderly to support continued independent living.

## Client/Family Teaching

- Teach the client and family signs of aspiration and precautions to prevent aspiration.
- Teach the client and family how to safely administer tube
  feeding.

# Risk for impaired parent/infant/child Attachment

## NANDA Definition

Disruption of the interactive process between parent/significant
other and infant/child that fosters the development of a protective and nurturing reciprocal relationship

The terms "bonding" and "attachment" are used to describe
the emotional connectedness that develops between the infant
and his/her parent/primary caregiver over the first months and
years of life. Bonding refers to the maternal process of emotional
connectedness, whereas attachment is the infant process of

● = Independent          ▲ = Collaborative

emotionally connecting with the mother (Box II-3). The two unfolding processes describe the foundation of the mother-infant relationship that allows attachment to evolve.

### Risk Factors

Physical barriers; anxiety associated with the parent role; substance abuse; premature infant, ill infant/child who is unable to effectively initiate parental contact as a result of altered behavioral organization; lack of privacy; inability of parents to meet personal needs; separation

| BOX II-3 | Parent/Infant/Child Attachment Behaviors | |
|---|---|---|
| **Securely Attached** | **Avoidantly Attached** | **Ambivalently Attached** |
| Mother (primary or caregiver) is warm, sensitively attuned, consistent. Quickly responds to baby's cries. | Mother is often emotionally unavailable or rejecting. Dislikes "neediness," may applaud independence. | Mother is unpredictable or chaotic. Often attentive but out of synch with baby. Most mothers tune in to baby's fear. |
| Baby readily explores, using mother as secure base. Cries least of three groups, most compliant with mother, and most easily put down after being held. | By end of first year, baby seeks little physical contact with mother, randomly angry with her, unresponsive to being held, but often upset when put down. | Baby cries a lot, is clingy and demanding, often angry, upset by small separations, chronically anxious in relation to mother, limited in exploration. |
| Preschool: Easily makes friends. Popular. Flexible and resilient under stress. Spends more time with peers. Good self-esteem. | Preschool: Often angry, aggressive, defiant. May be isolated, disliked. Hangs around teachers. Withdraws when in pain. | Preschool: Fretful and easily overwhelmed by anxiety. Immature, overly dependent on teacher. May be victimized by bullies. |

Adapted from Karen R: *Becoming attached, first relationships and how they shape our capacity to love*, p 444, New York and Oxford, 1998, Oxford University Press.

• = Independent      ▲ = Collaborative

## Parent

Maternal ambivalence toward pregnancy; unplanned/unwanted pregnancy; traumatic prenatal experience/birth trauma; unprepared for responsibility of parenting; poor parenting role models; history of abuse and neglect; substance abuse; insecure attachments within family of origin; social/emotional instability; homeless; maternal isolation, maternal depression; significant family stressors; prolonged separation from infant; hospitalization; teenage pregnancy; poverty; unsafe environment; low maternal education; use of corporal punishment; lack of empathy; lack of maternal sensitivity, unable to provide mutually satisfying interactions, lack of father's involvement/support, unstable/abusive relationship

## Infant/Child

Feeding difficulties; premature birth; prolonged hospitalization; colicky, episodes of prolonged, unexplained crying; genetic disposition-difficult temperament; unclear readable cues; disorganized behavior; inconsolable or difficult to console; frequent moves and placement homes; failed adoptions; inconsistent or inadequate day care, sudden maternal separation (illness, abandonment, death, prolonged hospitalization)

## Attachment Behaviors

Eye contact; smiles; exchange of gentle touching/caressing; engages in positive reciprocal interactions; exchange of vocalizations/vocal play (coos, babbles pleasurably, responds, initiates and imitates infant); looks/reaches/touches parent(s) for comfort when distressed; can be comforted with touch; comfortable with physical closeness, watches each other's face for sustained periods of time; relaxed in presence of each other; speaks positively of child

## Client Outcomes

### Parent(s) Will (Specify Time Frame):

- Display enjoyment with their infant/child.
- Be able to provide a safe environment free of hazards.

• = Independent          ▲ = Collaborative

A

- Provide nurturing environment responding to infant/child's need for nutrition/feeding, sleeping, comfort, and social play.
- Read and respond contingently to infant/child's behavioral cues (approach/engagement, avoidance/disengagement).
- Be able to calm and relieve their infant/child's distress.
- Engage in mutually satisfying interactions that provide an opportunity for attachment.
- Engage in nurturing tactile/kinesthetic/vestibular communication (such as holding, cuddling, stroking, and rocking).
- Demonstrate an awareness of developmentally appropriate activities that are interesting to the infant and growth-fostering.
- Not punish (inflict harm on) child for misbehavior.
- Be knowledgeable of appropriate community resources and support services.

## Nursing Interventions

- Establish a trusting relationship with the parents.
- Nurture parents so that they in turn can nurture their infant/child.
- Allow parents to verbalize their childhood fears: "ghosts in the nursery."
- Be an empathetic listener to parents' stories of childhood memories that may influence their struggle to attach with their child.
- Offer parent-to-parent support to parents of NICU-hospitalized infants.
- Assist parents in learning to accurately read infant's physical states (sleep/wake) and behavioral cues that communicate, approach/engagement and avoidance/disengagement, and respond in a contingent and sensitive way. When infants experience joyful and soothing responses from the parents to basic needs, infants experience satisfaction and emotional connectedness that

• = Independent        ▲ = Collaborative

evolves in building a secure relationship allowing for formation of an attachment bond.

- Support parents' ability to respond and relieve distress of infant/child.
- Assist parents with recognizing how their infant/child learns through sensory motor experiences (sights/visual, sounds/auditory, touch/tactile, vestibular/movement, and body awareness).
- Guide parents in adapting their behaviors and activities with infant/child cues and changing needs.
- Identify factors related to depressive symptoms and offer appropriate interventions.
- Offer anticipatory developmental guidance including interactive play activities that are interesting to the child. The unrealistic expectations of parents regarding infant/child abilities can negatively influence the parent-child relationship by expecting too much too soon.
- Attend to both the parents and infant/child in an effort to strengthen high-quality parent-infant interactions.
- Encourage parents of hospitalized infants to "personalize" their infant by bringing in baby clothes, pictures of themselves, toys, and tapes of their voices.
- Encourage physical closeness using skin-to-skin experiences for parents and infants as appropriate. Mothers have perceived skin-to-skin contact with their very immature infants as a positive and helpful intervention.
- Encourage parents and caregivers to massage their infants and children.
- Assist parents in developing new caregiving practice competencies and/or revising and extending old ones. One model to consider for use with parents is guided participation, a process in which an experienced person helps another with less experience to become competent in practices that are personally and socially meaningful for everyday life.
- Plan ways for parents to interact with/assist with caregiving for their infant/child.

• = Independent          ▲ = Collaborative

## Infant

- Provide lyrical, soothing music in the nursery and home as appropriate (with premature infants, visual and auditory stimulation must be designed as appropriate with post-conceptual age [PCA] and contingent with state and behavioral cues).
- Recognize and support attention capabilities of infant/child.
- Encourage opportunities for mutually satisfying interactions between infant and parent.
- Encourage opportunities for physical closeness.
- Provide therapeutic touch for children with anxiety.

## Multicultural

- Discuss cultural norms with families to provide care that is appropriate for enhancing attachment with the infant/child.
- Encourage a reciprocal attachment process.
- Promote the attachment process by providing a treatment environment that is culturally based and women centered.
- Empower family members to draw on personal strengths in which multiple worldviews and values of individual members are recognized, incorporated, and negotiated.
- Encourage positive involvement and relationship development between children and noncustodial fathers to enhance health and development.

## Home Care

- Above interventions may be adapted for home care use.
- Assess quality of interaction between parent and infant/child.
- ▲ Assess mother for depressive symptoms and initiate referral for mental health care as needed. Referral to psychiatric home health care, if available, can be helpful.
- Use interaction coaching: teach mother about infant's behavioral cues and how to match infant's preferences; have mother position infant in direct line of sight; dem-

• = Independent          ▲ = Collaborative

onstrate responsive behaviors that can be modulated
(e.g., facial expression, voice, touch); encourage practice
by trial and error; reinforce sensitive responsiveness as
it occurs; give positive reinforcement for success.

# Autonomic dysreflexia

## NANDA Definition

Life-threatening, uninhibited sympathetic response of the nervous system to a noxious stimulus after spinal cord injury at T7 or above

## Defining Characteristics

Pallor (below the injury); paroxysmal hypertension (sudden, periodic elevated blood pressure where systolic pressure is >140 mm Hg and diastolic pressure is >90 mm Hg); red splotches on skin (above the injury); bradycardia or tachycardia (pulse rate <60 or >100 beats/min); diaphoresis above the injury; headache (diffuse pain in different parts of the head, not confined to any nerve distribution area); blurred vision; chest pain; chilling; conjunctival congestion; Horner syndrome (contraction of pupil on one side, partial ptosis of the eyelid, recession of eyeball into the head, occasional loss of sweating over the affected side of the face); metallic taste in mouth; nasal congestion; paresthesia; pilomotor reflex (gooseflesh formation when skin is cooled)

## Related Factors (r/t)

Bladder distention; bowel distention; skin irritation; lack of client and caregiver knowledge

## Client Outcomes

**Client Will (Specify Time Frame):**

- Maintain normal vital signs.
- Remain free of dysreflexia symptoms.
- Explain symptoms, prevention, and treatment of dysreflexia.

● = Independent          ▲ = Collaborative

A

## Nursing Interventions

- Monitor the client for symptoms of dysreflexia. See Defining Characteristics.
- ▲ Observe with physician the cause of dysreflexia (e.g., distended bladder, impaction, pressure ulcer, urinary calculi, bladder infection, acute condition in the abdomen, penile pressure, ingrown toenail, or other source of noxious stimuli).
- ▲ If symptoms of dysreflexia are present, place client in high Fowler's position, remove all support hoses or binders, and immediately determine the identity of the noxious stimuli causing the response. If blood pressure cannot be decreased within 1 minute, notify the physician STAT.
- ▲ To determine the stimulus for dysreflexia:
  - ■ First, assess bladder function. Check for distention, and if present catheterize using an anesthetic jelly as a lubricant. Do not use Valsalva maneuver or Credé's method to empty the bladder. Ensure existing catheter patency. Also note signs of urinary tract infection.
  - ■ Second, assess bowel function. Numb the bowel area with a topical anesthetic as ordered, and once agent is effective (5 minutes), check for impaction.
  - ■ Third, assess the skin, looking for any points of pressure.
- ▲ Initiate antihypertensive therapy as soon as ordered.
- ▲ Be careful not to increase noxious sensory stimuli. If numbing agent is ordered, use it on anus and 1 inch of rectum before attempting to remove a fecal impaction. Also spray pressure ulcer with it. If necessary to replace an obstructed catheter, use an anesthetic jelly as ordered.
- Monitor vital signs every 3 to 5 minutes during acute event; continue to monitor vital signs after event is resolved.
- Watch for complications of dysreflexia, including signs of cerebral hemorrhage, seizures, myocardial infarction (MI), or intraocular hemorrhage.

• = Independent          ▲ = Collaborative

A

- Accurately and completely record any incidences of dysreflexia; especially note the precipitating stimuli.
- Use the following interventions to prevent dysreflexia:
  - Ensure that drainage from Foley catheter is good and that bladder is not distended.
  - Ensure a regular pattern of defecation to prevent fecal impaction.
  - Frequently change position of client to relieve pressure and prevent the formation of pressure ulcers.
  - If ordered, apply an anesthetic agent to any wound below level of injury before performing wound care.
- ▲ Because episodes can reoccur, notify all health care team members of the possibility of a dysreflexia episode.

## Home Care

- Above interventions may be adapted for home care use.
- Instruct the client with any known proclivity toward dysreflexia to wear a Medic Alert bracelet and carry a Medic Alert wallet card when not in a safe environment (i.e., not with someone who knows client has the condition and can respond appropriately).
- ▲ Establish an emergency plan: obtain physician orders for medications to be used in situations in which first aid does not work (e.g., nifedipine).
- ▲ If orders have not been obtained or client does not have medications, use emergency medical services.
- If episode of dysreflexia is resolved, monitor blood pressure every 30 to 60 minutes for next 4 to 5 hours or admit to institution for observation.
- ▲ Institute case management of frail elderly to support continued independent living.

## Client/Family Teaching

- Teach recognition of the earliest symptoms of dysreflexia, the actions that should be taken when they occur, and the need to summon help immediately. Give client a written card that contains this information.
- Teach steps to prevent dysreflexia episodes: care of blad-

• = Independent                    ▲ = Collaborative

A

der, bowel, and skin and prevention of other forms of noxious stimuli (i.e., not wearing clothing that is too tight).

# Risk for Autonomic dysreflexia

## NANDA Definition

At risk for life-threatening, uninhibited response of the sympathetic nervous system; post spinal shock; in an individual with spinal cord injury or lesion at T6 or above (has been demonstrated in clients with injuries at T7 or T8)

## Defining Characteristics and Risk Factors

An injury/lesion at T6 or above and at least one of the following noxious stimuli:

- Neurological stimuli: Painful/irritating stimuli below the level of injury
- Urological stimuli: Bladder distention; detrusor sphincter dyssynergia; bladder spasms; instrumentation or surgery; epididymitis; urethritis; urinary tract infection; calculi; cystitis; catheterization
- Gastrointestinal stimuli: Bowel distention; fecal impaction; digital stimulation; suppositories; hemorrhoids; difficult passage of feces; constipation; enemas; gastrointestinal system pathology; gastric ulcers; esophageal reflux; gallstones
- Reproductive stimuli: Menstruation; sexual intercourse; pregnancy; labor and delivery; ovarian cyst; ejaculation
- Regulatory stimuli: Temperature fluctuations; extreme environmental temperatures
- Musculoskeletal-integumentary stimuli: Cutaneous stimulations (e.g., pressure ulcer, ingrown toenail, dressings, burns, rash); heterotrophic bone; pressure over bony prominences or genitalia; spasm; fractures; range-of-motion exercises; wounds; sunburns
- Situational stimuli: Positioning; drug reactions (e.g., decon-

• = Independent          ▲ = Collaborative

gestants, sympathomimetics, vasoconstrictors, narcotic withdrawal); constrictive clothing (e.g., straps, stockings, shoes);
surgical procedures

• Cardiac/pulmonary problems: Pulmonary emboli; deep vein
thrombosis

## Client Outcomes, Nursing Interventions, and Client/Family Teaching

Refer to care plan for **Autonomic dysreflexia.**

## Disturbed Body image

## NANDA Definition

Confusion in mental picture of one's physical self

## Defining Characteristics

Verbalization of feelings that reflect an altered view of one's body
in appearance, structure, or function; verbalization of perceptions
that reflect an altered view of one's body in appearance, structure,
or function; nonverbal response to actual or perceived change in
body structure and/or function; behaviors of avoidance, monitoring, or acknowledgment of one's body

## Objective

Missing body part; trauma to nonfunctioning part; not touching
body part; hiding or overexposing body part (intentional or
unintentional); actual change in structure and/or function;
change in social involvement; change in ability to estimate spatial
relationship of body to environment; extension of body boundary
to incorporate environmental objects; not looking at body part

## Subjective

Refusal to verify actual change; preoccupation with change or
loss; personalization of part or loss by name; depersonalization of
part or loss by impersonal pronouns; extension of body boundary
to incorporate environmental objects

• = Independent        ▲ = Collaborative

## Related Factors (r/t)

B

Psychosocial, biophysical, cognitive/perceptual, cultural, spiritual, or developmental changes; illness; trauma or injury; surgery; illness treatment

## Client Outcomes

### Client Will (Specify Time Frame):

- State or demonstrate acceptance of change or loss and an ability to adjust to lifestyle change.
- Call body part or loss by appropriate name.
- Look at and touch changed or missing body part.
- Care for changed or nonfunctioning part without inflicting trauma.
- Return to previous social involvement.
- Correctly estimate relationship of body to environment.

## Nursing Interventions

- Use a tool such as the Body Image Instrument (BII) to identify clients who have concerns about changes in body image. The five BII subscales—General Appearance, Body Competence, Others' Reaction to Appearance, Value of Appearance, and Body Parts—exhibit moderate to high internal reliability and concurrent validity.
- ▲ Assess for body dysmorphic disorder (BDD) and make appropriate referrals. The severity of BDD varies. Some youth experience manageable distress about their appearance and are able to function well, although not up to their potential. Psychiatric treatment is often effective in decreasing BDD symptoms and the suffering they cause.
- Observe client's usual coping mechanisms during times of extreme stress and reinforce their use in the current crisis.
- Explore opportunities to assist the client to develop a realistic perception of his/her body image.
- Acknowledge denial, anger, or depression as normal feelings when adjusting to changes in body and lifestyle.

• = Independent          ▲ = Collaborative

B

- Identify clients at risk for body image disturbance (e.g., body builders, cancer survivors).
- Clients should not be rushed into sharing their feelings.
- Do not ask clients to explore feelings unless they have indicated a need to do so.
- Explore strengths and resources with client. Discuss possible changes in weight and hair loss; select a wig before hair loss occurs.
- Encourage the client to purchase clothes that are attractive and that deemphasize their disability.
- Allow client and others gradual exposure to the body change. Begin by having the client touch the affected area; then use a mirror to look at it. Go to a hospital shop with a nurse or support person and discuss feelings associated with the reaction of others to the body change.
- Encourage the client to discuss interpersonal and social conflicts that may arise.
- Encourage the client to make own decisions, participate in plan of care, and accept both inadequacies and strengths.
- ▲ Aid client in accepting help from others; provide a list of appropriate community resources (e.g., Reach to Recovery, Ostomy Association).
- Help client describe self-ideal, identify self-criticisms, and be accepting of self.
- Encourage the client to write a narrative description of their changes.
- Avoid looks of distaste when caring for clients who have had disfiguring surgery or injuries. Provide privacy; care should be completed without unnecessary exposure.
- Encourage the client to continue same personal care routine that was followed before the change in body image. It is preferable that this care be completed in the bathroom and not in bed.

## Geriatric

- Focus on remaining abilities. Have client make a list of strengths.

• = Independent          ▲ = Collaborative

B

## Multicultural

- Assess for the influence of cultural beliefs, norms, and values on the client's body image.
- Validate the client's feelings with regard to the impact of health status on disturbances in body image.
- Acknowledge that body image disturbances can affect all individuals regardless of culture, race, or ethnicity.
- Assess for the presence of conflicting cultural demands.
- Assess for the presence of depressive symptoms.

## Home Care

- Above interventions may be adapted for home care use.
- Assess client's stage of grieving or acceptance of body change on return to home setting. Include the future role of sexuality in the psychological assessment of acceptance as appropriate.
- Assess family/caregiver level of acceptance of client's body changes.
- Recognize that older women may continue their younger preoccupation with weight and recurrent dieting, despite being at normal weight. Assess source of low weight or weight loss with this in mind.
- Be accepting of body changes in all interactions with client and family/caregivers.
- Help client to see new or changing roles in family. Point out ways in which the community can help support client and family strengths.
- ▲ Refer to medical social services to address level of acceptance and possible financial impact of changes.
- Teach all aspects of care. Involve client and caregivers in self-care as soon as possible. Do this in stages if client still has difficulty looking at or touching changed body part.
- Teach family and client complications of medical condition and when to contact physician.
- ▲ Refer to occupational therapy if necessary to evaluate home setting for safety and adaptive equipment and to assist client with return to normal activities.

• = Independent          ▲ = Collaborative

▲ If appropriate, provide home health aide support to help the client and family through ADL transition.

▲ Refer to physical therapy if necessary to build range-of-joint motion, flexibility, and strength, to prevent contractures, to assist with transfer/ambulation safety, or to obtain use of a prosthetic device in the home setting.

• Assess for and promote good nutrition and sleep patterns. Adapt nutrition to specific physiological situations (e.g., client with ostomy).

• Assist family with obtaining needed supplies.

• Be alert to the differential body image found in clients with schizophrenia that may contribute to the need for assisted living and avoidance of competitive situations. Refer to care plan for **Powerlessness.**

▲ Refer for psychiatric home health care services for client reassurance and implementation of a therapeutic regimen. Psychiatric home health care nurses can address issues relating to client's distorted body image.

## Client/Family Teaching

• Teach appropriate care of surgical site (e.g., mastectomy site, amputation site, ostomy site).

• Inform client of available community support groups; offer to make initial phone call.

• Provide printed material and didactic information for significant others.

• Encourage significant others to offer support.

• Direct social support as follows: (1) instruct regarding practical care (bandaging); (2) encourage appraisal support (listening); (3) encourage self-esteem support (favorable comparisons between client's and others' appearance); (4) encourage sense of belonging (assist with socializing). The preceding are four categories of support recognized in the body-image care model.

▲ Refer an interdisciplinary team to clients with ostomies who are having difficulty with personal acceptance, personal and social body-image disruption, sexual con-

---

• = Independent          ▲ = Collaborative

cerns, reduced self-care skills, and the management of surgical complications.

**B**

## Risk for imbalanced Body temperature

### NANDA Definition

At risk for failure to maintain body temperature within a normal range

### Risk Factors

Altered metabolic rate; extremes of age or weight; exposure to cool/cold or hot/warm environments; dehydration; inactivity or vigorous activity; medications that cause vasoconstriction or vasodilation; sedation; clothing inappropriate for environmental temperature; illness or trauma that affects body temperature regulation

### Related Factors (r/t)

See Risk Factors.

### Client Outcomes

**Client Will (Specify Time Frame):**

- Maintain temperature within normal range of 97° to 99° F in the adult.
- Explain measures needed to maintain normal temperature.
- Identify symptoms of hypothermia or hyperthermia.

### Nursing Interventions

- Monitor temperature every 1 to 4 hours or use continuous temperature monitoring as appropriate.
- If client is awake, take the temperature orally in the adult, instead of using a tympanic thermometer or an axillary temperature reading.
- Take vital signs every 1 to 4 hours, noting changes associated with hypothermia: first, increased blood pres-

• = Independent        ▲ = Collaborative

sure, pulse, and respirations; then, decreased values as
hypothermia progresses.
- Monitor the client for signs of hypothermia (e.g., shivering, cool skin, piloerection, pallor, slow capillary refill,
  cyanotic nailbeds, decreased mentation, dysrhythmias).
- Note changes in vital signs associated with hyperthermia:
  rapid, bounding pulse; increased respiratory rate; and
  decreased blood pressure with orthostatic hypotension
  present.
- Monitor the client for signs of hyperthermia (e.g., headache, nausea and vomiting, weakness, absence of
  sweating, delirium, and coma).
- Maintain a consistent room temperature (72° F).
- Promote adequate nutrition and hydration.
- Adjust clothing to facilitate passive warming or cooling
  as appropriate.
- See Nursing Interventions for **Hypothermia** or **Hyperthermia** as appropriate.

## Geriatric

- Do not allow geriatric clients to become chilled. Keep
  covered when giving a bath or doing a procedure. Offer
  socks to wear when in bed and a head covering if desired.
- ▲ Assess medication profile for potential risk of drug-
  related altered body temperature.
- ▲ Ensure that elderly clients receive sufficient fluids during
  hot days and stay out of the sun.

## Pediatric

- Recognize that pediatric clients have a decreased ability
  to adapt to temperature extremes. Take the following ac-
  tions to maintain body temperature in the infant/child:
  - Keep the head covered.
  - Use blankets to keep the client warm.
  - Keep client covered during procedures, transport, and
    diagnostic testing.
  - Maintain a consistent room temperature of 72° F.
- Recognize that the infant and small child are vulnerable

<br>

• = Independent          ▲ = Collaborative

to develop heat stroke in hot weather and ensure they receive sufficient fluids and are protected from hot environments.

## Home Care
- Above interventions may be adapted for home care use.

## Prevention of Hypothermia in Cold Weather
- Avoid prolonged exposure outside. Wear a hat and gloves. Wool or fleece clothing can help to maintain body heat.
- Keep room temperature at 68° to 72° F.
- Ensure adequate source of heat; refer to social services if client is low income and heat could be turned off.
- Help elderly client determine a warm environment they can go to for safety in cold weather if his or her home environment is no longer warm.

## Prevention of Hyperthermia in Hot Weather
- Encourage the client to wear lightweight loose-fitting cotton clothing. Help the elderly remove their usual sweaters.
- Ensure that client drinks adequate amounts of fluids (2000 ml/day), avoiding caffeine and alcohol.
- ▲ Help client obtain a fan to increase evaporation, or an air conditioner as needed, using social services if necessary.
- Take the temperature of the elderly in hot weather.
- Help elderly client determine a cool environment they can go to for safety in hot weather.

## Client/Family Teaching
- Teach the client and family the signs of hypothermia and hyperthermia and the appropriate actions they should take if either condition develops.
- Teach the client and family the proper method for taking temperature.
- Impress upon the client the reasons for avoidance of alcohol and medications that depress cerebral function.

• = Independent          ▲ = Collaborative

# Bowel incontinence

## NANDA  Definition

Change in normal bowel elimination habits characterized by involuntary passage of stool

## Defining Characteristics

Constant dribbling of soft stool, fecal odor; inability to delay defecation; rectal urgency; self-report of inability to feel rectal fullness or presence of stool in bowel; fecal staining of underclothing; recognition of rectal fullness but reported inability to expel formed stool; inattention to urge to defecate; inability to recognize urge to defecate; irritation of perianal skin

## Related Factors (r/t)

Change in stool consistency (diarrhea, constipation, fecal impaction); abnormal motility (metabolic disorders, inflammatory bowel disease, infectious disease, drug-induced motility disorders, food intolerance); defects in rectal vault function (low rectal compliance from ischemia, fibrosis, radiation, infectious proctitis, Hirschsprung's disease, local or infiltrating neoplasm, severe rectocele); sphincter dysfunction (obstetric or traumatic induced incompetence, fistula or abscess, prolapse, third-degree hemorrhoids, high tone pelvic floor muscle dysfunction); neurological disorders impacting gastrointestinal motility, rectal vault function, and sphincter function (cerebrovascular accident, spinal injury, traumatic brain injury, central nervous system tumor, advanced stage dementia, encephalopathy, profound mental retardation, multiple sclerosis, myelodysplasia and related neural tube defects, gastroparesis of diabetes mellitus, heavy metal poisoning, chronic alcoholism, infectious or autoimmune neurological disorders, myasthenia gravis)

## Client Outcomes

### Client Will (Specify Time Frame):

* Have regular, complete evacuation of fecal contents from the

• = Independent          ▲ = Collaborative

rectal vault (pattern may vary from every day to every 3 to 5 days).

**B**
- Have regulation of stool consistency (soft, formed stools).
- Reduce or eliminate frequency of incontinent episodes.
- Demonstrate intact skin in the perianal/perineal area.
- Demonstrate the ability to isolate, contract, and relax pelvic muscles (when incontinence related to sphincter incompetence or high tone pelvic floor dysfunction).
- Increase pelvic muscle strength (when incontinence related to sphincter incompetence).

## Nursing Interventions

- In a reasonably private setting, directly question any client at risk about the presence of fecal incontinence. If the client reports altered bowel elimination patterns, problems with bowel control, or "uncontrollable diarrhea," complete a focused nursing history including previous and present bowel elimination routines, dietary history, frequency and volume of uncontrolled stool loss, and aggravating and alleviating factors.
- Complete a focused physical assessment including inspection of perineal skin, pelvic muscle strength assessment, digital examination of the rectum for presence of impaction and anal sphincter strength, and evaluation of functional status (mobility, dexterity, visual acuity).
- Complete an assessment of cognitive function.
- Document patterns of stool elimination and incontinent episodes via a bowel record including frequency of bowel movements, stool consistency, frequency and severity of incontinent episodes, precipitating factors, dietary and fluid intake.
- Assess stool consistency and its influence on risk for stool loss.
- Identify conditions contributing to or causing fecal incontinence.
- Improve access to toileting:
  - Identify usual toileting patterns among persons in the acute care or long-term care facility and plan opportunities for toileting accordingly.

• = Independent          ▲ = Collaborative

- Provide assistance with toileting for clients with limited access or impaired functional status (mobility, dexterity, access).
- Institute a prompted toileting program for persons with impaired cognitive status (retardation, dementia).
- Provide adequate privacy for toileting.
- Respond promptly to requests for assistance with toileting.
- Counsel clients with fecal incontinence associated with liquid stools (diarrhea) about methods to normalize stool consistency via dietary fiber or fiber supplements.
- For the client with intermittent episodes of fecal incontinence related to acute changes in stool consistency, begin a bowel reeducation program consisting of:
  - Cleansing the bowel of impacted stool if indicated.
  - Normalizing stool consistency by adequate intake of fluids (30 ml/kg of body weight/day) and dietary or supplemental fiber.
  - Establishing a regular routine of fecal elimination based on established patterns of bowel elimination (patterns established before onset of incontinence).
- Begin a prompted defecation program for the adult with dementia, mental retardation, or related learning disabilities.
- Begin a scheduled, stimulation defecation program for persons with neurological conditions causing fecal incontinence including the following steps:
  - Cleanse the bowel of impacted fecal material before beginning the program.
  - Implement strategies to normalize stool consistency including adequate intake of fluid and fiber and avoidance of foods associated with diarrhea.
  - Determine a regular schedule for bowel elimination (typically every day or every other day) based on prior patterns of bowel elimination whenever feasible.
  - Provide a stimulus before assisting the client to a position on the toilet; digital stimulation, a stimulat-

• = Independent          ▲ = Collaborative

ing suppository, a "mini-enema," or a pulsed evacuation enema may be used for stimulation.

▲ Begin a reeducation or pelvic floor muscle exercise program for persons with sphincter incompetence or high tone pelvic floor muscle dysfunction of the pelvic muscles, or refer persons with fecal incontinence related to sphincter dysfunction to a nurse specialist or other therapist with clinical expertise in these techniques of care.

• Begin a pelvic muscle biofeedback program among clients with urgency to defecate and fecal incontinence related to recurrent diarrhea.

• Thoroughly cleanse and dry the perianal and perineal skin daily using a cleanser capable of removing irritants (including urine, stool, and materials). Select a product with a slightly acidic pH designed to preserve its acid mantle. Select a product that is designed to remove irritants from the skin with minimal physical force. Avoid vigorous scrubbing with water, soap, and a washcloth. Consider selection of a product with a moisturizer.

• Cleanse the perineal and perianal skin following each episode of fecal incontinence.

• Apply a moisture barrier containing dimethicone or zinc oxide to patients with severe urinary incontinence or those with double urinary and fecal incontinence.

• When cleansing a client with a moisture barrier containing zinc oxide, avoid vigorous scrubbing or use of a traditional washcloth to remove the paste. Instead, cleanse fecal materials away from the skin, leaving a clean layer of zinc oxide paste when cleansing after a single episode or gently removing the paste with mineral oil.

▲ Consult the physician concerning use of a moisture barrier with active healing ingredients when perineal dermatitis exists. Apply and teach caregivers to use the product sparingly when applying to affected areas.

• Assist the client to select and apply a containment device for occasional episodes of fecal incontinence.

• Teach the caregiver of a client who has frequent episodes of fecal incontinence and limited mobility to regularly

• = Independent          ▲ = Collaborative

monitor the sacrum and perineal area for pressure ulcerations.
▲ Teach the client with more frequent stool loss to apply an anal continence plug in consultation with the physician.
• Apply a fecal pouch to the client with frequent stool loss, particularly when fecal incontinence produces altered perianal skin integrity.
▲ For the patient with acute fecal incontinence and liquid stools, consult with a nurse practitioner or physician concerning initiation of a specialized bowel management system.

## Geriatric
• Evaluate all elderly clients for established or acute fecal incontinence when the elderly client enters the acute or long-term care facility and intervene as indicated.
• Evaluate cognitive status in the elderly person with a NEECHAM confusion scale for acute cognitive changes, a Folstein Mini-Mental Status, or other tools as indicated.

## Home Care
• Above interventions may be adapted for home care use.
• Assess and teach a bowel management program to support continence. Address timing, diet, fluids, and actions taken independently to deal with bowel incontinence.
• Instruct caregiver to provide clothing that is nonrestrictive, can be manipulated easily for toileting, and can be changed with ease.
• Assist the family in arranging care in a way that allows the client to participate in family or favorite activities without embarrassment.
▲ If the client is limited to bed (or bed and chair), provide a commode or bedpan that can be easily accessed. If necessary, refer the client to physical therapy services to learn side transfers and to build strength for transfers.
▲ If the client is frequently incontinent, refer for home health aide services to assist with hygiene and skin care.

• = Independent        ▲ = Collaborative

B

- Teach the client and family to perform a bowel reeducation program; a scheduled, stimulated program; or other strategies to manage fecal incontinence.
- Teach the client and family about common dietary sources for fiber, as well as supplemental fiber or bulking agents as indicated.
- ▲ Refer the family to support services to assist with in-home management of fecal incontinence as indicated.
- Teach nursing colleagues and nonprofessional care providers the importance of providing toileting opportunities and adequate privacy for the client in an acute care or long-term care facility.

NOTE: Refer to nursing diagnoses **Diarrhea** and **Constipation** for detailed management of these related conditions.

# Effective Breastfeeding

## NANDA Definition

Mother-infant dyad/family exhibits adequate proficiency and satisfaction with the breastfeeding process

## Defining Characteristics

Effective mother/infant communication patterns; regular and sustained suckling/swallowing at the breast; appropriate infant weight pattern for age; infant content after feeding; mother able to position infant at breast to promote a successful latch-on response; signs and/or symptoms of oxytocin release; adequate infant elimination patterns for age; eagerness of infant to nurse; maternal verbalization of satisfaction with the breastfeeding process

## Related Factors (r/t)

Infant gestational age >34 weeks; support source; normal infant oral structure; maternal confidence; basic breastfeeding knowledge; normal breast structure

• = Independent          ▲ = Collaborative

## Client Outcomes

### Client Will (Specify Time Frame):

B

- Maintain effective breastfeeding.
- Maintain normal growth patterns (infant).
- Verbalize satisfaction with breastfeeding process (mother).

## Nursing Interventions

- Encourage and facilitate early skin-to-skin contact (SSC) (position includes contact of the naked baby with the mother's bare chest within 2 hours after birth).
- Encourage rooming-in and breastfeeding on demand.
- Monitor the breastfeeding process.
- Identify opportunities to enhance knowledge and experience regarding breastfeeding. Support and teaching must be individualized to the client's level of understanding.
- Give encouragement/positive feedback related to breastfeeding mother-infant interactions.
- Monitor for signs and symptoms of nipple pain and/or trauma.
- Discuss prevention and treatment of common breastfeeding problems. This permits the nurse to identify the need for information and clarification.
- Monitor infant responses to breastfeeding.
- Identify current support person network and opportunities for continued breastfeeding support.
- Avoid supplemental bottle feedings and do not provide samples of formula on discharge.
- ▲ Provide follow-up contact; provide home visits and/or peer counseling, as available.

## Multicultural

- Assess for the influence of cultural beliefs, norms, and values on current breastfeeding practices.
- Assess mother's timing preference to begin breastfeeding.
- Validate the client's concerns about the amount of milk taken.

• = Independent          ▲ = Collaborative

**B**

## Home Care

- Above interventions may be adapted for home care use.

## Client/Family Teaching

- Include the father and other family members in education about breastfeeding.
- Teach the client the importance of maternal nutrition.
- Reinforce the infant's subtle hunger cues (e.g., quiet-alert state, rooting, sucking, hand-to-mouth activity) and encourage the client to nurse whenever signs are apparent.
- Review guidelines for frequency (every 2 to 3 hours, or 8–12 feedings per 24 hours) and duration (until sucking and swallowing slow down and satiety is reached) of feeding times.
- Provide anticipatory guidance about common infant behaviors.
- Provide information about additional breastfeeding resources.

# Ineffective Breastfeeding

## NANDA Definition

Dissatisfaction or difficulty a mother, infant, or child experiences with the breastfeeding process

## Defining Characteristics

Unsatisfactory breastfeeding process; nonsustained suckling at the breast; resisting latching-on; unresponsive to comfort measures; persistence of sore nipples beyond first week of breastfeeding; observable signs of inadequate infant intake; insufficient emptying of each breast per feeding; infant inability to latch-on to maternal breast correctly; infant arching and crying at the breast; infant exhibiting fussiness and crying within the first hour after breastfeeding; actual or perceived inadequate milk supply; no observable signs of oxytocin release; insufficient opportunity for suckling at the breast

• = Independent      ▲ = Collaborative

## Related Factors (r/t)

Nonsupportive partner/family; previous breast surgery; infant receiving supplemental feedings with artificial nipple; prematurity; previous history of breastfeeding failure; poor infant sucking reflex; maternal breast anomaly; maternal anxiety or ambivalence; interruption in breastfeeding; infant anomaly; knowledge deficit

## Client Outcomes

### Client Will (Specify Time Frame):

- Achieve effective breastfeeding (dyad).
- Verbalize/demonstrate techniques to manage breastfeeding problems (mother).
- Manifest signs of adequate intake at the breast (infant).
- Manifest positive self-esteem in relation to the infant feeding process (mother).
- Explain alternative method of infant feeding if unable to continue exclusive breastfeeding (mother).

## Nursing Interventions

- Identify women with risk factors for lower breastfeeding initiation and continuation rates (age <20 years, low socioeconomic status) as well as factors contributing to ineffective breastfeeding as early as possible in the perinatal experience.
- Use valid and reliable tools to measure breastfeeding performance and to predict early discontinuance of breastfeeding whenever possible/feasible.
- Encourage and facilitate early skin-to-skin contact (SSC) (position includes contact of the naked baby with the mother's bare chest within 2 hours after birth).
- Encourage rooming-in and feeding on demand.
- Evaluate the breast and nipple structures and provide appropriate measures as needed.
- Observe a full breastfeeding session (every 8 hours in the early postpartum and once per visit on follow-up).
- Provide evidence-based teaching and breastfeeding assis-

• = Independent          ▲ = Collaborative

B

tance appropriate to the client's individualized needs (see Client/Family Teaching).
- Promote comfort and relaxation to reduce pain and anxiety.
- Provide time for clients to express expectations and concerns and give emotional support.
- Avoid supplemental feedings.
- Monitor infant behavioral cues and responses to breastfeeding.
- Collect data and monitor signs of adequate infant intake/nutrition.
- Provide necessary equipment/instruction/assistance for milk expression as needed.
- Provide anticipatory guidance in relation to home management of breastfeeding.
- Assist the client to identify and use a support network.
- Do not provide samples of formula on discharge.
- Initiate breastfeeding follow-up after hospital discharge.
▲ Provide referrals and resources.
- If unsuccessful in achieving effective breastfeeding, help client accept and learn an alternate method of infant feeding.

## Multicultural
- Assess for the influence of cultural beliefs, norms, and values on breastfeeding attitudes. Assess whether the client's concerns about the amount of milk taken during breastfeeding are contributing to dissatisfaction with the breastfeeding process.
- Assess the influence of family support on the decision to continue or discontinue breastfeeding.
- Assess for the influence of mother's weight on attempts to initiate and sustain breastfeeding.
- Validate the client's feelings regarding the difficulty or dissatisfaction with breastfeeding.

## Home Care
- Above interventions may be adapted for home care use.
▲ Investigate availability and refer to public health depart-

• = Independent          ▲ = Collaborative

ment, hospital home follow-up breastfeeding program, or other postdischarge support.

- Monitor for specific difficulties contributing to bonding difficulties between mother and infant. Refer to care plan for **Risk for impaired parent/infant/child Attachment.**

**B**

## Client/Family Teaching

- Review maternal and infant benefits of breastfeeding.
- Instruct the client on maternal breastfeeding behaviors/ techniques (preparation for, positioning, initiation of/ promoting latch-on, burping, completion of session, and frequency of feeding).
- Teach the client self-care measures for the breastfeeding woman (e.g., breast care, management of breast/nipple discomfort, nutrition/fluid, rest/activity).
- Provide information regarding infant cues and behaviors related to breastfeeding and appropriate maternal responses (e.g., cues that infant is ready to feed, behaviors during feeding that contribute to effective breastfeeding, measures of infant feeding adequacy).
- Provide education to father/family/significant others as needed.

# Interrupted Breastfeeding

## NANDA Definition

Break in the continuity of the breastfeeding process as a result of inability or inadvisability of placing the infant at the breast for feeding

## Defining Characteristics

Infant does not receive nourishment at the breast for some or all feedings; maternal desire to maintain lactation and provide (or eventually provide) her breast milk for her infant's nutritional needs; lack of knowledge regarding expression and storage of breast milk; separation of mother and infant

● = Independent          ▲ = Collaborative

## Related Factors (r/t)

Contraindications to breastfeeding; maternal employment; maternal or infant illness; need to abruptly wean infant; prematurity

## Client Outcomes

### Client Will (Specify Time Frame):

### Infant
- Receive mother's breast milk if not contraindicated by maternal conditions (e.g., certain drugs, infections) or infant conditions (e.g., true breast milk jaundice).

### Maternal
- Maintain lactation.
- Achieve effective breastfeeding or satisfaction with the breastfeeding experience.
- Demonstrate effective methods of breast milk collection and storage.

## Nursing Interventions

- Discuss mother's desire/intention to begin or resume breastfeeding.
- Provide anticipatory guidance to the mother/family regarding potential duration of the interruption when possible/feasible.
- Reassure mother/family that early measures to sustain lactation and promote parent-infant attachment can make it possible to resume breastfeeding when the condition/situation requiring interruption is resolved.
- Reassure the mother/family that the infant will benefit from any amount of breast milk provided.
- Provide time for mother/family to express their expectations and concerns and give emotional support. Emotional responses regarding events leading to the interruption that may arise include feelings of grief/loss, guilt, anxiety, and failure.
- ▲ Collaborate with the mother/family/health care provid-

• = Independent          ▲ = Collaborative

ers/employers (as needed) to develop a plan for expression of breast milk/infant feeding/and kangaroo care/skin-to-skin contact (KC).

- • Monitor for signs indicating infant's ability to breastfeed and interest in breastfeeding.
- • Provide evidence-based teaching and practical assistance with milk expression, storage, temporary feeding techniques, and breastfeeding techniques appropriate to the client's individualized needs (see Client/Family Teaching).
- • Observe mother performing psychomotor skills (expression, storage, alternative feeding, KC, and/or breastfeeding) and assist as needed.
- ▲ Provide and/or assist with arrangements and/or necessary equipment.
- ▲ Use supplementation only as medically indicated.
- • Provide anticipatory guidance for common problems associated with interrupted breastfeeding (e.g., incomplete emptying of milk glands, diminishing milk supply, infant difficulty with resuming breastfeeding, or infant refusal of alternative feeding method).
- ▲ Initiate follow-up and make appropriate referrals.
- • Assist the client to accept and learn an alternative method of infant feeding if effective breastfeeding is not achieved.

## Multicultural

- • Assess for the influence of cultural beliefs, norms, and values on current decision to stop breastfeeding.
- • Assess the influence of family support on the decision to continue or discontinue breastfeeding.
- • Assess whether the client's concerns about the amount of milk taken during breastfeeding are contributing to decision to stop breastfeeding.
- • Teach culturally appropriate techniques for maintaining lactation.
- • Validate the client's feelings with regard to the difficulty of or dissatisfaction with breastfeeding.

• = Independent          ▲ = Collaborative

B

## Home Care
- Above interventions may be adapted for home care use.

## Client/Family Teaching
- Teach mother effective methods to express breast milk.
- Teach mother/parents about kangaroo care.
- Instruct mother on safe breast milk handling techniques.
- Provide education to father/family/significant others as needed.

# Ineffective Breathing pattern

## NANDA Definition

Inspiration and/or expiration that does not provide adequate ventilation

## Defining Characteristics

Decreased inspiratory/expiratory pressure; decreased minute ventilation; use of accessory muscles to breathe; nasal flaring; dyspnea; altered chest excursion; shortness of breath; assumption of a three-point position; pursed-lip breathing; prolonged expiration phases; increased anteroposterior diameter; respiratory rate/min: infants = <25 or >60, ages 1–4 = <20 or >30, ages 5–14 = <14 or >25, adults over 14 = <11 or >24; depth of breathing: adult tidal volume = 500 ml at rest, infant tidal volume = 6–8 ml/kg; timing ratio; decreased vital capacity

## Related Factors (r/t)

Hyperventilation; hypoventilation syndrome; bony deformity; pain; chest wall deformity; anxiety; decreased energy/fatigue; neuromuscular dysfunction; musculoskeletal impairment; perception/cognitive impairment; obesity; spinal cord injury; body position; neurological immaturity; respiratory muscle fatigue

• = Independent          ▲ = Collaborative

## Client Outcomes

### Client Will (Specify Time Frame):

B

- Demonstrate a breathing pattern that supports blood gas results within the client's normal parameters.
- Report ability to breathe comfortably.
- Demonstrate ability to perform pursed-lip breathing and controlled breathing and use relaxation techniques effectively.
- Identify and avoid specific factors that exacerbate episodes of ineffective breathing patterns.

### Nursing Interventions

- Monitor respiratory rate, depth, and ease of respiration. Normal respiratory rate is 12 to 16 breaths/min in the adult.
- Note pattern of respiration. If client is dyspneic, note what seems to cause the dyspnea, the way in which the client handles the condition, and how the dyspnea resolves or worsens. Note amount of anxiety associated with the dyspnea.
- Attempt to determine if client's dyspnea is physiological or psychological in etiology.

### Psychological Dyspnea—Hyperventilation

- Assess cause of hyperventilation by asking client about current emotions and psychological state.
- Ask the client to breathe with you to slow down respiratory rate. Maintain eye contact and give reassurance.
- ▲ If pain is the cause of hyperventilation, provide medication routinely as ordered to prevent severe pain. Use distraction techniques to help client deal with pain. See interventions for **Acute Pain.**
- ▲ If client has chronic problems with hyperventilation, numbness and tingling in extremities, dizziness, and other signs of panic attacks, refer for counseling.

● = Independent          ▲ = Collaborative

**Physiological Dyspnea**

B

- Ensure that client in acute dyspneic state has received medications, oxygen, and any other treatment needed.
- Determine severity of dyspnea using a rating scale such as the modified Borg scale, rating dyspnea from 0 (best) to 10 (worst) in severity. An alternative scale is the visual analog scale (VAS), with dyspnea rated from 0 (best) to 100 (worst).
- Note abdominal breathing, use of accessory muscles, nasal flaring, retractions, irritability, confusion, or lethargy.
- Observe color of tongue, oral mucosa, and skin.
- Auscultate breath sounds, noting decreased or absent sounds, crackles, or wheezes.
- ▲ Monitor client's oxygen saturation and blood gases.
- ▲ Monitor for presence of pain and provide pain medication for comfort as needed.
- Use shoulder touching to coach clients to decrease their respiratory rate by demonstrating slower respirations; make eye contact with the client and communicate in a calm, supportive fashion.
- Support the client in using pursed-lip and controlled breathing techniques.
- Position the client in an upright or semi-Fowler's position. See nursing interventions for **Impaired Gas exchange** for further information on positioning.
- ▲ Administer oxygen as ordered.
- Increase client's activity to walking three times per day as tolerated. Assist the client to use oxygen during activity as needed.
- Schedule rest periods before and after activity.
- ▲ Evaluate the client's nutritional status. Refer to a dietitian if needed. Use nutritional supplements to increase nutritional level if needed.
- Provide small, frequent feedings.
- Offer a fan to move the air in the environment.
- Encourage the client to take deep breaths at prescribed intervals and do controlled coughing.
- Help the client with chronic respiratory disease evaluate the dyspnea experience to determine if it was similar

• = Independent          ▲ = Collaborative

to previous incidences of dyspnea and to recognize that
he or she survived those incidences. Encourage the client
to be self-reliant if possible, use problem-solving skills,
and maximize use of social support.

- See **Ineffective Airway clearance** if client has a problem
with increased respiratory secretions.
▲ Refer COPD client for pulmonary rehabilitation.

## Geriatric
- Encourage ambulation as tolerated.
- Encourage elderly clients to sit upright or stand and to
avoid lying down for prolonged periods during the day.

## Home Care
- Above interventions may be adapted for home care use.
- Assist the client and family with identification of other
factors that precipitate or exacerbate episodes of ineffective breathing patterns (i.e., stress, allergens, stairs, activities that have high energy requirements).
- Assess client knowledge of and compliance with medication regimen.
- Teach client and family the importance of maintaining
regimen and having necessary drugs easily accessible
at all times.
- Provide the client with emotional support in dealing with
symptoms of respiratory difficulty. Provide family with
support for care of a client with chronic or terminal
illness. Refer to care plan for **Powerlessness.**
- When respiratory procedures (e.g., apneic monitoring for
an infant) are being implemented, explain equipment
and procedures to family members, and provide needed
emotional support.
- When electrically based equipment for respiratory support is being implemented, evaluate home environment for electrical safety and proper grounding, for example. Ensure that notification is sent to the local utility
company, the emergency medical team, and the police
and fire departments.
- Refer to GOLD and ACP-ASIM/ACCP guidelines for

• = Independent          ▲ = Collaborative

B

COPD for management of home care and indications of hospital admission criteria.
- Support client's efforts at self-care. Ensure he or she has all the information needed to participate in care.
- Identify an emergency plan including when to call the physician or dial 911.
▲ Refer the client to an outpatient pulmonary rehabilitation program or a home-based training program for COPD.
▲ Refer to occupational therapy for evaluation and teaching of energy conservation techniques.
▲ Refer to home health aide services as needed to support energy conservation.
▲ Institute case management of frail elderly to support continued independent living. Respiratory difficulties represent and can lead to increasing need for assistance in using the health care system effectively. Case management combines nursing activities of client and family assessment, planning and coordination of care among all health care providers, delivery of direct nursing care, and monitoring of care and outcomes.

## Client/Family Teaching

- Teach pursed-lip and controlled breathing techniques.
- Using a prerecorded tape, teach client progressive muscle relaxation techniques.
- Teach about dosage, actions, and side effects of medications.
- Teach the client to identify and avoid specific factors that exacerbate ineffective breathing patterns, such as exposure to other sources of air pollution (especially smoking).

• = Independent          ▲ = Collaborative

# Decreased Cardiac output

## NANDA Definition

Inadequate blood pumped by the heart to meet metabolic demands of the body

## Defining Characteristics

**Altered heart rate/rhythm:** Dysrhythmias (tachycardia, bradycardia); palpitations; electrocardiographic changes

**Altered preload:** Jugular vein distention; fatigue; edema; murmurs; increased/decreased central venous pressure (CVP); increased/decreased pulmonary artery wedge pressure (PAWP); weight gain

**Altered afterload:** Cold/clammy skin; shortness of breath/dyspnea; oliguria; prolonged capillary refill; decreased peripheral pulses; variations in blood pressure readings; increased/decreased systemic vascular resistance (SVR); increased/decreased pulmonary vascular resistance (PVR); skin color changes

**Altered contractility:** Crackles; cough; orthopnea/paroxysmal nocturnal dyspnea; cardiac output less than 4 L/min; cardiac index less than 2.5 L/min; decreased ejection fraction; decreased stroke volume index (SVI); decreased left ventricular stroke work index (LVSWI); $S_3$ or $S_4$ sounds

**Behavioral/emotional:** Anxiety; restlessness

## Related Factors (r/t)

Altered heart rate/rhythm; altered stroke volume: altered preload, altered afterload, altered contractility

## Client Outcomes

**Client Will (Specify Time Frame):**

• Demonstrate adequate cardiac output as evidenced by blood pressure and pulse rate and rhythm within normal parameters for client; strong peripheral pulses; and an ability to tolerate activity without symptoms of dyspnea, syncope, or chest pain.

● = Independent          ▲ = Collaborative

- Remain free of side effects from the medications used to achieve adequate cardiac output.
- Explain actions and precautions to take for cardiac disease.

## C Nursing Interventions

- Monitor for symptoms of heart failure and decreased cardiac output; listen to heart sounds and lung sounds; note symptoms including dyspnea, orthopnea, paroxysmal nocturnal dyspnea, Cheyne-Stokes respirations, fatigue, weakness, third and fourth heart sounds, crackles in lungs, increased venous pressure greater than 16 cm $H_2O$, and positive hepatojugular reflex.
- Recognize the importance of cardiac index estimated by thermodilution in the ICU patient.
- Be aware of the use of impedance cardiography in noninvasive hemodynamic monitoring of heart failure.
- Recognize the effect of sleep-disordered breathing in heart failure.
- Observe for chest pain or discomfort; note location, radiation, severity, quality, duration, and associated manifestations such as nausea, indigestion, and diaphoresis; also note precipitating and relieving factors.
- ▲ If chest pain is present, have client lie down, monitor cardiac rhythm, give oxygen, check vital signs, run a monitor strip, medicate for pain, and notify the physician.
- Monitor intake and output. If client is acutely ill, measure hourly urine output and note decreases in output.
- Note results of electrocardiography and chest radiography.
- Note results of diagnostic imaging studies such as echocardiogram, radionuclide imaging, or dobutamine stress echocardiography.
- Watch laboratory data closely, especially arterial blood gases, electrolytes including potassium, and B-type natriuretic peptide (BNP assay).
- Monitor lab work such as complete blood count, sodium level, and serum creatinine level.
- ▲ Administer oxygen as needed per physician's order.

• = Independent          ▲ = Collaborative

- Place client in semi-Fowler's position or position of comfort.
▲ Check blood pressure, pulse, and condition before administering cardiac medications such as angiotensin-converting enzyme (ACE) inhibitors, digoxin, calcium channel blockers, and beta-blockers such as carvedilol. Notify physician if heart rate or blood pressure is low before holding medications.
- During acute events, ensure client remains on short-term bed rest or maintains activity level that does not compromise cardiac output.
- Gradually increase activity when client's condition is stabilized by encouraging slower paced activities or shorter periods of activity with frequent rest periods following exercise prescription; observe for symptoms of intolerance. Take blood pressure and pulse before and after activity and note changes. See care plan for **Activity intolerance.**
- Serve small sodium-restricted, low-cholesterol meals.
- Serve only small amounts of coffee or caffeine-containing beverages if requested (no more than 4 cups in 24 hours) if no resulting dysrhythmia.
- Monitor bowel function. Provide stool softeners as ordered. Caution client not to strain when defecating.
- Have clients use a commode or urinal for toileting and avoid use of a bedpan.
- Provide a restful environment by minimizing controllable stressors and unnecessary disturbances. Schedule rest periods after meals and activities.
- Weigh client at same time daily (after voiding).
- Apply graduated compression stockings as ordered. Ensure proper fit by measuring accurately. Remove the stocking at least twice a day, in the morning with the bath and in the evening, to assess the condition of the extremity; then reapply.
- Assess for presence of anxiety. Consider using music to decrease anxiety and improve cardiac function. See Nursing Interventions for **Anxiety** to facilitate reduction of anxiety in clients and family.

• = Independent          ▲ = Collaborative

▲ Refer for treatment if anxiety is present.
▲ Closely monitor fluid intake, including intravenous lines. Maintain fluid restriction if ordered.
▲ Observe for symptoms of cardiogenic shock including impaired mentation, hypotension with blood pressure lower than 90 mm Hg, decreased peripheral pulses, cold clammy skin, and signs of pulmonary congestion and decreased organ function. If present, notify physician immediately.
• If shock is present, monitor hemodynamic parameters for an increase in pulmonary wedge pressure, an increase in systemic vascular resistance, or a decrease in cardiac output and index.
• Titrate inotropic and vasoactive medications within defined parameters to maintain contractility, preload, and afterload per physician's order.
▲ Refer to heart failure program or cardiac rehabilitation program for education, evaluation, and guided support to increase activity and rebuild life.

**Geriatric**
• Observe for atypical pain; the elderly often have jaw pain instead of chest pain or may have silent myocardial infarctions (MIs) with symptoms of dyspnea or fatigue.
▲ If client has heart disease causing activity intolerance, refer for cardiac rehabilitation.
• Consider the use of graphic feedback with the elderly in exercise adherence.
▲ Observe for syncope, dizziness, palpitations, or feelings of weakness associated with an irregular heart rhythm.
▲ Observe for side effects from cardiac medications.

**Home Care**
• Some of the above interventions may be adapted for home care use.
▲ Begin discharge planning as soon as possible with case manager or social worker to assess home support systems and the need for community or home health services. Consider referral for advanced practice nurse

• = Independent          ▲ = Collaborative

(APN) follow-up. Support services may be needed to assist with home care, meal preparations, housekeeping, personal care, transportation to doctor visits, or emotional support.

- Adopt a clinical pathway to address focused interventions with congestive heart failure (CHF) or coronary artery bypass graft (CABG) surgery.
- ▲ Assess or refer to case manager or social worker to evaluate client's ability to pay for prescriptions.
- Continue to monitor client closely for exacerbation of heart failure when discharged home.
- Monitor women for differential symptoms of MI and institute emergency treatment measures as indicated.
- Instruct women in the differential symptoms of MI in women, and the need to take symptoms seriously, seeking help as indicated.
- Assess client for understanding of and compliance with medical regimen, including medications, activity level, and diet. Client/family may need repetition of instructions received at hospital discharge, and may require reiteration as fear of a recent crisis decreases.
- ▲ Assess and monitor for signs of depression (particularly in adults age 65 years or older) or social isolation. Refer for mental health treatment as indicated.
- Assess for signs/symptoms of cognitive impairment.
- Assess for fatigue and weakness frequently. Assess home environment for safety as well as resources/obstacles to energy conservation. Instruct client and family members on need for behavioral pacing and energy conservation.
- Instruct family and client about the disease process, complications of the disease process, information on medications, need for daily weighing, and when it is appropriate to call doctor.
- Help family adapt daily living patterns to establish life changes that will maintain improved cardiac functioning in the client. Take the client's perspective into consideration, and use a holistic approach in assessing and responding to client planning for the future.

• = Independent          ▲ = Collaborative

- Assist client to recognize and exercise power in using self-care management to adjust to health change.
- Support client self-efficacy to increase physical activity by creating a supportive environment, offering encouragement, providing anticipatory guidance, and supplying a realistic assessment of the client's abilities.
▲ Explore barriers to medical regimen adherence. Review medications and treatment regularly for needed modifications. Take complaints of side effects seriously and serve as client advocate to address changes as indicated.
▲ Refer for cardiac rehabilitation, strengthening exercises if client is not involved in outpatient cardiac rehabilitation. Refer to agency cardiac care program if available.
▲ Refer to medical social services as necessary for counseling about the impact of severe or chronic cardiac disease.
▲ Institute case management of frail elderly to support continued independent living.
▲ As client condition warrants, refer to hospice.
▲ Provide specific written materials and self-care plan for client/caregivers to use for reference. Consult dietitian or assist client in understanding the need for a sodium-restricted diet. Provide alternatives for salt such as spices, herbs, lemon juice, or vinegar.
- Identify emergency plan, including use of CPR. Encourage family members to become certified in cardiopulmonary resuscitation.

## Client/Family Teaching

- Teach symptoms of heart failure and appropriate actions to take if client becomes symptomatic.
- Teach importance of smoking cessation and avoidance of alcohol intake.
- Teach stress reduction techniques (e.g., imagery, controlled breathing, muscle relaxation techniques).
- Explain necessary restrictions, including consumption of a sodium-restricted diet, guidelines on fluid intake, and the avoidance of Valsalva maneuver. Teach the importance of pacing activities, work simplification tech-

• = Independent        ▲ = Collaborative

niques, and the need to rest between activities to prevent becoming overly fatigued.

▲ Assist the client in understanding the need for and how to incorporate lifestyle changes. Refer to cardiac rehabilitation for assistance with coping and adjustment.

▲ Teach the client actions, side effects, and importance of consistently taking cardiovascular medications.

• Provide client/family with advance directive information to consider. Allow client to give advance directions about medical care or designate who should make medical decisions if he or she should lose decision-making capacity.

• Instruct the client on importance of getting a pneumonia shot (usually one per lifetime) and yearly flu shots as prescribed by physician.

• Instruct client/family on the need to weigh daily and keep a weight log. Ask if client has a scale at home; if not, assist in getting one. Instruct on establishing baseline weight on own scale when client gets home.

• Provide specific written materials and self-care plan for client/caregivers to use for reference.

▲ Consult dietitian or assist client in understanding the need for a sodium-restricted diet. Provide alternatives for salt such as spices, herbs, lemon juice, or vinegar.

• Instruct family regarding cardiopulmonary resuscitation.

# Caregiver role strain

## NANDA Definition

Difficulty in performing family caregiver role

### Defining Characteristics

### Caregiving Activities

Difficulty performing/completing required tasks; preoccupation with care routine; apprehension about the future regarding care receiver's health and the caregiver's ability to provide care;

• = Independent          ▲ = Collaborative

apprehension about care receiver's care if caregiver becomes ill or dies; dysfunctional change in caregiving activities; apprehension about possible institutionalization of care receiver

### Caregiver Health Status—Physical
Gastrointestinal upset (e.g., mild stomach cramps, vomiting, diarrhea, recurrent gastric ulcer episodes); weight change; rash; hypertension; cardiovascular disease; diabetes; fatigue; headaches

### Caregiver Health Status—Emotional
Impaired individual coping; feeling depressed; disturbed sleep; anger; stress; somatization; increased nervousness; increased emotional lability; irritability; impatience; lack of time to meet personal needs; frustration

### Caregiver Health Status—Socioeconomic
Withdrawal from social life; changes in leisure activities; low work productivity; refuses career advancement

### Caregiver-Care Receiver Relationship
Grief/uncertainty regarding changed relationship with care receiver; difficulty watching care receiver go through the illness

### Family Processes
Family conflict; concerns about family members

## Related Factors (r/t)

### Care Receiver Health Status
Illness severity; illness chronicity; increasing care needs/dependency; unpredictability of illness course; instability of care receiver's health; problem behaviors; psychological or cognitive problems; addiction or codependency

### Caregiving Activities
Amount of activities; complexity of activities; 24-hour care responsibilities; ongoing changes in activities; discharge of family members to home with significant care needs; years of caregiving; unpredictability of care situation

• = Independent          ▲ = Collaborative

## Caregiver Health Status

Physical problems; psychological or cognitive problems; addiction or codependency; marginal coping patterns; unrealistic expectations of self; inability to fulfill one's own or others' expectations

## Socioeconomic Factors

Isolation from others; competing role commitments; alienation from family, friends, and coworkers; insufficient recreation

## Caregiver-Care Receiver Relationship

History of poor relationship; presence of abuse or violence; unrealistic expectations of caregiver by care receiver; mental status of elder inhibiting conversation

## Family Processes

History of marginal family coping; history of family dysfunction

## Resources

Inadequate physical environment for providing care (e.g., housing, temperature, safety); inadequate equipment for providing care; inadequate transportation; inadequate community resources (e.g., respite services, recreational resources); insufficient finances; lack of support; caregiver is not developmentally ready for caregiver role; inexperience with caregiving; insufficient time; lack of knowledge about or difficulty assessing community resources; lack of caregiver privacy; emotional strength; physical energy; assistance and support (formal and informal)

## Client Outcomes

- Caregiver will feel supported.
- Caregiver will report low or no feelings of burden or distress.
- Caregiver will maintain physical and psychological/emotional health.
- Caregiver will identify resources available to help in giving care.
- Caregiver will verbalize mastery of the care situation.
- Care receiver will obtain appropriate care.

• = Independent      ▲ = Collaborative

## Nursing Interventions

- Use an evaluation tool to determine caregiver burden and role strain. Various instruments have been developed, including the Burden Interview, the Caregiver Strain Index, the Caregiver Burden Inventory, the Caregiver Reaction Assessment, the Screen for Caregiver Burden, and the Subjective and Objective Burden Scale.
- Use an evaluation tool to determine potential caregiver resources such as mastery, social support, optimism, positive aspects of care.
- Screen for caregiver role strain at the onset of the care situation, at regular intervals throughout the care situation, and with changes in care recipient status and care transitions.
- Watch for signs of depression and deteriorating health in the caregiver, especially if the marital relationship is poor, the care recipient has cognitive or neuropsychiatric symptoms, there is little social support available, the caregiver becomes enmeshed in the care situation, the caregiver is elderly, female, or has poor preexisting physical or emotional health. Intervene to provide support and to help the caregiver obtain counseling to cope. If signs are present, refer to the care plan for **Hopelessness.**
- Watch for caregivers who become enmeshed in the care situation (for example, becoming overinvolved or unable to disentangle themselves from the caregiver role).
- Monitor the quality of care by the caregiver for adequacy and need for improvement.
- Arrange for intervals of respite care for the caregiver; encourage use if available.
- Help the caregiver to identify support systems and be assertive in using them.
- Encourage the caregiver to grieve over changes in the care receiver's condition. Give the caregiver permission to share angry feelings in a safe environment. Refer to Nursing Interventions for **Grieving.**
- Identify with the caregiver the factors that can and cannot be controlled.

• = Independent          ▲ = Collaborative

C

- Help the caregiver find personal time to meet his or her own needs, learn stress management techniques, schedule regular health screenings, and schedule regular respite time.
- Encourage the caregiver to schedule and keep routine health care appointments (i.e., annual physicals and screening tests).
- Support the caregiver in setting boundaries and determining the legitimate caregiving role.
- Encourage the caregiver to use humor to cope when appropriate, including cartoons, stories, and jokes.
- Encourage the caregiver to talk about feelings, concerns, uncertainties, and fears. Acknowledge the frustration associated with caregiver responsibilities.
- Observe for any evidence of caregiver or care receiver violence or abuse; if evidence is present, speak with the caregiver and care receiver separately.
▲ Involve the family in care transitions; use a multidisciplinary team to provide medical and social serves for instruction and planning.
- Give the caregiver permission to arrange custodial care in an extended care facility if necessary; support both caregiver and care receiver during this difficult transition.
- Help the caregiver deal with elements of placing the care receiver in a long-term care facility, planning for stress, and seeking solace in support from others.
- Encourage regular communication with the care recipient and with the health care team.
- Help caregiver assess his/her socioeconomic status (services reimbursed by insurance, available support through community and religious organizations).
- Help the caregiver identify competing occupational demands and potential ways to modify the work role in order to provide care (use the Family Medical Leave Act, change from full-time to part-time employment, work from home, take a leave of absence or early retirement).
- Validate the family's feelings regarding the impact of caregiving on family and personal lifestyle.

• = Independent          ▲ = Collaborative

C

## Geriatric

- Monitor the caregiver for psychological distress and signs of depression, especially if caring for a mentally impaired elder or if there was an unsatisfactory marital relationship before caregiving.
- Assess the health of caregivers at intervals, especially if they have their own chronic illness in addition to caregiving role.
- Recognize that it is hard for the elderly to accept a change in caregivers or in the environment.
- Assess social support and encourage the use of secondary carers in elderly caregivers.
- Provide skills' training related to direct care, such as performing complex monitoring tasks, interpreting patient symptoms, assisting with decision making, providing emotional support and comfort, and coordinating care.
- Teach symptom management techniques (assessment, potential causes, aggravating factors, potential alleviating factors, reassessment), particularly for fatigue, constipation, anorexia, and pain.

## Multicultural

- Assess for the influence of cultural beliefs, norms, values, and expectations on the family's experience of caregiving.
- Assess for conflicts between the caregiver's cultural obligations to provide care and competing factors such as employment, time management and arrangements, their own health, competing role demands, and low rewards.
- Assess and identify the impact of the caregiver's own health on role overload.
- Negotiate with the client regarding the aspects of caregiving that can be modified while still honoring cultural beliefs.
- ▲ Refer the family to social services or other supportive services to assist with the impact of caregiving.
- ▲ Assist the family/caregiver in identifying barriers that would prevent the use of social services or other supportive services that could help reduce the impact of caregiving.

● = Independent          ▲ = Collaborative

▲ Encourage the family to use support groups or other service programs.

• Encourage caregiver use of spirituality or religion as a source of support for the caregiver.

• Validate the family's feelings regarding the impact of caregiving on family and personal lifestyle.

## Home Care

• Identify client and caregiver factors that necessitated the use of formal home care services, and that may affect provision of care or that need to be addressed before the client can be safely discharged from home care.

• Assess the level of caregiver strain; use of a measurement tool may be helpful.

• Assess caregiver levels of optimism or pessimism.

• Assess the client and caregiver at every visit for quality of care provided, functional disability of care recipient, caregiver coping, and signs of caregiver stress. Document all observations objectively.

• Assess the client and caregiver at every visit for quality of relationship, and for the quality of caring that exists.

• Assess family caregiving skill. The identification of caregiver difficulty with any of a core set of processes highlights areas for intervention.

• Assess perceived level of power experienced by the caregiver in ability to complete daily activities.

• Assess preexisting strengths and weaknesses the caregiver brings to the situation, as well as current responses, depression, and fatigue levels.

• Identify and support strengths of the caregiver and efforts to gain control of unpredictable situations.

• Help the caregiver to stay connected with the client who may be behaving differently than usual, to make life as routine as possible, to help the client set goals and sustain hope, and to allow the client space to experience progress.

• Recognize that caregiver disabilities may not prevent them from providing care; assess each situation individually.

• = Independent        ▲ = Collaborative

- Form a trusting and supportive relationship with the caregiver. Allow the caregiver to verbalize frustrations.
- Assist the caregiver in identifying sources of concern and areas of stress in dealing with the client's illness.
- Instruct the caregiver in the care needs of the client, disease processes, medications, and expectations; use a variety of instructional techniques (e.g., explanations, demonstrations, visual aids) until the caregiver is able to express a degree of comfort with care delivery.
- Assist the caregiver and client in arranging care so that it is compatible with other household patterns.
- Explore the state of the relationship between the client and the caregiver before the onset of chronic illness or dementia; identify the strengths and weaknesses of each party. Formulate a plan to assist the couple in dealing with likely worsening of dementia.
- Explore with the spouse the process of understanding the client's behavior; assist the spouse in trying to be as realistic and positive as possible. Consider use of the Progressively Lowered Stress Threshold psychoeducational nursing intervention to help the spouse understand and handle the behavioral changes associated with Alzheimer's disease.
- ▲ Refer the client to home health aide services for assistance with ADLs and light housekeeping. Allow the caregiver to gain confidence in the respite provider.
- ▲ Identify appropriate individual and group interventions for the caregiver; assess for appropriateness of referrals given the caregiver's needs and mobility.
- ▲ Refer to a caregivers support group if available or recommend an online support group.
- Assess the caregiver for overinvolvement with the client and client's illness. Encourage the caregiver to address an enmeshed relationship with the client prompted by concerns over the client's illness and altered quality of life by discussing the issue, seeking respite, and attending support groups. Assist with identification of the spouse's needs and verbalization of the caregiving experience.
- ▲ Refer to case managers as necessary for community re-

• = Independent              ▲ = Collaborative

source assistance, financial planning, and supportive counseling for both client and caregiver.

▲ Refer for homemaker or psychiatric home health care services for respite, client reassurance, and implementation of a therapeutic regimen.

• As indicated by client status, assist the caregiver in examining the option of adult day care and maintaining realistic expectations of adult day care.

▲ As indicated by deterioration of the client's condition, assist the caregiver in examining options for institutional placement.

• Assess the caregiver's emotional response to placement of the client and provide support, cognitive interventions, and problem solving as needed.

• Be aware that physical demands on the caregiver tend to increase during the last 3 months of a care recipient's life, and more assistance with ADLs foretells greater risk of caregiver burden. Both emotional and instrumental support of the caregiver may increase toward recipient's end of life.

## Caregiver/Family Teaching

• Assess the caregiver's need for information (i.e., information on symptom management, disease progression, specific skills, available support).

• Teach the caregiver warning signs for burnout, depression, and anxiety. Help them to identify a resource in case they begin to feel overwhelmed.

• Teach the caregiver methods for managing disruptive behavioral symptoms if present. Refer to the care plan for **Chronic Confusion.**

• Teach the caregiver how to provide the physical care needed.

• Provide information and problem-solving techniques for symptom management in the care receiver.

• Provide ongoing support and evaluation of care skills as the care situation and care demands change.

• Provide information regarding the care recipient's diagnosis, treatment regimen, and expected course of illness.

• = Independent          ▲ = Collaborative

▲ Refer to counseling or support groups to assist in adjusting to the caregiver role.

C

# Risk for Caregiver role strain

## NANDA Definition

Caregiver vulnerability for perceived difficulty in performing family caregiver role

## Risk Factors

Caregiver not developmentally ready for caregiver role (e.g., a young adult needing to provide care for a middle-aged person); inadequate physical environment for providing care (e.g., housing, transportation, community services, equipment); unpredictable illness course or instability in care receiver's health; psychological or cognitive problems in care receiver; presence of situational stressors that normally affect families (e.g., significant loss, disaster, or crisis; economic vulnerability; major life events); presence of abuse or violence; premature birth/congenital defect; past history of poor relationship between caregiver and care receiver; marginal family adaptation or dysfunction prior to the caregiving situation; marginal caregiver's coping patterns; lack of respite and recreation for caregiver; inexperience with caregiving; caregiver is female; addiction or codependency; care receiver exhibits deviant, bizarre behavior; caregiver's competing role commitments; caregiver health impairment; illness severity of care receiver; caregiver is spouse; developmental delay or retardation of care receiver or caregiver; complexity/amount of caregiving tasks; discharge of family member with significant home care needs; duration of caregiving required; family/caregiver isolation

## Client Outcomes

### Client/Caregiver Will (Specify Time Frame):

- Maintain physical and psychological health.

● = Independent          ▲ = Collaborative

- Identify resources available to help in giving care.
- Obtain appropriate care.

**Nursing Interventions and Client/Family Teaching**

See care plan for **Caregiver role strain.**

C

---

## Impaired Comfort*

### Definition

State in which an individual experiences an uncomfortable sensation in response to a noxious stimulus; unpleasant sensation of being physically ill-at-ease that may be localized or generalized but is not described in terms of tissue damage

### Defining Characteristics

Verbalization of discomfort (specific examples include aches, pruritus, photophobia); observed behaviors indicative of discomfort; shifting and/or restlessness; tenseness; shivering and covering up or removing of covers; avoidance of particular stimuli; malaise; aching; stiffness; distention; hunger and thirst; reduced mobility; itching; reddened, irritated skin (pruritus)

### Related Factors (r/t)

Reaction to chemical irritants (including allergies); dry skin; illness and/or immobility; unmet physical needs (food, fluid, bathing, for example); fever; disease processes; pregnancy; immobility; musculoskeletal disorders; inflammation; intestinal gas, colic; medication side effects; contagious diseases (for example, chickenpox, meningitis)

### Client Outcomes

**Client Will (Specify Time Frame):**

- State he or she is comfortable.

---

*Impaired Comfort is not a NANDA-I-approved nursing diagnosis.

• = Independent      ▲ = Collaborative

- State that his or her uncomfortable sensations (aches, itching, for example) are relieved or diminished to an acceptable level.
- Explain methods to decrease own discomfort.
- Display improved physical mobility.
- Appear less restless and more at ease.

## Nursing Interventions

- Assess client needs holistically. Physical discomfort often coexists with and is exacerbated by emotional and spiritual discomfort; therefore addressing nonphysical needs can improve the client's perception of physical comfort. The nurse's therapeutic approach and demeanor can have a profound impact on perception of comfort.
- ▲ Consult with the physician for medication to reduce discomforting symptoms such as aching.
- Provide distraction techniques such as music, television, or games.
- Encourage early mobilization and provide routine position changes to decrease physical discomforts associated with bed rest.
- Position the client to maximize comfort.
- Provide simple massage.
- Provide gentle, soothing touch, which may be well suited for clients who cannot tolerate more stimulating interventions such as simple massage.
- Skin-to-skin contact and selection of the most effective method improve the comfort of newborns during routine blood draws.
- Inform the client of options for control of discomfort such as self-hypnosis and guided imagery, and provide these interventions if appropriate.
- Individualize the timing and type of bathing for each client; bathing may be distressing or comforting.
- Limit potentially uncomfortable interventions. Implement only when clearly needed and include the impetus for or timing of discontinuation in the plan of care.
- Tailor uncomfortable interventions to individual client needs or responses to therapy. Be aware of current

• = Independent        ▲ = Collaborative

research on alternatives to uncomfortable therapies that may benefit specific client groups or subgroups.
- Use careful, safe techniques when transferring patients in and out of beds or chairs.
- Offer acupressure either with the finger technique or with antinausea wrist bands for clients experiencing or at risk for nausea.
▲ Lower fevers with medication rather than sponging alone or in combination with medication unless there is a clear need to rapidly lower the client's temperature.

## Geriatric
- Comforting touch is helpful for elders because they respond to touch more than to verbal comforting.
- Frail elderly clients should be protected from cold discomfort, and can be offered warmed blankets to decrease discomfort.

## Multicultural
- Assess for the influence of cultural beliefs, norms, and values on the client's perceptions of skin and/or hair status and practices.
- Identify and clarify cultural language used to describe skin and hair.
- Assess skin for ashy appearance.
- Encourage the use of lanolin-based lotions for African-American clients with dry skin.
- Offer hair oil and lanolin-based lotion for dry scalp and skin.
- Use soap sparingly if the skin is dry.

## Home Care
- Assist the client and family in identifying and providing comfort measures that are effective and safe for the condition and situation.
- Encourage mobilization as frequently as is appropriate for the client.
- Keep the temperature of the home moderate to warm for frail clients.

• = Independent          ▲ = Collaborative

## Client/Family Teaching

- Teach techniques to use when the client is uncomfortable, including relaxation techniques, guided imagery, hypnosis, and music therapy.
- Instruct the client and family on prescribed medications and therapies that improve comfort.
- ▲ Teach the client to follow-up with the physician or other practitioner if discomfort persists.

## Pruritus

- Perform a complete assessment to determine the cause of pruritus (e.g., dry skin, contact with irritating substance, medication side effect, insect bite, infection, healing burns, underlying systemic disease).
- Assess for sleep disturbances.
- Implement soaks with cool or cold washcloths or offer cool baths if appropriate.
- Keep the client's fingernails short; have the client wear mitts if necessary.
- Leave pruritic area open to the air if possible.
- Use nonallergenic mild soap and use it sparingly.
- Keep skin well lubricated. After bathing, while the skin is still moist, apply nonallergenic moisturizers such as Medilan that are alcohol-free and available in cream or ointment form. Apply moisturizers daily.
- Provide simple massage for select client groups, such as those recovering from burns.
- Behavioral modification may reduce self-injury due to scratching and improve quality of life.
- ▲ Advocate for altering or substituting medications if pruritus is potentially a side effect of the current regimen.
- ▲ Consult with the physician for appropriate medications to relieve itching. Be aware of current research regarding medications best suited to relieving the pruritus associated with different causes.

## Geriatric

- Limit the number of complete baths to no more than one every other day. Consider the use of no-rinse skin cleansers as a bathing alternative for select clients.
- Use a superfatted soap such as Dove, Tone, Basis, or Caress.
- Increase fluid intake within cardiac or renal limits to a minimum of 1500 ml/day.
- Use a humidifier or place a container of water on a heat source to increase humidity in the environment, especially during winter.

## Home Care

- Assist the client and family in identifying and avoiding irritants that exacerbate pruritus (e.g., wool, cleansers, allergens).
- Teach the family to use mild, nonscented, and non–bleach-containing laundry products.
- Keep the temperature of the home moderate to cool. Use a humidifier.
- Support the use of the client's preferred body lotion, as long as it has not been found to exacerbate pruritus. Have the client apply lotion after bathing before blotting skin dry.

## Client/Family Teaching

- Teach techniques to use when the client is uncomfortable, including relaxation techniques, guided imagery, hypnosis, and music therapy.
- Teach the client with pruritus and the family to substitute rubbing, massage, pressure, or vibration for scratching when itching is severe and irrepressible.
- Teach the client and the family correct application or administration of prescribed medications or therapies.
- ▲ Instruct the client to see the primary care practitioner if itching persists and no cause is found.

• = Independent        ▲ = Collaborative

C

## Readiness for enhanced Communication

### NANDA Definition

Pattern of exchanging information and ideas with others that is sufficient for meeting one's needs and life's goals and can be strengthened

### Defining Characteristics

Expresses willingness to enhance communication; able to speak or write a language; forms words, phrases, and language; expresses thoughts and feelings; uses and interprets nonverbal cues appropriately; expresses satisfaction with ability to share information and ideas with others

### Related Factors (r/t)

To be developed

### Client Outcomes

**Client Will (Specify Time Frame):**

- Express willingness to enhance communication.
- Demonstrate ability to speak or write a language.
- Form words, phrases, and language.
- Express thoughts and feelings.
- Use and interpret nonverbal cues appropriately.
- Express satisfaction with ability to share information and ideas with others.

### Nursing Interventions

- Establish a good nurse-client relationship: provide appropriate education for the client, demonstrate caring by being present for the client.
- Carefully assess the client's readiness to communicate.
- Assess the client's literacy level.
- Listen attentively and provide a comfortable environment for communicating; use these practical guidelines to assist in communication:
  - Slow down and listen to the client's story.

• = Independent          ▲ = Collaborative

- Use "living room" language.
- Use pictures and stories to illustrate important points.
- Repeat instructions; limit the amount of information given.
- Have the client "teach back" to confirm understanding.
- Avoid asking, "Do you understand?"
- Be respectful, caring, and sensitive.

▲ Provide communication with specialty nurses who have knowledge about the client's situation.

▲ Refer couples in maladjusted relationships to psychosocial intervention and social support to strengthen communication; consider nurse specialists.

• Consider using music to enhance communication between client and family of a client who is dying and having difficulty expressing feelings and emotions.

## Pediatric

▲ All individuals involved in the care and everyday life of children with learning difficulties need to have a collaborate approach to communication.

## Geriatric

▲ Assess for hearing and vision impairments and make appropriate referrals for hearing aids.

• Use touch if culturally acceptable when communicating with older clients and their families.

• Caregivers may sing when delivering care and instructions.

▲ Use reminiscence therapy as a way to promote self-esteem and self-healing, to elevate mood, and to relieve stress and aid in communication.

## Multicultural

• Nurses should become more sensitive to the meaning of a culture's nonverbal communication modes, such as eye contact, facial expression, touching, or body language. Nurses should realize that their good intentions and their usual nonverbal communication style may

• = Independent          ▲ = Collaborative

sometimes be interpreted as offensive and insulting by a specific cultural group.

- Assess for the influence of cultural beliefs, norms, and values on the client's communication process.
- Assess personal space needs, acceptable communication styles, acceptable body language, interpretation of eye contact, perception of touch, and use of paraverbal modes when communicating with the client.
- Assess for how language barriers contribute to health disparities among ethnic and racial minorities.
- Take extreme care when using touch.
- Modify and tailor the communication approach in keeping with the client's particular culture.
- Use an interpreter if the client speaks a different language.
- Use therapeutic communication techniques that emphasize acceptance, offer the self, validate the client's concerns, and convey respect.
- Use reminiscence therapy as a language intervention.
- Utilization of standards on culturally and linguistically appropriate services (CLAS) in health care from the Office of Minority Health (OMH) of the U.S. Department of Health and Human Services (DHHS) should be adopted as needed.

## Home Care

- The interventions described previously may be used in home care.
- Refer to the care plan **Impaired verbal Communication**.

## Impaired verbal Communication

### NANDA Definition

Decreased, delayed, or absent ability to receive, process, transmit, and use a system of symbols

• = Independent          ▲ = Collaborative

## Defining Characteristics

Willful refusal to speak; disorientation in the three spheres of time, space, and person; inability to speak dominant language; does not or cannot speak; speaks or verbalizes with difficulty; inappropriate verbalizations; difficulty forming words or sentences (e.g., aphonia, dyslalia, dysarthria); difficulty expressing thoughts verbally (e.g., aphasia, dysphasia, apraxia, dyslexia); stuttering; slurring; dyspnea; absence of eye contact or difficulty in selectively attending; difficulty in comprehending and maintaining usual communication pattern; partial or total visual deficit; inability to use or difficulty in using facial or body expressions

## Related Factors (r/t)

Decrease in circulation to brain; cultural differences; psychological barriers (e.g., psychosis, lack of stimuli); physical barrier (e.g., tracheostomy, intubation); anatomical defect (e.g., cleft palate; alteration of neuromuscular visual system, auditory system, phonatory apparatus); brain tumor; differences related to developmental age; side effects of medication; environmental barriers; absence of significant others; altered perceptions; lack of information; stress; alteration of self-esteem or self-concept; physiological conditions; alteration of central nervous system; weakening of musculoskeletal system; emotional conditions

## Client Outcomes

### Client Will (Specify Time Frame):

- Use effective communication techniques.
- Use alternative methods of communication effectively.
- Demonstrate congruency of verbal and nonverbal behavior.
- Demonstrate understanding even if not able to speak.
- Express desire for social interactions.

## Nursing Interventions

▲ When the client is having difficulty communicating, assess and refer for consultation for hearing problems. Suspect hearing loss when:

• = Independent          ▲ = Collaborative

- Client frequently complains that people mumble or people's speech is not clear, or they hear only parts of conversations when people are talking.
- Client often asks people to repeat what they said.
- Client's friends or relatives tell them that they do not seem to hear very well.
- Client does not laugh at jokes because they miss too much of the story.
- Client needs to ask others about the details of a meeting that they just attended.
- Others say that the client plays the TV or radio too loudly.
- Client cannot hear the doorbell or the telephone.
- Client finds that looking at the person that is speaking to them makes it somewhat easier to understand, especially when they are in a noisy place or where there are competing conversations.

• Involve a familiar person when attempting to communicate with a person who has difficulty with communication.

▲ Identify the language spoken; obtain a language dictionary or interpreter if possible and accepted by the client.

• Listen carefully. Validate verbal and nonverbal expressions particularly when dealing with pain.

• Spend time communicating with the client.

• Use simple communication; speak in a well-modulated voice, smile, and show concern for the client.

• Maintain eye contact at the client's level.

• When working with the hearing impaired, remove masks and reduce background noise whenever possible.

• Use touch as appropriate.

• Use presence. Spend time with the client, allow time for responses, and make the call light readily available.

• Explain all health care procedures.

• Obtain communication equipment such as electronic devices, letter boards, picture boards, and magic slates.

• Consider electronic voice output communication aids for intubated clients.

• Establish an alternative method of communication such

• = Independent          ▲ = Collaborative

as writing or pointing to letters, word phrases, picture cards, or simple drawings of basic needs.

▲ Consider use of an intelligent keyboard to facilitate communication for clients unable to express themselves verbally.

▲ Consultation with a speech therapist may be helpful. Supplement the work of the speech therapist with appropriate exercises.

• Encourage the family to bring in familiar pictures or calendars.

• Establish an understanding of the client's symbolic speech (especially with schizophrenic clients). Ask the client to clarify particular statements.

• If a comprehension deficit is present, keep the environment quiet when communicating and get the client's attention before attempting to communicate (e.g., touch the client's shoulder, call the client's name).

• Do not raise your voice or shout at the client.

## Pediatric

• Observe behavioral communication cues in infants.

• Identify and define variations of communication that may be used by children with significant disabilities. Teach at least two new forms of socially acceptable communication techniques to teach as alternatives when communication breaks down. For example, teach use of one-word requests or teach the child to point; reinforce appropriate responses.

• Teach children with severe disabilities functional communication skills related to requesting and rejecting.

▲ Refer children with primary speech and language delay/disorder for speech and language therapy interventions.

## Geriatric

• Carefully assess all clients for hearing difficulty using an audiometer.

• Avoid use of "elderspeak."

• Initiate communication with the client with dementia.

• Encourage the client to wear hearing aids.

• = Independent          ▲ = Collaborative

- When communicating with a client, face toward his or her unaffected side or better ear.
- Provide sufficient light and remove distractions such as glare and background noise.
- Use low voice tones and recognize that perception of the sounds *f, s, th, ch, sh, b, t, p, k,* and *d* is impaired with age-related hearing loss.
- Facilitate communication and reminiscing with remembering boxes—boxes that contain objects, photographs, and writings that have meaning for the client.
- Use touch as culturally appropriate.

## Multicultural

- Nurses should become more sensitive to the meaning of a culture's nonverbal communication modes, such as eye contact, facial expression, touching, body language. Nurses should realize that their good intentions and their usual nonverbal communication style may sometimes be interpreted as offensive and insulting by a specific cultural group.
- Assess for the influence of cultural beliefs, norms, and values on the client's communication process.
- Assess personal space needs, acceptable communication styles, acceptable body language, interpretation of eye contact, perception of touch, and use of paraverbal modes when communicating with the client.
- Assess for how language barriers contribute to health disparities among ethnic and racial minorities.
- Take extreme care when using touch.
- Modify and tailor the communication approach in keeping with the client's particular culture.
- Use an interpreter if the client speaks a different language.
- Use therapeutic communication techniques that emphasize acceptance, offer the self, validate the client's concerns, and convey respect.
- Use reminiscence therapy as a language intervention.
- Utilization of standards on culturally and linguistically

• = Independent          ▲ = Collaborative

appropriate services (CLAS) in health care from the Office of Minority Health (OMH) of the U.S. Department of Health and Human Services (DHHS) should be adopted as needed.

## Home Care

- The interventions described previously may be adapted for home care use.
- ▲ Begin discharge planning as soon as possible with the case manager or social worker to assess the need for home support systems, assistive devices, and community or home health services.
- ▲ Continue with speech therapy services per the physician's order. Support the speech therapy plan of care.
- ▲ Assess the cause of communication difficulty and the psychological response to communication difficulty. Refer for mental health assessment as indicated.
- Use an understanding of the client's specific physiological changes to implement actions that will assist client communication, provide support, and decrease stress.
- Assess the family for possible role changes resulting from communication impairment of a family member.
- When possible, encourage the family to include the client in family activities using enhanced communication techniques with sensitivity.
- ▲ Refer to medical social services as necessary for help in obtaining funds for communication devices and counseling for dealing with the long-term impact of the communication changes in the family.
- ▲ Institute case management of the frail elderly to support continued independent living.
- ▲ Refer for psychiatric home health care services for client reassurance and implementation of a therapeutic regimen.

## Client/Family Teaching

- Teach the client and family techniques to increase communication.

• = Independent          ▲ = Collaborative

- Encourage significant others to use touch, such as holding the client's hand or stroking the arm.
- Teach the client how to use communication devices.
▲ Refer the client to a speech-language pathologist or audiologist.
▲ Refer to a specialist for possible surgical intervention when clients have surgical defects caused by cancer of the maxillary sinus and alveolar ridge.

# Decisional Conflict (specify)

## NANDA Definition

Uncertainty about course of action to be taken when choice among competing actions involves risk, loss, or challenge to personal life values

## Defining Characteristics

Verbalization of uncertainty about choices; verbalization of undesired consequences of alternative actions being considered; vacillation between alternative choices; delayed decision making; verbalization of feelings of distress while attempting to make a decision; self-focusing; physical signs of distress or tension (e.g., increased heart rate, increased muscle tension, restlessness); questioning of personal values and beliefs while attempting to make a decision

## Related Factors (r/t)

Support system deficit; perceived threat to value system; lack of experience or interference with decision making; multiple or divergent sources of information; lack of relevant information; unclear personal values/beliefs

## Client Outcomes

### Client Will (Specify Time Frame):

- State the advantages and disadvantages of choices.

• = Independent          ▲ = Collaborative

- Share fears and concerns regarding choices and responses of others.
- Make an informed choice.

## Nursing Interventions

- Observe for factors causing or contributing to conflict (e.g., value conflicts, fear of outcome, poor problem-solving skills).
- Work with and allow the client to make decisions in a way that is comfortable for the client, such as deferring (allowing others to decide), delaying (choosing an alternative that meets basic requirements), or deliberating (looking at all alternatives).
- Give the client time and permission to express feelings associated with decision making.
- Demonstrate reassurance with unconditional respect for and acceptance of the client's values, spiritual beliefs, and cultural norms.
- ▲ Use decision aids or computer-based decision aids to assist clients in making decisions.
- ▲ Initiate health teaching and referrals when needed.
- Facilitate communication between the client and family members regarding the final decision; offer support to the person actually making the decision.
- Provide detailed information on benefits and risks using functional terms and probabilities tailored to clinical risk, plus steps for considering the issues and means for making a decision, including values' clarification and decision aids, when clients are faced with difficult treatment choices.

### Geriatric

- Carefully assess clients with dementia for ability to make decisions: In evaluating reasoning, it may be helpful to take the client through the reasoning process. First learn about the social and situational context for the health care decision and then ask about the consequences of treatment alternatives for those contexts. Check if information is excluded because it was not re-

● = Independent          ▲ = Collaborative

membered or because it was not important to the
individual.
- If end-of-life discussions are being avoided, describe the
possible consequences.
- Discuss the purpose of a living will and advance
directives.
- Discuss choices or changes to be made (e.g., moving in
with children, moving into a nursing home, or moving into an adult foster care home).
- Teach family members how to be supportive of the final
decision or how to refrain from being destructive if they
are unable to be supportive.

## Multicultural
- Assess for the influence of cultural beliefs, norms, and
values on the client's decision-making conflict.
- Identify who will be involved in the decision-making
process.
- Use cross-cultural decision aids whenever possible to enhance an informed decision-making process.
- Validate the client's feelings regarding the decisional
conflict.

## Home Care
NOTE: Before addressing decisional conflict, nurses should be
aware of their existing biases and preconceptions, and avoid
superimposing them on the client's decision-making process. For
example, clients making end-of-life decisions must process multiple issues regarding their choices; nurses' discomfort with
end-of-life issues could interfere with clients' ability to reflect on
choices.
- The interventions described previously may be adapted
for home care use.
▲ Before providing any home care, assess the client plan for
advance directives (living will and power of attorney). If
a plan exists, place a copy in the client file. If no plan
exists, offer information on advance directives according
to agency policy. Refer for assistance in completing

• = Independent        ▲ = Collaborative

advance directives as necessary. Do not witness a living will.

- Determine the relevance of the decisional conflict to the plan of care.
- Assess the client and family for consensus (or lack thereof) regarding the issue of conflict. When the conflict involves end-of-life decisions, work to shift the client's and family's expectations from curative to palliative.
▲ If a decision is relevant to the plan of care, the primary nurse or medical social services may evaluate the need for a family conference and call such a conference. If a consensus cannot be reached, continue efforts to resolve the conflict. Clients, unless medically incompetent (by legal guidelines) or under authorized power of attorney, may make their own decisions.
- Assist the client and family in initiating problem solving and in identifying options, pros and cons, and consequences of choices. Refer to the care plan for **Anxiety** as indicated.
▲ If the decision is not relevant to the plan of care, refer to community support services appropriate to the type of decision and client need.

## Client/Family Teaching

▲ Instruct the client and family members to provide advance directives in the following areas:
  - Person to contact in an emergency
  - Preference (if any) to die at home or in the hospital
  - Desire to sign a living will
  - Desire to donate an organ
  - Funeral arrangements (i.e., burial, cremation)
- Inform the family of treatment options; encourage and defend self-determination.
- Identify reasons for family decisions regarding care. Explore ways in which family decisions can be respected.
- Recognize and allow the client to discuss the selection of complementary therapies available, such as spiritual

• = Independent          ▲ = Collaborative

support, relaxation, imagery, exercise, lifestyle changes, diet (e.g., macrobiotic, vegetarian), and nutritional supplementation.

▲ Provide the POLST form (Physician Orders for Life-Sustaining Treatment) for clients and families faced with end-of-life choice across the health continuum.

# Parental role Conflict

## NANDA Definition

Parent's experience of role confusion and conflict in response to crisis

## Defining Characteristics

Expresses concerns about changes in parental role, family functioning, family communication, family health; expresses concerns/feelings of inadequacy with regard to providing for child's physical and emotional needs during hospitalization or at home; reluctant to participate in usual caregiving activities, even with encouragement and support; demonstrates disruption in caretaking routines; expresses concern about perceived loss of control regarding decisions relating to child; verbalizes or demonstrates feelings of guilt, anger, fear, anxiety, and frustration concerning effect of child's illness on family processes

## Related Factors (r/t)

Change in marital status; home care of child with special needs (e.g., apnea monitoring, postural drainage, hyperalimentation); interruptions of family life as a result of home care regimens (e.g., treatments, caregivers, lack of respite); specialized care center policies; separation from child as a result of chronic illness; intimidation by invasive or restrictive modalities (e.g., isolation, intubation)

● = Independent          ▲ = Collaborative

## Client Outcomes

### Client Will (Specify Time Frame):

* Express feelings and perceptions regarding impacts of illness, disability, and/or hospitalization on parental role.
* Participate in hospital and home care as much as possible given the availability of resources and support systems.
* Exhibit assertiveness and responsibility in active family decision making regarding care of the child.
* Describe and select available resources to support parental management of the child's and family's needs.

## Nursing Interventions

* Assess and support parents' previous coping behaviors.
* Explore parent/family sources of stress, usual methods of coping, and perceptions of illness/condition. Capitalize on the strengths identified.
* Evaluate the family's perceived strength of its social support system. Encourage the family to use social support to increase its resiliency and to moderate stress.
* Determine the older-than-average mother's support systems and self-expectations for motherhood.
* Consider the use of family theory as a framework to help guide interventions (e.g., family stress theory, role theory, social exchange theory).
* Sustain parental involvement in shared decision making with regard to care by using the following steps:
  - Incorporate parents' information concerning the child's typical routines, behaviors, fears, likes, and dislikes.
  - Provide clear and direct first-hand information concerning the child's condition and progress.
  - Normalize the home/hospital environment as much as possible.
  - Collaborate in care by providing choices when possible.
* Seek and support parental participation in care.

• = Independent          ▲ = Collaborative

- Provide support for each parent's primary coping strategies.
- Offer respite care to assist parents in maintaining sufficient energy and personal resources to continue caregiving responsibilities.
- Be available to discuss concerns and be a good listener.
- Encourage the parent to meet his or her own needs for rest, nutrition, and hygiene. Provide facilities so that the parent may stay with the sick child (e.g., cot, reclining chair).
- Provide family-centered care: Demonstrate safe places where the parent may touch or stroke the child. Encourage the parent to talk or sing to the child. Adjust equipment so that the parent is able to hold the child, and provide a comfortable chair, preferably a rocking chair. Provide opportunities and offer praise for successful caregiving.
- ▲ Refer parents to available telephone counseling services.
- ▲ Support young grandmothers of teen mothers in areas of mother-daughter conflict such as child-rearing decisions, time with friends, household chores, and teens' choices/priorities with appropriate community referrals.

## Multicultural

- Acknowledge racial/ethnic differences at the onset of care.
- Assess for the influence of cultural beliefs, norms, and values on the client's perceptions of the parental role.
- Acknowledge that value conflicts arising from acculturation stresses may contribute to increased anxiety and significant conflict with the parental role.
- Promote the female parenting role by providing a treatment environment that is culturally based and woman centered.
- Validate the client's feelings with regard to parental role confusion and conflict.

● = Independent          ▲ = Collaborative

## Home Care

- The interventions described previously may be adapted for home care use.
- Assess family adjustment prenatally and postpartum; assist new parents to renegotiate behavior around issues such as amount of time spent together, sexual relationship, resolution of disagreements, and provision of sufficient time for leisure/recreational activities. Encourage the father to take an active role in infant care.
- ▲ Assess interference with family functioning. Refer for family counseling as indicated.

## Client/Family Teaching

- Furnish clear explanations about condition, disease or disability, associated treatments, and prognosis. Describe circumstances involving emotional and physical reactions of the child and types of family member reactions that might be anticipated in response to the condition or crisis. Provide ample time for skill practice.
- For parents of children with chronic disabilities, tailor educational opportunities based on the experiential phase of the parents (protection, survival, or development of the parent as a central person) as parents develop an identity as the central caregivers for their child.
- ▲ Refer parents of children with behavioral problems to parenting programs.
- ▲ Involve parents in formal and/or informal social support situations, such as Internet support groups.
- ▲ Teach the client about available community resources (e.g., therapists, ministers, counselors, self-help groups).
- ▲ Encourage parents with HIV/AIDS to implement custody plans for their children.

# Acute Confusion

## NANDA Definition

Abrupt onset of a cluster of global, transient changes and disturbances in attention, cognition, psychomotor activity level, level of consciousness, and/or sleep/wake cycle

## Defining Characteristics

Lack of motivation to initiate and/or follow through with goal-directed or purposeful behavior; fluctuation in psychomotor activity; misperceptions; fluctuation in cognition; increased agitation or restlessness; fluctuation in level of consciousness; fluctuation in sleep/wake cycle, hallucinations

## Related Factors (r/t)

Over 60 years of age; alcohol abuse; delirium; dementia; drug abuse

## Client Outcomes

### Client Will (Specify Time Frame):

- Demonstrate restoration of cognitive status to baseline.
- Obtain adequate amount of sleep.
- Demonstrate appropriate motor behavior.
- Maintain functional capacity.
- Optimize hydration and nutrition.

## Nursing Interventions

- Assess the client's behavior and cognition systematically and continually throughout the day and night, as appropriate.
- Perform an accurate mental status examination that includes the following:
  - Overall appearance, manner, and attitude
  - Behavioral characteristics and level of psychomotor behavior
  - Mood and affect (presence of suicidal or homicidal ideation as observed by others and reported by the client)
  - Insight and judgment
  - Cognition as evidenced by level of consciousness, orientation (to time, place, and person), and thought process and content (perceptual disturbances such as

• = Independent        ▲ = Collaborative

        illusions and hallucinations, paranoia, delusions, abstract thinking)
- ■ Attention
▲ Assess and report possible physiological alterations (e.g., sepsis, hypoglycemia, hypoxia, hypotension, infection, changes in temperature, fluid and electrolyte imbalance, use of medications with known cognitive and psychotropic side effects).
▲ Treat the underlying causes of delirium in collaboration with the health care team:
  - ■ Establish/maintain normal fluid and electrolyte balance; establish/maintain normal nutrition, normal body temperature, normal oxygenation (if the client experiences low oxygen saturation, deliver supplemental oxygen), normal blood glucose levels, normal blood pressure.
  - ■ Communicate client status, cognition, and behavioral manifestations to all necessary providers.
  - ■ Monitor for any trends occurring in these manifestations.
▲ Laboratory results should be closely monitored and physiological support given as appropriate.
- • Establish or maintain elimination patterns.
- • Plan care that allows for an appropriate sleep/wake cycle.
- • Conduct a medication review.
- • Modulate sensory exposure and establish a calm environment.
- • Manipulate the environment to make it as familiar to the client as possible. Use a large clock and calendar. Encourage visits by family and friends. Place familiar objects in sight.
- • Identify yourself by name at each contact even if you have met the client before; call the client by his or her preferred name.
- • Use appropriate communication techniques for clients at risk for confusion, including communicating clearly and providing simple explanations as needed.
- • Use orientation techniques. If the client becomes distressed or argumentative about what is real, however, do

    • = Independent        ▲ = Collaborative

C

not argue with the client. Rather, explore the emotion behind the client's non–reality-based statements.
- Offer reassurance to the client and use therapeutic communication at frequent intervals.
- Provide supportive nursing care including meeting of basic needs such as feeding, toileting, and hydration.
- Identify, evaluate, and treat pain quickly (see **Acute Pain** or **Chronic Pain**).
▲ Anticipate pain-producing conditions and treat pain with around-the-clock medications.
- Facilitate appropriate sensory input by having clients use aids (e.g., glasses, hearing aids) as needed.
- Recognize that delirium is frequently treated with an antipsychotic medication. Watch for side effects of the medications.

### Geriatric
- Mobilize the client as soon as possible; provide active and passive range-of-motion exercises.
▲ Provide sufficient medication to relieve pain.
- Explain hospital routines and procedures slowly and in simple terms; repeat information as necessary.
- Provide continuity of care when possible (e.g., provide the same caregivers, avoid room changes).
- If clients know that they are not thinking clearly, acknowledge the concern.
- Do not use the intercom to answer a call light.
- Keep the client's sleep/wake cycle as normal as possible (e.g., avoid allowing the client take daytime naps, avoid waking the client at night, give sedatives but not diuretics at bedtime, provide pain relief and back rubs).
- Maintain normal sleep/wake patterns (treat with bright light for 2 hours in the early evening).

### Home Care
- Some of the interventions described previously may be adapted for home care use.
- Assess and monitor for acute changes in cognition and behavior. An acute change in cognition and behavior

• = Independent          ▲ = Collaborative

is the classic presentation of delirium. It should be considered a medical emergency.

- Delirium is reversible but can become chronic if untreated, and the client may be discharged from the hospital to home care in a state of undiagnosed delirium.
- Use brief self-report measures to improve identification and clinical management of at-risk cases.
- Assess for treatable causes of changes in cognition and behavior.
- Assess fluid intake, dementia status, and occurrence of a fall within the past 30 days in evaluating confusion.
- Avoid preconceptions about the source of acute confusion; assess each occurrence on the basis of available evidence.
▲ Institute case management of frail elderly clients to support continued independent living.

## Client/Family Teaching

▲ Teach the family to recognize signs of early confusion and seek medical help.
- Counsel the client and family regarding the symptoms of delirium and its management and sequelae.

# Chronic Confusion

## NANDA Definition

Irreversible, long-standing, and/or progressive deterioration of intellect and personality characterized by decreased ability to interpret environmental stimuli; decreased capacity for intellectual thought processes; manifested by disturbances of memory, orientation, and behavior

## Defining Characteristics

Altered interpretation/response to stimuli; clinical evidence of organic impairment; progressive/long-standing cognitive impair-

• = Independent          ▲ = Collaborative

ment; altered personality; impaired memory (short- and long-term); impaired socialization; no change in level of consciousness

### Related Factors (r/t)

Multi-infarct dementia; Korsakoff's psychosis; head injury; Alzheimer's disease; cerebral vascular accident

### Client Outcomes

#### Client Will (Specify Time Frame):

- Remain content and free from harm.
- Function at maximal cognitive level.
- Participate in activities of daily living at the maximum of functional ability.
- Have minimal episodes of agitation since agitation occurs in up to 70% of patients with dementia.

### Nursing Interventions

- Determine the client's cognitive level using a screening tool such as the Mini-Mental State Exam (MMSE). The Mini-Cog is also a useful screening tool to be used in a busy setting.
- Gather information about the client's predementia functioning, including social situation, physical condition, and psychological functioning.
- Assess the client for signs of depression: insomnia, poor appetite, flat affect, and withdrawn behavior.
- Place an identification bracelet on client.
- Avoid as much as possible exposing the client to unfamiliar situations and people. Maintain continuity of caregivers. Maintain routines of care by observing established eating, bathing, and sleeping schedules. Send a familiar person with the client when the client goes for diagnostic testing or into unfamiliar environments.
- Keep the environment quiet. Avoid or minimize sights and sounds that have a high potential for misinterpretation, such as buzzers, alarms, and overhead paging systems.
- Begin each interaction with the client by identifying

• = Independent          ▲ = Collaborative

yourself and calling the client by name. Approach the client with a caring, loving, and accepting attitude and speak calmly and slowly.

- Give one simple direction at a time and repeat it as necessary. Use verbal and physical prompts, and model the desired action if needed and possible.
- Break down self-care tasks into simple steps (e.g., instead of saying, "Take a shower," say to the client, "Please follow me. Sit down on the bed. Take off your shoes. Now take off your socks").
- Keep questions simple; yes or no questions are often preferable. Use positive statements and actions and avoid negative communication.
- If eating in the dining room increases agitation, let the client leave and eat in a quieter environment with a smaller number of people.
- Provide finger food if the client has difficulty using eating utensils or is unable to sit to eat.
- Provide boundaries by placing red or yellow tape on the floor or by using a stop sign.
- Assess the cause of wandering rather than or before attempting to control the wandering.
- Write the client's name in large block letters in the room and on the client's clothing and possessions.
- Use symbols rather than words to identify areas such as the bathroom or kitchen. Utilize environmental cues such as clocks and a sign with mealtimes to decrease common mealtime questions and thus decrease agitation around mealtimes.
- Limit visitors to two and provide them with guidelines on what are appropriate topics to discuss with the client and how to best communicate with the client. (See how to converse with a memory-impaired person in the Client/Family Teaching section.)
- Set up scheduled quiet periods in a recliner or room. Use blankets and environmental cues to define rest periods.
- Provide quiet activities such as listening to music of the client's preference or introduce other cues that promote relaxation in the afternoon or early evening.

• = Independent          ▲ = Collaborative

C

- Provide simple activities for the client, such as folding washcloths and sorting or stacking activities. Avoid misleading and frightening stimuli, which may include the television, mirrors, and pictures of people or animals.
- If the client becomes increasingly confused and agitated, perform the following steps:
  ▲ Assess the client for physiological causes, including acute hypoxia, pain, medication effects, malnutrition, infections such as urinary tract infection, fatigue, electrolyte disturbances, and constipation. An acute change in behavior is a medical emergency and should be evaluated.
  ■ Assess for psychological causes, including changes in the environment, caregiver, and routine; demands to perform beyond capacity; multiple competing stimuli (including discomfort).
  ■ Avoid confrontations with the client; allow the client to dissipate energy by performing repetitive tasks or by pacing.
  ■ If the client is delusional or hallucinating, do not confront him or her with reality.
- Use validation therapy to verbally reflect back the emotions that the client appears to be feeling. Use statements such as, "It must be frightening to see a fire at the end of your bed," "I can see you are afraid," "I will stay with you," or "Tell me more about what is going on right now."
- Reality orientation (RO) techniques may be used if individualized. For some people with dementia, RO may enhance a sense of understanding of one's environment and hence their self-esteem, but in others it may negatively affect self-esteem.
- Decrease stimuli in the environment (e.g., turn off the television, take the client to a quiet place). Institute activities associated with pleasant emotions, such as playing soft music the client likes, looking through a photo album, providing favorite food, or using simulated presence therapy.

• = Independent          ▲ = Collaborative

- Avoid using restraints if at all possible.
- When bathing a patient with dementia, minimize patient discomfort by using the Bag Bath (if available). Bath time is an opportunity to emphasize person-centered nursing.

▲ Use as-necessary or low-dose regular dosing of psychotropic or antianxiety drugs only as a last resort. They are effective in managing symptoms of psychosis and aggressive behavior. Start with the lowest possible dose.

▲ Avoid the use of anticholinergic medications such as Benadryl.

- For predictable difficult times, such as during bathing and grooming, try the following:
  - Massage the client's hands lovingly or use therapeutic touch to relax the client.
  - Avoid questioning the client or highlighting situations in which the client is unable to remember since this can result in frustration and contribute to agitation.
  - Approach the client in a "patient-centered framework" because this offers a sense of control and promotes self-esteem.
  - Use positive behavioral reinforcement for each small step of bathing, such as praising the client for walking toward the shower, sitting in the shower chair, and removing items of clothing.
  - Treat the client with the utmost respect and give individualized care.
- For care of early dementia clients with primarily symptoms of memory loss, see the care plan for **Impaired Memory.**
- For care of clients with self-care deficits, see the appropriate care plan **(Feeding Self-care deficit; Dressing Self-care deficit;** and **Toileting Self-care deficit).**

## Geriatric

NOTE: Most of the aforementioned interventions apply to the geriatric client.

- Assess and treat pain.

• = Independent                    ▲ = Collaborative

**C**

## Multicultural

- Assess for the influence of cultural beliefs, norms, and values on the family's or caregiver's understanding of chronic confusion or dementia.
- Inform the client's family or caregiver of the meaning of and reasons for common behavior observed in clients with dementia.
- Assist the family or caregiver in identifying barriers that would prevent the use of social services or other supportive services that could help reduce the impact of caregiving.
- Assess the client for the presence of an instrumental activity of daily living (IADL) disability and chronic health conditions.
- ▲ Refer the family to social services or other supportive services to assist in meeting the demands of caregiving for the client with dementia.
- ▲ Encourage the family to make use of support groups or other service programs.
- Validate the family members' feelings with regard to the impact of the client's behavior on family lifestyle.
- African-American and Latino community-dwelling patients with moderate to severe dementia have a higher prevalence of dementia-related behaviors than Caucasians. Therefore as the aging minority population grows, it will be especially important to target caregiver education, in-home support, and resources to minority communities.

## Home Care

NOTE: Keeping the client as independent as possible is important. Because community-based care is usually less structured than institutional care, however, in the home setting the goal of maintaining safety for the client takes on primary importance.

- The interventions described previously may be adapted for home care use.
- Assess and monitor the client for acute changes in cognition and behavior.

● = Independent          ▲ = Collaborative

- Use brief self-report measures to improve identification and clinical management of at-risk cases.
- Assess for treatable causes of changes in cognition and behavior.
▲ Before providing any home care, assess the client plan for advance directives (living will and power of attorney). If a plan exists, place a copy in the client file. If no plan exists, offer information on advance directives according to agency policy. Refer for assistance in completing advance directives as necessary. Do not witness a living will.
- Assess the client's memory and executive function deficits before assuming the inability to make any medical decisions.
▲ Assess the home for safety features and client needs for assistive devices. Explore with the client and family areas of concern. Refer to an occupational therapist for adaptive measures. Problem-solve personal and environmental solutions for client protection.
- Elements of reality orientation therapy may be applied in the home, incorporating person-centered respect, reminiscence, validation, and sensory-motor stimulation.
▲ Evaluate the client's use or history of use of alcohol or drugs; continued use should be stopped if the client can be persuaded. Instruct the client and family regarding the influence of substance use on cognition and behavior. Assess for the potential for withdrawal; refer to a physician for withdrawal protocol as indicated.
- Provide support to the family of the client with a chronic and disabling condition; be prepared to offer support and information to family members who live at a distance as well.
- Use familiar aspects of the environment (smells, music, foods, pictures) to cue the client, capitalizing on habit to remind the client of activities in which the client can participate (e.g., cooperating with medication administration).
- Instruct the caregiver to provide a balanced activity

• = Independent          ▲ = Collaborative

**C**

schedule that neither stresses the client nor deprives the client of stimulation; avoid sustained low- or high-stimulation activity.

▲ If the client will require extensive supervision on an on-going basis, evaluate the client for day care programs. Refer the family to medical social services to assist with this process if necessary. Day care programs provide safe, structured care for the client and respite for the family.

• Encourage the family to include the client in family activities when possible. Reinforce the use of therapeutic communication guidelines (see Client/Family Teaching) and sensitivity to the number of people present.

• Assess family caregivers for caregiver stress, loneliness, and depression.

• Refer to the care plan for **Caregiver role strain.**

• Explore the state of the relationship that existed between the client and caregiver before the onset of dementia, including the strengths and weaknesses of each party. Formulate a plan to assist the couple to deal with the likely worsening of dementia.

• Explore with the spouse the process he or she is undergoing to understand the client's behavior; assist the spouse in being as realistic and positive as possible.

▲ Refer the client to medical social services as necessary to evaluate financial resources and initiate benefits or access to providers.

▲ Institute case management for frail elderly clients to support continued independent living.

▲ Refer for homemaker or psychiatric home health care services for respite, client reassurance, and implementation of a therapeutic regimen.

## Client/Family Teaching

• In the early stages of confusion (e.g., initial period following stroke), provide the caregiver with information on illness processes, needed care, and likely trajectory of progress.

• Recommend that the family develop a memory aid wallet

•  = Independent          ▲ = Collaborative

or booklet for the client, which contains pictures and text
that chronicle the client's life.
- Teach the family how to converse with a memory-
  impaired person. Guidelines include the following:
  - Ask the client to have a conversation with you.
  - Guide the conversation to specific, nonthreatening
    topics and redirect the conversation back on topic
    when the client begins to ramble.
  - Reassure and help out when the client gets stuck or
    cannot find the right words.
  - Smile and act interested in what the client is saying
    even if unsure what it means.
  - Thank the client for talking.
  - Avoid quizzing the client or asking a lot of specific
    questions.
  - Avoid correcting or contradicting something that was
    stated even if it is wrong.
- Teach the family how to set up the environment and use
  the care techniques/interventions listed so that cognitive and functional impairments that interact with the
  client's progressively lowered stress threshold (PLST)
  will be addressed. Identify stressors and initiate compensatory modifications of the environment.
- Instruct the family and care providers that faith, humor,
  patience, and contact with friends and family have been
  identified as positive approaches in keeping a client
  with dementia engaged in their care.
- Discuss with the family what to expect as the dementia
  progresses.
▲ Counsel the family about resources available regarding
  end-of-life decisions and legal concerns.
▲ Inform the family that, as dementia progresses, hospice
  care may be available in the home in the terminal
  stages to help the caregiver.

NOTE: The nursing diagnoses **Impaired Environmental interpretation syndrome** and **Chronic Confusion** are very similar in
definition and interventions. **Impaired Environmental interpre-**

**C**

**tation** must be interpreted as a syndrome when other nursing diagnoses would also apply. **Chronic Confusion** may be interpreted as the human response to a situation or situations that require a level of cognition of which the individual is no longer capable. Further research is under way to make this distinction clear to the practicing nurse.

## Constipation

### NANDA Definition

Decrease in normal frequency of defecation, accompanied by difficult or incomplete passage of stool and/or passage of excessively hard, dry stool

### Defining Characteristics

Change in bowel pattern; bright red blood with stool; presence of soft, pastelike stool in rectum; distended abdomen; dark, black, or tarry stool; increased abdominal pressure; percussed abdominal dullness; pain with defecation; decreased volume of stool; straining with defecation; decreased frequency of stool; dry, hard, formed stool; palpable rectal mass; feeling of rectal fullness or pressure; abdominal pain; inability to pass stool; anorexia; headache; change in abdominal growling (borborygmi); indigestion; atypical presentation in older adults (e.g., change in mental status, urinary incontinence, unexplained falls, elevated body temperature); severe flatus; generalized fatigue; hypoactive or hyperactive bowel sounds; palpable abdominal mass; abdominal tenderness with or without palpable muscle resistance; nausea and/or vomiting; oozing of liquid stool

### Related Factors (r/t)

#### Functional

Recent environmental changes; habitual denial or ignoring of urge to defecate; insufficient physical activity; irregular defecation habits; inadequate toileting (e.g., timeliness, positioning for defecation, privacy); abdominal muscle weakness

● = Independent        ▲ = Collaborative

### Psychological
Depression; emotional stress; mental confusion

### Pharmacological
Antilipemic agents; overdose of laxatives; calcium carbonate; aluminum-containing antacids; nonsteroidal anti-inflammatory drugs (NSAIDs); opiates; anticholinergics; diuretics; iron salts; phenothiazines; sedatives; sympathomimetics; bismuth salts; antidepressants; calcium channel blockers

### Mechanical
Rectal abscess or ulcer; pregnancy; rectal anal fissure; tumor; megacolon (Hirschsprung's disease); electrolyte imbalance; rectal prolapse; prostate enlargement; neurological impairment; rectal anal stricture; rectocele; postsurgical obstruction; hemorrhoids; obesity

### Physiological
Poor eating habits; decreased motility of gastrointestinal tract; inadequate dentition or oral hygiene; insufficient fiber intake; insufficient fluid intake; change in usual foods and eating patterns; dehydration

## Client Outcomes

### Client Will (Specify Time Frame):

- Maintain passage of soft, formed stool every 1 to 3 days without straining.
- State relief from discomfort of constipation.
- Identify measures that prevent or treat constipation.

## Nursing Interventions

- Assess usual pattern of defecation, including time of day, amount and frequency of stool, consistency of stool; history of bowel habits or laxative use; diet including fluid intake; exercise patterns; personal remedies for constipation; obstetrical/gynecological history; surgeries; alterations in perianal sensation; present bowel regimen.
- Have the client or family keep a diary of bowel habits us-

• = Independent          ▲ = Collaborative

C

ing a Management of Constipation Assessment Inventory, including information such as time of day; usual stimulus; consistency, amount, and frequency of stool; fluid consumption; and use of any aids to defecation.

▲ Review the client's current medications.

▲ If the client is receiving opioids, request an order for stool softeners from the primary care practitioner and institute a bowel regimen before the onset of constipation.

• If new onset of constipation, determine if the client has recently stopped smoking.

• Palpate for abdominal distention, percuss for dullness, and auscultate bowel sounds.

▲ Check for impaction; if present, perform digital removal per physician's order.

▲ If the client is uncomfortable or in pain due to constipation or has acute or chronic constipation that does not respond to increased fiber, fluid, activity, and appropriate toileting, refer the client to the primary care practitioner for an evaluation of bowel function and health status.

• Provide privacy for defecation. Help the client to the bathroom and close the door if possible. Toileting is recommended 5 to 15 minutes after meals, especially after breakfast when the gastrocolic reflex is strongest.

• Ask the client to keep a food log of the foods eaten during the last 24 hours. If needed, instruct the client in the need to eat five to nine fruits and vegetables per day, and at least three servings of whole-grain foods.

• Encourage fiber intake of 25–30 g/day for adults. Emphasize foods such as fresh fruits, beans, vegetables, and bran cereals. Add fiber to diet gradually with increased intake of fluids.

▲ Use a mixture of 1 cup of Kellogg's All-Bran cereal, 1 cup of applesauce, and 1 cup of prune juice; begin administration in small amounts and gradually increase amount. Refer to references for dosing. Keep refrigerated. Always check with the primary care practitioner before initiating this intervention. It is important that the client also ingest sufficient fluids.

• = Independent          ▲ = Collaborative

▲ If client would prefer to increase fiber intake using a pill, recommend that client use a tablet that contains methylcellulose.

• Encourage a fluid intake of 1.5 to 2 L/day (6 to 8 glasses of liquids per day). If oral intake is low, gradually increase fluid intake.

• Encourage the client to be out of bed as soon as possible and to perform the activities of daily living himself or herself as able. Encourage exercises such as turning and changing positions in bed, lifting the hips off the bed, performing range-of-motion exercises, alternately lifting each knee to the chest, doing wheelchair lifts, doing waist twists, stretching the arms away from the body, and pulling in the abdomen while taking deep breaths.

• Initiate a regular schedule for defecation, using the client's normal evacuation time whenever possible. Offer hot coffee, hot lemon water, or prune juice before breakfast, or while the client sits on the toilet if necessary. An optimal time for many individuals is 30 minutes after breakfast because of the gastrocolic reflex.

• Help the client onto a bedside commode or toilet with the client's hips flexed and feet flat.

• Have the client deep breathe through the mouth to encourage relaxation of the pelvic floor muscle and use the abdominal muscles to help evacuation.

▲ Provide laxatives, suppositories, and enemas only as needed if other more natural interventions are not effective, and as ordered only; establish a client goal of eliminating laxative use.

• Avoid the use of both soapsuds and tap water enemas if possible, or use a low concentration of castile soap only. If enemas are ordered, measure the amount of fluid given and the amount expelled.

▲ For the stable neurological client, consider use of a bowel routine of a Therevac enema instead of suppositories every other day. For persistent constipation, refer to a physician for evaluation.

• = Independent          ▲ = Collaborative

C

## Geriatric

- Explain the importance of adequate fiber and fluid intake, activity, and established toileting routines to ensure soft, formed stool.
- Determine the client's perception of normal bowel elimination; promote adherence to a regular schedule. Misconceptions regarding the frequency of bowel movements can lead to anxiety and overuse of laxatives.
- Explain the Valsalva maneuver and the reason it should be avoided.
- Respond quickly to the client's call for help with toileting.
- Avoid regular use of enemas in the elderly.
- ▲ Use opioids cautiously. If they are ordered, use stool softeners and bran mixtures to prevent constipation.
- Position the client on the toilet or commode and place a small footstool under the feet.

## Home Care

- The interventions described previously may be adapted for home care use.
- Take complaints seriously and evaluate claims of constipation in a matter-of-fact manner.
- Assess the self-care management activities the client is already using.
- The following treatment recommendations have been offered:
  - Acknowledge the client's life-long experience of bowel function; respect beliefs, attitudes, and preferences; avoid patronizing responses.
  - Make available comprehensive, useful written information about constipation and possible solutions.
  - Make available empathetic and accessible professional care to provide treatment and advice; a multidisciplinary approach (including physician, nurse, and pharmacist) should be used.
  - Institute a bowel management program.

• = Independent          ▲ = Collaborative

C

- Consider affordability when suggesting solutions to constipation; discuss cost-saving strategies.
- Discuss a range of solutions to constipation and allow the client to choose the preferred options.
- Have orders in place for a suppository and enema as the need may occur.

- Although the use of a bedside commode may be necessitated by the client's condition, allow the client to use the toilet in the bathroom when possible and provide assistance.
- In older clients, routinely advise consumption of fluids, fruits, and vegetables as part of the diet, and ambulation if the client is able. Introduce a bowel management program at the first sign of constipation.
- ▲ Refer for consideration of the use of polyethylene glycol 3350 (PEG-3350) for constipation.
- Advise the client against attempting to remove impacted feces on his or her own.
- Instruct the client and family in appropriate expectations for having bowel movements.
- When using a bowel program, establish a pattern that is very regular and allows the client to be part of the family unit.

## Client/Family Teaching

- Instruct the client on normal bowel function and the need for adequate fluid and fiber intake, activity, and a defined toileting pattern in a bowel program.
- Encourage the client to pay attention to defecation warning signs and develop a regular schedule of defecation by using a stimulus such as a warm drink or prune juice.
- Encourage the client to avoid long-term use of laxatives and enemas and to gradually withdraw from their use if they are used regularly.
- If not contraindicated, teach the client how to perform bent-leg sit-ups to increase abdominal tone; also encourage the client to contract the abdominal muscles fre-

• = Independent          ▲ = Collaborative

quently throughout the day. Help the client develop a
daily exercise program to increase peristalsis.

C

## Perceived Constipation

### NANDA Definition

State in which individual makes a self-diagnosis of constipation
and ensures daily bowel movement through abuse of laxatives,
enemas, and suppositories

### Defining Characteristics

Expectation of a daily bowel movement that results in overuse of
laxatives, enemas, and suppositories; expectation of a bowel
movement at same time every day

### Related Factors (r/t)

Cultural or family beliefs; faulty appraisals; impaired thought
processes

### Client Outcomes

**Client Will (Specify Time Frame):**

- Regularly defecate soft, formed stool without using any aids.
- Explain the need to decrease or eliminate the use of stimu-
  lant laxatives, suppositories, and enemas.
- Identify alternatives to stimulant laxatives, enemas, and sup-
  positories for ensuring defecation.
- Explain that defecation does not have to occur every day.

### Nursing Interventions

- Have the client keep a diary of bowel habits using a
  Management of Constipation Assessment Inventory, including information such as time of day; usual stimulus; consistency, amount, and frequency of stool; fluid
  consumption; and use of any aids to defecation.

• = Independent          ▲ = Collaborative

- Determine the client's perception of an appropriate defecation pattern.
- Monitor the use of laxatives, suppositories, or enemas and suggest replacing them with increased fiber intake along with increased fluids to 2 L/day.
- Ask the client to keep a food log of the foods eaten for the last 24 hours or recall the usual foods eaten. If necessary, teach the client the need to eat at least five and preferably nine servings of fruits and vegetables per day, and at least three servings of whole-grain foods.
▲ Use a mixture of 1 cup of Kellogg's All-Bran cereal, 1 cup of applesauce, and 1 cup of prune juice; begin administration in small amounts and gradually increase amount. Refer to references for dosing. Keep refrigerated. Always check with the primary care practitioner before initiating this intervention. It is important that the client also ingest sufficient fluids.
- If client would prefer to increase fiber intake using a pill, recommend that client use a tablet that contains methylcellulose.
- Encourage the client to respond promptly to the defecation reflex.
▲ If the client is uncomfortable or in pain due to constipation or has chronic constipation that does not respond to increased fiber and fluid intake, activity, and appropriate toileting, refer the client to a gastroenterologist for an evaluation of bowel function and health status.
▲ Obtain a dietary referral for analysis of the client's diet and input on how to improve the diet to ensure adequate fiber intake and nutrition.
▲ Assess for signs of depression, a sedentary lifestyle, a history of sexual abuse, and obesity. Refer for counseling as appropriate.
- Encourage the client to increase activity, walking for at least 30 minutes at least 5 days a week as tolerated.
▲ Observe for the presence of an eating disorder, the use of laxatives to control or decrease weight; refer for counseling if needed.

● = Independent          ▲ = Collaborative

**Home Care**

- The interventions described previously may be adapted for home care use.
- Take complaints seriously and evaluate claims of constipation in a matter-of-fact manner.
- Obtain family and client histories of bowel or other patterned behavioral problems.
- Observe family cultural patterns related to eating and bowel habits.
- Encourage a mindset and program of self-care management. Elicit from the client the self-talk he or she uses to describe body perceptions; correct catastrophizing interpretations.
- Instruct the client in a healthy lifestyle that supports normal bowel function (e.g., activity, fluid intake, diet) and encourage progressive inclusion of these elements into daily activities.
- Discuss the client's self-image. Help the client to reframe the self concept as capable.
- Instruct the client and family in appropriate expectations for having bowel movements.
- Offer instruction and reassurance regarding explanations for variation from the previous pattern of bowel movements.
- Contract with the client and/or a responsible family member regarding the use of laxatives. Have the client maintain a bowel pattern diary. Observe for diarrhea or frequent evacuation.
- ▲ Teach the family to carry out the bowel program per the physician's orders.
- ▲ Refer for home health aide services to assist with personal care, including the bowel program, if appropriate.
- Identify a contingency plan for bowel care if the client is dependent on outside persons for such care.

**Client/Family Teaching**

- Explain normal bowel function and the necessary ingre-

• = Independent          ▲ = Collaborative

dients for a regular bowel regimen (e.g., fluid, fiber, activity, and regular schedule for defecation).

- Work with the client and family to develop a diet that fits the client's lifestyle and includes increased fiber.
- Teach the client that it is not necessary to have daily bowel movements and that the passage of anywhere from three stools each day to three stools each week is considered normal.
- Explain to the client the harmful effects of the continual use of defecation aids such as laxatives and enemas.
- Encourage the client to gradually decrease the use of laxatives and/or enemas, and to recognize that this process may take months.
- Determine a method of increasing the client's fluid intake and fit this practice into the client's lifestyle.
- Explain what the Valsalva maneuver is and why it should be avoided.
- Work with the client and family to design a bowel training routine that is based on previous patterns (before laxative or enema abuse) and incorporates the consumption of warm fluids, increased fiber, and increased fluids; privacy; and a predictable routine.

## Additional Nursing Interventions, Client/Family Teaching

See care plan for **Constipation**.

# Risk for Constipation

## NANDA Definition

At risk for a decrease in normal frequency of defecation accompanied by difficult or incomplete passage of stool and/or passage of excessively hard, dry stool

• = Independent          ▲ = Collaborative

## Risk Factors (r/t)

### Functional
Habitual denial/ignoring urge to defecate; recent environmental changes; inadequate toileting (e.g., timeliness, positioning for defecation, privacy); irregular defecation habits; insufficient physical activity; abdominal muscle weakness

### Psychological
Depression; emotional stress; mental confusion

### Physiological
Insufficient fiber intake; dehydration; inadequate dentition or oral hygiene; poor eating habits; insufficient fluid intake; change in usual foods and eating patterns; decreased motility of gastrointestinal tract

### Pharmacological
Anticonvulsants; phenothiazines; nonsteroidal anti-inflammatory agents; sedatives; aluminum-containing antacids; laxative overuse; iron salts; anticholinergics; antidepressants; antilipemic agents; calcium channel blockers; calcium carbonate; diuretics; sympathomimetics; opiates; bismuth salts

### Mechanical
Rectal abscess or ulcer; pregnancy; rectal anal structure; postsurgical obstruction; rectal and anal fissures; megacolon (Hirschsprung's disease); electrolyte imbalance; tumors; prostate enlargement; rectocele; rectal prolapse; neurological impairment; hemorrhoids; obesity

## Client Outcomes

### Client Will (Specify Time Frame):
- Maintain passage of soft, formed stool every 1 to 3 days without straining.
- Identify measures that prevent constipation.
- Explain rationale for not using laxatives and enemas.

## Nursing Interventions and Client/Family Teaching
See care plan for **Constipation.**

• = Independent          ▲ = Collaborative

# Ineffective Coping

## NANDA Definition

Inability to form a valid appraisal of internal or external stressors, inadequate choices of practiced responses, and/or inability to access or use available resources

## Defining Characteristics

Lack of goal-directed behavior or resolution of problem, including inability to attend; difficulty with organized information; sleep disturbance; abuse of chemical agents; decreased use of social support; use of forms of coping that impede adaptive behavior; poor concentration; fatigue; inadequate problem solving; verbalized inability to cope or ask for help; inability to meet basic needs; destructive behavior toward self or others; inability to meet role expectations; high illness rate; change in usual communication patterns; risk-taking behavior

## Related Factors (r/t)

Gender differences in coping strategies; inadequate level of confidence in ability to cope; uncertainty; inadequate social support created by characteristics of relationships; inadequate level of perception of control; inadequate resource availability; high degree of threat; situational crises; maturational crises; disturbance in pattern of tension release; inadequate opportunity to prepare for stressor; inability to conserve adaptive energies; disturbance in pattern of appraisal of threat

## Client Outcomes

### Client Will (Specify Time Frame):

- Verbalize ability to cope and ask for help when needed.
- Demonstrate ability to solve problems related to current needs.
- Remain free of destructive behavior toward self or others.
- Communicate needs and negotiate with others to meet needs.

• = Independent        ▲ = Collaborative

- Discuss how recent or ongoing life stressors have overwhelmed normal coping strategies.
- Demonstrate new effective coping strategies.
- Have illness and accident rates not excessive for age and developmental level.

## Nursing Interventions

- Observe for causes of ineffective coping such as poor self-concept, grief, lack of problem-solving skills, lack of support, or recent change in life situation.
- Observe for strengths such as the ability to relate the facts and to recognize the source of stressors.
- Assess the risk of the client's harming self or others and intervene appropriately. See the care plan for **Risk for Suicide.**
- Help the client set realistic goals and identify personal skills and knowledge.
- Use empathetic communication and encourage the client and family to verbalize fears, express emotions, and set goals.
- Encourage the client to make choices and participate in the planning of care and scheduled activities.
- Provide mental and physical activities within the client's ability (e.g., reading, television, radio, crafts, outings, movies, dinners out, social gatherings, exercise, sports, games).
- If the client is physically able, encourage moderate aerobic exercise.
- Provide information regarding care before care is given.
- Discuss changes with the client before making them.
- Discuss the client's and family's power to change a situation or the need to accept a situation.
- Use active listening and acceptance to help the client express emotions such as sadness, guilt, and anger (within appropriate limits).
- Encourage the client to describe previous stressors and the coping mechanisms used.
- Be supportive of coping behaviors; allow the client time to relax.

● = Independent    ▲ = Collaborative

- Help the client to define the meaning of his or her symptoms.
- Encourage the use of cognitive behavioral relaxation (e.g., music therapy, guided imagery).
- Use distraction techniques during procedures that cause the client to be fearful.
- ▲ Refer for counseling as needed.

## Geriatric

- Engage the client in reminiscence.
- ▲ Assess and report possible physiological alterations (e.g., sepsis, hypoglycemia, hypotension, infection, changes in temperature, fluid and electrolyte imbalances, and use of medications with known cognitive and psychotropic side effects).
- Determine if the individual is displaying a change in personality as a manifestation of difficulty with coping.
- Increase and mobilize the support available to the elderly client. Encourage interaction with family and friends.
- Actively listen to complaints and concerns.

## Multicultural

- Assess for the influence of cultural beliefs, norms, and values on the client's perceptions of effective coping.
- Assess the influence of fatalism on the client's coping behavior.
- Assess the influence of cultural conflicts that may affect coping abilities.
- Assess for intergenerational family problems that can overwhelm coping abilities.
- Encourage spirituality as a source of support for coping.
- Negotiate with the client with regard to the aspects of coping behavior that will need to be modified.
- Identify which family members the client can count on for support.
- Support the inner resources that clients use for coping.
- Use an empowerment framework to redefine coping strategies.

• = Independent          ▲ = Collaborative

**Home Care**

- The interventions described previously may be adapted for home care use.
- Observe the family for coping behavioral patterns. Obtain family and client history as possible.
▲ Assess for suicidal tendencies. Refer for mental health care immediately if indicated.
- Identify an emergency plan should the client become suicidal. Refer to the care plan for **Risk for Suicide**.
▲ Assess for affective symptoms after cerebrovascular accident (CVA) in the elderly, particularly emotional lability and depression. Refer for evaluation and treatment as indicated.
- Encourage the client to use self-care management to increase the experience of personal control. Identify with the client all available supports and sense of attachment to others. Refer to the care plan for **Powerlessness.**
▲ Refer to medical social services for evaluation and counseling, which will promote adequate coping as part of the medical plan of care. If no primary medical diagnosis has been made, request medical social services to assist with community support contacts.
▲ Refer the client and family to support groups.
▲ If monitoring medication use, contract with the client or solicit assistance from a responsible caregiver.
▲ Institute case management for frail elderly clients to support continued independent living.
▲ If the client is homebound, refer for psychiatric home health care services for client reassurance and implementation of a therapeutic regimen.

NOTE: All of the previously mentioned interventions may be applied in the home setting. Home care may offer psychiatric nursing or the services of a licensed clinical social worker under special programs. Traditionally, insurance does not reimburse for counseling that is not related to a medical plan of care unless it falls under one of the programs just described. Public health agencies generally do not have the clinical support needed to offer

• = Independent          ▲ = Collaborative

psychiatric nursing services to clients. Clients are usually treated in the ambulatory mental health system.

## Client/Family Teaching

- Teach the client to problem solve. Have the client define the problem and cause, and list the advantages and disadvantages of the options.
- Provide the seriously ill client and his or her family with needed information regarding the condition and treatment.
- Teach relaxation techniques.
- Work closely with the client to develop appropriate educational tools that address individualized needs.
- ▲ Teach the client about available community resources (e.g., therapists, ministers, counselors, self-help groups).

# Readiness for enhanced Coping

## NANDA Definition

Pattern of cognitive and behavioral efforts to manage demands that is sufficient for well-being and can be strengthened

## Defining Characteristics

Defines stressors as manageable; seeks social support; uses a broad range of problem-oriented and emotion-oriented strategies; uses spiritual resources; acknowledges power; seeks knowledge of new strategies; is aware of possible environmental changes

## Client Outcomes

### Client Will (Specify Time Frame):

- Verbalize ability to cope and ask for help when needed.
- Demonstrate ability to solve problems related to current needs.

● = Independent          ▲ = Collaborative

- Communicate needs and negotiate with others to meet needs.
- State that stressors are manageable.
- Demonstrate new effective coping strategies.
- Seek social support for problems associated with coping.
- Seek spiritual support of personal choice.

## Nursing Interventions

- Observe for strengths such as the ability to relate the facts and to recognize the source of stressors.
- Use empathetic communication and encourage the client and family to verbalize fears, express emotions, and set goals.
- Help the client set realistic goals and identify personal skills and knowledge.
- Encourage expression of positive thoughts and emotions.
- Encourage the use of cognitive behavioral relaxation (e.g., music therapy, guided imagery).
- ▲ Refer for cognitive behavioral therapy.
- Encourage the client to use spiritual coping mechanisms such as faith and prayer.
- Help the client with depression to maintain social support networks or assist in building new ones.
- ▲ Consider a workplace stress management program to enhance coping skills.
- ▲ Refer the client with breast cancer to a psychosocial group intervention for coping skills' training, stress management, relaxation exercises, and psychosocial support.
- Refer to the care plans for **Readiness for enhanced Communication** and **Readiness for enhanced Spiritual well-being.**

## Pediatric

- Encourage exercise for children and adolescents to promote positive self-esteem to enhance coping and to prevent behavioral and psychological problems.

• = Independent          ▲ = Collaborative

## Geriatric

▲ Consider the use of telephone support for caregivers of family members with dementia.

▲ Refer the client with Alzheimer's disease who is terminally ill to hospice care.

▲ Refer the widowed older client to self-help support groups.

## Multicultural

• Assess for the influence of cultural beliefs, norms, and values on the client's perceptions of effective coping.

• Encourage spirituality as a source of support for coping.

• Identify which family members the client can count on for support.

• Support the inner resources that clients use for coping.

• Use an empowerment framework to redefine coping strategies.

## Home Care

• The interventions described previously may be adapted for home care use.

• Observe the family for coping behavioral patterns. Obtain family and client history as possible.

• Encourage the client to use self-care management to increase the experience of personal control. Identify with the client all available support groups and sense of attachment to others.

▲ Refer the client and family to support groups.

## Client/Family Teaching

• Teach relaxation techniques.

▲ Teach the client about available community resources (e.g., therapists, ministers, counselors, self-help groups).

• = Independent          ▲ = Collaborative

**C**

# Ineffective community Coping

## NANDA  Definition

Pattern of community activities (for adaptation and problem solving) that is unsatisfactory for meeting the demands or needs of the community

## Defining Characteristics

Expressed community powerlessness; failure of community to meet its own expectations; deficits of community participation; deficits in communication methods; excessive community conflicts; expressed vulnerability; high illness rates; stressors perceived as excessive; increased social problems (e.g., homicides, vandalism, arson, terrorism, robbery, infanticide, abuse, divorce, unemployment, poverty, militancy, mental illness)

## Related Factors (r/t)

Natural or man-made disasters; ineffective or nonexistent community systems (e.g., lack of emergency medical, transportation, or disaster planning systems); deficits in community social support services and resources; inadequate resources for problem solving

## Community Outcomes

**A Broad Range of Community Members Will (Specify Time Frame):**

- Participate in community actions to improve power resources.
- Develop improved communication among community members.
- Participate in problem solving.
- Demonstrate cohesiveness in problem solving.
- Develop new strategies for problem solving.
- Express power to deal with change and manage problems.

• = Independent          ▲ = Collaborative

## Nursing Interventions

NOTE: The diagnosis of **Ineffective Coping** does not apply and should not be used when stress is being imposed by external sources or circumstances. If the community is a victim of circumstances, using the nursing diagnosis **Ineffective Coping** is equivalent to blaming the victim. See the care plans for **Ineffective community Therapeutic regimen management** and **Readiness for enhanced community Coping.**

C

- Establish a collaborative partnership with the community (see the care plan for **Ineffective community Therapeutic regimen management** for references).
- Assist the community with team building.
- Participate with community members in the identification of stressors and assessment of distress; for example, observe and participate in community meetings and task forces.
- Identify community strengths with community members.
- Identify the health services and information resources that are currently available in the community.
- Work with community members to increase awareness of ineffective coping behaviors (e.g., conflicts that prevent community members from working together, anger and hate that paralyze the community).
- Provide support to the community and help community members to identify and mobilize additional sources of support.
- Use focus group methods to evaluate and strengthen interventions.
- Use mentoring strategies for community members.
- Advocate for the community in multiple arenas (e.g., television, newspapers, and governmental agencies).
- Work with community groups to improve the economic status and reduce unemployment.
- Write grant proposals to help community members obtain funds for programs that reduce stress or improve coping.
- Work with members of the community to identify and develop coping strategies that promote a sense of power (e.g., obtaining sources for funding, collaborating with other communities).

• = Independent          ▲ = Collaborative

C

- Obtain police support for community partnerships aimed at healthy coping.
- Support positive attitudes and feelings as a basis for change.
- Protect children from exposure to community conflicts.

## Multicultural

- Acknowledge the stressors unique to racial/ethnic communities.
- Work with members of the community to prioritize and target health goals specific to the community.
- Approach community leaders and members of color with respect, warmth, and professional courtesy.
- Establish and sustain partnerships with key individuals within communities when developing and implementing programs.
- Use community church settings as a forum for advocacy, teaching, and program implementation.
- Ask political leaders to become part of the partnership process.

## Community Teaching

- Teach strategies for stress management.
- Explain the relationship between enhancing power resources and coping.

# Readiness for enhanced community Coping

## NANDA Definition

Pattern of community activities for adaptation and problem solving that is satisfactory for meeting the demands or needs of the community but that can be improved for management of current and future problems/stressors

## Defining Characteristics

One or more of the following characteristics that indicate

• = Independent        ▲ = Collaborative

effective coping: positive communication between community/aggregates and larger community; availability of programs for recreation and relaxation; sufficiency of resources for managing stressors; agreement that community is responsible for stress management; active planning by community for predicted stressors; active problem solving by community when faced with issues; positive communication among community members

## Related Factors (r/t)

Community has sense of power to manage stressors; social supports available; resources available for problem solving

## Community Outcomes

### Community Will (Specify Time Frame):

- Develop enhanced coping strategies.
- Maintain effective coping strategies for management of stress.

## Nursing Interventions

NOTE: Interventions depend on the specific aspects of community coping that can be enhanced (e.g., planning for stress management, communication, development of community power, community perceptions of stress, community coping strategies). Nursing interventions are conducted in collaboration with key members of the community, community/public health nurses, and members of other disciplines.

- Describe the roles of community/public health nurses in working with healthy communities.
- Help the community to obtain funds for additional programs.
- Encourage positive attitudes toward the community through the media and other sources.
- Help community members to collaborate with one another for power enhancement and coping skills.
- Encourage critical thinking.
- Demonstrate optimal use of the power resources.
- Reduce poverty whenever possible.

● = Independent                ▲ = Collaborative

▲ Collaborate with community members to improve educational levels within the community.

## Multicultural

• Acknowledge the stresses unique to racial/ethnic communities.
▲ Identify health services and information that are currently available in the community.
• Work with members of the community to prioritize and target health goals specific to the community.
• Approach community leaders and members of color with respect, warmth, and professional courtesy.
• Establish and sustain partnerships with key individuals within communities when developing and implementing programs.
• Use community church settings as a forum for advocacy, teaching, and program implementation.

## Community Teaching

• Review coping skills, power for coping, and the use of power resources.

# Defensive Coping

## NANDA Definition

Repeated projection of falsely positive self-evaluations based on self-protective pattern that defends against underlying perceived threats to positive self-regard

## Defining Characteristics

Grandiosity; rationalization of failures; hypersensitivity to slight/criticism; denial of obvious problems/weaknesses; projection of blame/responsibility; lack of follow-through or participation in treatment or therapy; superior attitude toward others; hostile laughter or ridicule of others; difficulty in perception of reality/reality testing; difficulty establishing/maintaining relationships

• = Independent          ▲ = Collaborative

## Related Factors (r/t)

To be developed

## Client Outcomes

### Client Will (Specify Time Frame):

- Acknowledge need for change in coping style.
- Accept responsibility for own behavior.
- Establish realistic goals with validation from caregivers.
- Solicit caregiver validation in decision making.

## Nursing Interventions

- Assess for the presence of denial as a coping mechanism.
- Do not confront denial if its consequences are not a significant threat to health.
- Determine whether the client has a positive or negative overall appraisal of a given event.
- Develop a trusting, therapeutic relationship with the client and family.
- Ask appropriate questions using an assessment tool such as the Fast Alcohol Screening Test (FAST) to assess whether denial is being used in association with alcoholism. For each question, the client is asked to circle the appropriate response: Less than Monthly, Monthly, Weekly, Daily, or Almost Daily.

  1. MEN: How often do you have EIGHT or more drinks on one occasion?
     WOMEN: How often do you have SIX or more drinks on one occasion?
  2. How often during the last year have you been unable to remember what happened the night before because you had been drinking?
  3. How often during the last year have you failed to do what was normally expected of you because of drinking?
  4. In the last year has a relative or friend, a doctor, or a health worker been concerned about your drinking or suggested you decrease your alcohol consumption?

- Determine the client's perception of the problem and

C

then provide reality-based examples of the true situation (e.g., witnesses to an accident, blood alcohol levels, problems caused by alcohol).

- Help the client identify patterns of response that may be maladaptive.
- ▲ Promote the client's feelings of self-worth by using group or individual therapy, role playing, one-to-one interactions, and role modeling.
- Support strengths and normal observations with, "I note that" or "I want you to notice." Tell clients when they do something well.
- Teach the client to use positive thinking by blocking negative thoughts with the word "Stop!" and inserting positive thoughts (e.g., "I'm a good [person, friend, student]").
- ▲ Provide feedback regarding others' perceptions of the client's behavior through group or milieu therapy or one-to-one interactions.
- Encourage the client to use "I" statements and to accept responsibility and consequences of actions.
- Refer to the care plans for **Ineffective Denial** and **Dysfunctional Family processes: alcoholism**.

## Geriatric

- Assess the client for anger and identify previous outlets for anger.
- Explore new outlets for anger, including physical activities within the client's capabilities (e.g., hitting a pillow, woodworking, sanding, scrubbing floors).
- Utilize the CAGE tool with this population and include drug use along with drinking. An affirmative answer to two or more of the following questions is considered a basis for suspicion of alcohol abuse:

  **C:** Have you ever felt you ought to **Cut down** on drinking?

  **A:** Have people **Annoyed** you by criticizing your drinking?

  **G:** Have you ever felt bad or **Guilty** about your drinking?

• = Independent          ▲ = Collaborative

**E:** Have you ever had a drink the first thing in the morning to steady your nerves or get rid of a hangover **(Eye opener)**?

- Assess the client for dementia or depression.
- If a traumatic event has occurred, support positive religious coping behaviors.

## Multicultural

- Assess for the influence of cultural beliefs, norms, and values on the client's feelings of defensiveness.
- Acknowledge racial/ethnic differences at the onset of care.
- Use therapeutic communication techniques that emphasize acceptance, offer the self, validate the client's concerns, and convey respect.
- Give a rationale when assessing ethnically diverse clients for alcohol use/misuse or other sensitive behaviors.

## Home Care

- The interventions described previously may be adapted for home care use.
- Include in the initial assessment client and family histories of mental health problems.
- Observe family dynamics for dysfunctional and supportive communication.
- ▲ Refer to a mental health professional for possible psychodrama therapy, especially if the client experiences difficulty in coping with a traumatic event.
- ▲ In the absence of primary medical diagnoses, refer to medical social services for assistance in contacting appropriate community services.
- ▲ If medical diagnoses coexist with defensive coping, confirm and validate the client's mental health plan and progress.
- ▲ Refer to a therapist for debriefing if a traumatic or critical event has occurred.
- ▲ Refer for psychiatric home health care services for client reassurance and implementation of a therapeutic regimen.

• = Independent          ▲ = Collaborative

## Client/Family Teaching

▲ Teach the client the actions and side effects of medications and the importance of taking them as prescribed, even when the client is feeling good.
▲ Work with the client's support group to identify harmful behaviors and to seek help for the client if he or she is unable to control behavior.
• Support family efforts using religious coping behaviors.

# Compromised family Coping

## NANDA Definition

Situation in which usually supportive primary person (family member or close friend) provides insufficient, ineffective, or compromised support, comfort, assistance, or encouragement that may be needed by client to manage or master adaptive tasks related to health challenge

## Defining Characteristics

### Objective

Significant person attempts assistive or supportive behaviors with less than satisfactory results; significant person displays protective behavior disproportionate (too little or too much) to client's abilities or need for autonomy; significant person withdraws or enters into limited or temporary personal communication with client at time of need

### Subjective

Client expresses or confirms a concern or complaint about significant other's response to his or her health problem; significant person describes or confirms an inadequate understanding or knowledge base, which interferes with effective assistance or supportive behaviors; significant person describes preoccupation with personal reaction (e.g., fear, anticipatory grief, guilt, or anxiety) to client's illness, disability, or other situational or developmental crisis

• = Independent          ▲ = Collaborative

## Related Factors (r/t)

Temporary preoccupation of a significant person who tries to manage emotional conflicts and personal suffering and is unable to perceive or act effectively with regard to client's needs; temporary family disorganization and role changes; prolonged disease or disability progression that exhausts supportive capacity of significant people; other situational or developmental crises or problems significant person may be facing; inadequate or incorrect information or understanding by primary person; little support provided by client, in turn, for primary person

## Client Outcomes

### Family/Significant Person Will (Specify Time Frame):

- Verbalize internal resources to help deal with the situation.
- Verbalize knowledge and understanding of illness, disability, or disease.
- Provide support and assistance as needed.
- Identify need for and seek outside support.

## Nursing Interventions

- Assess the strengths and deficiencies of the family system.
- Assess how family members interact with each other; observe verbal and nonverbal communication and individual and group responses to stress.
- Establish rapport with families by providing accurate communication.
- Consider the use of family theory as a framework to help guide interventions (e.g., family stress theory, role theory, social exchange theory).
- Help family members recognize the need for help and teach them how to ask for it.
- Encourage expression of positive thoughts and emotions.
- Encourage family members to verbalize feelings. Spend time with them, sit down and make eye contact, and offer coffee and other nourishment.
- Provide opportunities for families to discuss spirituality.

• = Independent          ▲ = Collaborative

- Mothers may require additional support in their role of caring for chronically ill children.
- Provide privacy during family visits. If possible, maintain flexible visiting hours to accommodate more frequent family visits. If possible, arrange staff assignments so the same staff members have contact with the family. Familiarize other staff members with the situation in the absence of the usual staff member.
- Determine whether the family is suffering from additional stressors (e.g., child care issues, financial problems).
▲ Refer the family with ill family members to appropriate resources for assistance as indicated (e.g., counseling, psychotherapy, financial or spiritual support).

## Pediatric

- Assess the adolescent's perception of support from family and friends during crisis.
- Provide educational interventions and psychosocial interventions such as coping skills training in treatment for families and their adolescents who have type 1 diabetes.
- Encourage the use of family rituals such as connection, spirituality, love, recreation, celebration, and evolving, especially in single parent families.
- Encourage laughing, playing, singing, talking, and praying with seriously injured children.
▲ Link trained volunteers with "vulnerable" first-time parents. Provide social support and information related to age-appropriate expectations of infants.

## Geriatric

- Perform a holistic assessment of all needs of informal spousal caregivers.
- Help caregivers to establish one's priorities and concentrate on them, believe in one's self and one's ability to handle the situation, take life one day at a time, look for positive aspects in each situation, and rely on one's own expertise and experience.

• = Independent          ▲ = Collaborative

▲ Refer caregivers of Alzheimer's clients to a monthly psychoeducational support group.
▲ Consider the use of telephone support for caregivers of family members with dementia.
• Assist in finding transportation to enable family members to visit.

## Multicultural

• Acknowledge racial/ethnic differences at the onset of care.
• Approach families of color with respect, warmth, and professional courtesy.
• Assess for the influence of cultural beliefs, norms, and values on the family's perceptions of coping.
• Give a rationale when assessing families with regard to sensitive issues.
• Use a family-centered approach when working with Latino, Asian, African-American, and Native-American clients.
• Facilitate modeling and role playing for family regarding healthy ways to communicate and interact.
• Validate the family's feelings regarding the impact of the client's illness on the family's lifestyle.
• Work to provide caregivers who understand the importance of the family's cultural beliefs and values.

## Home Care

• The interventions described previously may be adapted for home care use.
• Assess the reason behind the breakdown of family coping.
• During the time of compromised coping, increase visits to ensure safety of the client, support of the family, and assistance with coping strategies. Provide reassurance regarding expectations for prognosis as appropriate.
▲ Assess the needs of the caregiver in the home. Intervene to meet needs as appropriate to total case management and explore all available resources that may be used to

• = Independent          ▲ = Collaborative

C

provide adequate home care (e.g., parish nursing as an effective adjunct, home health aide services to relieve caregiver's fatigue). Encourage caregivers not to neglect their own physical, mental, and spiritual health and provide more specific information about the client's needs and ways to meet them.

▲ Refer the family to medical social services for evaluation and supportive counseling. Dedicating time for nurturing the caregivers and reassuring the client allows the clients/ caregivers to express feelings and feel hope.

▲ Serve as an advocate, mentor, and role model for caregiving. Write down or contract for the care needed by the client.

▲ When a terminal illness is the precipitating factor for ineffective coping, offer hospice services and support groups as possible resources.

· With a cancer client, encourage family discussion of stressors (including the meaning of the illness, fear of recurrence, the client's employment status) and resources (family social support).

· Encourage the client and family to discuss changes in daily functioning and routines created by the client's illness. Validate discomfort resulting from changes.

· Support positive individual and family coping efforts.

▲ If compromised family coping interferes with the ability to support the client's treatment plan, refer for psychiatric home health care services for family counseling and implementation of a therapeutic regimen.

## Client/Family Teaching

· Provide truthful information and support for the family and significant persons regarding the client's specific illness or condition.

▲ Refer women with recurrent breast cancer and their family caregivers to a FOCUS program (Family involvement, Optimistic attitude, Coping effectiveness, Uncer-

• = Independent          ▲ = Collaborative

tainty reduction, and Symptom management), a family-based program of care.
- Promote individual and family relaxation and stress reduction strategies.
▲ For families of children in residential care, provide a parent support and education group to give opportunities for parents to access support, learn new parenting skills, and, ultimately, optimize their relationships with their children.

# Disabled family Coping

## NANDA Definition

Behavior of significant person (family member or other primary person) that disables his/her capacity and the client's capacity to effectively address tasks essential to either person's adaptation to the health challenge

## Defining Characteristics

Intolerance; agitation, depression, aggression, hostility; adaptation of illness behavior of client; rejection; psychosomaticism; neglectful relationships with other family members; neglectful care of client with regard to basic human needs and/or illness treatment; distortion of reality regarding client's health problem, including extreme denial about its existence or severity; impaired restructuring of meaningful life for self; impaired individualization, prolonged overconcern for client; desertion; decisions and actions that are detrimental to economic or social well-being; carrying on usual routines, disregarding client's needs; abandonment; client's development of helpless, inactive dependence; disregarding needs

## Related Factors (r/t)

Significant person with chronically unexpressed feelings such as guilt, anxiety, hostility, and despair; arbitrary handling of family's

• = Independent          ▲ = Collaborative

resistance to treatment, which tends to solidify defensiveness by dealing inadequately with underlying anxiety; dissonant or discrepant coping styles for dealing with adaptive tasks by significant person and client or among significant people; highly ambivalent family relationships

## Client Outcomes

### Family/Significant Person Will (Specify Time Frame):

- Express realistic understanding and expectations of the client.
- Participate positively in the client's care within the limits of his or her abilities.
- Identify responses that are harmful.
- Acknowledge and accept the need for assistance with circumstances.
- Express feelings openly, honestly, and appropriately.

## Nursing Interventions

- Assess the strengths and deficiencies of the family system.
- Identify current behaviors of family members, such as withdrawal (e.g., not visiting, briefly visiting, ignoring client when visiting), anger and hostility toward the client and others, or expression of guilt.
- Note other stressors in the family (e.g., financial, job related).
- ▲ Evaluate the family's perceived strength of its social support system. Encourage the family to use social support to increase its resiliency and to moderate stress.
- Consider the use of family theory as a framework to help guide interventions (e.g., family stress theory, role theory, social exchange theory).
- Encourage family members to verbalize feelings by discussing ways to solve problems associated with the client's condition.
- Encourage expression of positive thoughts and emotions.
- Mothers may require additional support in their role of caring for chronically ill children.

• = Independent          ▲ = Collaborative

▲ Encourage family members to participate in appropriate support programs (e.g., chronic obstructive pulmonary disease [COPD] support groups, Arthritis I Can Cope groups, Alzheimer's support groups).

▲ Observe for any symptoms of elder or child abuse or neglect.

**Pediatric**

• Assess the adolescent's perception of support from family and friends during crisis.

• Encourage the use of family rituals such as connection, spirituality, love, recreation, celebration, and evolving, especially in single parent families.

• Encourage laughing, playing, singing, talking, and praying with seriously injured children.

▲ Link trained volunteers with "vulnerable" first-time parents. Provide social support and information related to age-appropriate expectations of infants.

**Geriatric**

• Perform a holistic assessment of all needs of informal spousal caregivers.

• Help caregivers to establish one's priorities and concentrate on them, believe in one's self and one's ability to handle the situation, take life one day at a time, look for positive aspects in each situation, and rely on one's own expertise and experience.

▲ Refer caregivers of Alzheimer's clients to a monthly psychoeducational support group.

▲ Consider the use of telephone support for caregivers of family members with dementia.

▲ Refer the family to appropriate senior community resources (e.g., senior centers, Medicare assistance, meal programs, parish nursing services, charitable organizations).

▲ If actual or potential abuse or neglect is an issue, report it to the appropriate agency.

▲ Encourage the family member to participate in appropriate support groups (e.g., COPD support groups,

• = Independent          ▲ = Collaborative

Arthritis I Can Cope groups, Alzheimer's support groups).
- Work with the family to manage common challenges related to normal aging.

## Multicultural
- Work to provide caregivers who understand the importance of a family's cultural beliefs and values.
- Acknowledge racial/ethnic differences at the onset of care.
- Approach families of color with respect, warmth, and professional courtesy.
- Assess for the influence of cultural beliefs, norms, and values on the family's perceptions of coping.
- Use a family-centered approach when working with Latino, Asian, African-American, and Native-American clients.
- Facilitate modeling and role playing for the family regarding healthy ways to communicate and interact.
- Validate the feelings of family members or significant caregivers regarding the impact of the client's illness on family lifestyle.

## Home Care
NOTE: This diagnosis presents the complex and difficult problem of securing an appropriate response by the family to a client's illness and caregiving needs. The same problem in the home setting creates an unusually high risk for abuse of the client. The nurse is cautioned that the margin of time for planning and effectively supporting the family unit to avoid abuse may be minimal or even negligible. Suspected or actual abuse should be reported to adult protective services.
- The interventions described previously may be adapted for home care use.
- If the client has been in an institution, establish empathetic contact with the client and family before discharge.
- Assess the family member's ability and willingness to assist in client care. Determine if the family member is an appropriate source of support for the client.

• = Independent          ▲ = Collaborative

C

- Assess the family member's understanding of the client's illness and behavior. Instruct in appropriate expectations of the client and correct any misconceptions.
- During the time of compromised coping, increase visits to assess the safety of the client and family, provide assistance with coping strategies, identify dysfunctional coping mechanisms, and intervene as necessary.
- Identify any changes in skills needed for client care and support caregiving efforts. Assess the needs of the caregiver in the home. Intervene to meet needs as appropriate to total case management and explore all available resources that may be used to provide adequate home care (e.g., add home health aide services; coordinate services with mental health agencies; encourage caregivers not to neglect their own physical, mental, and spiritual health; and give more specific information about the client's needs and ways to meet them).
- ▲ Serve as an advocate, mentor, and role model for appropriate behavior. Write down or contract for the care needed by the client.
- ▲ When a terminal illness is the precipitating factor for ineffective coping, offer hospice services and support groups as possible resources.
- Support positive individual and family coping efforts.
- ▲ If disabled family coping interferes with the family member's ability to support the client's treatment plan, refer for psychiatric home health care services for family and client counseling and implementation of a therapeutic regimen.

## Client/Family Teaching

- Encourage family members to ask for a break in caregiving and to spend time away from the client.
- Provide truthful information and support for the family and significant persons regarding the client's specific illness or condition.
- Involve the client and family in the planning of care as often as possible; mutual goal-setting is often an effective strategy.

• = Independent          ▲ = Collaborative

- Discuss with the family appropriate ways to demonstrate feelings.
- Help the family identify the health care needs of the client and family; teach the skills necessary to address health care needs.
- Promote individual and family relaxation and stress reduction strategies.

# Readiness for enhanced family Coping

## NANDA Definition

Effective management of adaptive tasks by family member involved with client's health challenge, who now exhibits desire and readiness for enhanced health and growth with regard to self and in relation to client

## Defining Characteristics

Individual expresses interest in making contact on a one-to-one basis or through mutual aid group with another person who has experienced a similar situation; attempts to describe growth impact of the crisis on his or her own values, priorities, goals, or relationships; moves in the direction of health promotion and health-enriching lifestyle that supports and monitors maturational processes; audits and negotiates treatment programs and generally chooses experiences that optimize wellness

## Related Factors (r/t)

Needs sufficiently gratified and adaptive tasks effectively addressed to enable goals of self-actualization to surface

## Client Outcomes

### Family Will (Specify Time Frame):

- State a plan for growth.
- Perform tasks needed for change.
- State positive effects of changes made.

• = Independent          ▲ = Collaborative

## Nursing Interventions

- Assess how family members interact with each other; observe verbal and nonverbal communication and individual and group responses to stress.
- Evaluate the family's perceived strength of its social support system. Encourage the family to use social support to increase its resiliency and to moderate stress.
- Consider the use of family theory as a framework to help guide interventions (e.g., family stress theory, role theory, social exchange theory).
- Establish rapport with families by providing accurate communication.
- Provide opportunities for families to discuss spirituality.
- When a client is undergoing surgery, give the family a 5- to 10-minute progress report about halfway through the surgical procedure.
- Allow the family to be present during invasive procedures and resuscitation efforts.
- Encourage setting aside leisure time free of obligatory tasks for family members to enjoy each other's company; because everyone is busy, family members may need to set up a schedule for leisure time.
- ▲ Identify support groups that discuss problems and concerns similar to those of the family (e.g., Al-Anon, Arthritis I Can Cope). Such groups allow family members to discuss issues and concerns with others who share the same lived experience.

## Pediatric

- Encourage the use of family rituals such as connection, spirituality, love, recreation, celebration, and evolving, especially in single parent families.
- Encourage laughing, playing, singing, talking, and praying with seriously injured children.
- Provide educational interventions and psychosocial interventions such as coping skills' training in treatment for families and their adolescents who have type 1 diabetes.
- ▲ Link trained volunteers with "vulnerable" first-time par-

ents. Provide social support and information related to age-appropriate expectations of infants.

## Geriatric

- Perform a holistic assessment of all needs of informal spousal caregivers.
- Help caregivers to establish one's priorities and concentrate on them, believe in one's self and one's ability to handle the situation, take life one day at a time, look for positive aspects in each situation, and rely on one's own expertise and experience.
- ▲ Consider the use of telephone support for caregivers of family members with dementia.
- ▲ Refer caregivers of Alzheimer's clients to a monthly psychoeducational support group.
- Encourage family members to reminisce with the older family member.
- Start and maintain a log of anecdotal stories about the older family member.
- Encourage children in the family to spend time with and share activities with the older family member.
- ▲ Refer the family to parenting classes and classes for coping with the needs of older parents.

## Multicultural

- Acknowledge racial/ethnic differences at the onset of care.
- Approach families of color with respect, warmth, and professional courtesy.
- Assess for the influence of cultural beliefs, norms, and values on the family's perceptions of coping.
- Use a family-centered approach when working with Latino, Asian, African-American, and Native-American clients
- Facilitate modeling and role playing for family with regard to healthy ways to communicate and interact.
- Validate family members' feelings regarding the impact of the client's illness on family lifestyle.

• = Independent          ▲ = Collaborative

## Home Care

- The nursing interventions described previously for **Readiness for enhanced Family processes** should be used in the home environment with adaptations as necessary.
- Provide a videophone network for peer support for frail elderly people living at home.
- Encourage families to assist women caring for husbands with chronic obstructive pulmonary disease (COPD) to provide respite care so the women may have recreation time.

## Client/Family Teaching

- Provide truthful information and support for the family and significant persons regarding the client's specific illness or condition.
- Promote individual and family relaxation and stress reduction strategies.
- ▲ Refer women with recurrent breast cancer and their family caregivers to a FOCUS program (Family involvement, Optimistic attitude, Coping effectiveness, Uncertainty reduction, and Symptom management), a family-based program of care.

# Risk for sudden infant Death syndrome

## NANDA Definition

Presence of risk factors for sudden death of an infant under 1 year of age

## Risk Factors

**Modifiable:** Infants placed to sleep in the prone or side-lying position; prenatal and/or postnatal infant smoke exposure; infant overheating/overwrapping; soft underlayment/loose articles in the sleep environment; delayed or nonattendance of prenatal care

• = Independent            ▲ = Collaborative

**Potentially Modifiable:** Low birth weight; prematurity; young maternal age

**Nonmodifiable:** Male gender; ethnicity (e.g., African-American or Native-American race of mother); seasonality of sudden infant death syndrome (SIDS) deaths (higher in winter and fall months); SIDS mortality peaks for infant age of 2 to 4 months

## Related Factors (r/t)

See Risk Factors.

## Client Outcomes

**Client Will (Specify Time Frame):**

- Explain appropriate measures to prevent SIDS.
- Demonstrate correct techniques for positioning the infant, protecting the infant from harm.

## Nursing Interventions

- Position infants on their back to sleep; do not position in the prone position.
- Avoid use of loose bedding such as blankets and sheets for sleeping. If blankets are used, they should be tucked in around the crib mattress so the infant's face is less likely to become covered by bedding.
- Avoid overheating the infant by lightly clothing the child for sleep, and avoid overbundling. The infant should not feel hot to touch.
- Provide the infant a certain amount of time in prone position or "tummy time" while the infant is awake and observed.
- Use electronic respiratory or cardiac monitors to detect cardiorespiratory arrest only if ordered.

## Home Care

- Most of the interventions above are relevant.
- Evaluate home for potential safety hazards such as inappropriate cribs, cradles, or strollers.

● = Independent        ▲ = Collaborative

- Determine where and how the child sleeps and provide instructions on safe sleeping positions and environments as needed.

## Multicultural

- Discuss cultural norms with families in order to provide care that is appropriate for promoting safety for the infant in sleeping arrangements.
- Encourage Native-American mothers to avoid drinking and to avoid wrapping infants in excessive blankets or clothing.
- Encourage African-American mothers to find alternatives to bed-sharing and to avoid placing pillows, soft toys, and soft bedding in the sleep environment.

## Client/Family Teaching

- Teach families to position the infant on their back to sleep; do not position in the prone position.
- Teach the parents to place the infant supine to sleep with the head rotated to one side for a week, and then to the other side for a week. Parents should also change the orientation of the crib at intervals so the infant turns the head in alternate directions.
- Recommend the following infant care practices to parents:
  - Infants should not be put to sleep on soft surfaces such as waterbeds, sofas, or soft mattresses.
  - Avoid placing soft materials in the infant's sleeping environment such as pillows, quilts, and comforters. Do not use sheepskins under a sleeping infant.
  - Avoid placing soft objects such as stuffed toys and other gas-trapping objects in an infant's sleeping environment.
  - Avoid the use of loose bedding, such as blankets and sheets. If blankets are to be used, they should be tucked in around the crib mattress so the infant's face is less likely to become covered by bedding.
- Teach parents the need to obtain a crib that conforms to

the safety standards of the Consumer Product Safety Commission.

D

- Teach parents not to place the infant in an adult bed to sleep, or a sofa or chair. Infants should sleep in a crib.
- Teach parents not to sleep with an infant, especially if alcohol or medications/illicit drugs are used by the parents.
- Recommend an alternative to sleeping with an infant; parents might consider placing the infant's crib near their bed to allow for more convenient breastfeeding and parent contact.
- Teach parents to avoid overheating the infant by lightly clothing the child for sleep and avoiding overbundling. The infant should not feel hot to touch. The bedroom temperature should be comfortable to an adult wearing light bedclothing.
- Question parents regarding following recommendations for the prevention of SIDS at each well-baby visit or at visit with health care practitioner for illness. Strongly encourage compliance with precautions to prevent SIDS.
- Teach the need to stop smoking during pregnancy and to refrain from smoking around the infant; inform parents that smoking is a risk factor for SIDS.
- Recommend parents with infants in child care make it very clear to the employees that the infant must be placed in the supine position *only* to sleep, not prone or side-lying.
- Teach child care employees how best to position infants for sleeping and the dangers of a too soft environment.
- ▲ Teach precautions to prevent SIDS to parents living in deprived areas.
- ▲ Involve family members in learning and practicing rescue techniques, including treatment of choking, breathing, and CPR. Initiate referral to formal training classes. Family members need adequate preparation to deal with emergency situations and should take part in the AHA Basic Lifesaving Course or the American Red Cross Infant/Child CPR Course.

• = Independent          ▲ = Collaborative

# Ineffective Denial

## NANDA Definition

The conscious or unconscious attempt to reduce anxiety or fear by disavowing the knowledge or meaning of an event, leading to the detriment of health

## Defining Characteristics

Delays seeking or refuses health care attention to the detriment of health; does not perceive personal relevance of symptoms or danger; displaces source of symptoms to other organs; displays inappropriate affect; does not admit fear of death or invalidism; makes dismissive gestures or comments when speaking of distressing events; minimizes symptoms; unable to admit impact of disease on life pattern; uses home remedies (self-treatment) to relieve symptoms; displaces fear of impact of condition

## Related Factors (r/t)

Fear of consequences; chronic or terminal illness; actual or perceived fear of possible losses (e.g., job, significant other); refusal to acknowledge substance abuse problem; fear of the social stigma associated with disease

## Client Outcomes

**Client Will (Specify Time Frame):**

- Seek out appropriate health care attention when needed.
- Use home remedies only when appropriate.
- Display appropriate affect and verbalize fears.
- Remain substance-free.
- Actively engage in treatment program related to identified "substance" of abuse.
- Demonstrate alternate adaptive coping mechanism.

## Nursing Interventions

- Assess the client's understanding of symptoms and illness.
- Spend time with the client; allow time for responses.

• = Independent          ▲ = Collaborative

**D**

- Assess whether the use of denial is helping or hindering the patient's care. Provide support for clients who are using denial as a way of coping.
- Allow the client to express and use denial as a coping mechanism.
- Assess for subtle signs of denial (e.g., unrealistic display of optimism, downplaying of symptoms, inability to admit one's own fear).
- Avoid confrontation.
- Support the client's spiritual coping measures.
- Develop a trusting, therapeutic relationship with the client/family.
- Encourage individual family members to share their concerns and worries.
- Ask appropriate questions using an assessment tool such as FAST to determine whether denial is being used in association with alcoholism or drug use. The client is asked to circle the appropriate response for each question: Less than Monthly; Monthly; Weekly; Daily; Almost Daily.
  1. MEN: How often do you have EIGHT or more drinks on one occasion?
     WOMEN: How often do you have SIX or more drinks on one occasion?
  2. How often during the last year have you been unable to remember what happened the night before because you had been drinking?
  3. How often during the last year have you failed to do what was normally expected of you because of drinking?
  4. In the last year, has a relative or friend, a doctor, or other health worker been concerned about your drinking or suggested you decrease your alcohol consumption?
- Sit at eye level.
- Use touch if appropriate and with permission. Touch the client's hand or arm.
- Explain signs and symptoms of illness; as necessary, reinforce use of prescribed treatment plan.

● = Independent        ▲ = Collaborative

- Have the client make choices regarding treatment and actively involve the client in the decision-making process.
- Help the client recognize existing and additional sources of support; allow time for adjustment.
- Encourage the client/family to describe prior crises and methods of coping.
- ▲ If appropriate, refer family to a skilled mental health counselor for help in planning an intervention to observe whether denial has been or is being used as a coping mechanism in other areas of life.
- Refer to care plans **Defensive Coping** and **Dysfunctional Family processes: alcoholism.**

## Geriatric

- Identify recent losses of the client, because grieving may prolong denial. Encourage the client to take one day at a time.
- Encourage the client to verbalize feelings.
- Encourage communication among family members.
- Recognize denial.
- Use reality-focusing techniques. Wherever possible, provide realistic feedback, allowing the client to validate his or her perceptions.

## Multicultural

- Assess for the influence of cultural beliefs, norms, and values on the client's understanding of and ability to acknowledge health status.
- Discuss with the client those aspects of his or her health behavior/lifestyle that will remain unchanged by health status.
- Negotiate with the client regarding the aspects of health behavior that will need to be modified as a result of health status.
- Assess the role of fatalism on the client's ability to acknowledge health status.
- Validate the client's feelings of anxiety and fear related to health status.

• = Independent          ▲ = Collaborative

D

## Home Care

- Observe family interaction and roles. Assess whether denial is being used to meet the needs of another family member.
- ▲ Refer the client and family to psychiatric clinical nurse specialist or medical social services for evaluation and treatment as indicated per physician order.
- ▲ Refer the client/family for follow-up if prolonged denial is a risk.
- ▲ Identify an emergency plan, including how to contact hotlines and receive emergency services.
- Encourage communication between family members, particularly when dealing with the loss of a significant person.

## Client/Family Teaching

- Teach signs and symptoms of illness and appropriate responses (e.g., taking medication, going to the emergency department, calling the physician). Provide a list of important names and numbers.
- Teach family members that denial may continue throughout the adjustment period; instruct family members not to be confrontational.
- ▲ If the problem is substance abuse, refer to an appropriate community agency (e.g., Alcoholics Anonymous).
- Teach families of clients with brain injuries that denial has been associated with damage to the right hemisphere.
- Inform family of available community support resources.

## Impaired Dentition

## NANDA Definition

Disruption in tooth development/eruption patterns or structural integrity of individual teeth

• = Independent          ▲ = Collaborative

## Defining Characteristics

Excessive plaque; crown or root caries; halitosis; tooth enamel discoloration; toothache; loose teeth; excessive calculus; incomplete eruption for age (may be primary or permanent teeth); malocclusion or tooth misalignment; premature loss of primary teeth; worn down or abraded teeth; tooth fracture(s); missing teeth or complete absence; erosion of enamel; asymmetrical facial expression

**D**

## Related Factors (r/t)

Ineffective oral hygiene; sensitivity to heat or cold; barriers to self-care; nutritional deficits; dietary habits; genetic predisposition; selected prescription medications; premature loss of primary teeth; excessive intake of fluorides; chronic vomiting; chronic use of tobacco, coffee, tea, red wine; lack of knowledge regarding dental health; excessive use of abrasive cleaning agents; bruxism

## Client Outcomes

**Client Will (Specify Time Frame):**

- Have clean teeth, healthy pink-colored gums, and pleasant odor in mouth.
- Demonstrate ability to masticate foods without difficulty.
- State no pain originating from teeth.
- Demonstrate measures that can be taken to improve dental hygiene.

## Nursing Interventions

- ▲ Inspect oral cavity/teeth at least once daily and note any discoloration; presence of debris; amount of plaque buildup; presence of lesions, edema, or bleeding; intactness of teeth. Refer to a dentist or periodontist as appropriate.
- • Monitor the client's nutritional and fluid status to determine if adequate. Recommend the client eat a balanced diet and limit snacks between meals.
- • Recommend the client decrease or preferably stop intake of soft drinks.

• = Independent          ▲ = Collaborative

▲ Assess the client for underlying medical condition that may be causing halitosis.

• Determine the client's mental status and manual dexterity; if the client is unable to care for self, dental hygiene must be provided by nursing personnel. The nursing diagnosis **Bathing/hygiene Self-care deficit** is then also applicable.

• Determine the client's usual method of oral care. Whenever possible, build on the client's existing knowledge base and current practices to develop an individualized plan of care.

• If the client is free of bleeding disorders and is able to swallow, encourage the client to brush teeth after each meal with a soft toothbrush using fluoride-containing toothpaste and to floss teeth daily.

• If the client is unable to brush own teeth, follow this procedure:
    1. Use a soft bristle baby toothbrush.
    2. Use fluoride toothpaste and tap water or saline as a solution.
    3. Brush teeth in an up-and-down manner.
    4. Suction as needed.

• Avoid using foam sticks to clean teeth; use only to swab out the oral cavity.

• Tell the client to direct the toothbrush vertically toward the tooth surfaces.

• Instruct the client to clean the tongue when performing oral hygiene. Brush tongue with soft toothbrush and follow with a mouth rinse. Use tap water or saline only for a mouth rinse. Avoid the use of hydrogen peroxide, lemon-glycerin swabs, or alcohol-based mouthwashes.

• If the client does not have a bleeding disorder, encourage the client to floss daily with approximately 18 inches of floss using a gentle rubbing up-and-down motion.

▲ Recommend client see a dentist at prescribed intervals, generally two times per year if teeth are in satisfactory condition.

• = Independent          ▲ = Collaborative

- If platelet numbers are decreased, or if the client is edentulous, use moistened toothettes or a specially made very soft toothbrush for oral care.
- Provide scrupulous dental care to critically ill clients.
- If teeth are nonfunctional for chewing, modification of oral intake (e.g., edentulous diet, soft diet) may be necessary. The nursing diagnosis **Imbalanced Nutrition: less than body requirements** may apply.
- If the client is unable to swallow, keep suction nearby when providing oral care.
- See care plan for **Impaired Oral mucous membrane.**

**D**

### Geriatric
- Consider recommending use of an ultrasonic toothbrush if any impairment of manual dexterity exists.
- Carefully observe oral cavity and lips for abnormal lesions when providing dental care.
- ▲ Consider professional oral health care for the elderly in nursing homes.
- Ensure that dentures are removed and cleaned regularly, preferably after every meal and before bedtime; select appropriate adhesives to improve breath. Dentures left in the mouth at night impede circulation to the palate and predispose the client to oral lesions.
- ▲ Recognize that halitosis in older adults is a common condition that may have oral or non-oral sources.

### Pregnant Client
- Encourage the expectant mother to eat a healthy, balanced diet that is rich in calcium.

### Infant Oral Hygiene
- Gently wipe baby's gums with a washcloth or sterile gauze at least once a day.
- Never allow child to fall asleep with a bottle containing milk, formula, fruit juice, or sweetened liquids. If child needs a comforter between regular feedings, at night, or during naps, fill a bottle with cool water or give the

child a clean pacifier recommended by your dentist or physician. Never give the child a pacifier dipped in any sweet liquid. Avoid filling child's bottle with liquids such as sugar water and soft drinks.

- When multiple teeth appear, brush with small toothbrush with small (pea-sized) amount of fluoride toothpaste. Recommend that child use either a fluoride gel or a fluoride varnish.

## Older Children

▲ Encourage family to talk with the dentist about dental sealants, which can help prevent cavities in permanent teeth.

- Recommend the child use dental floss to help prevent gum disease. The dentist will provide guidelines on when to start using floss. Talk to your dentist about when to start flossing.
- Recommend to parents that they not permit the child to smoke or chew tobacco, and stress the importance of setting a good example by not using tobacco products themselves.
- Recommend the child drink fluoridated water when possible.

▲ If a child has halitosis, consider the presence of parasites in the gastrointestinal system as a cause.

## Multicultural

- Assess for the influence of cultural beliefs, norms, and values on the client's understanding of dental care.
- Assess for barriers to access to dental care such as lack of insurance.
- Instruct mothers on the danger of feeding infants bottles filled with soda, juice, or milk when the infant goes to sleep.
- Assess for dental anxiety.
- Validate the client's feelings with regard to dental health and access to dental care.

• = Independent          ▲ = Collaborative

- Introduce the dental home concept to improve families' access to dental care.

## Home Care

- Assess client patterns for daily and professional dental care and related patterns (e.g., smoking, nail biting). Assess for environmental influences on dental status (e.g., fluoride).
- Assess client facilities and financial resources for providing dental care.
- Request dietary log from the client, adding a column for type of food (e.g., soft, pureed, regular).
- Observe a typical meal to assess first-hand the impact of impaired dentition on nutrition.
- Identify mechanical needs for food preparation and ease of ingestion/digestion to meet the client's dental/nutritional needs.
- Assist the client with accessing financial or other resources to support optimal dental and nutritional status.

## Client/Family Teaching

- Teach how to inspect the oral cavity and monitor for problems with the teeth and gums.
- Teach how to implement a personal plan of dental hygiene, including appropriate brushing of teeth and tongue and use of dental floss.
- Teach the client the value of having an optimal fluoride concentration in drinking water, and to brush teeth twice daily with fluoride toothpaste.
- Teach clients of all ages the need to decrease intake of sugary foods and to brush teeth regularly.
- Suggest chewing gum with sugar to reduce oral malodor.
- Inform individuals who are considering tongue piercing of the potential complications such as chipping and cracking of teeth and possible trauma to the gingiva. If piercing is done, teach the client how to care for the wound and prevent complications.

• = Independent        ▲ = Collaborative

# Risk for delayed Development

## NANDA Definition

At risk for delay of 25% or more in one or more of the areas of social or self-regulatory behavior or cognitive, language, gross, or fine motor skills

## Risk Factors

### Prenatal

Maternal age <15 or >35 years; substance abuse; infections; genetic or endocrine disorders; unplanned or unwanted pregnancy; lack of, late, or poor prenatal care; inadequate nutrition; illiteracy; poverty

### Individual

Prematurity; seizures; congenital or genetic disorders; positive drug screening test; brain damage (e.g., hemorrhage in postnatal period, shaken baby, abuse, accident); vision impairment; hearing impairment or frequent otitis media; chronic illness; technology dependence; failure to thrive, inadequate nutrition; foster or adopted child; lead poisoning; chemotherapy; radiation therapy; natural disaster; behavior disorders; substance abuse

### Environmental

Poverty; violence

### Caregiver

Abuse; mental illness; mental retardation or severe learning disability

## Client Outcomes

### Client/Parents/Primary Caregiver Will (Specify Time Frame):

- Describe realistic, age-appropriate patterns of development.
- Promote activities and interactions that support age-related developmental tasks.

• = Independent        ▲ = Collaborative

## Nursing Interventions

- Refer to care plan for **Delayed Growth and development.**

NOTE: Determination of the etiology for delayed development is critical because it will direct the selection of interventions for treating the diagnosis. Parenting skill deficits, lack of consistency between caregivers, and hospitalization versus a chronic medical condition/developmental disability will necessitate different strategies. A hospitalization experience with regressive behaviors can be a transient occurrence as opposed to a chronic situation, which may have more severe and longer delays requiring more in-depth intervention. Parenting skills and consistent expectations between multiple caregivers can be addressed by more intensive education efforts.

- Avoid exposure to organic solvents during pregnancy.

## Multicultural

- Acknowledge racial/ethnic differences at the onset of care.
- Assess for the influence of cultural beliefs, norms, and values on the client's perceptions of child development.
- Use a neutral, indirect style when addressing areas in which improvement is needed (such as a need for verbal stimulation) when working with clients.
- Assess whether exposure to community violence is contributing to developmental problems.
- Validate the client's feelings and concerns related to child's development.

## Home Care

- Assess for the presence of substances that could cause developmental delay.
- Assist family to identify appropriate skill-building activities for child.
- Provide emotional support for family members' reactions to evidence of developmental delay.

• = Independent        ▲ = Collaborative

▲ If possible, refer family to a program of animal-assisted therapy.

## Client/Family Teaching

▲ Encourage mothers to abstain from alcohol and cocaine use during pregnancy; refer to treatment programs for substance abuse.

▲ Provide support groups and education on human immunodeficiency virus (HIV) and caring for infants with this diagnosis.

• Provide developmental care interventions to preterm infants to improve neurodevelopmental outcomes.

• Provide neonatal positioning procedures for preterm infants to prevent extremity malalignment, skull deformities, and gross motor delay.

• Encourage adequate antepartum and postpartum care for both mother and child.

• Counsel parents, siblings, and caregivers about the importance of smoking cessation and the necessity of eliminating all second-hand smoke exposure.

• Teach caregivers of children appropriate developmental interactions; use anticipatory guidance to facilitate preparation for developmental milestones.

# Diarrhea

## NANDA Definition

Passage of loose, unformed stools

## Defining Characteristics

Hyperactive bowel sounds; at least three loose liquid stools per day; urgency; abdominal pain; cramping

## Related Factors (r/t)

### Psychological
High stress levels and anxiety

• = Independent          ▲ = Collaborative

## Situational

Alcohol abuse; toxins; laxative abuse; radiation; tube feedings; adverse effects of medications; contaminants; travel

## Physiological

Inflammation; malabsorption; infectious processes; irritation; parasites

## Client Outcomes

### Client Will (Specify Time Frame):

- Defecate formed, soft stool every day to every third day.
- Maintain a rectal area free of irritation.
- State relief from cramping and decreased diarrhea or no diarrhea.
- Explain cause of diarrhea and rationale for treatment.
- Maintain good skin turgor and keep body weight at usual level.
- Contain stool appropriately (if previously incontinent).

## Nursing Interventions

- Assess pattern of defecation or have the client keep a diary that includes the following: time of day defecation occurs; usual stimulus for defecation; consistency, amount, and frequency of stool; type of, amount of, and time food consumed; fluid intake; history of bowel habits and laxative use; diet; exercise patterns; obstetrical/gynecological, medical, and surgical histories; medications; alterations in perianal sensations; and present bowel regimen.
- Assess stool consistency and its influence on risk for stool loss.
- ▲ Identify cause of diarrhea if possible based on history (e.g., rotavirus exposure, HIV infection, seafood ingestion, medication effect, radiation therapy, protein malnutrition, laxative abuse, stress). See Related Factors (r/t).
- ▲ If the client has watery diarrhea, a low-grade fever, abdominal cramps, and a history of antibiotic therapy, consider possibility of *Clostridium difficile* infection.

• = Independent          ▲ = Collaborative

▲ If the client has diarrhea associated with antibiotic therapy, consult with primary care practitioner regarding the use of probiotics, such as yogurt with active cultures, to treat diarrhea or also use probiotics to prevent diarrhea when first beginning antibiotic therapy.

• Use Standard Precautions when caring for clients with diarrhea to prevent spread of infectious diarrhea; use gloves and hand washing.

▲ Obtain stool specimens as ordered to either rule out or diagnose an infectious process (e.g., ova and parasites, *C. difficile* infection, bacterial cultures).

• Observe and record number and consistency of stools per day; if desired, use a fecal incontinence collector for accurate measurement of output.

• Inspect, palpate, percuss, and auscultate abdomen; note whether bowel sounds are frequent.

• Assess for dehydration by observing skin turgor over sternum and inspecting for longitudinal furrows of the tongue. Watch for excessive thirst, fever, dizziness, lightheadedness, palpitations, excessive cramping, bloody stools, hypotension, and symptoms of shock.

• Observe for symptoms of sodium and potassium loss (e.g., weakness, abdominal or leg cramping, dysrhythmia). Note results of electrolyte laboratory studies.

• Monitor and record intake and output; note oliguria and dark, concentrated urine.

• Measure specific gravity of urine if possible.

• Weigh the client daily and note decreased weight.

• Give diluted clear fluids as tolerated (e.g., clear soda, Jell-O), serving at lukewarm temperature.

▲ If diarrhea is associated with cancer or cancer treatment, once infectious cause of diarrhea is ruled out, provide medications as ordered to stop diarrhea.

▲ If the client has chronic diarrhea causing fecal incontinence at intervals, consider suggesting use of dietary fiber from psyllium or gum arabic after consultation with primary practitioner.

▲ If diarrhea is chronic and there is evidence of malnutrition, consult with primary care practitioner for a di-

• = Independent          ▲ = Collaborative

etary consult and possible use of a hydrolyzed formula (a clear liquid supplement containing increased protein) to maintain nutrition while the gastrointestinal system heals.

- Encourage the client to eat small, frequent meals and to consume foods that are easy to digest (e.g., bananas, crackers, pretzels, rice, potatoes, clear soups, applesauce).
- Encourage the client to avoid milk products, foods high in fiber, and caffeine (dark sodas, tea, coffee, chocolate).
- Provide a readily available bedpan, commode, or bathroom.
- If the client has diarrhea and incontinence, consider use of a perineal assessment tool to measure the risk for perineal skin injury.
- Thoroughly cleanse and dry the perianal and perineal skin daily and as necessary using a cleanser capable of stool removal. Select a product with a slightly acidic pH designed to preserve its acid mantle, and designed to remove irritants from the skin with minimal physical force. Avoid vigorous scrubbing with water, soap, and a washcloth. Consider selection of a product with a moisturizer.
- If the client is receiving a tube feeding, do not assume it is the cause of diarrhea. Perform a complete assessment to rule out other causes such as medication effects, sorbitol in medications, or an infection.
- If the client is receiving a tube feeding, note rate of infusion, and prevent contamination of feeding by rinsing container every 8 hours and replacing it every 24 hours.
- If the client is receiving a tube feeding, suggest formulas that contain a bulking agent such as Jevity, or add soluble dietary fiber to the feeding per physician/dietitian orders.

## Pediatric

▲ Recommend the parents give the child oral rehydration fluids to drink in the amounts specified by the physician, especially during the first 4 to 6 hours to replace fluid losses. Once the child is rehydrated, an orally adminis-

• = Independent          ▲ = Collaborative

tered maintenance solution should be used along with food.

- Recommend the mother resume breastfeeding as soon as possible.
- Recommend parents not give the child decarbonated soda, fruit juices, Jell-O, or Kool-Aid.
- Recommend parents give children foods with complex carbohydrates such as potatoes, rice, bread, cereal, yogurt, fruits, and vegetables. The BRAT diet is often advocated: bananas, rice, applesauce, and toast. Avoid fatty foods and foods high in simple sugars.

## Geriatric

- ▲ Evaluate medications the client is taking. Recognize that many medications can result in diarrhea, including digitalis, propranolol, angiotensin-converting enzyme (ACE) inhibitors, histamine-receptor antagonists, NSAIDs, anticholinergic agents, oral hypoglycemia agents, antibiotics, and others.
- ▲ Monitor the client closely to detect whether an impaction is causing diarrhea; remove impaction as ordered.
- ▲ Seek medical attention if diarrhea is severe or persists for more than 24 hours, or if the client has symptoms of dehydration or electrolyte disturbances such as lassitude, weakness, or prostration.
- Provide emotional support for clients who are having trouble controlling unpredictable episodes of diarrhea.

## Home Care

- Above interventions may be adapted for home care use.
- Assess the home for general sanitation and methods of food preparation. Reinforce principles of sanitation for food handling.
- Assess for methods of handling soiled laundry if the client is bed-bound or has been incontinent. Instruct or reinforce Universal Precautions with family and bloodborne pathogen precautions with agency caregivers.
- ▲ When assessing medication history, include over-the-counter drugs, both general and those currently being

• = Independent          ▲ = Collaborative

used to treat the diarrhea. Instruct clients not to mix over-the-counter medications when self-treating.

▲ Evaluate current medications for indication that specific interventions are warranted.

▲ Consult with physician regarding need for blood work or stool specimens.

▲ Evaluate need for home health aide or homemaker service referral.

▲ Evaluate need for durable medical equipment in the home.

## Client/Family Teaching

- Encourage avoidance of coffee, spices, milk products, and foods that irritate or stimulate the gastrointestinal tract.
- Teach appropriate method of taking ordered antidiarrheal medications; explain side effects.
- Explain how to prevent the spread of infectious diarrhea (e.g., careful hand washing, appropriate handling and storage of food).
- Help the client to determine stressors and set up an appropriate stress reduction plan.
- Teach signs and symptoms of dehydration and electrolyte imbalance.
- Teach perirectal skin care.

# Risk for Disuse syndrome

## NANDA Definition

At risk for a deterioration of body systems as the result of prescribed or unavoidable musculoskeletal inactivity

## Risk Factors

Paralysis; altered level of consciousness; mechanical immobilization; prescribed immobilization; severe pain (NOTE: Complications from immobility can include pressure ulcer, constipation,

• = Independent          ▲ = Collaborative

stasis of pulmonary secretions, thrombosis, urinary tract infection and/or retention, decreased strength or endurance, orthostatic hypotension, decreased range of joint motion, disorientation, disturbed body image, and powerlessness.)

## D  Related Factors (r/t)

See Risk Factors.

## Client Outcomes

### Client Will (Specify Time Frame):

- Maintain full range-of-motion in joints.
- Maintain intact skin, good peripheral blood flow, and normal pulmonary function.
- Maintain normal bowel and bladder function.
- Express feelings about imposed immobility.
- Explain methods to prevent complications of immobility.

## Nursing Interventions

- Use a functional assessment instrument to evaluate abilities including instruments such as the Barthel Index, the Katz Index of Activities of Daily Living, or the FIM instrument.
- Have the client do exercises in bed if not contraindicated (e.g., flexing and extending feet and quadriceps, performing gluteal and abdominal sitting exercises, lifting small weights to maintain muscle strength).
- ▲ If not contraindicated by the client's condition, obtain referral to physical therapy for use of tilt table to provide weight-bearing on long bones.
- Perform range-of-motion exercises for all possible joints at least twice daily, perform passive or active range-of-motion exercises as appropriate.
- Use high-top sneakers or specialized boots from the occupational therapy department to prevent footdrop; remove shoes twice daily to provide foot care.
- Position the client so that joints are in normal anatomical alignment at all times.

• = Independent        ▲ = Collaborative

D

- If client is immobile, consider use of a transfer chair—a chair that becomes a stretcher.
- Assist the client to walk as soon as medically possible.
- Consider use of a continuous lateral rotation therapy bed.
▲ If at all possible, help the client begin a walking program, using a physical therapist as needed.
- Be very careful when helping the client into a chair and when transferring. Be sure to lock beds and wheelchairs. Recognize that there is a high probability for falls.
- Minimize cardiovascular deconditioning by positioning clients as close to the upright position as possible several times daily. The hazards of bed rest in the elderly are multiple, serious, quick to develop, and slow to reverse.
- When getting the client up after bed rest, do so slowly and watch for signs of postural hypotension, tachycardia, nausea, diaphoresis, or syncope. Take the blood pressure lying, sitting, and standing, waiting 2 minutes between each reading.
- Obtain assistive devices such as braces, crutches, or canes to help the client reach and maintain as much mobility as possible.
- Turn the client at least every 2 hours and carefully observe skin condition, especially bony prominences.
- Provide the client with a pressure-relieving horizontal support surface. For further interventions on skin care, see **Impaired Skin integrity.**
▲ Request a physical therapy referral to help the client learn how to move self in bed, including bridging, and also how to transfer out of bed.
▲ Apply graduated compression stockings as ordered. Ensure proper fit by measuring client; remove stockings at least twice daily, in the morning with bath and in the evening, to assess condition of extremity; then reapply.
- Monitor peripheral circulation and especially note color, pulse, and calf or thigh swelling; check Homans' sign, but recognize that it is an unreliable sign of deep venous thrombosis (DVT).

• = Independent          ▲ = Collaborative

D

- Have the client cough and deep breathe or use incentive spirometry every 2 hours while awake.
- Monitor respiratory functions, noting breath sounds and respiratory rate. Percuss for new onset of dullness in lungs.
- Note bowel function daily. Provide increased fluids, fiber, and natural laxatives such as prune juice as needed.
- Increase fluid intake to 2000 mL/day within the client's cardiac and renal reserve.
- Encourage intake of a balanced diet with adequate amounts of fiber and protein.

## Geriatric
- Help the mostly immobile client achieve mobility as soon as possible, depending on physical condition.
- Use the Outcome Expectation for Exercise scale to determine client's self-efficacy expectations and outcome expectations toward exercise.
- For a client who is mostly immobile, minimize cardiovascular deconditioning by positioning the client in an upright position several times daily.
- If client is frail, ensure good nutrition, appropriate medications, attention to vision and hearing deficits, and increase social support along with exercise.
- If the client is mostly immobile, encourage him or her to attend a low-intensity aerobic chair exercise class that includes stretching and strengthening chair exercises.
- Refer the client to physical therapy for resistance exercise training as able, including abdominal crunch, leg press, leg extension, leg curl, calf press, and more.
▲ If client is geriatric or is scheduled for an elective surgery that will result in admission into the ICU and immobility, such as recovery from a total knee replacement surgery, initiate a prehabilitation program that includes a warm-up, aerobic strength, flexibility, and functional task work.
▲ Refer to physical therapy for an individualized strength training program.

• = Independent          ▲ = Collaborative

- Monitor for signs of depression: flat affect, poor appetite, insomnia, many somatic complaints.
- Keep careful track of bowel function in the elderly; do not allow the client to become constipated.

## Home Care

D

NOTE: Care for all body systems because the immobilized or otherwise at risk client must continue in the home as stated in the previously mentioned interventions. The primary nurse monitors and adjusts the plan of care accordingly per physician orders.

- Some of the above interventions may be adapted for home care use.
- ▲ Begin discharge planning as soon as possible with case manager or social worker to assess need for home support systems and community or home health services.
- ▲ Become oriented to all programs of care for the client before discharge from institutional care.
- ▲ Confirm the immediate availability of all necessary assistive devices for the home.
- Perform complete physical assessment and recent history at initial visit.
- ▲ Refer to physical and occupational therapies for immediate evaluations of the client's potential for independence and functioning in the home setting and for follow-up care.
- Allow the client to have as much input and control of the plan of care as possible.
- Assess knowledge of all care with caregivers. Review as necessary.
- ▲ Support the family of the client in assumption of caregiver activities. Refer for home health aide services for assistance and respite as appropriate. Refer to medical social services as appropriate.
- ▲ Institute case management of frail elderly to support continued independent living.

• = Independent        ▲ = Collaborative

## Client/Family Teaching

- Teach how to perform range-of-motion exercises in bed if not contraindicated.
- Teach the family how to turn and position the client and provide all care necessary.

NOTE: Nursing diagnoses that are commonly relevant when the client is on bed rest include **Constipation, Risk for impaired Skin integrity, Disturbed Sensory perception, Disturbed Sleep pattern, Adult Failure to thrive,** and **Powerlessness.**

# Deficient Diversional activity

## NANDA Definition

Decreased stimulation from or interest or engagement in recreational or leisure activities

## Defining Characteristics

Usual hobbies cannot be undertaken in hospital; patient's statements reflect boredom and the wish for something to do or to read, for example

## Related Factors (r/t)

Environmental lack of diversional activity as a result of long-term hospitalization or frequent or lengthy treatments

## Client Outcomes

### Client Will (Specify Time Frame):
- Engage in personally satisfying diversional activities.

## Nursing Interventions

- Observe for signs of deficient diversional activity: restlessness, unhappy facial expression, and statements of boredom and discontent.

● = Independent         ▲ = Collaborative

- Observe ability to engage in activities that require good vision and use of hands.
- Discuss activities with clients that are interesting and feasible in the present environment.
- Encourage the client to share feelings about situation of inactivity instead of usual life activities.
- Encourage a mix of physical and mental activities (e.g., crafts, videotapes). Provide activities that are entertaining, such as videotapes, joke books, or a "humor room."
- Use "bread therapy"—have clients bake bread with a bread maker two times per day or as needed.
▲ Arrange animal-assisted therapy; have the client interact with or care for a dog or cat.
- Encourage the client to schedule visitors so that they are not all present at once or at inconvenient times.
- Provide reading material, television, radio, and books on tape.
- If clients are able to write, have them keep journals; if clients are unable to write, have them record thoughts on tape.
▲ Request recreational or art therapist to assist with providing diversional activities.
▲ Request an order for a child life specialist or, if not available, a play therapist for children.
- Provide a change in scenery; get the client out of the room if possible.
- Help the client to experience nature through looking at a nature scene from a window, or walking through a garden if possible.
- Structure the environment as needed to promote optimal comfort and sensory diversity (e.g., have family bring in posters, banners, or a sound system; change lighting; change direction bed faces).
- Recommend activities in which the client can watch movement of animals and develop involvement (e.g., bird-watching, keeping a fish tank).

• = Independent          ▲ = Collaborative

- Work with family to provide music that is enjoyable to the client.
- Structure the client's schedule around personal wishes for time of care, relaxation, and participation in fun activities.
- Spend time with the client when possible or arrange for a friendly visitor.

## Pediatric

- ▲ Provide activities such as video projects and use of computer-based support groups for children, such as Starbright World—a computer network where children interact virtually, sharing their experiences and escaping hospital routines.
- Provide virtual reality experiences for children, which can be used as distraction techniques during chemotherapy treatments, for example. Recommend programs such as Magic Carpet, Sherlock Holmes Mystery, and Seventh Guest.

## Geriatric

- If possible, arrange for the client to attend a group senior citizen exercise session for progressive strength training, even if exercise can only be done while seated.
- Encourage involvement in senior citizen activities (e.g., AARP, YMCA, church groups). Arrange transportation to activities as needed.
- Encourage clients to use their ability to help others by volunteering.
- Provide an environment that promotes activity (e.g., one that has adequate lighting for crafts, large-print books); allow periods of solitude and privacy.
- ▲ Use reminiscence therapy in conjunction with the expression of emotions. Refer to a reminiscence group if available.
- ▲ Use the Eden Alternative with the elderly: bring in appropriate plants for the elderly client to care for; pro-

• = Independent          ▲ = Collaborative

vide animals such as birds, fish, dogs, and cats as appropriate for the client; and allow children to visit.
- For clients in assisted living facilities, provide leisure educational programs.
- Provide recreational therapy exercises in the morning for clients with dementia in the extended care facility.

D

## Multicultural
▲ Assess for the influence of cultural beliefs, norms, and values on the client's leisure activity interests.
▲ Validate the client's feelings and concerns related to lack of stimulation or interest in leisure activities.

## Home Care
NOTE: Many of the previously listed interventions should be administered in the home setting (e.g., modifying the environment to stimulate the client, scheduling visitors to allow for rest and activity). Some adaptations will be necessary.

- Explore with the client previous interests; consider related activities that are within the client's capabilities.
▲ Assess the client for depression. Refer for mental health services as indicated.
- Assess the family's ability to respond to the client's psychosocial needs for stimulation. Assist as able.
▲ Refer to occupational therapy to assist the client and family with identifying diversional activities within the capability of the client and family.
▲ Introduce (or continue) friendly volunteer visitors if the client is willing and able to have the company. If transportation is an issue or if the client does not want visitors in the home, consider alternatives (e.g., telephone contacts, computer messaging).
▲ In the presence of a psychiatric disorder, refer for psychiatric home health care services for client reassurance and implementation of therapeutic regimen.

• = Independent          ▲ = Collaborative

## Client/Family Teaching

- Work with the client and family in learning diversional activities that the client is interested in (e.g., knitting, hooking rugs, writing memoirs).
- If the client is in isolation, give the client complete information on why isolation is needed and how it should be accomplished, especially guidelines for visitors.

**E**

# Disturbed Energy field

## NANDA Definition

Disruption of the flow of energy surrounding a person's being, resulting in disharmony of the body, mind, and/or spirit

### Defining Characteristics

Perceptions of changes in patterns of energy flow, such as: movement (wave, spike, tingling, dense, flowing); sounds (tone, words); temperature change (warmth, coolness); visual changes (image, color); disruption of the field (deficit, hole, spike, bulge, obstruction, congestion, diminished flow in energy field)

### Related Factors

Slowing or blocking of energy flows secondary to: pathophysiological factors; illness (specify); pregnancy; injury; treatment-related factors; immobility; labor and delivery; perioperative experience; chemotherapy; situational factors (personal, environmental); pain; fear; anxiety; grieving; maturational factors; age-related developmental difficulties or crisis (specify)

### Client Outcomes

**Client Will (Specify Time Frame):**

- State sense of well-being.
- State feeling of relaxation.
- State decreased pain.

● = Independent     ▲ = Collaborative

- State decreased tension.
- Demonstrate evidence of physical relaxation (e.g., decrease in blood pressure, pulse, respiration rate, and muscle tension).

## Nursing Interventions

- Refer to care plans for **Anxiety, Acute Pain,** and **Chronic Pain.**
- Consider using therapeutic touch (TT) for clients with anxiety, tension, pain, and other conditions that indicate a disruption in the flow of energy.
- Consider use of treatments for clients with psychological depression and self-perceived stress.
- Administer TT as described in the following discussion (may also include healing touch and reiki practice).

## Guidelines for Therapeutic Touch

- TT may be practiced by anyone with the requisite preparation, desire, and commitment. Required preparation is the completion of a minimum 12 contact hour basic workshop by a TT practitioner who meets the criteria as a "NH-PAI, Inc. (Nurse Healer-Professional Associates International) qualified TT teacher." Health care professionals need to have practiced TT on a consistent basis for at least 1 year under the direction of a mentor (during the mentorship year, at the discretion and under the supervision of a mentor, the health care professional can begin using TT in a health care/hospital setting). A further requirement of the practitioner is the completion of a 14 contact hour intermediate level course of instruction by a qualified TT teacher.
- Those who are not licensed health care professionals may practice TT within their families, religious or spiritual community, and friends. Investigation of state licensing laws and regulations is necessary before accepting fees for practicing TT to ensure lawful practices. Those who are licensed to perform specific or general health-related services, including counseling or massage therapy, need to clarify roles and scope of practice parameters with

their respective state regulatory entity or board or with an attorney.

NOTE: Nurses who are not trained in TT should consider spending quiet time with clients, listening to their concerns.

- TT practitioners adhere to a code of ethics in the practice of TT. Keeping client information confidential, using TT only with permission of the client, charging reasonable fees for services, and practicing responsible use of other interventions in conjunction with the TT process are important elements of that code.
- TT is conducted according to the standards for its practice developed by Dr. Dolores Krieger and Dora Kunz and in accordance with the above guidelines.

## Administer TT by Performing the Following Steps:

- Centering in the present moment: Shift awareness from the physical environment to an inner focus on the center within self, a center of calm and balance through which nurses perceive themselves and the client as a unitary whole.
- Assessment: Pass palmar surface of hands 2 to 4 inches over the client's body from head to toe.
- Treatment (unruffling): Use hands to brush or smooth out the energy flow. Sweep the hands downward and out of the field from head to toe, and concentrate on the areas of disturbance that were identified during the assessment.
- Direction and modulation of energy: Rest hands on or near the body area where a block of congestion is detected or in other areas of energy imbalance. Facilitate transfer of energy to these areas.
- Finish: Finish when it is judged that the appropriate amount of change has taken place (e.g., for an infant, 1 to 2 minutes; for an adult, 5 to 7 minutes), keeping in mind the importance of gentleness. The procedure may also be stopped when the client indicates it is time to

stop. Note whether the client has experienced a relaxation response and any related outcomes.

## Pediatric

- Consider using TT or healing touch for pediatric clients with adjunct therapies to decrease stress, anxiety, and pain.
- Teach that when working with the very young, old, or ill or when working in the head area, TT should be gentle and used only for short periods.

## Geriatric

- Consider therapeutic touch for agitated clients with Alzheimer's disease.

## Multicultural

- Assess for the influence of cultural beliefs, norms, and values on the client's sense of disharmony of mind and spirit.
- Assess for the presence of specific culture-bound syndromes that may manifest as disturbances in energy or spirit.
- Validate the client's feelings and concerns related to sense of disharmony or energy disturbance.

## Home Care

- See Guidelines for Therapeutic Touch.
- ▲ Help the client and family accept TT as a healing intervention. Consultation and collaboration with a specialist may be the best approach to nursing care. Numerous studies have reported positive outcomes of healing touch as a noninvasive complementary therapy.
- Assist the family with providing an appropriate space in which TT can be administered.
- ▲ Assess clients with bipolar disorder for the occurrence of social rhythm disruption, particularly during periods of stressful life events. Refer for mental health treatment.

• = Independent        ▲ = Collaborative

▲ In the presence of a psychiatric disorder, refer for psychiatric home health care services for client reassurance and implementation of therapeutic regimen.

## Client/Family Teaching

- Teach the TT process to clients and family members.
- Teach that when working with the very young, old, or ill or when working in the head area, TT should be gentle and used only for short periods.
- Teach the client how to use guided imagery.
- Teach the client to use deep breathing to relax. Ask the client to have the disease, affected organ, or symptom assume an image. After the image has been identified, ask the client to speak to the image to address an unresolved issue.

# Impaired Environmental interpretation syndrome

## NANDA Definition

Consistent lack of orientation to person, place, and time, or circumstances for more than 3 to 6 months, necessitating a protective environment

## Defining Characteristics

Chronic confusional states; consistent disorientation in known and unknown environments; loss of occupation or social functioning resulting from memory decline; slow to respond to questions; inability to follow simple directions/instructions, concentrate, or reason

## Related Factors (r/t)

Depression; dementia (e.g., Alzheimer's disease, multi-infarct, Pick's disease, AIDS, Parkinson's disease, alcoholism)

• = Independent          ▲ = Collaborative

## Client Outcomes

### Client Will (Specify Time Frame):

- Remain content and free from harm.
- Function at maximal cognitive level.
- Participate in ADLs at the maximum of functional ability.

## Nursing Interventions, Client/Family Teaching

See care plan for **Chronic Confusion.**

# Adult Failure to thrive

## NANDA Definition

Progressive functional deterioration of a physical and cognitive nature with remarkably diminished ability to live with multisystem diseases, cope with ensuing problems, and manage care

## Defining Characteristics

Anorexia—does not eat meals when offered; states does not have an appetite, is not hungry, or "I don't want to eat"; inadequate nutritional intake—eating less than body requirements; consumption of minimal to no food at most meals (i.e., consumes less than 75% of normal requirements); weight loss (from baseline weight)—5% unintentional weight loss in 1 month or 10% unintentional weight loss in 6 months; physical decline (decline in bodily function)—evidence of fatigue, dehydration, incontinence of bowel and bladder; frequent exacerbations of chronic health problems (e.g., pneumonia, urinary tract infections); cognitive decline (decline in mental processing) as evidenced by problems with responding appropriately to environmental stimuli, demonstrated difficulty in reasoning, decision making, judgment, memory, and concentration; decreased perception; decreased social skills; social withdrawal—noticeable decrease from usual past behavior in attempts to form or participate in cooperative and interdependent relationships (e.g., decreased verbal communication with staff, family, friends); decreased participation in ADLs that the older person once enjoyed; self-care deficit—no longer looks after or takes charge of physical cleanliness or appearance; difficulty performing simple self-care tasks; neglect of home environment and/or financial responsibilities; apathy as evidenced by lack of observable feeling or emotion in terms of normal ADLs and environment; altered mood state—expresses feelings of sadness, being low in spirit; expresses loss of interest in pleasurable outlets such as food, sex, work, friends, family, hobbies, or entertainment; verbalizes desire for death

## Related Factors (r/t)

Depression; apathy; fatigue

## Client Outcomes

### Client Will (Specify Time Frame):

- Resume highest level of functioning possible.
- Express feelings.
- Participate in ADLs.
- Participate in social interactions.
- Consume adequate dietary intake for weight and height.
- Maintain usual weight.
- Have adequate fluid intake with no signs of dehydration.
- Maintain personal cleanliness and clean home environment.

## Nursing Interventions

### Psychosocial

- Elderly clients who have failure to thrive (FTT) should be evaluated by review of the patient's ADLs, cognitive function, and mood; a targeted history and physical examination; and selected laboratory studies.
- Assess for depression using a geriatric depression scale. Be alert for depression in clients newly admitted to nursing homes.
- ▲ Carefully assess for elderly abuse and refer for treatment.

• = Independent          ▲ = Collaborative

- Screen for depression in persons with adult macular degeneration (AMD) and low vision or vision loss.
- Provide reality orientation for clients with mild dementia.
- Provide music for clients with dementia.
▲ Consider the use of "light therapy."
- Instill hope and encourage the expression of positive thoughts.
- Provide opportunities for interaction with the natural environment.
- Provide opportunities for visitation from animals.
- Encourage clients to reminisce and to share and compile life histories.
- Encourage clients to pray if they desire.
- Encourage elderly clients to take part in activities and social relationships according to their capacity and wishes.
- Assist clients to participate in activities by assessing motivation and helping them to identify reasons to participate such as better mobility, more independence, feelings of well-being.
- Provide physical touch for clients. Touch their hand or arm when speaking with them; offer hugs with permission.
- Administer TT.

## Physiological

▲ Assess possible causes for adult FTT and treat any underlying problems such as malnutrition, diarrhea, renal failure, and illnesses that are caused by physical and cognitive changes.
▲ Assess for signs of dehydration. Administer 1600 mL of fluid in 24 hours. Offer fluids regularly to bedridden clients.
- Assess for signs of fatigue and sensory changes that may indicate an infection is present that may be related to undetected diabetes mellitus or HIV.
- Assess how frequently the frail elder living at home goes outdoors. (Ask the client how often they go outside the

house, for example, shopping, taking a walk, going out to work in garden.)

- Assess grip strength.
- Monitor weight loss, leaving 25% or more of food uneaten at most meals, psychiatric/mood diagnoses, and deteriorated ability to participate in activities of daily living.
- Offer nutrient-dense foods such as dairy and fruit products: vanilla custard, strawberry yogurt, vanilla/apple yogurt, orange/peach juice, apple/berry/grape juice, and applesauce. (Adopt appropriate foods for the individual tastes of the elderly client.)
- Play soothing music during mealtimes to increase the amount of food eaten.
- Decrease noise and increase lighting in the dining area.
- Serve "family style meals."
- Provide appropriate nutrition for the client whose obesity may be affecting physical performance and thus has limited ability to perform ADLs, which leads to functional dependence.
- Frail elderly clients should also participate in carefully supervised group exercise and balance and gait programs accompanied by music. (An exercise program that has been used in research consisted of a 45-minute group session conducted twice weekly; it involved walking, stooping, and chair stands under the supervision of skilled trainers. Exercises were moderate but gradually increased in intensity and included different materials, such as balls, ropes, weights, and elastic bands.) (Another exercise treatment used a wheelchair bicycle, combining small group activity therapy and one-on-one bike rides with a staff member.)
- ▲ Refer for possible pharmacological intervention.
- Refer to care plans for **Imbalanced Nutrition: less than body requirements, Hopelessness,** and **Disturbed Energy field.**

## Multicultural

- Assess for the influence of cultural beliefs, norms, and

values on the family's or care-giver's understanding of
FTT.
▲ Refer culturally diverse patients to appropriate social,
  medical, mental health, and long-term care services.
• Validate the family's feelings and concerns related to
  FTT symptoms.

## Home Care

• Above interventions may be adapted for home care use.
▲ Begin discharge planning as soon as possible with case
  manager or social worker to assess need for home
  support systems, assistive devices, and community or
  home health services.
• Assess client's willingness to eat; fashion interventions
  accordingly.
• Assess and track areas of decreased functioning resulting
  from failure to thrive. Ensure that all symptomatology
  is considered for necessary action.
• Give permission for role activity changes. Negotiate and
  clarify role expectations and reevaluate as necessary.
• Provide support for family/caregivers.
• If FTT is due to a dementing illness, refer to care plan
  for **Chronic Confusion.**
• Assess nutritional status for multiple potential influences
  of malnutrition, including chronic and acute disorders,
  loss of self-sufficiency, malabsorption disorders, changes
  in sense of taste, dental problems, reduced physical activity, problems with appropriate medication use, and
  economic or psychological factors.
▲ Refer to medical social services or mental health counseling, resource identification, and/or community support
  groups. If necessary, contract with the client to attend sessions.
▲ Refer to home health aide services for assistance with
  ADLs throughout the duration of decreased
  participation.
▲ Institute case management of frail elderly to support
  continued independent living. Failure to thrive

• = Independent          ▲ = Collaborative

represents and can lead to increasing needs for assistance in using the health care system effectively.
▲ Refer for homemaker or psychiatric home health care services for respite, client reassurance, and implementation of therapeutic regimen.

## Client/Family Teaching

▲ Refer for medical evaluation when cognitive changes are noticed.
• Encourage family to provide social interaction with the client.
• Instruct the family to monitor the elder person's weight.
▲ Provide referral for evaluation of hearing and appropriate hearing aids.
▲ Refer for psychotherapy and possible medication if the etiology is depression.
▲ Refer for possible medication therapy when the diagnosis is dementia.

# Risk for Falls

## NANDA Definition

Increased susceptibility to falling that may cause physical harm

### Risk Factors

#### Adults
History of falls; wheelchair use; 65 years of age or older; female (if elderly); lives alone; lower limb prosthesis; use of assistive devices (e.g., walker, cane)

#### Physiological
Presence of acute illness; postoperative conditions; visual difficulties; hearing difficulties; arthritis; orthostatic hypotension; sleeplessness; faintness when turning or extending neck; anemias; vascular disease; neoplasms (i.e., fatigue/limited mobility, urgency and/or incontinence, diarrhea, decreased lower extremity

• = Independent          ▲ = Collaborative

strength, postprandial blood sugar changes, foot problems, impaired physical mobility, impaired balance, difficulty with gait, unilateral neglect, proprioceptive deficits, neuropathy); diminished mental status (e.g., confusion, delirium, dementia, impaired reality testing)

## Medication
Antihypertensive agents; ACE inhibitors; diuretics; tricyclic antidepressants; alcohol use; antianxiety agents; opiates; hypnotics or tranquilizers

**F**

## Environment
Restraints; weather conditions (e.g., wet floors/ice); throw/scatter rugs; cluttered environment; unfamiliar, dimly lit room; no antislip material in bath and/or shower

## Children (<2 Years of Age)
Male gender when younger than 1 year; lack of auto restraints; lack of gate on stairs; lack of window guard; bed located near window; unattended infant on bed/changing table/sofa; lack of parental supervision

## Related Factors (r/t)

See Risk Factors.

## Client Outcomes

### Client Will (Specify Time Frame):

- Remain free of falls.
- Change environment to minimize the incidence of falls.
- Explain methods to prevent injury.

## Nursing Interventions

- Determine risk of falling by using an evaluation tool such as the Fall Risk Assessment, the Conley scale, or the FRAINT tool for fall risk assessment.
- Screen all clients for stability and mobility skills (supine to sitting, sitting supported and unsupported, sitting to standing, standing, walking and turning around, trans-

• = Independent       ▲ = Collaborative

ferring, stooping to floor and recovering, and sitting down). Use tools such as the Balance scale or the Get Up and Go scale.

- Recognize that when people attend to another task while walking, such as carrying a cup of water, clothing, or supplies, they are more likely to fall.
- Be careful when getting a mostly immobile client up. Be sure to lock the bed and wheelchair and have sufficient personnel to protect the client from falls.
- Identify clients likely to fall by placing a "Fall Precautions" sign on the doorway and by keying the Kardex and chart. Use a "high-risk fall" arm band and room sign to alert staff for increased vigilance and mobility assistance.
- ▲ If the client must be placed in a wrist or vest restraint because of physician orders, use increased vigilance and watch for falls.
- ▲ Evaluate the client's medications to determine whether medications increase the risk of falling; consult with physician regarding the client's need for medication if appropriate.
- Thoroughly orient the client to environment. Place the call light within reach and show how to call for assistance; answer call light promptly.
- Use ¼- to ½-length side rails only, and maintain the bed in a low position. Ensure that wheels are locked on both bed and commode. Keep dim light in room at night.
- Routinely assist the client with toileting on his or her own schedule. Always take the client to bathroom on awakening, before bedtime, and before administering sedatives
- Keep the path to the bathroom clear, label the bathroom, and leave the door open.
- ▲ Avoid use of restraints if at all possible. Obtain a physician's order if restraints are necessary.
- In place of restraints, use the following:
  - Well-staffed and educated nursing personnel with frequent client contact.

• = Independent          ▲ = Collaborative

F

- Nursing units designed to care for clients with cognitive or functional impairments.
- Nonskid footwear.
- Alarm systems with ankle, above the knee, or wrist sensors.
- Bed or wheelchair alarms.
- Increased observation of the client.
- Locked doors to unit.
- Low or very low height beds.
- Border-defining pillow/mattress to remind the client to stay in bed.

▲ If the client has a new onset of confusion (delirium), recognize that the cause is usually physiological and is a medical emergency. Provide reality orientation when interacting.

· Have family bring in familiar items, such as clocks and watches from home, to maintain orientation.

· If the client has chronic confusion with dementia, use validation therapy that reinforces feelings but does not confront reality. See interventions for **Chronic Confusion.**

· Ask family to stay with the client to prevent the client from accidentally falling or pulling out tubes.

· If the client is unsteady on feet, use a walking belt or two nursing staff members when ambulating the client.

· Place a fall-prone client in a room that is near the nurses' station.

· Help clients sit in a stable chair with arm rests. Avoid use of wheelchairs and geri-chairs except for transportation as needed.

· Ensure that the chair or wheelchair fits the build, abilities, and needs of the client to ensure propulsion with legs or arms and ability to reach the floor, eliminating footrests and minimizing problems with shearing.

· Avoid use of wheelchairs as much as possible because they can serve as a restraint device. Most people in wheelchairs do not move.

▲ Refer to physical therapy for strengthening exercises, gait training, and help with balance to increase mobility.

● = Independent          ▲ = Collaborative

## Geriatric

- Assess ability to move using the "Up & Go" test. Ask the client to rise from a sitting position, walk 10 feet, turn, and return to the chair to sit.
- If client exhibits new onset of falling, check blood pressure and pulse rate supine, sitting, and standing for orthostatic hypotension.
- Encourage the client to wear glasses and use walking aids when ambulating.
- Help the client obtain and wear a specially designed hip protector when ambulating. Hip protectors are worn in a specially designed stretchy undergarment containing a pocket on each side for placement of the protector.
- If the client experiences dizziness because of orthostatic hypotension when getting up, teach methods to decrease dizziness, such as rising slowly, remaining seated several minutes before standing, flexing feet upward several times while sitting, sitting down immediately if feeling dizzy, and trying to have someone present when standing.
- ▲ If the client is experiencing syncope, determine symptoms that occur before syncope, and note medications that the client is taking. Refer for medical care. The circumstances surrounding syncope often suggest the cause.
- ▲ Observe client for signs of anemia, and refer to primary care practitioner for testing if appropriate.
- ▲ Evaluate client for chronic alcohol intake, as well as mental health and neurological function.
- ▲ Refer to physical therapy for strength training, using free weights or machines.
- ▲ If an elderly woman has symptoms of urge incontinence, refer to a urologist for evaluation and ensure the path to the bathroom is well lighted and free of obstructions.

## Home Care

- Some of the above interventions may be adapted for home care use.
- If the client was identified as a fall risk in the hospital,

• = Independent          ▲ = Collaborative

recognize that there is a high incidence of falls after discharge, and use all measures possible to reduce the incidence of falls.

- Assess and monitor for acute changes in cognition and behavior.
- Assess for additional factors leading to risk for falls.
- Assess home environment for threats to safety: clutter, slippery floors, scatter rugs, unsafe stairs and stairwells, blocked entries, extension cords (across pathway), high beds, pets, and pet excrement. Use antiskid acrylic floor wax, nonskid rugs, stair rails, and skid-proof strips near the bed to prevent slippage. Evaluate need for safety devices in bathing area (e.g., hand grip, shower chair, hand-held showerhead).
- ▲ Institute a home-based, nurse-delivered exercise program to reduce falls or refer to physical therapy services for client and family education of safe transfers and ambulation and for strengthening exercises (for the client).
- ▲ Instruct the client and family/caregivers on how to correct identified hazards. Refer to occupational therapy services for assistance if needed.
- ▲ Use a multifactorial assessment along with interventions targeted to the identified risk factors. Key components of the interventions include evaluating need for all medications; balance, gait and strength training; use of strategies to deal with postural hypotension if present; home safety evaluation with needed modifications; and any needed cardiovascular treatment.
- Encourage balanced diet, with particular inclusion of vitamin D and calcium.
- If the client lives alone or spends a lot of time alone, teach the client what to do if he or she falls and cannot get up, and make sure he or she has a personal emergency response system or a cellular phone that is available from the floor.
- If the client is at risk for falls, use gait belt and additional persons when ambulating.
- Ensure appropriate nonglare lighting in the home. Ask the client to install indoor strip or "runway" type of light-

• = Independent        ▲ = Collaborative

ing to baseboards to help client balance. Install motion-sensitive lighting that turns on automatically when the client gets out of bed to go to the bathroom.
- Have the client wear supportive low-heeled shoes with good traction when ambulating.
- Consider the use of external hip protectors for clients at risk for falls.
▲ Refer to physical therapy services for the client and family education of safe transfers and ambulation and for strengthening/balance exercises (for the client) for ambulation and transfers.
  ■ Provide a signaling device for clients who wander or are at risk for falls.
  ■ Provide medical identification bracelets for clients at risk for injury from dementia, seizures, or other medical disorders.
  ■ Suggest a t'ai chi class designed for the elderly to selected clients who have sufficient balance to participate.

## Client/Family Teaching

- Teach the client how to safely ambulate at home, including using safety measures such as hand rails in the bathroom and avoiding carrying things or performing other tasks while walking.
- Teach the client the importance of maintaining a regular exercise program such as walking.

# Dysfunctional Family processes: alcoholism

## NANDA Definition

The state in which the psychosocial, spiritual, and physiological functions of the family unit are chronically disorganized, leading to conflict, denial of problems, resistance to change, ineffective problem solving, and a series of self-perpetuating crises

● = Independent          ▲ = Collaborative

## Defining Characteristics

### Roles and Relationships

Inconsistent parenting/low perception of parental support; ineffective spouse communication/marital problems; intimacy dysfunction; deterioration in family relationships/disturbed family dynamics; altered role function/disruption of family roles; closed communication systems; chronic family problems; family denial; lack of cohesiveness; neglected obligations; lack of skills necessary for relationships; reduced ability of family members to relate to each other for mutual growth and maturation; family unable to meet security needs of its members; disrupted family rituals; economic problems; family does not demonstrate respect for individuality and autonomy of its members; triangulating family relationships; pattern of rejection

### Behavioral

Refusal to get help/inability to accept and receive help appropriately; inadequate understanding or knowledge of alcoholism; ineffective problem-solving skills; loss of control of drinking; manipulation; rationalization/denial of problems; blaming; inability to meet emotional needs of its members; alcohol abuse; broken promises; criticizing; dependency; impaired communication; difficulty with intimate relationships; enabling to maintain drinking; expression of anger inappropriately; isolation; inability to meet spiritual needs of its members; inability to express or accept wide ranges of feelings; inability to deal with traumatic experiences constructively; inability to adapt to change; immaturity; harsh self-judgment; lying; lack of dealing with conflict; lack of reliability; nicotine addiction; orientation toward tension relief rather than achievement of goals; seeking approval and affirmation; difficulty having fun; agitation; chaos; contradictory, paradoxical communication; diminished physical contact; disturbances in academic performance in children; disturbances in concentration; escalating conflict; failure to accomplish current or past developmental tasks/difficulty with life cycle transitions; family special occasions are alcohol centered; controlling communication/power struggles; self-blaming; stress-related physical illnesses; substance abuse other than alcohol; unresolved grief; verbal abuse of spouse or parent

• = Independent          ▲ = Collaborative

## Feelings

Insecurity; lingering resentment; mistrust; vulnerability; rejection; repressed emotions; responsibility for alcoholic's behavior; shame/embarrassment; unhappiness; powerlessness; anger/suppressed rage; anxiety, tension, or distress; emotional isolation/loneliness; frustration; guilt; hopelessness; hurt; decreased self-esteem/worthlessness; hostility; lack of identity; fear; loss; emotional control by others; misunderstood; moodiness; abandonment; being different from other people; being unloved; confused love and pity; confusion; failure; depression; dissatisfaction

## Related Factors (r/t)

Abuse of alcohol; genetic predisposition; lack of problem-solving skills; family history of alcoholism; resistance to treatment; biochemical influences; addictive personality

## Client Outcomes

### Family/Client Will (Specify Time Frame):

- Develop relationship with nurse that demonstrates at least minimal level of trust.
- Demonstrate an understanding of alcoholism as a family illness and the severity of the threat to emotional and physical health of family members.
- Develop and state a belief in feasibility and effectiveness of efforts to address alcoholism.
- Demonstrate change from dysfunctional patterns by moving from inappropriate to appropriate role relationships, improving cohesion among family members, decreasing conflict and social isolation, and improving coping behaviors.
- Maintain improvements.

## Nursing Interventions

- When completing a family assessment, assess behaviors of alcohol abuse, loss of control of drinking, denial, nicotine addiction, impaired communication, inappropriate expression of anger, and enabling behaviors.
- Screen clients for at-risk drinking during routine primary

• = Independent          ▲ = Collaborative

care visits. At-risk drinking is defined as consuming an average of two or more drinks per day (chronic drinking), or two or more occasions of consuming five or more drinks in the past month (binge drinking), or, in the past month, one or more occasion of driving after consuming three or more drinks (drinking and driving).

- Ask appropriate questions using an assessment tool such as FAST to determine whether denial is being used in association with alcoholism or drug use. The client is asked to circle the appropriate response for each question: Less than Monthly; Monthly; Weekly; Daily; Almost Daily.

  1. MEN: How often do you have EIGHT or more drinks on one occasion?
     WOMEN: How often do you have SIX or more drinks on one occasion?
  2. How often during the last year have you been unable to remember what happened the night before because you had been drinking?
  3. How often during the last year have you failed to do what was normally expected of you because of drinking?
  4. In the last year has a relative or friend, a doctor, or other health worker been concerned about your drinking or suggested you decrease your alcohol consumption?

- Demonstrate high levels of empathy and expectancy of positive outcomes in interactions with family members.
- Stress individual self-focus as a first step in problem resolution.
- Help family to restructure family patterns of interaction and function to support the development of consistency, a predictable environment, emotional nurturance, and positive modeling.
- Assist with stabilization and maintenance of positive change in the family. Instruct the alcoholic's family members before the client's discharge to give verbal messages that convey concern about the alcoholic's problem drinking, their observations of the alcoholic's past

F

• = Independent          ▲ = Collaborative

episodes of drinking, and wishes and support for abstinence.
- Instill hope and encourage the expression of positive thoughts.
- Monitor family closely for return to old patterns of behavior.
- Provide activities that are physical in nature, such as adventure therapy and therapeutic camping, as part of a substance abuse treatment program.
▲ Consider alternative therapies such as acupuncture.
▲ Refer for possible use of medications such as naltrexone and acamprosate to control problem drinking.
- Refer to care plans **Ineffective Denial** and **Defensive Coping.**

## Pediatric

▲ Educate family members about available educational and support programs.
▲ Use close-ended questions when questioning adolescents about drinking behavior.
▲ Provide a brief motivational interviewing and cognitive-behavioral–based alcohol intervention group (AIG) program for young people at risk of developing a problem with alcohol.
- Encourage parent involvement with adolescents: supervision and emotional support.
- Work at strengthening adolescents' relationships in and out of the home.
▲ Provide school-based prevention programs using peer leaders at an early age.
▲ Provide a school-based drug-prevention program to junior high students.

## Geriatric

- Include assessment of possible alcohol abuse when assessing elderly family members.
- Use CAGE tool with this population and include drug use along with drinking. An affirmative answer to two or

• = Independent          ▲ = Collaborative

more of the following questions is considered a basis for suspicion of alcohol abuse:

**C:** Have you ever felt you ought to **Cut down** on drinking?

**A:** Have people **Annoyed** you by criticizing your drinking?

**G:** Have you ever felt bad or **Guilty** about your drinking?

**E:** Have you ever had a drink first thing in the morning to steady your nerves or get rid of a hangover (**Eye opener**)?

▲ Provide alcohol treatment programs for geriatric clients in primary care settings.

## Multicultural

- Acknowledge racial/ethnic differences at the onset of care.
- Approach families of color with respect, warmth, and professional courtesy.
- Give rationale when assessing African-American families about alcohol use and misuse.
- Use a family-centered approach when working with Latino, Asian-American, African-American, and Native-American clients.
- When working with Asian-American clients, provide opportunities for the family to save face.
- Some less acculturated Latino families may be unwilling to discuss family issues with health care providers until they perceive a close relationship with the provider.
- Utilize family strengthening interventions, e.g., behavioral parent training, family skills training, in-home family support, brief family therapy, and family education when working with culturally diverse families.
- Work with families in a way that incorporates cultural elements.

## Home Care

NOTE: In the community setting, alcoholism as an etiology for dysfunctional family processes must be consid-

F

• = Independent          ▲ = Collaborative

ered in two categories. The first is when the client suffers personally from the illness; the second is when a significant other suffers from the illness; that is, the client is not the active alcoholic but may be dependent on the alcoholic for caregiving. The listed considerations apply to both situations with appropriate adaptation for the circumstances.

- Above interventions may be adapted for home care use.
- Identify client/family expectations of the home care nurse and nurse expectations of the client/family by use of a well-defined contract. Be specific and realistic. Adjust the contract only with clear consent and understanding of the client/family.
- Work with family members to support a sense of valued fit on their part; include them in treatment planning, and identify the importance of their roles in the client's care. At the same time, encourage their pursuit of positive outside activities that enhance their sense of belonging.
- ▲ Establish well-defined contingency and emergency plans for the care of the client.
- Request concrete, measurable tasks of the client and family for caregiving and provide concrete, nonjudgmental instruction to the client/family regarding the interactions of alcohol use with medications, therapeutic regimen.
- ▲ Observe for abuse of other medications. Notify physician of problems noted.
- ▲ If the client is a recovering alcoholic, extreme care must be taken in the use of psychoactive or pain medications. Notify physician if inappropriate medications have been inadvertently ordered.
- ▲ Refer for medical social work services at outset of care.
- ▲ Provide information regarding available substance abuse treatment programs and support groups.
- Acknowledge without judgment when resolution of alcoholism is not a goal of care.
- ▲ Refer for psychiatric home health care services for client reassurance and implementation of therapeutic regimen.

• = Independent          ▲ = Collaborative

## Client Family Teaching

- Suggest client do a confidential Internet self-screening test for identification of problems and suggestions for treatment if a problem with alcohol is suspected. There are many tools available.

# Readiness for enhanced Family processes    F

## NANDA Definition

A pattern of family functioning that is sufficient to support the well-being of family members and can be strengthened

## Defining Characteristics

Expresses willingness to enhance family dynamics; family functioning meets physical, social, and psychological needs of family members; activities support the safety and growth of family members; communication is adequate; relationships are generally positive; interdependent with community; family tasks are accomplished; family roles are flexible and appropriate for developmental stages; respect for family members is evident; family adapts to change; boundaries of family members are maintained; energy level of family supports activities of daily living; family resilience is evident; balance exists between autonomy and cohesiveness

## Client Outcomes

### Family/Client Will (Specify Time Frame):

- Identify ways to cope effectively and use appropriate support systems (family).
- Meet physical, psychosocial, and spiritual needs of members or seek appropriate assistance (family).
- Demonstrate knowledge of potential environmental, lifestyle, and genetic risks to health and use appropriate measures to decrease possibility of risk (family).

• = Independent          ▲ = Collaborative

- Focus on wellness, disease prevention, and maintenance (family and individual).
- Seek balance among exercise, work, leisure, rest, and nutrition (family and individual).

## Nursing Interventions

F

- Assess the family's stress level and coping abilities during the initial nursing assessment.
- Consider the use of family theory as a framework to help guide interventions (e.g., family stress theory, role theory, social exchange theory).
- Use family-centered care, and role modeling for holistic care of families.
- Discuss with the family members how they have handled previous crises.
- Support family empowerment: strength and resourcefulness.
- Spend time with family members; allow them to verbalize their feelings.
- Encourage family members to find meaning in a serious illness such as cancer.
- Have family members participate in client conferences that involve all members of the health care team.
- ▲ Provide family-centered care to explore and use all available resources appropriate for situation (e.g., counseling, social services, self-help groups, pastoral care).
- ▲ Consider referral for walk-in family therapy.

## Pediatric

- Provide a parenting class series based on individual and couple changes in meaning/identity, roles, and relationship/interaction during the transition to parenthood. Address mother/father roles, infant communication abilities, and patterns of the first 3 months of life in a mutually enjoyable, possibility-focused way.
- Encourage families with adolescents to have family meals.

• = Independent          ▲ = Collaborative

▲ Consider the use of adventure therapy for adolescents with cancer.

## Geriatric

- Carefully listen to residents and family members in the long-term care facility.
- Support caregivers' awareness of the positive effects of their contribution to the well-being of parents.
- Teach family members about impact of developmental events (e.g., retirement, death, change in health status, and change in household composition).
- Encourage social networks, social integration, and social engagement with friends, children, and relatives for the elderly.

## Multicultural

- Assess for the influence of cultural beliefs, norms, and values on the family's perceptions of normal functioning.
- With the client's consent, facilitate a group meeting for family members to discuss how the family is functioning.
- Facilitate modeling and role-playing for the client and family regarding healthy ways to start a discussion about the client's prognosis.
- Identify and acknowledge the stresses unique to racial/ethnic families.
- Offer frequent gestures of support to family members.
- Encourage family mealtimes.

## Home Care

- The nursing interventions described previously for **Readiness for enhanced Family processes** should be used in the home environment with adaptations as necessary.
- Provide a videophone network for peer support for frail elderly people living at home.
- Encourage families to assist women caring for husbands with chronic obstructive pulmonary disease (COPD) to provide respite care so the women may have recreation time.

• = Independent        ▲ = Collaborative

## Client/Family Teaching

- Refer to Client/Family Teaching in **Readiness for enhanced family Coping** for suggestions that may be used with minor adaptations.

# Interrupted Family processes

F

## NANDA Definition

Change in family relationships and/or functioning

## Defining Characteristics

Changes in power alliances; assigned tasks; effectiveness in completing assigned tasks; mutual support; availability for effective responsiveness and intimacy; patterns and rituals, participation in problem solving; participation in decision making; communication patterns; availability for emotional support; satisfaction with family; stress-reduction behaviors; expressions of conflict with and/or isolation from community resources; somatic complaints; expressions of conflict within family

## Related Factors (r/t)

Power shift of family members; shift in family roles; shift in health status of a family member; developmental transition and/or crisis; situational transition and/or crisis; informal or formal interaction with community; modification in family social status; modification in family finances

## Client Outcomes

### Family/Client Will (Specify Time Frame):

- Express feelings (family).
- Identify ways to cope effectively and use appropriate support systems (family).
- Treat impaired family member as normally as possible to avoid overdependence (family).

• = Independent            ▲ = Collaborative

- Meet physical, psychosocial, and spiritual needs of members or seek appropriate assistance (family).
- Demonstrate knowledge of illness or injury, treatment modalities, and prognosis (family).
- Participate in the development of a plan of care to the best of ability (significant person).

## Nursing Interventions

- Assess the family's stress level and coping abilities during the initial nursing assessment.
- Establish rapport with families by providing accurate communication.
- Use family-centered care and role modeling for holistic care of families.
- ▲ Provide family-centered care to explore and use all available resources appropriate for situation (e.g., counseling, social services, self-help groups, pastoral care).
- Acknowledge the range of emotions and feelings that may be experienced when there is a change of health status in a family member; counsel family members that it is normal to be angry or afraid, for example.
- Encourage family members to list their personal strengths.
- Involve family members in the care and information/patient teaching sessions with the client.
- Encourage family to visit the client; adjust visiting hours to accommodate family's schedule (e.g., schedule around work, school, babysitting needs). Assist with sleeping arrangements if family is spending the night; provide a place to lie down, pillows, and blankets.
- Allow and encourage family to assist in the client's care. Allow family presence during invasive procedures and resuscitation.
- ▲ Consider use of video home training as a method of early support in problems of family life control.

## Pediatric

- Allow and encourage family to assist in the client's care.

• = Independent          ▲ = Collaborative

▲ Carefully assess potential for reunifying children placed in foster care with their birth parents.

## Geriatric

- Teach family members about the impact of developmental events (e.g., retirement, death, change in health status, and change in household composition).
- Encourage family members to be involved in the care of relatives who are in residential care settings.
- Support group problem solving among family members and include the older member.
- ▲ Refer family for counseling with a psychotherapist who is knowledgeable about gerontology.
- Refer to care plan for **Readiness for enhanced family Coping.**

## Multicultural

- Assess for the influence of cultural beliefs, norms, and values on the family's perceptions of normal functioning.
- With the client's consent, facilitate a group meeting for family members to discuss how the family is functioning.
- Facilitate modeling and role-playing for the client and family regarding healthy ways to start a discussion about the client's prognosis.
- Identify and acknowledge the stresses unique to racial/ethnic families.
- Offer frequent gestures of support to family members.
- Encourage the family members to demonstrate and offer caring and support to each other.
- Validate the family's feelings regarding concerns about current crisis and family functioning.
- Encourage family mealtimes.

## Home Care

- The nursing interventions described previously for **Compromised family Coping** should be used in the home environment with adaptations as necessary.
- Encourage help from the family when communicating

• = Independent          ▲ = Collaborative

F

with clients in advanced stages of cancer who are no longer able to communicate their illness and symptom needs.

## Client/Family Teaching

- Refer to Client/Family Teaching in **Compromised family Coping** and **Readiness for enhanced family Coping** for suggestions that may be used with minor adaptations.

F

# Supportive Family role performance*

## Definition

Patterns of family behavior and expression consistent with expectations and normal role functioning of the family unit in support of an ill or incapacitated family member

## Defining Characteristics

Stated or observed desire of family to be part of the therapy provided to a family member, to provide support to that person during therapy, or to help the person endure the therapy; stated or observed desire of family to be present at the time of family member's death

## Related Factors (r/t)

Family member undergoing therapeutic treatments, including: cardiopulmonary resuscitation, invasive procedures, discomforting diagnostic tests, induction of or emergence from general anesthesia; health care crisis

---

*Note: **Supportive Family role performance** is a wellness-oriented diagnosis. It is not currently an official NANDA-I nursing diagnosis, but it is included because the authors believe that the desire of families to provide support to their members is a normal human response to health care crises and that nurses can use interventions to assist families in meeting this role expectation.

• = Independent          ▲ = Collaborative

## Client Outcomes

### Client Will (Specify Time Frame):

- Express appropriate concern for ill member and ask how they may assist or support (family).
- Request information about process/procedure/therapy and about client condition/status (family).
- Maintain communication among all members of family unit, including contacting family members not present as desired by ill member, and provide accurate information to other family members (family).
- Identify level of participation/presence and collaboration in determining care desired and appropriate for client needs (individual and family).
- Provide encouragement, comforting touch, and emotional support to ill member (family).
- Seek social and/or spiritual support appropriate for ill member (family and individual).
- Verbalize meaning and significance of health crisis (family and individual).
- State that his or her sense of support is adequate (individual).
- Express feeling supported, able to cope (individual).
- Appear less anxious and/or exhibit improved cooperation with treatment activities (individual).
- State feeling of accomplishment or role fulfillment (family).

## Nursing Interventions

- When providing perioperative care for a pediatric client, offer the parents the option to be present during induction and recovery from anesthesia.
- Assess the anxiety level, temperament, and physical health of the child and parents before surgery to guide individualized care and to screen for those who may not benefit from this intervention.
- ▲ If you are not already part of the procedural or resuscitation team, introduce yourself to the staff responsible for treating the client and family.
- Assess the suitability of the client's physical location for family presence.

• = Independent          ▲ = Collaborative

- ▲ Obtain consensus from the staff for the family's presence and the timing of the family's presence.
- • Obtain information about the client's status, response to treatment, and likely ongoing needs and convey this information to the client's family in a timely manner. Assist the family in contacting family members not currently present, if requested.
- • Facilitate family involvement and presence in accordance with the client's and/or family's stated desires.
- • Advocate for the family's desire to be present during resuscitation if the prognosis is very grim.
- • Introduce yourself and other members of the support team to the family and client. Use the client's name when speaking to the family.
- • Make a holistic assessment of the client's and family's emotional, psychosocial, and spiritual support needs, taking into consideration developmental status.
- ▲ Determine the psychological burden of the prognosis and participation for the family, and inform the treatment team of the family's emotional reaction to the client's condition.
- • Treat the family as a cohesive unit and as participants in the client's care.
- • If client is undergoing resuscitation, assure the family that best possible care is being given to their relative. While conveying accurate information, foster realistic hope.
- • Inform the family of behavioral expectations and limits before entering the treatment area. Provide a dedicated staff person to ensure that family members are never left unattended at the bedside.
- • When the family indicates they wish to be present, accompany the family to and from the treatment area, and announce their presence to the treatment staff each time the family enters. Escort the family from the bedside if requested by the staff providing direct care.
- • Provide the opportunity for the family to ask questions and to see, touch, and speak to the client before transfers.
- • Offer families the opportunity to be present during pain-

F

• = Independent          ▲ = Collaborative

ful or distressing procedures to provide comfort, and demonstrate techniques that the family may employ to enhance the comfort of their ill family member.

- Families may request to be present during critical diagnostic procedures such as testing for brainstem death.
▲ In the event of a client death, offer and/or coordinate family bereavement follow-up at established intervals.
- If specific policies regarding family presence are not available for the care area or facility, advocate the development and adoption of such policies.

## Multicultural

- No specific multicultural studies have been performed for this diagnosis. Assess for the influence of cultural beliefs, norms, values, and expectations on the individual's and family's perception of appropriate family support and family presence during treatment.
- Cultural differences between organizations/associated professional staff and clients/families may limit clinician responses to crisis situations.
- See the care plan for **Readiness for enhanced family Coping.**

## Geriatric

- Current studies have not addressed the specific needs of geriatric clients and their families related to family presence during resuscitation and invasive procedures.
- Older clients may be less likely to prefer having family members present during resuscitation when compared with younger clients.
- See the care plan for **Readiness for enhanced Family processes.**
- See the care plan for **Anticipatory Grieving.**

## Home Care

- An increasing number of invasive procedures are being performed in the home setting. The client and family

• = Independent        ▲ = Collaborative

preferences regarding family presence during these procedures should be assessed.
- Above interventions may be adapted for home care use.
- See the care plan for **Readiness for enhanced Family processes**.

## Client/Family Teaching

- Provide education to parents regarding their role and expectations when they are present for induction and recovery from anesthesia.
- Prepare the family (and client, if conscious) before entering the treatment area, assuring they have been informed about what to expect, what they will see, hear, and/or smell.
- Provide information and explanations to the family and client regarding the interventions being performed or anticipated, medical or nursing jargon used during treatment, and expectations of the client's response to treatment.

# Fatigue

## NANDA Definition

An overwhelming, sustained sense of exhaustion and decreased capacity for physical and mental work at usual level

## Defining Characteristics

Inability to restore energy even after sleep; lack of energy or inability to maintain usual level of physical activity; increase in rest requirements; tired; inability to maintain usual routines; verbalization of an unremitting and overwhelming lack of energy; lethargic or listless; perceived need for additional energy to accomplish routine tasks; compromised concentration; disinterest in surroundings, introspection; decreased performance; compromised libido; drowsy; feelings of guilt for not keeping up with responsibilities; inability to concentrate; weakness

• = Independent          ▲ = Collaborative

### Related Factors (r/t)

**Psychological**
Stress; anxiety; depression; boring lifestyle

**Environmental**
Humidity; lights; noise; temperature

**Situational**
Negative life events; occupation

**Physiological**
Sleep deprivation; pregnancy; poor physical condition; disease states (e.g., cancer, HIV, multiple sclerosis); increased physical exertion; malnutrition; anemia; metabolic imbalance

### Client Outcomes

**Client Will (Specify Time Frame):**

- Identify potential factors that aggravate and relieve fatigue.
- Describe ways to assess and track patterns of fatigue.
- Verbalize increased energy and improved well-being.
- Explain energy conservation plan to offset fatigue.
- Explain energy restoration plan to offset fatigue.

### Nursing Interventions

- Assess severity of fatigue on a scale of 0 to 10 (average fatigue, worst and best levels); assess frequency of fatigue (number of days per week and time of day), activities and symptoms associated with increased fatigue (i.e., pain), ability to perform activities of daily living (ADLs) and instrumental activities of daily living (IADLs), interference with social and role function, times of increased energy, ability to concentrate, mood, and usual pattern of activity. Consider use of an instrument such as the Profile of Mood State Short Form Fatigue subscale, the Multidimensional Assessment of Fatigue, the Lee Fatigue scale, the Multidimensional Fatigue Inventory, the HIV-Related Fatigue scale, the Brief Fatigue Inventory, or the Dutch Fatigue scale to accurately assess fatigue.

- Evaluate adequacy of nutrition and sleep patterns (napping throughout the day, inability to fall asleep or stay asleep). Encourage the client to get adequate rest, limit naps (particularly in the late afternoon or evening), use a routine sleep/wake schedule, and eat a well-balanced diet with at least eight glasses of water a day. Refer to **Imbalanced Nutrition: less than body requirements** or **Disturbed Sleep pattern** if appropriate.

▲ Determine with help from the primary care practitioner whether there is a physiological or psychological cause of fatigue that could be treated, such as anemia, pain, electrolyte imbalance (i.e., altered potassium levels), hypothyroidism, depression, or medication effect.

▲ Work with the physician to determine if the client has chronic fatigue syndrome.

- Encourage the client to express feelings about fatigue, including the client's perception of potential causes of fatigue and possible interventions to alleviate fatigue; use active listening techniques and help identify sources of hope.

- Encourage the client to keep a journal of activities, symptoms of fatigue, and feelings, including how fatigue impacts the client's normal activities and roles.

- Help the client set small, easily achieved short-term goals such as writing two sentences in a journal daily or walking to the end of the hallway twice daily to increase activity tolerance.

- Help the client identify essential and nonessential tasks and determine those tasks that can be delegated. Give the client permission to limit social and role demands if needed (e.g., switch to part-time employment, hire cleaning service).

- Assist the client with ADLs and IADLs as necessary; encourage independence and activity without causing exhaustion.

- Encourage walking exercise.

• = Independent          ▲ = Collaborative

F

▲ With the physician's approval, refer to physical therapy for carefully monitored aerobic exercise program and possible physical aids, such as a walker or cane.

• Patients may desire multiple strategies to relieve fatigue, rather than one single intervention, particularly when there are multiple potential etiologies present.

▲ Refer the client to diagnosis-appropriate support groups such as National Chronic Fatigue Syndrome Association, Multiple Sclerosis Association, or cancer fatigue websites (such as the Oncology Nurses Association).

▲ For a cardiac client, recognize that fatigue is common following a myocardial infarction. Refer to cardiac rehabilitation for a carefully prescribed and monitored exercise program.

• For fatigue with multiple sclerosis, encourage energy conservation, "recharging efforts," and excellent self-care, and consider use of a cooling suit for clients with multiple sclerosis whose fatigue increases in a warm environment.

• For attentional fatigue, suggest restorative activities using nature such as sitting outside, bird-watching, and gardening.

▲ Consider referring for cognitive therapy to help deal with symptoms of fatigue and help change negative thought patterns.

• For fatigue associated with cancer, monitor lab values for potential anemia, evaluate treatment regimen (chemotherapy and/or radiation) and tumor burden, and suggest energy conservation intervention.

• If fatigue is associated with cancer or cancer-related treatment, assess for other symptoms that may enhance fatigue (e.g., pain or depression). Fatigue in patients with cancer may manifest itself as the inability to direct attention necessary to perform usual activities ("attentional fatigue").

▲ Refer the client to occupational therapy to learn new energy-conserving and energy-restoring ways to perform tasks.

• = Independent          ▲ = Collaborative

## Geriatric

- Review comorbid conditions that may contribute to fatigue, such as congestive heart failure, arthritis, and cancer.
- Identify recent losses; monitor for depression as a possible contributing factor to fatigue.
- ▲ Review medications for side effects.

## Home Care

- Above interventions may be adapted for home care use.
- Assess the client's history and current patterns of fatigue as they relate to the home environment; determine environmental and behavioral triggers of increased fatigue.
- ▲ Refer to occupational therapy if substantial intervention is needed to assist the client in adapting to home and daily patterns.
- Assist the client with identifying or creating a safe, restful place within the home that can be used routinely (e.g., a room with familiar, nonthreatening, or nonfrightening belongings).
- For clients receiving chemotherapy, intervene to:
  - Relieve symptom distress (negative mood, nausea, difficulty sleeping).
  - Encourage as much physical activity as possible.
  - Support a positive attitude for the future.
  - Support adequate recovery time between treatments.
- ▲ Refer cancer clients to a community-based pain and fatigue management program, such as the I Feel Better program, if available.
- Teach the client/family the importance of and methods for setting priorities for activities, especially those having a high energy demand (e.g., home/family events). Instruct in realistic expectations and behavioral pacing.
- Assess effect of fatigue on the client's relatedness; recognize that the client's fatigue affects the whole family. Initiate the following interventions:
  - Avoid dismissing reports of fatigue; validate the cli-

• = Independent          ▲ = Collaborative

ent's experience and foster hope for eventual treatment, if not resolution, of the fatigue.

- Identify with the client ways in which he or she continues to be a valued part of his or her social environment.
- Identify with the client ways in which he or she continues to participate in equitable exchange with others.
- Encourage the client to maintain regular family routines (e.g., meals, sleep patterns) as much as possible.
- Initiate cognitive restructuring to refute the client's guilt-producing and negative thought patterns.
- Assess and intervene with family/friends' contributions to guilt-inducing self-talk.
- Work with the client to inoculate against the negative thinking of others.
- Explore family life and demands to identify accommodations.
- Support the client's efforts at limit-setting on the demands of others.
- Assist the client to move toward a state of parallelism by working to identify and relieve sources of physical or emotional discomfort. Degree of involvement, limited by fatigue, need not be changed.
▲ Refer for family therapy in the event the client's fatigue interferes with normal family functioning.
▲ If fatigue has affected the client's ability to participate in relationships effectively, refer for psychiatric home health care services for client reassurance and implementation of therapeutic regimen.

## Client/Family Teaching

- Help client to do cognitive reframing: Share information about fatigue and how to live with it, including need for positive self-talk.
- Teach strategies for energy conservation (e.g., sitting instead of standing during showering, storing items at waist level).

• = Independent          ▲ = Collaborative

- Teach the client to carry a pocket calendar, make lists of required activities, and post reminders around the house.
- Teach the importance of following a healthy lifestyle with adequate nutrition, fluids, and rest; pain relief; relief of insomnia; and appropriate exercises to decrease fatigue (i.e., energy restoration).
- Teach stress-reduction techniques such as controlled breathing, imagery, and use of music.
- See **Anxiety** care plan if appropriate; anxiety is correlated with increased fatigue.

F

# Fear

## NANDA Definition

Response to perceived threat that is consciously recognized as a danger

## Defining Characteristics

Report of apprehension; increased tension; decreased self-assurance; excitement; being scared; jitteriness; dread; alarm; terror; panic

### Cognitive
Identifies object of fear, stimulus believed to be a threat; diminished productivity, learning ability, problem-solving ability

### Behaviors
Increased alertness; avoidance or attack behaviors; impulsiveness; narrowed focus on "it" (i.e., the focus of the fear)

### Physiological
Increased pulse; anorexia; nausea; vomiting; diarrhea; muscle tightness; fatigue; increased respiratory rate and shortness of breath; pallor; increased perspiration; increased systolic blood pressure; pupil dilation; dry mouth

• = Independent          ▲ = Collaborative

## Related Factors (r/t)

Natural/innate origin (e.g., sudden noise, acrophobia, pain, loss of physical support); learned response (e.g., conditioning, modeling from or identification with others); separation from support system in potentially stressful situation (e.g., hospitalization, hospital procedures); unfamiliarity with environmental experience(s); language barrier; sensory impairment; innate releasers (neurotransmitters); phobic stimulus

## F  Client Outcomes

### Client Will (Specify Time Frame):

- Verbalize known fears.
- State accurate information about the situation.
- Identify, verbalize, and demonstrate those coping behaviors that reduce own fear.
- Report and demonstrate reduced fear.

## Nursing Interventions

- Assess source of fear with the client.
- Assess for a history of anxiety.
- Have the client draw the object of their fear.
- Discuss situation with the client and help distinguish between real and imagined threats to well-being.
- Encourage the client to explore underlying feeling that may be contributing to the fear.
- Stay with clients when they express fear; provide verbal and nonverbal (touch and hug with permission and if culturally acceptable) reassurances of safety if safety is within control.
- Explore coping skills used previously by the client to deal with fear; reinforce these skills and explore other outlets.
- Provide back rubs and massage for clients to decrease anxiety.
- Use TT and healing touch techniques.
- ▲ Refer for cognitive behavioral therapy.
- ▲ Animal-assisted therapy can be incorporated into the care of perioperative patients.

● = Independent         ▲ = Collaborative

- Encourage clients to express their fears in narrative form.
- Refer to care plans for **Anxiety** and **Death Anxiety.**

## Pediatric

- Instruct parents that nighttime fear is common in children.
- Explore coping skills used previously by the client to deal with fear. Children generally rate their coping behaviors as helpful.
- Teach parents to use cognitive-behavioral strategies such as positive coping statements ("I am a brave girl [boy]. I can take care of myself in the dark.") and rewards of bravery tokens for appropriate behavior.
- Screen for depression in clients who report social/school fears.
- Teach relaxation technique to children to induce calmness.

## Geriatric

- Establish a trusting relationship so that all fears can be identified.
- Monitor for dementia and use appropriate interventions.
- Provide a protective and safe environment, use consistent caregivers, and maintain the accustomed environmental structure.
- Observe for untoward changes if antianxiety drugs are taken.
- Assess for fear of falls in hospitalized patients with hip fractures to determine risk of poor health outcomes.
- Encourage exercises to improve physical skills and levels of mobility to decrease fear of falling.
- Assist the client in identifying and reducing risk factors of falls, including environmental hazards in and out of the home, the importance of good nutrition and activity, proper footwear, and how to stand up after a fall.

● = Independent          ▲ = Collaborative

## Multicultural

- Assess for the presence of culture-bound anxiety/fear states.
- Assess for the influence of cultural beliefs, norms, and values on the client's perspective of a stressful situation.
- Identify what triggers the fear response.
- Identify how the client expresses fear.
- Validate the client's feelings regarding fear.
- Assess for fears of racism in culturally diverse clients.

## Home Care

- Above interventions may be adapted for home care use.
- Assess to differentiate the presence of fear versus anxiety.
- Refer to care plan for **Anxiety.**
- During initial assessment, determine whether current or previous episodes of fear relate to the home environment (e.g., perception of danger in home or neighborhood or of relationships that have a history in the home).
- Identify with the client what steps may be taken to make the home "safe."
- ▲ Encourage the client to seek or continue appropriate counseling to reduce fear associated with stress or to resolve alterations in irrational thought processes.
- ▲ Encourage the client to have a trusted companion, family member, or caregiver present in the home for periods when fear is most prominent. Pending other medical diagnoses, a referral to homemaker/home health aide services may meet this need.
- ▲ Offer to sit with a terminally ill client quietly as needed by the client or family, or provide hospice volunteers to do the same.

## Client/Family Teaching

- Teach the client the difference between warranted and excessive fear.
- Teach stress management interventions to clients who experience emotions of fear.
- Teach families to share personal stories about an illness

• = Independent          ▲ = Collaborative

using the computer-based psychoeducational application experience journal.

- Teach clients to use guided imagery when they are fearful: have them use all senses to visualize a place that is "comfortable and safe" for them.
- ▲ Teach use of appropriate community resources in emergency situations (e.g., hotlines, emergency departments, law enforcement, judicial systems).
- ▲ Encourage use of appropriate community resources in nonemergency situations (e.g., family, friends, neighbors, self-help and support groups, volunteer agencies, churches, recreation clubs and centers, seniors, youths, others with similar interests). Teach the client appropriate use of ordered medications.
- ▲ In event of bioterrorism provide accurate information to ensure that health care personnel have appropriate training and preparation.

## Readiness for enhanced Fluid balance

### NANDA Definition

A pattern of equilibrium between fluid volume and chemical composition of body fluids that is sufficient for meeting physical needs and can be strengthened

### Defining Characteristics

Expresses willingness to enhance fluid balance; stable weight; moist mucous membranes; food and fluid intake adequate for daily needs; straw-colored urine with specific gravity within normal limits; good tissue turgor; no excessive thirst; urine output appropriate for intake; no evidence of edema or dehydration

### Related Factors (r/t)

Motivation to improve hydration status

● = Independent          ▲ = Collaborative

## Client Outcomes

### Client Will (Specify Time Frame):

- Maintain light yellow urine output.
- Maintain elastic skin turgor, moist tongue, and moist mucous membranes.
- Explain measures that can be taken to improve fluid intake.

## Nursing Interventions

- Discuss normal fluid requirements. A guideline is 1–1.5 mL of fluid per each calorie needed, so an average intake would be between 2000 and 3000 mL/day, or at least 8 cups of fluid.
- Recommend mainly intake of water, but milk or fruit juice can also be effective in maintaining good fluid balance.
- Recommend the client decrease the use of alcoholic beverages and beverages containing caffeine.
- Recommend the client avoid intake of carbonated beverages; instead, suggest the client drink water.

### Geriatric
- Encourage the elderly client to develop a pattern of drinking water regularly.

### Home Care
- Assess availability of clean drinking water in the home, or assess resources to acquire bottled water.
- ▲ Assess available and preferred fluids. Refer for social services if resources are needed to purchase adequate fluid.

### Client/Family Teaching
- Teach the client to drink water before and during participation in activities that can result in quick dehydration, such as distance running or gardening in hot weather.
- Caution the athletic client not to drink excessively during competition or training, to follow the dictates of thirst.
- Teach clients who work or exercise in hot environments to increase intake of both water and electrolyte-

• = Independent        ▲ = Collaborative

carbohydrate beverages; sports drinks are needed when exercise exceeds 1 hour in duration or during prolonged competitive games that require repeated intermittent activity.
- Ask the client to monitor the color of their urine to determine if adequately hydrated.

# Deficient Fluid volume

## NANDA Definition

Decreased intravascular, interstitial, and/or intracellular fluid (refers to dehydration, water loss alone without change in sodium level)

## Defining Characteristics

Decreased urine output; increased urine concentration; weakness; sudden weight loss (except in third-spacing); decreased venous filling; increased body temperature; decreased pulse volume/pressure; change in mental state; elevated hematocrit levels; decreased skin/tongue turgor; dry skin/mucous membranes; increased thirst; increased pulse rate; decreased blood pressure

## Related Factors (r/t)

Active fluid volume loss; failure of regulatory mechanisms

## Client Outcomes

### Client Will (Specify Time Frame):

- Maintain urine output of more than 1300 mL/day (or at least 30 mL/hr).
- Maintain normal blood pressure, pulse, and body temperature.
- Maintain elastic skin turgor; moist tongue and mucous membranes; and orientation to person, place, and time.
- Explain measures that can be taken to treat or prevent fluid volume loss.

• = Independent          ▲ = Collaborative

• Describe symptoms that indicate the need to consult with health care provider.

## Nursing Interventions

**F**

• Watch for early signs of hypovolemia, including restlessness, weakness, muscle cramps, headaches, inability to concentrate, and postural hypotension.
• Monitor for the existence of factors causing deficient fluid volume (e.g., vomiting, diarrhea, difficulty maintaining oral intake, fever, uncontrolled type 2 diabetes, diuretic therapy).
• Monitor daily weight for sudden decreases, especially in the presence of decreasing urine output or active fluid loss. Weigh the client on the same scale with the same type of clothing at the same time of day, preferably before breakfast.
• Monitor total fluid intake and output every 8 hours (or every hour for the unstable client). Recognize that urine output is not always an accurate indicator of fluid balance.
• Watch trends in urine output for 3 days; include all routes of intake and output and note color and specific gravity of urine.
• Monitor vital signs of clients with deficient fluid volume every 15 minutes to 1 hour for the unstable client (every 4 hours for the stable client). Observe first for tachycardia, tachypnea, and decreased pulse pressure; then monitor for hypotension, decreased pulse volume, and increased or decreased body temperature.
• Monitor for inelastic skin turgor, thirst, dry tongue and mucous membranes, longitudinal tongue furrows, speech difficulty, dry skin, sunken eyeballs, weakness (especially of upper body), headache, and confusion.
• Provide frequent oral hygiene, at least twice a day (if mouth is dry and painful, provide hourly while awake).
• Provide fresh water and oral fluids preferred by the client (distribute over 24 hours [e.g., 1200 mL during the day, 800 mL in the evening, and 200 mL during the night]); provide prescribed diet; offer snacks (e.g., frequent

• = Independent          ▲ = Collaborative

drinks, fresh fruits, fruit juice); instruct significant other
to assist the client with feedings as appropriate.
- Provide free water with tube feedings as appropriate
(50–100 mL every 4 hours) or 30 mL/kg of body weight.
- Institute measures to rest the bowel when the client is
vomiting or has diarrhea (e.g., restrict food or fluid intake when appropriate, decrease intake of milk products).
▲ Hydrate the client with ordered intravenous solutions if
prescribed (see care plan for **Diarrhea** or **Nausea**).
▲ Provide oral replacement therapy as ordered and tolerated with a hypotonic glucose- electrolyte solution when
the client has acute diarrhea or nausea/vomiting. Provide small, frequent quantities of slightly chilled
solutions.
▲ Administer antidiarrheals and antiemetics as appropriate.
▲ If the client requires intravenous fluid replacement,
maintain patent intravenous access, set an appropriate intravenous infusion flow rate, and administer at a constant flow rate as ordered.
- Assist with ambulation if the client has postural
hypotension.

## Critically Ill
- If a trauma client, check manual blood pressure until the
systolic pressure is 110 mm Hg. Do not rely on automatic blood pressure measurements.
▲ Monitor central venous pressure, right atrial pressure,
and pulmonary wedge pressure for decreases.
▲ Monitor serum and urine osmolality, serum sodium concentration, BUN/creatinine ratio, and hematocrit level
for elevations.
▲ Use a sublingual capnometry device if available to determine level of tissue hypoxia caused by lack of fluid
volume.
▲ Insert a Foley catheter if ordered and measure urine output hourly. Notify physician if less than 30 mL/hour.
▲ When ordered, initiate a fluid challenge of crystalloids
(0.9% normal saline or lactated Ringer's) for replacement
of intravascular volume; monitor the client's response

• = Independent          ▲ = Collaborative

to prescribed fluid therapy and fluid challenge, especially noting central venous pressure and pulmonary capillary wedge pressure readings, vital signs, urine output, blood lactate concentrations, and lung sounds.

- When the client is hypotensive, position the client supine with legs elevated, if not contraindicated.

▲ Monitor trends in serum lactic acid levels and base deficit obtained from blood gasses as ordered.

▲ Consult physician if signs and symptoms of deficient fluid volume persist or worsen.

**F**

## Pediatric

- Monitor the child for signs of deficient fluid volume, including capillary refill time, skin turgor, and respiratory patterns along with other symptoms.

▲ Reenforce the physician's recommendation for the parents to give the child oral rehydration fluids in the amounts specified, especially during the first 4 to 6 hours to replace fluid losses. Once the child is rehydrated, an orally administered maintenance solution should be used along with food.

- Recommend the mother resume breastfeeding as soon as possible.
- Recommend parents refrain from giving the child decarbonated soda, fruit juices, Jell-O, or Kool-Aid.
- Recommend parents give children foods with complex carbohydrates such as potatoes, rice, bread, cereal, yogurt, fruits, and vegetables. The BRAT diet is often advocated: bananas, rice, applesauce, and toast. Avoid fatty foods and foods high in simple sugars.

## Geriatric

- Monitor elderly clients for deficient fluid volume carefully, noting new onset of weakness, dizziness, or dry mouth with longitudinal furrows.
- Evaluate the risk for dehydration using the Dehydration Risk Appraisal Checklist.
- Check skin turgor of elderly client on the forehead, sternum, or inner thigh; also look for the presence of lon-

gitudinal furrows on the tongue and dry mucous membranes.

- Encourage fluid intake by offering fluids regularly to cognitively impaired clients.
- Incorporate regular hydration into daily routines (e.g., extra glass of fluid with medication or social activities). Consider use of a beverage cart and a hydration assistant to routinely offer increased beverages to clients in extended care.
- If client is identified as having chronic dehydration, flag the food tray to indicate to caregivers they should finish 75% to 100% of their food and fluids.
- Note the color of client's urine and compare against a urine color chart to monitor adequate fluid intake.
- Monitor elderly clients for excess fluid volume during the treatment of deficient fluid volume: listen to lung sounds, watch for edema, and note vital signs.

## Home Care

- Determine if it is appropriate to intervene for deficient fluid volume or to allow the client to die comfortably without fluids as desired.
- Teach family members how to monitor urine output in the home (e.g., use of commode "hat" in the toilet, urinal, or bedpan; or use of catheter and closed drainage system). Instruct family members to monitor both intake and output.
- When weighing the client, use the same scale each day. Be sure the scale is on a flat (not cushioned) surface. Do not weigh the client with the scale placed on any kind of rug. Use bed or chair scales for clients who are unable to stand.
- ▲ Teach family about complications of deficient fluid volume and when to call physician.
- ▲ If the client is receiving intravenous fluids, there must be a responsible caregiver in the home. Teach caregiver about administration of fluids, complications of intravenous administration (e.g., fluid volume overload, speed of medication reactions), and when to call for assistance.

• = Independent          ▲ = Collaborative

Assist caregiver with administration as long as necessary to maintain client safety.

▲ Identify an emergency plan, including when to call 911.

## Client/Family Teaching

- Instruct the client to avoid rapid position changes, especially from supine to sitting or standing.
- Teach the client and family about appropriate diet and fluid intake.
- Teach the client and family how to measure and record intake and output accurately.
- Teach the client and family about measures instituted to treat hypovolemia and to prevent or treat fluid volume loss.
- Instruct the client and family about signs of deficient fluid volume that indicate they should contact a health care provider.

# Excess Fluid volume

## NANDA Definition

Increased isotonic fluid retention

## Defining Characteristics

Jugular vein distention; decreased hemoglobin and hematocrit levels; weight gain over short time period; changes in respiratory pattern, dyspnea or shortness of breath; orthopnea; abnormal breath sounds (rales or crackles); pulmonary congestion; pleural effusion; intake exceeds output; $S_3$ heart sound; change in mental status; restlessness; anxiety; blood pressure changes; pulmonary artery pressure changes; increased central venous pressure; oliguria; azotemia; specific gravity changes; altered electrolytes; edema, may progress to anasarca; positive hepatojugular reflex

## Related Factors (r/t)

Compromised regulatory mechanism; excess fluid intake; excess sodium intake

• = Independent          ▲ = Collaborative

## Client Outcomes

### Client Will (Specify Time Frame):

- Remain free of edema, effusion, anasarca; maintain appropriate weight.
- Maintain clear lung sounds; display no evidence of dyspnea or orthopnea.
- Remain free of jugular vein distention, positive hepatojugular reflex, and gallop heart rhythm.
- Maintain normal central venous pressure, pulmonary capillary wedge pressure, cardiac output, and vital signs.
- Maintain urine output within 500 mL of intake with normal urine osmolality and specific gravity values.
- Explain measures that can be taken to treat or prevent excess fluid volume, especially fluid and dietary restrictions and medications.
- Describe symptoms that indicate the need to consult with a health care provider.

### Nursing Interventions

- Monitor location and extent of edema; use a millimeter tape measure in the same area at the same time each day to measure edema in extremities.
- Monitor daily weight for sudden increases; use same scale and type of clothing at same time each day, preferably before breakfast.
- Monitor lung sounds for crackles, monitor respirations for effort, and determine the presence and severity of orthopnea.
- With head of bed elevated 30 to 45 degrees, monitor jugular veins for distention in the upright position; assess for positive hepatojugular reflex.
- ▲ Monitor central venous pressure, mean arterial pressure, pulmonary artery pressure, pulmonary capillary wedge pressure, and cardiac output; note and report trends indicating increasing pressures over time.
- Monitor vital signs; note decreasing blood pressure, tachycardia, and tachypnea. Monitor for gallop

• = Independent          ▲ = Collaborative

rhythms. If signs of heart failure are present, see nursing care plan for **Decreased Cardiac output.**

▲ Monitor serum osmolality, serum sodium concentration, BUN/creatinine ratio, and hematocrit level for decreases.

• Monitor intake and output; note trends reflecting decreasing urine output in relation to fluid intake.

• Monitor the client's behavior for restlessness, anxiety, or confusion; use safety precautions if symptoms are present.

• Monitor for the development of conditions that increase the client's risk for excess fluid volume.

▲ Assist with CRRT (continuous renal replacement therapy) as ordered if the client is critically ill and excessive fluid must be removed.

▲ Provide a restricted-sodium diet as appropriate if ordered.

▲ Monitor serum albumin level and provide protein intake as appropriate.

▲ Administer prescribed diuretics as appropriate; check blood pressure before administration to ensure it is adequate. If diuretic is administered intravenously, note and record urine output following the dose.

▲ Monitor for side effects of diuretic therapy: orthostatic hypotension (especially if the client is also receiving ACE inhibitors), hypovolemia, and electrolyte imbalances (hypokalemia and hyponatremia). Observe for hyperkalemia in clients receiving a potassium-sparing diuretic, especially with the concurrent administration of an ACE inhibitor.

▲ Implement fluid restriction as ordered, especially when serum sodium concentration is low; include all routes of intake. Schedule fluids around the clock, and include the type of fluids preferred by the client.

• Maintain the rate of all intravenous infusions carefully.

• Turn clients with dependent edema frequently (i.e., at least every 2 hours).

• Provide for scheduled rest periods.

• = Independent          ▲ = Collaborative

- Promote a positive body image and good self-esteem. See the care plan for **Disturbed Body image**.
▲ Consult with physician if signs and symptoms of excess fluid volume persist or worsen.

## Geriatric

- Recognize that the presence of risk factors for excess fluid volume is particularly serious in the elderly.

## Home Care

F

- Assess client and family knowledge of disease process causing excess fluid volume.
- Teach about disease process and complications of excess fluid volume, including when to contact physician.
- Assess client and family knowledge and compliance with medical regimen, including medications, diet, rest, and exercise. Assist family with integrating restrictions into daily living.
- If the client is confined to bed rest or has difficulty reclining, follow previously mentioned positioning recommendations.
▲ Teach and reinforce knowledge of medications. Instruct the client not to use over-the-counter medications (e.g., diet medications) without first consulting the physician.
▲ Instruct the client to make the primary physician aware of medications ordered by other physicians.
▲ Identify emergency plan for rapidly developing or critical levels of excess fluid volume when diuresing is not safe at home.
▲ Teach about signs and symptoms of both excess and deficient fluid volume and when to call physician.

## Client/Family Teaching

- Describe signs and symptoms of excess fluid volume and actions to take if they occur.
- Teach client on diuretics to weigh self daily in the morn-

• = Independent          ▲ = Collaborative

F

ing, and notify the physician if there is a 3 pound or
more change in weight.

- Teach the importance of fluid and sodium restrictions.
  Help the client and family to devise a schedule for intake
  of fluids throughout entire day. Refer to dietitian concerning implementation of low-sodium diet.

- Teach how to take diuretics correctly: take one dose in
  the morning and second dose (if taken) no later than
  4 pm. Adjust potassium intake as appropriate for
  potassium-losing or potassium-sparing diuretics. Note
  the appearance of side effects such as weakness, dizziness, muscle cramps, numbness and tingling, confusion, hearing impairment, palpitations or irregular heart-
  beat, and postural hypotension.

- Caution the athletic client not to drink excessively during
  competition or training, to follow the dictates of thirst.

- For the client undergoing hemodialysis, spend time with
  the client to detect any factors that may interfere with
  the client's compliance with the fluid restriction or restrictive diet.

# Risk for deficient Fluid volume

## NANDA Definition

At risk for experiencing vascular, cellular, or intracellular
dehydration

## Risk Factors

Factors influencing fluid needs (e.g., hypermetabolic state);
extremes of age; extremes of weight; excessive losses of fluid
through normal routes (e.g., diarrhea); loss of fluids through
abnormal routes (e.g., indwelling tubes); deviations affecting
access, intake, or absorption of fluids (e.g., physical immobility);
knowledge deficiency regarding fluid volume; medication (e.g.,
diuretics)

• = Independent          ▲ = Collaborative

## Client Outcomes

### Client Will (Specify Time Frame):

- Maintain urine output of more than 1300 mL/day (or at least 30 mL/hr).
- Maintain normal blood pressure, pulse, and body temperature.
- Maintain elastic skin turgor; moist tongue and mucous membranes; and orientation to person, place, and time.
- Explain measures that can be taken to treat or prevent fluid volume loss.
- Describe symptoms that indicate the need to consult with health care provider.

F

## Nursing Interventions

- Watch for early signs of hypovolemia, including restlessness, weakness, muscle cramps, headaches, inability to concentrate, and postural hypotension.
- Monitor for the existence of factors causing deficient fluid volume (e.g., vomiting, diarrhea, difficulty maintaining oral intake, fever, uncontrolled type 2 diabetes, diuretic therapy).
- Monitor daily weight for sudden decreases, especially in the presence of decreasing urine output or active fluid loss. Weigh the client on the same scale with the same type of clothing at the same time of day, preferably before breakfast.
- Monitor total fluid intake and output every 8 hours (or every hour for the unstable client). Recognize that urine output is not always an accurate indicator of fluid balance.
- Check orthostatic blood pressures with the client lying, sitting, and standing.
- Monitor for inelastic skin turgor, thirst, dry tongue and mucous membranes, longitudinal tongue furrows, speech difficulty, dry skin, sunken eyeballs, weakness (especially of upper body), headache, and confusion.

• = Independent        ▲ = Collaborative

- Use appropriate preoperative fasting guidelines as ordered: "Allow the consumption of clear liquids up to two hours before elective surgery, a light breakfast (tea and toast, for example) six hours before the procedure, and a heavier meal eight hours beforehand."
- See care plan for **Deficient Fluid volume.**

## Geriatric

- Monitor elderly clients for deficient fluid volume carefully, noting new onset of weakness, dizziness, or dry mouth with longitudinal furrows.
- Evaluate the risk for dehydration using the Dehydration Risk Appraisal Checklist.
- Check skin turgor of elderly client on the forehead, sternum, or inner thigh; also look for the presence of longitudinal furrows on the tongue and dry mucous membranes.
- Encourage fluid intake by offering fluids regularly to cognitively impaired clients.
- Incorporate regular hydration into daily routines (e.g., extra glass of fluid with medication or social activities). Consider use of a beverage cart and a hydration assistant to routinely offer increased beverages to clients in extended care.
- Aim for 1500 mL of oral liquids per day unless contraindicated by a medical condition such as congestive heart failure.
- Allow adequate time for eating and drinking at meals.
- Note the color of the urine and compare against a urine color chart to monitor adequate fluid intake.

## Home Care

- Assess availability of clean drinking water in the home, or assess resources to acquire bottled water.
- Assess available and preferred fluids. Refer for social services if resources are needed to purchase adequate fluid.

## Client/Family Teaching

- Teach clients who work or exercise in hot environments to increase intake of both water and electrolyte-carbohydrate beverages.

# Risk for imbalanced Fluid volume

## NANDA Definition

At risk for decrease, increase, or rapid shift of intravascular, interstitial, and/or intracellular fluid (body fluid loss, gain, or both)

## Risk Factors

Major invasive procedures

## Client Outcomes

- Lung sounds clear, respiratory rate 12 to 20, and free of dyspnea postoperatively
- Urine output greater than 30 mL/hr
- Blood pressure, pulse rate, temperature, and pulse oximetry values within expected range
- Laboratory values within expected range
- Nonedematous extremities and dependent areas
- Mental orientation unchanged from preoperative status

## Nursing Interventions

- Monitor vital signs of clients with deficient fluid volume—every 15 minutes to 1 hour if unstable and every 4 hours if stable. Observe for tachycardia, tachypnea, and decreased pulse pressure, which will occur first, followed by hypotension, decreased pulse volume, and increased or decreased body temperature.
- Check the client's orthostatic blood pressures.
- Monitor for nonelastic skin turgor, thirst, dry tongue and mucous membranes, longitudinal tongue furrows, difficulty speaking, dry skin, sunken eyeballs, weakness (especially upper body), headache, and confusion, which are symptoms of decreased body fluids.

• = Independent          ▲ = Collaborative

F

- • Provide frequent oral hygiene at least twice daily. If the client's mouth is dry and painful, provide oral hygiene hourly while awake.
- ▲ Initiate measures to rest the bowel when the client is vomiting or has diarrhea; for example, restrict food or fluid intake when appropriate or decrease intake of milk products. Hydrate the client with any prescribed (ordered) intravenous solutions.
- ▲ Provide oral replacement therapy as ordered and tolerated, with a hypotonic glucose-electrolyte solution when the client has acute diarrhea or nausea/vomiting. Provide small, frequent quantities of slightly chilled solutions.
- ▲ Maintain patent intravenous access, if the client requires intravenous fluid replacement.
- • Monitor for the existence of factors causing deficient fluid volume, e.g., vomiting, diarrhea, difficulty maintaining oral intake, fever, uncontrolled type 2 diabetes, diuretic therapy, preoperative bowel preparation.
- ▲ When ordered, administer a fluid challenge giving a specified amount of IV fluid, such as 0.9% normal saline rapidly IV, for replacement of intravascular volume and monitor client's response; noting vital signs, lung sounds, and urine output, and pulmonary capillary wedge pressure or central venous pressures if applicable.
- ▲ Keep all IV fluids on a volumetric pump.
- • Monitor intake and output.
- ▲ Measure urine output hourly. If urine output is <30 mL/hr or 0.5 mL/kg/hr, notify the physician.
- • Observe for trends in output for 3 days; include all routes of intake and output and note color and specific gravity of urine.
- • Monitor daily weight for sudden decreases, especially in the presence of decreasing urine output or active fluid loss. Weigh the client on the same scale, in the same type clothing, at the same time of day, preferably before breakfast.
- ▲ Monitor trends in serum lactic acid levels and base deficit, obtained from blood gases as ordered.

• = Independent          ▲ = Collaborative

## Surgical Clients

- Perform a preoperative assessment to identify clients with increased risk for hemorrhage or hypovolemia such as those with recent traumatic injury; abnormal bleeding or clotting times; complicated renal/liver disease; major organ transplant; history of aspirin, nonsteroidal anti-inflammatory usage, or anticoagulant therapy; history of hemophilia, von Willebrand's disease, or disseminated intravascular coagulation.

- Monitor for signs of intraoperative hypovolemia, e.g., decreased urinary output, decreased central venous pressure, hypotension, increased pulse, and/or increased respirations.

- Monitor for signs of intraoperative hypervolemia, e.g., dyspnea, coarse crackles, increased pulse and respirations, decreased urinary output, all of which could progress to pulmonary edema.

- Monitor for signs of intraoperative third-spacing.

▲ In the critically ill surgical client with a pulmonary artery catheter, monitor pressures, especially wedge pressure.

- Monitor clients undergoing laparoscopic or hysteroscopic procedures for the development of pulmonary edema when dextran is used as the irrigation fluid.

▲ Monitor dextran infusion and recovery rates every 15 minutes.

▲ If large amounts of hypotonic irrigation solutions (e.g., glycine) are used during surgery, carefully keep track of fluid inflow and outflow.

▲ Monitor clients undergoing transurethral resection of the prostate (TURP) procedures for symptoms of TURP syndrome, e.g., headache, visual changes, agitation, lethargy, vomiting, muscle twitching, bradycardia, diminished pupillary reflexes, hypertension, and respiratory distress.

▲ Monitor clients undergoing percutaneous nephrolithotomy (PCNL) procedures for excessive fluid absorption and volume overload.

▲ If the client is undergoing endometrial ablation under general anesthesia, watch for symptoms of decreased

• = Independent          ▲ = Collaborative

body temperature, decreased oxygen saturation, dilated pupils, and tremulousness.
- Observe the surgical client for signs of hyperkalemia, e.g., cardiac dysrhythmias, heart block, asystole, abdominal distention, and weakness.
- Observe the client who has undergone bilateral thyroid surgeryfor hypocalcemia.
- Observe surgical clients closely for signs of hypokalemia.
- Recognize that the surgical client may develop hyponatremia related to inappropriate antidiuretic hormone (ADH) secretion, which can be caused by trauma, thrombosis, abscesses, hemorrhages, or hematomas.
- Monitor the surgical client for signs and symptoms of hyponatremia, e.g., nausea, confusion, disorientation, twitching, seizures, and/or hypotension.
- Accurately measure blood loss intraoperatively.

## Home Care
- Determine if it is appropriate to intervene for deficient fluid volume or to allow the client to die comfortably without fluids as desired.
- Family members should be taught how to monitor urine output in the home, e.g., commode "hat" in toilet, urinal, or bedpan; use of catheter, for example.

## Geriatric
- Be especially vigilant when monitoring vital signs and fluids in elderly surgical clients.
- Assess preoperatively for symptoms of dehydration, e.g., weakness, dizziness, dry mouth with longitudinal tongue furrows.
- Check skin turgor of the elderly client on the forehead, sternum, or inner thigh; also look for the presence of longitudinal tongue furrows and dry mucous membranes.
- Encourage fluid intake regularly to cognitively impaired clients.

• = Independent          ▲ = Collaborative

- Incorporate regular hydration into daily routines, such as providing an extra glass of fluid with medication or during social activities. Consider using a beverage cart and a hydration assistant to routinely offer beverages to clients in extended care facilities.
- Note the color of urine and compare against a urine color chart to monitor adequate fluid intake.
- Monitor elderly clients for excess fluid volume during the treatment of deficient fluid volume: listen to lung sounds, watch for edema, and note vital signs.

**Pediatric**

- Monitor pediatric surgical clients closely for signs of fluid loss.
- Administer fluids preoperatively until NPO status must be initiated, so that fluid deficit is decreased.

## Impaired Gas exchange

### NANDA Definition

Excess or deficit in oxygenation and/or carbon dioxide elimination at the alveolar-capillary membrane

### Defining Characteristics

Visual disturbances; decreased carbon dioxide; dyspnea; abnormal arterial blood gas levels; hypoxia; irritability; somnolence; restlessness; hypercapnia; tachycardia; cyanosis; abnormal skin color (pale, dusky); hypoxemia; hypercarbia; headache on awakening; abnormal rate, rhythm, depth of breathing; diaphoresis; abnormal arterial pH; nasal flaring

### Related Factors (r/t)

Ventilation-perfusion imbalance; alveolar-capillary membrane changes

• = Independent ▲ = Collaborative

## Client Outcomes

### Client Will (Specify Time Frame):

- Demonstrate improved ventilation and adequate oxygenation as evidenced by blood gas levels within normal parameters for that client.
- Maintain clear lung fields and remain free of signs of respiratory distress.
- Verbalize understanding of oxygen supplementation and other therapeutic interventions.

## Nursing Interventions

- Monitor respiratory rate, depth, and effort, including use of accessory muscles, nasal flaring, and abnormal breathing patterns.
- Auscultate breath sounds every 1 to 2 hours. The presence of crackles and wheezes may alert the nurse to airway obstruction, which may lead to or exacerbate existing hypoxia.
- Monitor the client's behavior and mental status for the onset of restlessness, agitation, confusion, and (in the late stages) extreme lethargy.
- ▲ Monitor oxygen saturation continuously using pulse oximetry. Note blood gas results as available.
- Observe for cyanosis of the skin; especially note color of the tongue and oral mucous membranes.
- Position clients in semi-Fowler's, with an upright posture at 45 degrees if possible.
- If the client has unilateral lung disease, alternate semi-Fowler's position in an upright posture with a lateral position (with 10- to 15-degree elevation and "good lung down" for 60 to 90 minutes). This method is contraindicated for clients with pulmonary abscess or hemorrhage or interstitial emphysema.
- If the client has bilateral lung disease, position the client in either semi-Fowler's or a side-lying position, which increases oxygenation as indicated by pulse oximetry (or, if the client has a pulmonary catheter, venous oxygen saturation).

• = Independent          ▲ = Collaborative

▲ Turn the client every 2 hours. Monitor mixed venous oxygen saturation closely after turning. If it drops below 10% or fails to return to baseline promptly, turn the client back into the supine position and evaluate oxygen status. If the client does not tolerate turning, consider use of a kinetic bed that rotates the client from side to side in a turn of at least 40 degrees.

• If the client is obese or has ascites, consider positioning the client in reverse Trendelenburg's position at 45 degrees for periods as tolerated.

▲ If the client has adult respiratory distress syndrome, or difficulty maintaining oxygenation, consider positioning the client prone with the upper thorax and pelvis supported, allowing the abdomen to protrude. Monitor oxygen saturation and turn back to supine position if desaturation occurs.

• If the client is acutely dyspneic, consider having the client lean forward over a bedside table, if tolerated.

• Help the client to deep breathe and perform controlled coughing. Have the client inhale deeply, hold the breath for several seconds, and cough two or three times with the mouth open while tightening the upper abdominal muscles as tolerated.

NOTE: If the client has excessive fluid in the respiratory system, see the interventions for **Ineffective Airway clearance.**

▲ Monitor the effects of sedation and analgesics on the client's respiratory pattern; use judiciously.

• Schedule nursing care to provide rest and minimize fatigue.

▲ Administer humidified oxygen through an appropriate device (e.g., nasal cannula or Venturi mask per the physician's order); aim for an $O_2$ saturation level of 90%.

• Watch for onset of hypoventilation as evidenced by increased somnolence.

▲ Assess nutritional status including serum albumin level and BMI.

• Assist the client to eat small meals frequently and use di-

• = Independent          ▲ = Collaborative

etary supplements as necessary. For some clients, drinking 30 mL of a supplement such as Ensure or Pulmocare every hour while awake can be helpful.

- If the client is severely debilitated from chronic respiratory disease, consider the use of a wheeled walker to help in ambulation.
- Watch for signs of psychological distress including anxiety, agitation, and insomnia. Refer for counseling as needed.
▲ Refer the COPD client to a pulmonary rehabilitation program.

NOTE: If the client becomes ventilator-dependent, see the care plan for **Impaired spontaneous Ventilation.**

### Geriatric

▲ Use central nervous system depressants carefully to avoid decreasing respiration rate.
▲ Maintain low-flow oxygen therapy.

### Home Care

- Assess the home environment for irritants that impair gas exchange. Help the client to adjust the home environment as necessary (e.g., install an air filter to decrease the level of dust).
▲ Refer the client to occupational therapy as necessary to assist the client in adaptation to the home and environment and in energy conservation.
- Assist the client with identifying and avoiding situations that exacerbate impairment of gas exchange (e.g., stress-related situations, exposure to pollution of any kind, proximity to noxious gas fumes such as chlorine bleach).
- Refer to GOLD and ACP-ASIM/ACCP guidelines for management of home care and indications of hospital admission criteria.
- Instruct the client to keep the home temperature above 20° C (68° F) and to avoid cold weather.

• = Independent        ▲ = Collaborative

- Instruct the client to limit exposure to persons with respiratory infections.
- Instruct the family in the complications of the disease and the importance of maintaining the medical regimen, including when to call a physician.
▲ Assess nutritional status. Instruct the client to eat several small meals and use dietary supplements as necessary. For some clients, drinking 30 mL of a supplement such as Ensure or Pulmocare every hour while awake can be helpful.
▲ Refer the client for home health aide services as necessary for assistance with activities of daily living.
- When respiratory procedures are being implemented, explain equipment and procedures to family members, and provide needed emotional support.
- When electrically based equipment for respiratory support is being implemented, evaluate home environment for electrical safety, proper grounding, etc. Ensure that notification is sent to the local utility company, the emergency medical team, and police and fire departments.
▲ Assess family role changes and coping ability. Refer the client to medical social services as appropriate for assistance in adjusting to chronic illness.
- Support the family of the client with chronic illness.

## Client/Family Teaching

- Teach the client how to perform pursed-lip breathing and controlled diaphragmatic breathing, and how to use the tripod position. Have the client watch the pulse oximeter to note improvement in oxygenation with these breathing techniques.
- Teach the client energy conservation techniques and the importance of alternating rest periods with activity. See nursing interventions for **Fatigue.**
▲ Teach the importance of not smoking:
  ■ Be very clear in approach, and ask the client to set a date for smoking cessation.

• = Independent          ▲ = Collaborative

▲ Recommend pharmacological support unless contra-indicated (nicotine replacement therapy or antidepressant).

▲ Refer the client to smoking-cessation programs.

■ Encourage clients who relapse to keep trying to quit.

▲ Instruct the family regarding home oxygen therapy if ordered (e.g., delivery system, liter flow, safety precautions).

• Teach the client the need to receive a yearly influenza vaccine.

• Teach the client relaxation techniques to help reduce stress responses and panic attacks resulting from dyspnea.

• Teach the client to use music, along with a rest period, to decrease dyspnea and anxiety.

## Grieving*

### NANDA Definition

State in which an individual or group of individuals reacts to an actual or perceived loss, which may be loss of a person, object, function, status, relationship, or body part

### Defining Characteristics

Verbal expression of distress at loss; anger; sadness; crying; difficulty in expressing loss; alterations in eating habits, sleep patterns, dream patterns, activity levels, or libido; reliving of past experiences; interference with life function; alterations in concentration or pursuit of tasks

### Related Factors (r/t)

Actual or perceived object loss, which may include loss of people,

---

*NOTE: **Grieving** is a wellness-oriented nursing diagnosis. It is not an official NANDA nursing diagnosis, but it is included because the authors believe that grieving is part of the normal human response to loss and that nurses can use interventions to help the client grieve.

• = Independent          ▲ = Collaborative

possessions, job, status, home, ideals, or parts and processes of
the body

## Client Outcomes

### Client Will (Specify Time Frame):

- Express feelings of guilt, fear, anger, or sadness.
- Identify problems associated with grief (e.g., changes in appetite, insomnia, loss of libido, decreased energy, alteration in activity level).
- Plan for the future one day at a time.
- Function at normal developmental level and perform activities of daily living.

## Nursing Interventions

- Use a grief instrument such as the Hogan Grief Reaction Checklist (HGRC) to evaluate the client with regard to the six factors in the normal trajectory of the grieving process: despair, panic behavior, blame and anger, detachment, disorganization, and personal growth.
- Allow family members to participate in care of the body of the deceased if desired. Help survivors say goodbye in the most loving and caring way possible.
- Allow the family "holding" behaviors, including taking photographs of the deceased or clipping a piece of hair.
- Help the bereaved client survive during times of acute grief. Ensure that the client maintains sufficient nutrition and help the client determine a routine to make it through each day.
- Encourage the client to share memories and tell stories of the person or object of loss by making comments such as, "Tell me about your wife [husband, parent]." Conduct an in-depth personal interview to learn about the client and loved one or loss.
- Consider the use of a "grief map." This allows the individual to conceptualize each phenomenon of grief and to visualize progress through the issues associated with the feelings.

• = Independent          ▲ = Collaborative

G

- Actively listen to the client's expression of grief; do not interrupt, do not tell your own story, and do not offer meaningless platitudes such as, "It will be better this way."
- Encourage the client to "cry out" his or her grief and express feelings, including sadness and anger.
- If the client or family members are expressing anger, try not to react in anger. Instead, allow feelings to be expressed, listen to the expressions of anger, and accept their right to those feelings. Try lowering your voice and slowing your rate of speech as you respond to the client and/or family.
- Help the client identify previous successful personal coping stratgies. Use music if appropriate.
- Encourage the client to follow comforting grief rituals such as interacting with nature, lighting votive candles, saying a rosary, prayer or whatever ritual brings spiritual comfort in dealing with the loss.
- Help the client realize that feelings of "why me" or "if only" may come with grieving.
- Warn the grieving client that when driving, they may experience overwhelming grief.
- ▲ Refer the client for spiritual counseling if desired.
- Provide information about the grief process, including the stages of grieving: denial, anger, bargaining, and acceptance.
- Help the client realize that spasms of grief can come at any time, that most people don't go through the stages in a predictable fashion, and that the grieving process takes time and is painful.
- Help the client determine the best way and place to find social support. Encourage the client to continue to use supports for 1 to 2 years.
- ▲ Assess for causes of dysfunctional grieving (e.g., sudden death, highly dependent or ambivalent relationship with the deceased, lack of coping skills, lack of social support, previous physical or mental health problems, death of a child, death of a wife, death of a loved one by

● = Independent          ▲ = Collaborative

suicide). Refer for counseling, starting 2 to 8 weeks after the loss and for up to 3 months following bereavement Refer to the care plan for **Dysfunctional Grieving.**

- Assess for signs of depression: feelings of worthlessness, inability to eat or sleep, or sleeping all the time.
- Encourage family members to set aside time to talk with one another about the loss without criticizing or belittling one another's feelings.
- ▲ Identify available community resources, including bereavement groups at local hospitals and hospice centers. Volunteers who provide bereavement support can also be effective.
- ▲ Recognize times when you as a nurse are affected by loss and need grief resolution. Attend a grief resolution group, ask for help from pastoral services, speak with a kind friend who is supportive, or seek counseling.

## Pediatric/Parent

- Treat children with respect, give them the opportunity to talk about their concerns, and answer questions honestly.
- Listen to the child's expression of grief.
- Consider giving the child a "Memory Bag" to have after experiencing a sudden death; contents include a teddy bear, a coloring book on working through grief for different ages, a journal for children to write in, and crayons.
- Help parents recognize that children do not have to be "fixed"; instead they need support going through an experience of grieving just as adults.
- Ask the child if he or she would like a photo of the deceased person or a lock of hair to keep.
- Encourage children to listen to music that they enjoy.
- ▲ Refer grieving children and parents to a program to help facilitate grieving if desired, especially if the death was traumatic.
- Help the adolescent determine sources of support and how to utilize them effectively.

• = Independent          ▲ = Collaborative

- Encourage parents to seek mental health services as needed, learn stress reduction, and take good care of their health.

## Geriatric

▲ Use reminiscence therapy in conjunction with the expression of emotions. Refer to a reminiscence group if available.
- Identify previous losses and assess the client for depression.
- Monitor an older adult who has been treated for bereavement-related depression for relapse or recurrence.
- Evaluate the social support system of the elderly client. If the support system is minimal, help the client determine how to increase available support.
- Provide support for the family when the loss is associated with dementia of the family member.

## Multicultural

- Assess for the influence of cultural beliefs, norms, and values on the client's grief and mourning practices.
- Assess for the influence of cultural beliefs, norms, and values on the client's expressions of grief.
- Identify whether the client had been notified of the deceased's health status and was able to be present at the deathbed.
- Teach patients to recognize grief responses.

## Home Care

NOTE: Grieving may be encountered as the client comes to terms with his or her own loss or death, or as the family reacts to the client's death.

- The interventions described previously may be adapted for home care use.
- Listen actively as the client grieves his or her own death or real or perceived loss. Normalize the client's expressions of grief for himself or herself. Demonstrate a caring and hopeful approach.

• = Independent        ▲ = Collaborative

- If the agency has served the deceased as a client, allow the primary caregivers to attend the services.
- Plan the first home visit within 10 days after the loss by the client; be guided by the type of loss and the family's schedule following the loss.
- If the loss is of a loved one, allow the client to express feelings about the loss through interaction with the home environment (e.g., looking at pictures, keeping special chairs or clothing). Symbols of the lost loved one can be comforting and allow the bereaved to accept the loss in stages.
- Do not react with shock or disbelief at family members' reports (e.g., feeling like the deceased is still there).
▲ Refer the client to medical social services as necessary for losses not related to death.
▲ Refer the bereaved to hospice bereavement programs.
▲ Refer the bereaved spouse to an Internet self-help group if desired.
- Assess caregiver reaction to bereavement issues and caregiver burden. Suggest preventive intervention for potential bereavement maladjustment if indicated.
- Modify expectations of the client's response according to the degree of anticipation of the loved one's death.
▲ After loss of a pregnancy, encourage the client to follow through on a counseling referral.

# Anticipatory Grieving

## NANDA Definition

Intellectual and emotional responses and behaviors by which individuals, families, and communities work through the process of modifying self-concept based on the perception of potential loss

## Defining Characteristics

Expression of distress at potential loss; sorrow; guilt; denial of potential loss; anger; altered communication patterns; potential

• = Independent          ▲ = Collaborative

loss of significant object (e.g., people, possessions, job, status, home, ideals, parts and processes of the body); denial of significance of the loss; bargaining; alteration in eating habits, sleep patterns, dream patterns, activity level, or libido; difficulty taking on new or different roles; resolution of grief before the reality of loss

## Related Factors (r/t)

Perceived or actual impending loss of people, objects, possessions, job, status, home, ideals, or parts and processes of the body

## Client Outcomes

### Client Will (Specify Time Frame):

- Express feelings of guilt, anger, or sorrow.
- Identify problems associated with anticipatory grief (e.g., changes in activity, eating, or libido).
- Seek help in dealing with anticipated problems.
- Plan for the future one day at a time.

## Nursing Interventions

- Actively listen to the client's and/or family's expression of grief; do not interrupt, do not tell your own story, and do not offer meaningless platitudes such as, "It will be better this way."
- If grief results from the impending death of a loved one:
  - Allow family members to stay with the loved one during the dying process if desired and help them determine appropriate times to take breaks if appropriate.
  - Spend time in the room with the dying client and family.
  - Check in frequently when you are not able to stay at the bedside.
  - Talk openly about the dying process and changes in condition that indicate death is near.
  - Caution families that the dying person can often hear, and encourage them to reminisce about the good times.

• = Independent          ▲ = Collaborative

- ■ Encourage family members to touch the dying client if they are comfortable doing so.
- • Encourage family members to listen carefully to messages given by the dying loved one; they may hear symbolic or obscure language referring to the dying process.
- • Ask the client if he or she is suffering, and take whatever measures possible to relieve suffering.
- • If the dying client or family is denying the seriousness of his or her condition, do not negate the denial. Instead listen to clients so they feel they have been understood, and know that they are supported in dealing with their situation.
- • Help the dying client to maintain hope by focusing on the moment, reviewing his or her assets, making decisions regarding care, and maintaining important relationships.
- • Help family members to let the loved one go if appropriate; give the loved one permission to die.
- • Use therapeutic communication with open-ended questions such as, "What are your thoughts and fears?"
- • Keep family members informed about the client's condition.
- • Encourage the client to "cry out" grief and express feelings, including sadness or anger.
- • Encourage the client to take care of any unfinished business if appropriate. Have the client make an advance directive with support.
- • Help the dying client build memories. This can be done a number of ways, including the following:
  - ■ Writing love letters—letters to be opened on family birthdays or other special days after death
  - ■ Making audiotape or videotape recordings—to share memories and say goodbye
  - ■ Writing a journal—an autobiography to be read by children and loved ones
  - ■ Planning his or her own funeral
  - ■ Writing his or her own obituary
  - ■ Leaving a legacy—designating money for favorite causes

G

• = Independent          ▲ = Collaborative

- Determine the need for sedation during the dying process if desired by the client.
▲ Assess for spiritual distress and refer the client for spiritual counseling if desired and appropriate.
- Help the client and/or family determine how best to obtain social support.
- Identify problems with eating or sleeping, and intervene with suggestions as appropriate.
- Encourage the caregiver of a dying person to live one day at a time and recognize that mourning is occurring while caring for the loved one. Help the caregiver express feelings of loss and encourage the caregiver to practice self-care. Refer to the care plan for **Caregiver role strain** if appropriate.

## Pediatric/Parent
- Treat children with respect, give them the opportunity to talk about their concerns, and answer questions honestly.
- Listen to the child's expression of grief.
- Help parents recognize that children do not have to be "fixed"; instead they need support going through an experience of grieving just as adults.
- Ask the child if he or she would like a lock of hair to keep.
- Encourage children to listen to music that they enjoy.
- Help the adolescent determine sources of support and how to utilize them effectively.

## Geriatric
- Assist the client with end-of-life decisions and advance directives.
- In extended care facilities, consider use of nurse "Bereavement Leaders" who are responsible to help dying clients and their families in the process of bereavement.

## Multicultural
- Assess for the influence of cultural beliefs, norms, and values on the client's grief and mourning practices.
- Encourage discussion of the grief process.

• = Independent          ▲ = Collaborative

- Assess for the influence of cultural beliefs, norms, and values on the client's expressions of grief.
- Teach patients to recognize grief responses.

## Home Care

NOTE: Hospice care encourages clients and families to experience the client's final days in the setting of choice. All of the previously mentioned interventions can and should be applied in the home setting when that is the setting selected.

G

- Listen actively; normalize the client's and family's expressions of grief for a loved one who is expected to die. Demonstrate a caring and hopeful approach.
- ▲ When the client has a history of loss of a pregnancy, assess the client's need for a counseling referral during subsequent pregnancies.

## Palliative Care

- When the potential loss is of a loved one, refer the grieving client to hospice volunteer services for support.
- Evaluate symptomatology of client in anticipation of planning for terminal care. Raise the issue with client and family; discuss advance care directives; determine wishes for remaining at home and contingency plans for terminal hospitalization.
- Assess caregiver reaction to bereavement issues and caregiver burden. Suggest preventive intervention for potential bereavement maladjustment if indicated.
- Encourage caregivers to ventilate feelings and concerns about their perceptions of the client's suffering, of loss and feelings of inadequacy, and of any physical or psychological symptoms they are having. Implement interventions in response to expressed powerlessness. Refer to care plan for **Powerlessness**.
- Assist client to optimize retention of as many usual activities and family/friends contacts as possible. Explain all elements of care to client. Refer to care plan for **Powerlessness.**

• = Independent          ▲ = Collaborative

- Focus on spiritual needs of client to insure a continued sense of connectedness. Refer to care plan for **Spiritual distress.**

### Client/Family Teaching

- Teach caregivers that they are doing anticipatory grieving as they care for their loved ones, which is part of the reason care can be so difficult. The grief can become more acute as death approaches.
- Teach families how to provide mouth care and other comfort measures for the dying client as desired.

G

# Dysfunctional Grieving

## NANDA Definition

Extended unsuccessful use of intellectual and emotional responses by which individuals, families, and communities attempt to work through the process of modifying self-concept based on the perception of loss

NOTE: It is now recognized that sometimes what was previously diagnosed as **Dysfunctional Grieving** might instead be **Chronic Sorrow,** in which grief lingers and is reactivated at intervals. Refer to the nursing diagnosis **Chronic Sorrow** if appropriate.

## Defining Characteristics

Repetitive use of ineffectual behaviors associated with attempts to reinvest in relationships; crying; sadness; reliving of past experiences with little or no reduction (diminishment) of intensity of grief; labile affect; expression of unresolved issues; interference with life functioning; verbal expression of distress at loss; idealization of lost object (e.g., people, possessions, job, status, home, ideals, parts and processes of the body); difficulty in expressing loss; denial of loss; anger; alterations in eating habits, sleep patterns, dream patterns, activity level, libido, concentration, and/or pursuit of tasks; developmental regression; expres-

• = Independent          ▲ = Collaborative

sion of guilt; prolonged interference with life functioning; onset or exacerbation of somatic or psychosomatic responses

## Related Factors (r/t)

Actual or perceived object loss (e.g., of people, possessions, job, status, home, ideals, parts and processes of the body)

## Client Outcomes

### Client Will (Specify Time Frame):

G

- Express appropriate feelings of guilt, fear, anger, or sadness.
- Identify problems associated with grief (e.g., changes in appetite, insomnia, nightmares, loss of libido, decreased energy, alteration in activity levels).
- Seek help in dealing with grief-associated problems.
- Plan for the future one day at a time.
- Identify personal strengths.
- Function at a normal developmental level and perform activities of daily living after an appropriate length of time.

## Nursing Interventions

- Assess the client's state of grieving. Use a tool such as the Hogan Grief to Personal Growth Model or the Grief Experience Inventory.
- Assess for the causes of dysfunctional grieving (suddenness, interpersonal violence, trauma, suicide, homicide, also highly dependent or ambivalent relationship with the deceased, inadequate coping skills, lack of social support, or previous physical or mental health problems).
- Identify problems of eating and sleeping; ensure that basic human needs are being met.
- Develop a trusting relationship with the client by using therapeutic communication techniques.
- Establish a defined time to meet and discuss feelings about the loss and to perform grief work. Encourage the client to "cry out" grief and to talk about feelings of anger, sadness, and guilt.

● = Independent          ▲ = Collaborative

▲ Assess for spiritual distress and refer the client to the appropriate spiritual leader.
- Help the client recognize that, although sadness will occur at intervals for the rest of his or her life, it will become bearable.
- Help the client complete the following "guilt work" exercises:
  - Identify "if onlys" and put them into perspective.
  - Deal with "I didn't do" by looking at what was accomplished.
  - Forgive himself or herself; say to the client, "You are being awfully hard on yourself; try not to hurt yourself over something you could not have controlled."
- Help the client review past experiences, role changes, and coping skills.
- Encourage the client to keep a journal and write about the bereavement experience.
- Help the client to identify his or her own strengths to use in dealing with loss; reinforce these strengths; consider the use of music.
- If the client or family members are expressing anger, try not to react in anger. Instead, allow feelings to be expressed, listen to the expressions of anger, and accept their right to those feelings. Try lowering your voice and slowing your rate of speech as you respond to the client and/or family.
- Expect the client to meet responsibilities; give positive reinforcement.
▲ Identify available community resources, including bereavement groups at local hospitals and hospice centers.
▲ Determine whether the client is experiencing depression, suicidal tendencies, or other emotional disorders. Refer the client for counseling as appropriate.

## Pediatric/Parent
- Treat children with respect, give them the opportunity to talk about their concerns, and answer questions honestly.

● = Independent          ▲ = Collaborative

- Listen to the child's expression of grief.
- Help parents recognize that children do not have to be "fixed"; instead they need support going through an experience of grieving just as adults.
- Encourage children to listen to music that they enjoy.
- ▲ Refer grieving children and parents to a program to help facilitate grieving if desired, especially if the death was traumatic.
- Help the adolescent determine sources of support and how to utilize them effectively.
- Encourage parents to seek mental health services as needed, learn stress reduction, find sources of support, and take good care of their health.
- If client is an adolescent exposed to a peer's suicide, watch for symptoms of traumatic grief as well as post traumatic stress disorder which include numbness, preoccupation with the deceased, functional impairment, and poor adjustment to the loss.

## Geriatric
- Use reminiscence therapy in conjunction with the expression of emotions. Refer to a reminiscence group if available.
- Identify previous losses and assess the client for depression.
- Monitor an older adult who has been treated for bereavement-related depression for relapse or recurrence.
- Evaluate the social support system of the elderly client. If the support system is minimal, help the client determine how to increase available support.

## Multicultural
- Assess for the influence of cultural beliefs, norms, and values on the client's grief and mourning practices.
- Assess for the influence of cultural beliefs, norms, and values on the client's expressions of grief.
- Encourage discussion of the grief process.
- Identify whether the client had been notified of the

• = Independent          ▲ = Collaborative

health status of the deceased and was able to be present
during illness and death.
- Validate the client's feelings regarding the loss.
- Teach patients to recognize grief responses.

## Home Care

- The interventions described previously may be adapted
  for home care use.
- Encourage the client to make choices about daily living and the home environment that acknowledge the
  loss.
- Evaluate the long-term support system of the bereaved
  client. Encourage the client to interact with the support system at defined intervals.
- Discourage the client from making any drastic life
  changes immediately.
- ▲ Refer the client to or encourage continued interaction
  with hospice volunteers and bereavement programs as
  continuing forms of support.
- ▲ Refer the client to medical social services, especially the
  hospice program social worker, for assistance with grief
  work.
- ▲ Evaluate the need for psychiatric referral.
- ▲ After loss of a pregnancy, encourage the client to follow
  through with a counseling referral.
- ▲ If the client is identified as having a psychiatric disorder,
  refer for psychiatric home health care services or "in-
  terapy" (online therapy) for client reassurance and implementation of a therapeutic regimen.

# Risk for Dysfunctional Grieving

## NANDA Definition

At risk for extended, unsuccessful use of intellectual and emotional responses and behaviors by an individual, family, or
community following a death or perception of loss

• = Independent          ▲ = Collaborative

## Risk Factors

### General

Preloss neuroticism; preloss psychological symptoms; frequency of major life events; predisposition for anxiety and feelings of inadequacy; past psychiatric or mental health treatment

### Perinatal

Later gestational age at time of loss; limited time since perinatal loss and subsequent conception; length of life of infant; absence of other living children; congenital anomaly; number of past perinatal losses; marital adjustment problems; viewing of ultrasound images of the fetus

G

## Related Factors (r/t)

See Risk Factors

## Client Outcomes

### Client Will (Specify Time Frame):

- Express appropriate feelings of guilt, fear, anger, or sadness.
- Identify problems associated with grief (e.g., changes in appetite, insomnia, nightmares, loss of libido, decreased energy, alteration in activity levels).
- Seek help in dealing with grief-associated problems.
- Plan for the future one day at a time.
- Identify personal strengths.
- Function at a normal developmental level and perform activities of daily living after an appropriate length of time.

## Nursing Interventions, Client/Family Teaching

Refer to care plan for **Dysfunctional Grieving.**

# Delayed Growth and development

## NANDA Definition

Deviations from age-group norms

• = Independent         ▲ = Collaborative

## Defining Characteristics

Altered physical growth; delay or difficulty in exercising skills (motor, social, expressive) typical of age group; inability to perform self-care or self-control activities appropriate for age; flat affect; listlessness; decreased responses

## Related Factors (r/t)

Prescribed dependence; indifference; separation from significant others; environmental and stimulation deficiencies; effects of physical disability; inadequate caretaking; inconsistent responsiveness; multiple caretakers

## Client Outcomes

### Client/Parents/Primary Caregiver Will (Specify Time Frame):

- Describe realistic, age-appropriate patterns of growth and development.
- Promote activities and interactions that support age-related developmental tasks.
- Display consistent, sustained achievement of age-appropriate behaviors (social, interpersonal, and/or cognitive) and/or motor skills.
- Achieve realistic developmental and/or growth milestones based on existing abilities, extent of disability, and functional age.
- Exhibit limited temporary behavioral regression that reverses shortly after episode of illness or hospitalization.
- Attain steady gains in growth patterns.

## Nursing Interventions

NOTE: Determination of the etiological basis for delayed growth and development is critical because it will direct the selection of interventions for treating the client. Parenting skill deficits, lack of consistency between caregivers, hospitalization, and a chronic medical condition or developmental disability will necessitate different strategies. A hospitalization experience with regressive behaviors can be a transient occurrence, whereas a chronic situation may

• = Independent        ▲ = Collaborative

result in more severe and longer delays requiring more in-depth intervention. Parenting skills and consistent expectations by multiple caregivers can be addressed by more intensive education efforts.

- To determine risk for or actual deviations in normal development, consider the use of a screening tool. Some tools are the Brigance Infant and Toddler Screens and PRAMS, the Pregnancy Risk Assessment Monitoring System.
- Provide skin-to-skin contact for newborns and moms. Place the naked baby prone on the mother's bare chest at birth or soon afterward (< 24 hours).
- Regularly compare height and weight measurements for the child or adolescent with established age-appropriate norms and previous measurements.
- ▲ Initiate referrals for a more comprehensive growth and/or development evaluation if indicated.
- ▲ Identify coexisting health or medical conditions that may be contributing to the alteration in growth and/or development, and refer the client to a specialist in the appropriate health care discipline for management.
- Examine parental/caregiver expectations of future learning, ability, and developmental achievements of children with developmental disabilities.
- Prepare children for hospitalization; Include hospital tours, film, books and play therapy, interventions all designed to increase knowledge and promote understanding of the hospitalization process.
- Provide support groups and education on HIV and caring for infants with this diagnosis.
- Provide meaningful stimulation for hospitalized infants and children.
- Provide opportunities for mother-infant skin-to-skin contact (kangaroo care or KC) for preterm infants.
- ▲ Engage the child in appropriate play activities. Refer the child to a play/recreational therapist (if available) for supplemental strategies.

G

• = Independent          ▲ = Collaborative

- Enlist and encourage involvement of the parents and/or family as participants in care, particularly for hospitalized infants, toddlers, preschoolers, or school-aged children, whenever possible without exceeding the parents'/family's emotional and physical limits.
- Model age-appropriate and cognitively appropriate caregiver skills by doing the following:
  - Communicating with the child in a manner appropriate to cognitive level of development
  - Giving the child tasks and responsibilities appropriate to age or functional age level
  - Instituting the use of safety devices such as assistive equipment
  - Encouraging the child to perform ADLs as appropriate
- Provide an environment that promotes additional sleep and rest opportunities.
- Provide developmental care interventions to preterm infants to improve neurodevelopmental outcomes.
- Provide neonatal positioning procedures for preterm infants to prevent extremity malalignment, skull deformities, and gross motor delay.

## Multicultural

- Acknowledge racial/ethnic differences at the onset of care.
- Assess for the influence of cultural beliefs, norms, and values on the client's perceptions of child development.
- Use a neutral, indirect style in addressing areas in which improvement is needed (such as a need for verbal stimulation) when working with Native-American clients.
- Assess whether exposure to community violence is contributing to developmental problems.
- Assess and identify for possible environmental conditions which may be a contributing factor to altered growth and development.

• = Independent          ▲ = Collaborative

- Validate the client's feelings and concerns related to the child's development.
- Provide information on the effects of environmental risk exposure on growth and development.

## Home Care

- The interventions described previously may be adapted for home care use.
- Assess for the presence of substances that could cause developmental delay. Children's access to substances that cause neurological deficits (e.g., lead-based paint) should be identified and eliminated.
- ▲ Refer maternal drug users to home intervention programs.
- Help the family to identify appropriate skill-building activities for the child.
- Provide emotional support for family members in their reactions to evidence of developmental delay.
- ▲ If possible, refer the family to a program of animal-assisted therapy.

## Client/Family Teaching

- Provide parents and/or caregivers realistic expectations for attainment of growth and development milestones. Clarify expectations and correct misconceptions.
- Have parents and/or caregivers rehearse coping strategies for approaching developmental milestones and acknowledge positive actions and behaviors.
- Teach methods of providing meaningful stimulation for infants and children.
- Instruct the client with regard to age-appropriate activities and play, nutrition, discipline, and safety, and support growth and development.
- ▲ Elicit the involvement of parents and caregivers in social support groups and parenting classes.
- ▲ Furnish information about community resources.

• = Independent          ▲ = Collaborative

## Risk for disproportionate Growth

### NANDA Definition

At risk for growth above the 97th percentile or below the 3rd percentile for age, crossing two percentile channels; disproportionate growth

### Risk Factors

**Prenatal**

Congenital/genetic disorders; maternal malnutrition; multiple gestation; teratogen exposure; substance use/abuse

**Individual**

Infection; prematurity; malnutrition; organic and inorganic factors; caregiver and/or individual maladaptive feeding behaviors; anorexia; insatiable appetite; infection; chronic illness; substance abuse

**Environmental**

Deprivation; teratogen exposure; lead poisoning; poverty; violence; natural disasters

**Caregiver**

Abuse; mental illness; mental retardation or severe learning disability

### Client Outcomes

**Client/Parents/Primary Caregiver Will (Specify Time Frame):**

- State information related to possible teratogenic agents.
- State information related to adequate nutrition.
- Seek help from appropriate professionals for nutritional needs.

### Nursing Interventions

NOTE: Management of a risk diagnosis necessitates the use of approaches incorporating primary and secondary

• = Independent          ▲ = Collaborative

prevention. Primary prevention interventions, which include activities such as nutrition counseling, focus on thwarting the development of a disease or condition. Secondary prevention is achieved through screening, monitoring, and surveillance.

- Consider the use of formula milk for preterm and low-birth-weight infants.
- Assess and limit exposure to all drugs (prescription, "recreational," and over-the-counter) and give the mother information on known teratogenic agents (Table II-1).
- Reduce the risk of TORCH infections (toxoplasmosis, other infections, rubella, cytomegalovirus [CMV] infection, and herpes simplex):
  - Varicella zoster and rubella viruses: vaccinate nonimmune women prior to conception.
  - CMV: practice meticulous hand washing and secretion control and limit exposure to large numbers of infants and children.
  - *Toxoplasma gondii:* avoid exposure to cat litter and avoid work in garden or areas where cat feces may be present; do not feed undercooked meats to cats.
  - Parvovirus: limit contact with persons with known fifth disease.
  - Herpes virus: practice meticulous hand washing and secretion control, especially in contact with young infants.
- ▲ Promote a team approach toward preconception and pregnancy glucose control for women with diabetes.
- ▲ Women with phenylketonuria (PKU) should be referred to a nutritionist experienced in the dietary implications of phenylalanine restriction. Since 40% of all pregnancies are unplanned, women with PKU are urged to maintain phenylalanine restriction throughout their childbearing years.
- Provide for adequate nutrition and nutritional monitoring in clients with developmental disorders.
- Adequate intake of vitamin D is set at 200 IU/day by the

• = Independent          ▲ = Collaborative

G

| TABLE II-I |
| --- |

**Teratogenic Agents**

| Drug | Risk/Effect |
| --- | --- |
| ACE inhibitors (captopril, enalapril, etc.) | Appear to be teratogenic when used in the 2nd and 3rd trimesters, causing fetal calvarial hypoplasia, oligohydramnios, and renal anomalies. |
| Alcohol | Risk is for FAS, alcohol-related birth defects, or alcohol-related neurodevelopmental abnormalities. FAS may be characterized by microcephaly, IUGR, and/or developmental delay. Chronic alcoholism is considered most harmful. Binge drinking may also confer significant risk. No safe limit for prenatal alcohol consumption has been established. |
| Anticonvulsants (hydantoin, valproic acid, carbamazepine, and primidone [Mysoline]) | Effects may include cardiac defects, microcephaly, IUGR, hypoplastic nails, depressed nasal bridge, cleft lip, hip dislocation, hypoplastic nose, low-set ears, small mandible; risk increases with number of anticonvulsants used concurrently. |
| Antineoplastics (alkylating agents) | Case reports show 10-50% of cases were malformed for different drugs in this class, including busulfan, chlorambucil, cyclophosphamide, and mechlorethamine. The malformation rate for first trimester exposure is quoted at 11.6%. Problems seen include IUGR, cleft palate, agenesis of kidney, malformations of digits, cardiac anomalies, and cloudy corneas. |
| Antineoplastics (antimetabolites) | Only case reports are available, but an average of 40% of cases were malformed. This class includes aminopterin, 5-fluorouracil, methotrexate, and methylaminopterin, which are strong folic acid antagonists. First trimester exposure produces risk for cleft lip and palate, low-set ears, cranial anomalies, and anencephaly. Fetal abnormalities with cyclophosphamide and vinblastine have also been noted. |
| Cocaine | Can cause vascular disruption anomalies (e.g., intestinal atresia, limb reductions), IUGR, microcephaly, genitourinary tract defects, irritability, and muscular rigidity in the newborn. |

*Continued*

• = Independent        ▲ = Collaborative

## TABLE II-I

### Teratogenic Agents—cont'd

| Drug | Risk/Effect |
|------|-------------|
| Fluconazole | Fetal anomalies have been observed only when high-dose parenteral therapy is used (e.g., treatment of the mother for coccidiomycosis meningitis). |
| Diethylstilbestrol | In female offspring, increases risk for cancer, uterine and cervical malformations, reduced fertility, preterm deliveries, perinatal mortality, and SABs; in male offspring, may cause cysts of epididymis, cryptorchidism, hypogonadism, and diminished spermatogenesis. |
| Lithium | Small increase in risk for cardiac defects (Ebstein's anomaly in particular). Important in this drug to consider benefits and risk potentials. |
| Methimazole | Antithyroid drug that may increase the risk for prematurity, small-for-gestational-age infants, and scalp defects. |
| Methylene blue | Reported to cause intestinal atresias when injected into amniotic fluid during amniocentesis. |
| Penicillamine | Increases risk for connective tissue defects, cerebral palsy, and hydrocephalus. |
| Retinoids (isotretinoin, etretinate, acitretin) | Use of systemic retinoids increases risk for SAB; deformities of cranium, ears, face, limbs, and liver; hydrocephalus; microcephalus; heart defects; and cognitive defects without dysmorphology. Quoted risk for adverse outcome with use of isotretinoin is 38%. These agents have a prolonged teratogen risk because they are stored in adipose tissue and can persist for months. |
| Tetracyclines | Use from the 20th gestational week on causes dental staining. |
| Thalidomide | High risk for limb defects, facial hemangiomas, microtia, and ocular and renal anomalies. Now back on the market. |

*Continued*

• = Independent        ▲ = Collaborative

### TABLE II-I

**Teratogenic Agents—cont'd**

| Drug | Risk/Effect |
|------|-------------|
| Warfarin (Coumadin) and indandiones (anisindione) anticoagulants | Increased risk for SAB, stillbirth, and prematurity as well as fetal warfarin syndrome (CNS defects, nasal hypoplasia, skull defects, abnormal ears, malformed eyes, microcephaly, skeletal deformities, mental retardation, etc.). Malformations are reported in 16% of exposed fetuses, hemorrhages in 3%, and stillbirths in 8%. |

G

*CNS*, central nervous system; *FAS*, fetal alcohol syndrome; *IUGR*, intrauterine growth retardation; *SAB*, spontaneous abortion.

National Academy of Sciences. Because adequate sunlight exposure is difficult to determine, a supplement of 200 IU/day is recommended for the following groups to prevent rickets and vitamin D deficiency in healthy infants and children:

- All breastfed infants unless they are weaned to at least 500 mL/day of vitamin D–fortified formula or milk
- All nonbreastfed infants who are ingesting less than 500 mL/day of vitamin D–fortified formula or milk
- Children and adolescents who do not receive regular sunlight exposure, do not ingest at least 500 mL/day of vitamin D–fortified milk, or do not take a daily multivitamin supplement containing at least 200 IU of vitamin D

• All women of childbearing age who are capable of becoming pregnant should take 400 mcg of folic acid daily.

• Provide for adequate nutrition for clients with active intestinal inflammation.

• Provide for adequate nutrition for pediatric and adolescent clients on long-term oral glucocorticoid therapy (e.g., those treated for chronic severe asthma).

▲ Provide tube feedings per physician's orders when appropriate for clients with neuromuscular impairment.

• Refer to the care plan for **Delayed Growth and development.**

• = Independent        ▲ = Collaborative

**Multicultural**

- Assess for the influence of cultural beliefs, norms, values, and expectations on parents' perceptions of normal growth and development.
- Assess for the influence of acculturation.
- Negotiate with clients regarding which aspects of healthy nutrition can be modified while still honoring cultural beliefs.
- Assess whether the parents are concerned about the amount of food eaten.
- Assess the influence of family support on patterns of nutritional intake.
- Encourage parental efforts at increasing physical activity and decreasing dietary fat for their children.
- Encourage limiting television viewing to 2 hours or less per day for children and discourage the consumption of sweetened soft drinks.

**Home Care**

- The interventions described previously may be adapted for home care use.
- Provide aids to assist in compliance with the care plan (e.g., prepare medication schedules and put a week's medication in daily containers).
- Provide sufficient outside supports (e.g., written notices, calendars, planned ride shares) to assist with follow-through of the agreed-upon actions.
- ▲ Include a health promotion focus for clients with disabilities, with the goals of reducing secondary conditions (e.g., obesity, hypertension, pressure sores), maintaining functional independence, providing opportunities for leisure and enjoyment, and enhancing overall quality of life.
- Encourage a mind-set and program of self-care management.
- Establish a written contract with the client to follow the agreed-upon health care regimen.
- Meet with the client following completion of the proposed actions to review the contract and determine

• = Independent          ▲ = Collaborative

the next course of action. Do this until the client is able to initiate and follow through independently.

- Using self-care management precepts, instruct the client in the multiple possible situations to which he or she may need to respond; include the use of role playing. Instruct the client in generating hypotheses from available evidence rather than solely from experience.

### Client/Family Teaching

- Provide anticipatory guidance for parents and caregivers regarding expectations for normal patterns of growth. Clarify expectations and correct misconceptions.
- ▲ Refer clients to a registered dietitian for nutritional counseling.
- Teach families the importance of taking measures to prevent lead poisoning: Wash the hands before preparing the child's food. Wash the child's hands before serving food. Wash bottle nipples and pacifiers frequently, especially if they fall on the floor. Wash the child's toys frequently. Stomp the feet before coming into the house to clean shoes of outside soil that may carry lead from exterior house paint. Damp mop frequently along baseboards, around door frames, under windowsills, and around iron radiators. Wash windowsills and window wells frequently. Move the crib away from window wells. Always damp mop before sweeping or vacuuming. Home vacuum cleaners do not trap lead dust; they blow it into the air.

## Ineffective Health maintenance

### NANDA Definition

Inability to identify, manage, or seek out help to maintain health

### Defining Characteristics

History of lack of health-seeking behavior; reported or observed

• = Independent          ▲ = Collaborative

lack of equipment, financial, and/or other resources; reported or observed impairment of personal support systems; expressed interest in improving health behaviors; demonstrated lack of knowledge regarding basic health practices; demonstrated lack of adaptive behaviors to internal and external environmental changes; reported or observed inability to take responsibility for following basic health practices in any or all functional pattern areas

## Related Factors (r/t)

Ineffective family coping; perceptual-cognitive impairment (complete or partial lack of gross or fine motor skills); lack of or significant alteration in communication skills (written, verbal, or gestural); unachieved developmental tasks; lack of material resources; dysfunctional grieving; disabling spiritual distress; inability to make deliberate and thoughtful judgments; ineffective coping

## Client Outcomes

### Client Will (Specify Time Frame):

- Discuss fear of or blocks to implementing health regimen.
- Follow mutually agreed upon health care maintenance plan.
- Meet goals for health care maintenance.

## Nursing Interventions

- Assess the client's feelings, values, and reasons for not following the prescribed plan of care. See Related Factors.
- Assess for family patterns, economic issues, and cultural patterns that influence compliance with a given medical regimen.
- Help the client determine how to arrange a daily schedule that incorporates the new health care regimen (e.g., taking pills before meals).
- ▲ Refer the client to social services for financial assistance if needed.
- ▲ Identify support groups related to the disease process

• = Independent          ▲ = Collaborative

(e.g., Reach to Recovery for a woman who has had a mastectomy).
• Help the client to choose a healthy lifestyle and to have appropriate diagnostic screening tests.
• Assist the client in reducing stress.
• Identify complementary healing modalities such as herbal remedies, acupuncture, healing touch, yoga, or cultural shamans that the client uses in addition to or instead of the prescribed allopathic regimen.
▲ Refer the client to community agencies for appropriate follow-up care (e.g., day treatment or adult day health program).
• Obtain or design educational material that is appropriate for the client; use pictures if possible.
• Ensure that follow-up appointments are scheduled before the client is discharged; discuss a way to ensure that appointments are kept.

## Geriatric

▲ Assess sensory deficits and psychomotor skills. Supply the appropriate assistive devices.
• Discuss "symptoms of daily living" in addition to the major illness.
• Recognize resistance to change in lifelong patterns of personal health care.
• Discuss with the client and support person realistic goals for changes in health maintenance.
• Instruct the client in the symptoms of myocardial infarction and the need for timeliness in seeking care.
• Consider the age of the client when suggesting screening for disease.

## Multicultural

• Assess for the influence of cultural beliefs, norms, and values on the client's ability to modify health behavior.
• Discuss with the client those aspects of health behavior and lifestyle that will remain unchanged by health status.

• = Independent        ▲ = Collaborative

- Assess the effect of fatalism on the client's ability to modify health behavior.
- Validate the client's feelings regarding the impact of health status on current lifestyle.
- Assess for access to health services.

## Home Care

- The interventions described previously may be adapted for home care use.
- Assessment of urologic, developmental, psychosocial, and sleep-related etiologies is important in evaluating the presence of enuresis as an unachieved developmental task.
- Provide aids to assist in compliance with the plan of care (e.g., prepare medication schedules and put a week's medication in daily containers).
- Provide sufficient outside supports (e.g., written notices, calendars, planned ride shares) to assist with follow-through on the agreed-upon actions.
- Include a health promotion focus for the client with disabilities, with the goals of reducing secondary conditions (e.g., obesity, hypertension, pressure sores), maintaining functional independence, providing opportunities for leisure and enjoyment, and enhancing overall quality of life.
- Encourage a mind-set and program of self-care management.
- Establish a written contract with the client to follow the agreed-upon health care regimen.
- Meet with the client following completion of the proposed actions to review the contract and determine the next course of action. Do this until the client is able to initiate and follow through independently.
- Using self-care management precepts, instruct the client about multiple possible situations to which he or she may need to respond; include the use of role playing. Instruct in generating hypotheses from available evidence rather than solely from experience.

• = Independent        ▲ = Collaborative

## Client/Family Teaching

- Provide the family with lists of addresses where information can be obtained from the Internet. (Most libraries have Internet access with printing capabilities.)
- Have the client and family demonstrate at least twice any procedures to be done at home.
- Teach the client about the symptoms associated with discontinuation of a selective serotonin reuptake inhibitor (SSRI) and consider dosage tapering.
- Explain nonthreatening aspects before introducing more anxiety-producing possible side effects of the disease or medical regimen.
- Treat tobacco use as a chronic problem. Acknowledge the pleasure associated with smoking. Encourage the client to work towards a goal of permanent abstinence. Advise the client about possible relapse.

H

# Health-seeking behaviors

## NANDA Definition

Active seeking (by individual in stable health) of ways to alter personal health habits and/or environment to move toward higher level of health

NOTE: Stable health is defined as the achievement of age-appropriate illness-prevention measures; report of good or excellent health from the client; and control of signs and symptoms of disease, if present.

## Defining Characteristics

Expressed or observed desire to seek higher level of wellness for self or family; demonstrated or observed lack of knowledge of health-promoting behaviors; stated or observed unfamiliarity with wellness community resources; expressed concern about effect of current environmental conditions on health status; expressed or observed desire for increased control of health practice

• = Independent        ▲ = Collaborative

## Related Factors (r/t)

Role change; change in developmental level (e.g., marriage, parenthood, empty-nest status, retirement); lack of knowledge regarding need for preventive health behaviors, appropriate health screenings, optimal nutrition, weight control, regular exercise program, stress management, supportive social network, and responsible role participation

## Client Outcomes

### Client Will (Specify Time Frame):

- Maintain ideal weight and be knowledgeable about nutritious diet.
- Demonstrate ways to fit newly prescribed change in health habits into lifestyle.
- List community resources available for assistance with achieving wellness.
- List ways to include wellness behaviors in current lifestyle.

## Nursing Interventions

- Discuss the client's beliefs about health and his or her ability to maintain health.
- Identify barriers and benefits to being healthy.
- Identify environmental and social factors that the client perceives as health promoting.

## Nutritional

- Determine the client's height and weight. Compare results with the standard weight for age and height.
- Assess the role that stress plays in overeating and weight-cycling.
- Encourage client to use the new nutritional guidelines as developed by the USDA.

## Adequate Nutrients Within Calorie Needs

- Encourage client to consume a variety of nutrient-dense foods and beverages within and among the basic food groups while choosing foods that limit the intake of satu-

• = Independent  ▲ = Collaborative

rated and *trans* fats, cholesterol, added sugars, salt, and alcohol.

- Meet recommended intakes within energy needs by adopting a balanced eating pattern, such as the U.S. Department of Agriculture (USDA) Food Guide or the Dietary Approaches to Stop Hypertension (DASH) Eating Plan.

## Weight Management

- To maintain body weight in a healthy range, balance calories from foods and beverages with calories expended.
- To prevent gradual weight gain over time, make small decreases in food and beverage calories and increase physical activity.

## Food Groups to Encourage

- Consume a sufficient amount of fruits and vegetables while staying within energy needs. Two cups of fruit and 2 1/2 cups of vegetables per day are recommended for a 2000-calorie intake, with higher or lower amounts depending on the calorie level.
- Choose a variety of fruits and vegetables each day. In particular, select from all five vegetable subgroups (dark green, orange, legumes, starchy vegetables, and other vegetables) several times a week.
- Consume 3 or more ounce-equivalents of whole-grain products per day, with the rest of the recommended grains coming from enriched or whole-grain products. In general, at least half the grains should come from whole grains.
- Consume 3 cups per day of fat-free or low-fat milk or equivalent milk products.

## Fats

- Consume less than 10 percent of calories from saturated fatty acids and less than 300 mg/day of cholesterol, and keep *trans* fatty acid consumption as low as possible.
- Keep total fat intake between 20 to 35 percent of calories, with most fats coming from sources of polyun-

• = Independent          ▲ = Collaborative

saturated and monounsaturated fatty acids, such as fish, nuts, and vegetable oils.
- When selecting and preparing meat, poultry, dry beans, and milk or milk products, make choices that are lean, low-fat, or fat-free.
- Limit intake of fats and oils high in saturated and/or *trans* fatty acids, and choose products low in such fats and oils.

## Carbohydrates
- Choose fiber-rich fruits, vegetables, and whole grains often.
- Choose and prepare foods and beverages with little added sugars or caloric sweeteners, such as amounts suggested by the USDA Food Guide and the DASH Eating Plan.
- Reduce the incidence of dental caries by practicing good oral hygiene and consuming sugar- and starch-containing foods and beverages less frequently.

## Sodium and Potassium
- Consume less than 2300 mg (approximately 1 teaspoon of salt) of sodium per day.
- Choose and prepare foods with little salt. At the same time, consume potassium-rich foods, such as fruits and vegetables.

## Alcoholic Beverages
- Those who choose to drink alcoholic beverages should do so sensibly and in moderation—defined as the consumption of up to one drink per day for women and up to two drinks per day for men.
- Alcoholic beverages should not be consumed by some individuals, including those who cannot restrict their alcohol intake, women of childbearing age who may become pregnant, pregnant and lactating women, children and adolescents, individuals taking medications that can interact with alcohol, and those with specific medical conditions.
- Alcoholic beverages should be avoided by individuals en-

• = Independent          ▲ = Collaborative

gaging in activities that require attention, skill, or coordination, such as driving or operating machinery. NOTE: The *Dietary Guidelines for Americans 2005* contains additional recommendations for specific populations. Their Web address is http://www.health.gov/dietaryguidelines/dga2005/recommendations.htm.

## Exercise

- Engage in regular physical activity and reduce sedentary activities to promote health, psychological well-being, and a healthy body weight.
  - To reduce the risk of chronic disease in adulthood: Engage in at least 30 minutes of moderate-intensity physical activity, above usual activity, at work or home on most days of the week.
  - For most people, greater health benefits can be obtained by engaging in physical activity of more vigorous intensity or longer duration.
  - To help manage body weight and prevent gradual, unhealthy body weight gain in adulthood: Engage in approximately 60 minutes of moderate- to vigorous-intensity activity on most days of the week while not exceeding caloric intake requirements.
  - To sustain weight loss in adulthood: Participate in at least 60 to 90 minutes of daily moderate-intensity physical activity while not exceeding caloric intake requirements. Some people may need to consult with a healthcare provider before participating in this level of activity.
  - Achieve physical fitness by including cardiovascular conditioning, stretching exercises for flexibility, and resistance exercises or calisthenics for muscle strength and endurance. NOTE: The *Dietary Guidelines for Americans 2005* contains additional recommendations for specific populations. Their Web address is www.health.gov/dietaryguidelines/dga2005/recommendations.htm.
- ▲ Advise the client to consult with a physician for testing to determine the ability to tolerate a specific regimen.

• = Independent          ▲ = Collaborative

- Explore with the client weightlifting options to increase muscle strength and stamina.
- Encourage exercise for cancer survivors.
- Help the client focus on the enjoyment of exercise. Set up a support and reward system.
- Consider using music with exercise.
- Encourage aerobic exercises that increase heart rate within the prescribed limit. Encourage the client to exercise at least three times per week for 20 or more minutes using exercises that the client prefers (e.g., walking, jogging, aerobics, swimming, bicycling, yoga, tai chi).

## Stress Management
- Ask the client to define stress in terms of lifestyle events and assign events a value on a scale from 1 to 5.
- Determine ways in which the client relieves stress and evaluate their effectiveness.
- Determine the client's social support network.
- Teach stress-relieving techniques (e.g., deep and slow breathing, progressive muscle relaxation, meditation, imagery, problem solving).

## Smoking, Drinking, Self-Medication
- Discuss the risk-taking behaviors of smoking, drinking, and self-medication.
- Discuss the frequency of risk-taking habits.
- ▲ Refer a client who smokes to Smoke Enders or a similar community-based program. Discuss ways in which the client can deal with a change in behavior.
- ▲ Refer a client who drinks alcohol excessively to Alcoholics Anonymous. Identify a support person to help the client into the organization.
- ▲ Identify patterns of self-medication with over-the-counter medications and herbal remedies, and excessive use of prescribed medications.
- Refer to the care plans for **Dysfunctional Family processes: alcoholism, Ineffective Denial**, and **Defensive Coping**.

• = Independent            ▲ = Collaborative

## Health-Seeking Behaviors
- Teach stress-relieving techniques (e.g., deep and slow breathing, progressive muscle relaxation, exercise, meditation, power strategies, problem solving, imagery, verbalization of feelings, spiritual practice [prayer]).
- Recognize and allow the client to discuss the choice of complementary therapies available, such as spiritual practice, relaxation, imagery, exercise, lifestyle, diet (e.g., macrobiotic, vegetarian), and nutritional supplementation.

## Health Screening, Appropriate Health Care
- Assess the frequency of illness-preventing practices, such as routine physical examinations, dental examinations, influenza immunization, breast self-examinations (and mammograms as recommended) for women, testicular self-examinations and prostate examinations for men, and screening for familial diseases such as glaucoma and elevated cholesterol level. See the care plan for **Ineffective Health maintenance.**
- Provide a phone call to remind the client of appointments.

## Pediatric
- Provide for appropriate nutrition for children. See Box II-4.
- ▲ Follow the recommended guidelines for childhood immunizations.

## Geriatric
- Assess the client's awareness of deficits that may result from normal aging (e.g., changes in sleep patterns or frequency of urination, loss of visual acuity in night driving, loss of hearing, dietary changes, memory changes, loss of significant others).
- Identify coping mechanisms that promote wellness and place control of life choices back with the client. Discuss ways to prepare for retirement security.
- ▲ Find suitable housing that provides support, safety, pro-

• = Independent          ▲ = Collaborative

| BOX  II-4 | Pediatric Nutrition Guidelines |
|---|---|

- Aim for five servings of fruits and vegetables each day. You can gradually build up to this amount. A good goal to try: eat fruit with each meal for a week.
- Reduce fat. Opt for low-fat substitutes:
  - Low-fat dairy—skim or 1% milk (after age 2), cheese with 2 to 6 grams of fat per ounce
  - Lean meats and poultry—95% lean ground beef or turkey; remove visible fat from meat; remove skin from poultry
  - Low-fat or fat-free salad dressings, mayonnaise and margarine
  - Desserts—angel food cake, low-fat ice cream or frozen yogurt, animal crackers, vanilla wafers, gingersnaps, graham crackers
- Eat sugary foods in moderation. If your child eats a healthy diet, one sweet a day is fine.
- Drink water, skim or 1% milk (after age 2) instead of high-calorie, sugary drinks.
- Check ingredients on nutrition labels. Foods with sugar listed as one of the first three or four ingredients may be high in sugar and should be eaten in moderation.
- Eat healthy snacks. Keep healthy foods on-hand for snacks. Good snack ideas include:
  - Fresh fruit
  - Cereal with low-fat milk
  - Low-fat cheese with low-fat crackers
  - Graham crackers with low-fat hot chocolate
  - Raw vegetables with low-fat dip
  - Applesauce

H

tection, meals, and social events. Consider in-home care by adult children when possible.
▲ Give the client information about community resources for the elderly (e.g., services providing transportation to appointments, Meals-on-Wheels, home visitation services, pets, American Association of Retired Persons, Elder Hostel, Internet addresses).
▲ Assess the environment for signs of elder abuse and report as appropriate.
• Teach health-protecting behaviors to the elderly: monitoring cholesterol intake, exercising, having the stool checked for occult blood, or undergoing a mammogram, Papanicolaou test, or prostate or skin evaluation.
• Teach the importance of exercise.

•  = Independent          ▲ = Collaborative

▲ Form collaborative multidisciplinary partnerships with nurse-managed clinics for health promotion and chronic disease care management for community-residing older adults.
• Consider the age of the client when suggesting screening for disease.

## Multicultural

• Assess for the influence of cultural beliefs, norms, and values on the client's beliefs about health behavior.
• Acknowledge and praise those aspects of the client's behavior and lifestyle that are health promoting.
• Negotiate with the client the aspects of health behavior that will require further modification.
• Validate the client's feelings regarding the impact of health behavior on current lifestyle.
• Utilize a community focus intervention.

## Home Care

NOTE: All the previously listed nursing interventions are applicable to the home care setting. For more information, see Home Care interventions in the care plan for **Ineffective Health maintenance.**

## Client/Family Teaching

• Discuss the role of environmental and social factors in supporting a healthy family life.
• Use written, verbal and video to provide information about health-seeking opportunities and wellness and provide the family with lists of addresses and where information can be found. Suggest use of the Internet. (Most libraries have Internet access with printing capabilities.)
• Teach the importance of receiving flu vaccine. Offer vaccinations in convenient locations free of charge, and discuss perceived barriers with patients.
• Identify physical and emotional threats to family security (e.g., domestic violence, child abuse, school violence).
• Teach women how to monitor ovarian health: monthly self-monitoring using a symptom checklist including

• = Independent          ▲ = Collaborative

personal and family risks and early symptoms of gastrointestinal symptoms.

# Impaired Home maintenance

## NANDA Definition

Inability to independently maintain a safe and growth-promoting
immediate environment

## Defining Characteristics

H

### Subjective

Household members express difficulty in maintaining their home
in a comfortable fashion; household members describe outstand-
ing debts or financial crises; household requests assistance with
home maintenance

### Objective

Disorderly surroundings; unwashed or unavailable cooking
equipment, clothes, or linen; accumulation of dirt, food wastes,
or hygienic wastes; offensive odors; inappropriate household
temperature; overtaxed family members (e.g., exhausted, anxious); lack of necessary equipment or aids; presence of vermin or
rodents; repeated hygienic disorders, infestations, or infections

## Related Factors (r/t)

Client/family member with disease or injury; unfamiliarity with
neighborhood resources; lack of role modeling; lack of knowledge; insufficient family organization or planning; inadequate
support systems; impaired cognitive or emotional functioning;
insufficient finances

## Client Outcomes

### Client Will (Specify Time Frame):

• Wear clean clothing, eat nutritious meals, and have a sanitary
  and safe home.

　　　• = Independent　　　▲ = Collaborative

- Have the resources to cope physically and emotionally with the chronic illness process.
- Use community resources to assist with treatment needs.

## Nursing Interventions

- Establish a plan of care with the client and family based on the client's needs and the caregiver's capabilities.
- Assess the concerns of family members, especially the primary caregiver, about long-term home care.
- Set up a system of relief for the main caregiver in the home and plan for sharing of household duties.
- Encourage social relationships with family and friends, even if by phone.
- ▲ Initiate referral to community agencies as needed, including housekeeping services, Meals-on-Wheels, wheelchair-compatible transportation services, and oxygen therapy services.
- ▲ Obtain adaptive equipment and telemedical equipment, as appropriate, to help family members continue to maintain the home environment.
- Consider the use of permethrin-impregnated mattress liners to control dust mites.
- ▲ Refer the client to social services to help with debt consolidation or financial concerns.
- ▲ Ask the family to identify support people who can help with home maintenance.

## Geriatric

- ▲ Explore community resources to assist with home care (e.g., senior centers, Department of Aging, hospital discharge planners, the Internet, or church parish nurse).
- Visit the client's home to assess safety features (e.g., no throw rugs, safety bars in the bathroom, stair borders that distinguish each step, adequate nonglare lighting).
- Encourage regular eye examinations.
- The following interventions should be considered for those with low or failing sight:
  - Reduce glare.

    ❏ Use nonglare light bulbs.
    ❏ Remove wax from floors to reduce glare.
    ❏ Encourage the client to wear sunglasses.
    ❏ Use sheer curtains or blinds.
- Use proper lighting.
    ❏ Use night lights in the bedroom, bathroom, and
       hallways.
    ❏ Use dimmer switches and three-way bulbs to con-
       trol light.
    ❏ Put bright lights at the top and bottom of a
       staircase.
    ❏ Use consistent lighting to minimize shadows.
- Enhance color contrast.
    ❏ Use colored tape to define steps.
    ❏ Paint walls and staircase to contrast with floor.
    ❏ Put glow-in-the-dark tape on light switches and
       door knobs.
    ❏ Use colored dishes.
- Encourage the client to use low-vision aids.
    ❏ Use magnifiers to improve near vision.
    ❏ Hang magnifiers around the neck for convenience
       when sewing, doing crafts, or reading.
    ❏ Request large-print medication labels, books, and
       phones.
    ❏ Use handrails on stairs.
    ❏ Keep flashlights in a convenient location.
▲ During the home visit, be alert for signs of elder abuse.
   Report any findings.
- See the care plan for **Risk for Injury.**

## Multicultural

- Acknowledge the stresses unique to racial/ethnic
   communities.
- Identify what services and information are currently
   available in the community to assist with housing
   needs.
- Approach families of color with respect, warmth, and
   professional courtesy.

        ● = Independent         ▲ = Collaborative

## Home Care

NOTE: By definition, this nursing diagnosis consists of primarily community-based interventions. Home care and public health nursing are two community resources that can help the family to restore or improve home management. The previous interventions incorporate these resources.

## Client/Family Teaching

- Teach the caregiver the need to set aside some personal time every day to meet his or her own needs.
- Encourage family members to perform home maintenance activities (e.g., cooking, cleaning, fire prevention).
▲ Identify support groups within the community to assist families in the caregiver role.
- Provide support when the family must move their family member to an assisted living facility (ALF).
▲ Provide written instructions for medication management and side effects, written instructions for equipment brought to the home, and resource phone numbers for emergency needs.
- Promote food safety. Instruct client to avoid microbial foodborne illness by observing the following:
  ■ Clean hands, food contact surfaces, and fruits and vegetables. Meat and poultry should not be washed or rinsed.
  ■ Separate raw, cooked, and ready-to-eat foods while shopping, preparing, or storing foods.
  ■ Cook foods to a safe temperature to kill microorganisms.
  ■ Chill (refrigerate) perishable food promptly and defrost foods properly.
  ■ Avoid raw (unpasteurized) milk or any products made from unpasteurized milk, raw or partially cooked eggs or foods containing raw eggs, raw or undercooked meat and poultry, unpasteurized juices, and raw sprouts.

• = Independent          ▲ = Collaborative

# Hopelessness

## NANDA Definition

Subjective state in which individual sees limited or unavailable alternatives or personal choices and is unable to mobilize energy for problem solving on his or her own behalf

## Defining Characteristics

Passivity; decreased verbalization; blunted or flat affect; verbal cues (e.g., saying "I can't," sighing, "I'll never . . . ," "There is no future"); closing of eyes; anorexia; decreased response to stimuli; increased/decreased sleep; lack of initiative; lack of involvement in care; passively allowing care; shrugging in response to speaker; turning away from speaker; reports feeling lost, unable to cope, or abandoned

## Related Factors (r/t)

Abandonment; prolonged activity restriction creating isolation; loss of beliefs in transcendent values/God; long-term stress; failing or deteriorating chronic physiological and/or psychological condition; negative life review; perception of demands that overwhelm personal resources

## Client Outcomes

### Client Will (Specify Time Frame):

- Verbalize feelings, participate in care.
- Make positive statements (e.g., "I can" or "I will try").
- Set goals.
- Make eye contact, focus on speaker.
- Maintain appropriate appetite for age and physical health.
- Sleep appropriate length of time for age and physical health.
- Express concern for another.
- Initiate activity.

## Nursing Interventions

▲ Monitor and document the potential for suicide. (Refer

• = Independent          ▲ = Collaborative

the client for appropriate treatment if a potential for suicide is identified.) See the care plan for **Risk for Suicide** for specific interventions.

- Explore the client's definition of hope.
- Assist in identifying sources of hope.
- Assist the client in identifying reasons for living.
- Provide realistic feedback.
- Assess for pain and respond with appropriate measures for pain relief.
- Assist with problem solving and decision making.
- Determine appropriate approaches based on the underlying condition or situation that is contributing to feelings of hopelessness.
- Assist the client in looking at alternatives and setting goals that are important to him or her.
- In dealing with possible long-term deficits, work with the client to set small, attainable goals.
- Spend one-on-one time with the client. Use empathy; try to understand what the client is saying and communicate this understanding to the client.
- Encourage decision making in the daily schedule.
- Encourage expression of feelings and acknowledge acceptance of them.
- Give the client time to initiate interactions. After an appropriate amount of time is allowed, approach the client in an accepting and nonjudgmental manner.
- Encourage the client to participate in group activities.
- Teach alternative coping strategies.
- Review the client's strengths with the client. Have the client list his or her own strengths on a note card and carry this list for future reference.
- Communicate clearly what the illness trajectory and/or course of treatment will involve.
- Use humor as appropriate.
- Involve family and significant others in the plan of care.
- Encourage the family and significant others to express care, hope, and love for the client.
- Assess for signs and symptoms of depression.
▲ Consider use of integrative therapies such as omega-3

• = Independent        ▲ = Collaborative

fatty acids, *Hypericum perforatum* (St. John's wort), S-adenosyl-methionine, folate, 5-hydroxytryptophan, acupuncture, exercise, and light therapy.

- Use touch to demonstrate caring, if culturally appropriate and with the client's permission, and encourage the family to do the same.
- Facilitate access to resources to support a positive spirituality.
- For additional interventions, see the care plans for **Spiritual distress, Readiness for enhanced Spiritual well-being,** and **Disturbed Sleep pattern.**

## Geriatric

H

- Assess for clinical signs and symptoms of depression; differentiate depression from organic dementia.
- ▲ If depression is suspected, confer with the primary physician regarding referral for mental health services.
- Take threats of self-harm or suicide seriously.
- Identify significant losses that may be leading to feelings of hopelessness.
- Discuss stages of emotional responses to multiple losses.
- Use reminiscence and life-review therapies to identify past coping skills.
- Express hope to the client and give positive feedback whenever appropriate.
- Identify the client's past and current sources of spirituality. Help the client explore life and identify those experiences that are noteworthy. The client may want to read the Bible or other religious text or have it read to him or her.
- Encourage visits from children.
- ▲ Administer medications as ordered and evaluate for possible drug interactions that may produce and/or exacerbate observed symptoms.
- Position the client by a window, take the client outside, or encourage activities such as gardening (if ability allows).
- Provide esthetic forms of expression such as dance, music, literature, pictures.

• = Independent          ▲ = Collaborative

- If possible, have the client perform daily regular exercise adapted to his or her abilities.

## Multicultural
- Assess for the influence of cultural beliefs, norms, and values on the client's feelings of hopelessness.
- Assess the effect of fatalism on the client's expression of hopelessness.
- Assess for depression and refer to appropriate services.
- Encourage spirituality as a source of support for hopelessness.
- Validate the client's feelings regarding the impact of health status on current lifestyle.

## Home Care
- Assess for isolation within the family unit. Encourage the client to participate in family activities. If the client cannot participate, encourage him or her to be in the same area and watch family activities. If possible, move the client's bed or primary sitting place to an active household area.
- ▲ If depression is suspected, confer with the primary health care provider regarding referral for mental health services.
- Reminisce with the client about his or her life.
- Identify areas in which the client can have control. Allow the client to set achievable goals in these areas. Assist the client when necessary to negotiate desirable outcomes.
- Clearly explain potential benefits and risks of a proposed intervention.
- If illness precipitated the hopelessness, discuss knowledge of and previous experience with the disease. Help the client to identify past coping strengths.
- ▲ Provide plant or pet therapy if possible.
- ▲ Provide a safe environment so that the client cannot harm himself or herself. (See also the no-suicide contract in the following section.) Provide one-to-one contact

when necessary. Refer the client for immediate mental health treatment if needed.

▲ If it is consistent with the client's religious beliefs, refer for spiritual counseling by clergy of the client's choice.

▲ In the presence of a psychiatric disorder, refer for psychiatric home health care services for client reassurance and implementation of a therapeutic regimen.

## Client/Family Teaching

• Provide information regarding the client's condition, treatment plan, and progress.

• Provide positive reinforcement, praise, and acknowledgment of the challenges of caregiving to family members.

• Teach the use of stress-reduction techniques, relaxation, and imagery. Many cassette tapes on relaxation and meditation are available. Assist the client and caregivers with relaxation based on their preference from the initial assessment.

• Encourage families to express love, concern, and encouragement, and allow the client to verbalize feelings.

▲ Refer the client to self-help groups such as I Can Cope and Make Today Count.

▲ Refer the family to community support groups targeted to the specific needs of the family caregivers.

# Hyperthermia

## NANDA Definition

Body temperature elevated above normal range

NOTE: Elevated body temperature can be either fever or hyperthermia. Fever is a normal response in which the core body temperature increases at least 0.8° to 1.1° C (1.5° to 2.0° F) above an individual's normal temperature (>38° C [>100.5° F]). This elevation is in response to a chemical signal (endogenous pyrogen) released as part of an inflammatory response, such as in

• = Independent        ▲ = Collaborative

infection or tissue injury. Because there is a proportional enhancement of the immune system for each degree of temperature elevation, fever is believed to be adaptive to 40° C (104° F). Hyperthermia is an abnormal increase in core body temperature, usually above 40° C (104° F), that occurs as a result of disorders of temperature control. Causes include brain trauma, heat stroke, drugs (e.g., cocaine, "ecstasy"), and malignant hyperthermia of anesthesia. Hyperthermia is not adaptive and should be treated as a medical emergency.

## Defining Characteristics

H

- Fever: core body temperature elevated at least 0.8° to 1.1° C (1.5° to 2.0° F) above individual's normal temperature (>38° C [>100.5° F])
- Hyperthermia: body temperature above 40° C (104° F) with flushed or hot skin, increased respiratory rate, and tachycardia

## Related Factors (r/t)

- Fever: Infection; tissue injury; illness or trauma; dehydration; blood transfusion; medication; neoplasm; increased metabolic rate
- Hyperthermia: Exposure to hot environment; vigorous activity; inappropriate clothing; inability or decreased ability to perspire; brain injury; medication; anesthesia; severe illness; trauma

## Client Outcomes

### Client Will (Specify Time Frame):

- Maintain oral temperature within adaptive levels (below 40° C [104° F]) or lower, depending on the presence of cardiopulmonary illness and client comfort.
- Remain free of dehydration.

## Nursing Interventions

▲ Assess an afebrile hospitalized client's temperature per institutional policy, upon assessment of signs or

• = Independent        ▲ = Collaborative

symptoms of infection, if the client has chills, or at least once a day between 5 PM and 7 PM.

- Measure and record a febrile client's temperature at least every 4 to 6 hours or whenever a change in condition occurs (e.g., chills, change in mental status).
- Temperature can be measured with acceptable accuracy using an electronic probe in the mouth or via the external auditory canal (tympanic membrane). Although inconvenient, rectal temperature measurement is highly accurate. Axillary measurements are inaccurate and should not be used. Where equipment is available in ICU settings, temperature measurement by intravascular or bladder thermistor is a highly accurate method. Measurement of brain temperature may be available for neurosurgical patients and is highly accurate but the relationship of brain temperature to core temperature has not yet been accurately determined.
- Use the same site and method (device) for temperature measurement for a given client so that temperature trends are assessed accurately.
- ▲ Notify the physician of temperature according to institutional standards or written orders, or when temperature reaches 38° C (100.5° F). Also notify the physician of the presence of a change in mental status.
- ▲ Administer antipyretic medication per physician orders, when infection-induced fever is above 40° C (104° F), and when the client cannot tolerate the increase in metabolic demand, such as the acutely ill or in advanced cardiac or respiratory disease. The antipyretic acetaminophen is preferred over aspirin.
- ▲ Assess fluid loss and facilitate oral intake or administer intravenous fluids to accomplish fluid replacement.
- When diaphoresis is present, assist the client with bathing and changing into dry clothing.
- Do not use external cooling measures such as ice packs, tepid water baths, or removal of blankets and clothing for fever management; these measures cause shivering and are ineffective.

H

• = Independent          ▲ = Collaborative

▲ Cooling blanket use is indicated for temperature reduction if the client's fever is above 40.6° C (105° F) and cannot be controlled with antipyretics and if a high body temperature is related to hyperthermia, a disorder of temperature regulation.

• When using a cooling blanket, choose a convective air-flow system, set the temperature regulator to 0.6° to 1.1° C (1° to 2° F) below the client's current temperature, and wrap the client's extremities with towels to prevent shivering.

• Use a non-steroidal antipyretic (e.g., acetaminophen) instead of or in conjunction with a cooling blanket to improve fever reduction and decrease the duration of cooling blanket use.

## Geriatric

• An increase in oral temperature of 0.8° to 1.1° C (1.5° to 2.0° F) above baseline or above 37.2° C (99° F) should be considered a fever in the elderly.

• Rectal temperature may be more accurate to diagnose fever in elderly clients. However, nursing judgment must be used to determine if rectal temperature measurement is acceptable to the client, especially a client with mental changes or dementia.

• Assess for other signs and symptoms of infection in addition to or in the absence of fever in the elderly. Suspect infection when there has been a decline in function, including new or increased confusion, incontinence, falling, decreased mobility, or failure to cooperate.

▲ Help the client seek medical attention immediately if fever is present. To diagnose the fever source, assess for possible precipitating factors, including changes in medication, environmental changes, and recent medical interventions or infectious exposures.

• In hot weather, encourage elderly clients to drink 8 to 10 glasses of fluid per day (within their cardiac and renal reserves) regardless of whether they are thirsty. Assess for the need for and presence of fans or air conditioning.

• = Independent          ▲ = Collaborative

- In hot weather, monitor the elderly client for signs of heat stroke: temperature of 37.8° C (100° F) to 38.9° C (102° F), orthostatic blood pressure drop, weakness, restlessness, mental status changes, faintness, thirst, nausea, and vomiting. If signs are present, move the client to a cool place, have the client lie down, give sips of water, check orthostatic blood pressure, spray with lukewarm water, cool with a fan, and seek medical assistance immediately.

## Home Care

- Some of the interventions described previously may be adapted for home care use.

- Assess whether the client or family has a thermometer. Instruct as needed in the type of thermometer (non–mercury containing preferred; sublingual or tympanic location rather than skin patches) and how to use and read it accurately.

- Teach the client and family that handwashing is the most effective way to prevent the transmission of viral and bacterial infections that may cause fever. However, it is not necessary to specifically purchase antibacterial household cleaning products, as these products have not been shown to decrease the incidence of infection among household members.

▲ Teach the client and family to use acetaminophen rather than aspirin or ibuprofen for fever reduction at home to prevent possible adverse effects. (NOTE: The maximum daily dose of acetaminophen is 4000 mg/day in a healthy adult. In clients with liver dysfunction, doses greater than 2000 mg/day, if taken on a regular basis, may be harmful. A client with kidney dysfunction should take acetaminophen no more often than every 6 hours.)

- Help the client and caregivers prevent and monitor for heat stroke/hyperthermia during times of high outdoor temperatures. Preventive measures include minimizing time spent outdoors, use of air conditioning

H

• = Independent            ▲ = Collaborative

or fan, increasing fluid intake, and taking frequent rest periods.

- To prevent heat-related injury in athletes, laborers, and military personnel instruct them to acclimate gradually to the higher temperatures, increase fluid intake, wear vapor-permeable clothing, and take frequent rests.

▲ In the event of temperature elevation above the adaptive range, institute measures to decrease temperature (e.g., get the client out of the sun and into a cool place, remove excess clothing, have the client drink fluids, spray the client with lukewarm water, and fan with cool air). Seek medical attention immediately if temperature is at or above 40° C (104° F).

▲ If the client is in hospice or is terminally ill, follow the client's wishes and the physician's orders in determining the management of fever.

## Client/Family Teaching

- Teach that infection-induced fever enhances the immune system (the beneficial effect occurs at oral temperatures of less than 40° C [104° F]), so the client can participate in the decision of whether to treat the fever. If treatment is elected or appropriate, instruct in the use of acetaminophen as the most effective means for fever reduction with fewer potential side effects than other antipyretics.

- Teach the client that shivering with infection-induced fever has detrimental effects and that activities that can cause shivering (e.g., blanket removal, lowering of room temperature, tepid water baths, ice packs) should be avoided.

- Instruct to increase fluids to prevent heat-induced hyperthermia and dehydration in the presence of fever, but to avoid liquids that contain alcohol, caffeine, or large amounts of sugar.

- Teach the client to stay in a cooler environment during periods of excessive outdoor heat or humidity. If the client does go out, instruct him or her to avoid vigorous

• = Independent          ▲ = Collaborative

physical activity, wear lightweight, loose-fitting clothing, and wear a hat to minimize sun exposure.

# Hypothermia

## NANDA Definition

Body temperature below normal range

## Defining Characteristics

Pallor; reduction in body temperature below normal range; shivering; cool skin; cyanotic nailbeds; hypertension and then hypotension; piloerection; slow capillary refill; tachycardia

## Related Factors (r/t)

Exposure to cool or cold environment; use of medications causing vasodilation; malnutrition; inadequate clothing; illness or trauma; evaporation from skin in cool environment; decreased metabolic rate; damage to hypothalamus; consumption of alcohol; aging; inability or decreased ability to shiver; inactivity

## Client Outcomes

### Client Will (Specify Time Frame):

- Maintain body temperature within normal range.
- Identify risk factors of hypothermia.
- State measures to prevent hypothermia.
- Identify symptoms of hypothermia and actions to take when hypothermia is present.

## Nursing Interventions

- Remove the client from the cause of the hypothermic episode (e.g., cold environment, cold or wet clothing). Ensure that the client is in a warm environment.
- Watch the client for signs of hypothermia: shivering, slurred speech, clumsy movements, fatigue, confusion.

• = Independent          ▲ = Collaborative

As hypothermia progresses, the skin becomes pale, numb, and waxy. Muscles are tense, fatigue and weakness can occur, and gradually there can be loss of consciousness with loss of a pulse and breathing.

- Cover the client with warm blankets and apply a covering to the head and neck to conserve body heat.
- Take the temperature at least hourly; if more than mild hypothermia is present (temperature lower than 35° C [95° F]), use a continuous temperature-monitoring device.
- ▲ Use a pulmonary artery catheter temperature-measuring device if available; if not, consider using a bladder catheter that measures temperature.
- If the client is awake, measure the oral temperature instead of the tympanic or axillary temperature.
- Monitor the client's vital signs every hour and as appropriate. Note changes associated with hypothermia, such as initially increased pulse rate, respiratory rate, and blood pressure with mild hypothermia, and then decreased pulse rate, respiratory rate, and blood pressure with moderate to severe hypothermia.
- ▲ Attach electrodes and a cardiac monitor. Watch for dysrhythmias.
- ▲ Monitor for signs of coagulopathy (e.g., oozing of blood from any open areas or from intravascular catheter sites or mucous membranes). Also note results of clotting studies as available.
- For mild hypothermia (core temperature of 35° C [95° F]), rewarm client passively:
  - Set room temperature to 21° to 24° C (70° to 75° F).
  - Keep the client dry, remove any damp or wet clothing.
  - Layer clothing and blankets and cover the client's head; use insulated metallic blankets.
  - Offer warm fluids, no alcohol or caffeine.
- For moderate hypothermia (core temperature 32° to 28° C [89.6° to 82.4° F]) use active external rewarming methods. The rewarming rate should not exceed 1° C (1.8° F) per hour. Methods include the following:

• = Independent          ▲ = Collaborative

- Forced-air warming systems
- Carbon-fiber blanket
- Electric blankets
- Radiant heat lights
- For severe hypothermia (core temperature below 28° C [82.4° F]) use active core-rewarming techniques:
    - Recognize that continuous arteriovenous extracorporeal blood rewarming is most effective. Note: this requires cardiopulmonary bypass and not all facilities have this capability.
    - Administer heated and humidified oxygen through the ventilator as ordered.
    - Administer heated IV fluids at prescribed temperature.
    - Perform peritoneal lavage, bladder irrigations.
- Check blood pressure frequently when rewarming; watch for hypotension.
- ▲ Administer IV fluids, using a rapid infuser IV fluid warmer as ordered.
- Determine the factors leading to the hypothermic episode; see Related Factors.
- ▲ Request a social service referral to help the client obtain the heat, shelter, and food needed to maintain body temperature.
- ▲ Encourage proper nutrition and hydration. Request a referral to a dietitian to identify appropriate dietary needs.

**Pediatric**
- Recognize that pediatric clients have a decreased ability to adapt to temperature extremes. Take the following actions to maintain body temperature in the infant/child:
    - Keep the head covered.
    - Use blankets to keep the client warm.
    - Keep the client covered during procedures, transport, and diagnostic testing.
    - Keep the room temperature at 22.2°C (72° F).
- For the preterm or low-birth-weight baby, utilize specially designed bags, skin-to-skin care and trans-warmer mattresses to keep preterm infants warm.

• = Independent            ▲ = Collaborative

## Geriatric

- Assess neurological signs frequently, watching for confusion and decreased level of consciousness.
- Recognize that the elderly can develop indoor hypothermia from air conditioning or ice baths. Clients present with vague complaints of mental and/or other skill deterioration.

## Home Care

NOTE: Hypothermia is not a symptom that appears in the normal course of home care. When it occurs, it is a clinical emergency and the client/family should access emergency medical services immediately.

H

- Some of the interventions described earlier may be adapted for home care use.
- Before a medical crisis occurs, confirm that the client or family has a thermometer and can read it. Instruct as needed. Verify that the thermometer registers accurately.
- Instruct the client or family to take the temperature when the client displays cyanosis, pallor, or shivering.
- Monitor temperature every hour, as noted previously.
- ▲ If temperature continues to drop, activate the emergency system and notify a physician. Hypothermia is a clinically acute condition that cannot be managed safely at home.
- ▲ If the client is in hospice care or is terminally ill, follow advance directives, client wishes, and the physician's orders. Keep the client free of pain.

## Client/Family Teaching

- Teach the client and family signs of hypothermia and the method of taking the temperature (age-appropriate).
- Teach the client methods to prevent hypothermia: wearing adequate clothing, including a hat and mittens; heating the environment to a minimum of 20° C (68° F); and ingesting adequate food and fluid.

● = Independent          ▲ = Collaborative

▲ Teach the client and family about medications such as sedatives, opioids, and anxiolytics that predispose the client to hypothermia (as appropriate).

# Disturbed personal Identity

## NANDA Definition

Inability to distinguish between self and nonself

## Defining Characteristics

Withdrawal from social contact; change in ability to determine relationship of the body to the environment; inappropriate or grandiose behavior

## Related Factors (r/t)

Situational crisis; psychological impairment; chronic illness; pain

## Client Outcomes

### Client Will (Specify Time Frame):

- Show interest in surroundings
- Respond to stimuli with appropriate affect
- Perform self-care and self-control activities appropriate for age
- Acknowledge personal strengths
- Engage in interpersonal relationships
- Verbalize willingness to change lifestyle and use appropriate community resources

## Nursing Interventions

- Assess carefully for a history of abuse.
- Assess for any history of seizure disorder; adhere to the diagnostic criteria for dissociative disorder in the *Diagnostic and Statistical Manual of Mental Disorders*, fourth edition *(DSM-IV)* and conduct a structured clinical interview.

• = Independent          ▲ = Collaborative

- Avoid labeling the client with terms such as multiple personality disorder (MPD).
- Spend time communicating with the client.
- Work with the client on setting personal goals.
- Address the client by name. Let the client know who is approaching and orient the client to the surroundings.
- Provide communication, clear rules and aims, and safety procedures.
- Work with the client to utilize his or her senses to deescalate problem behavior.
- Give the client permission to share his or her experiences, such as if the client has always lived in secrecy and is not sure how much is safe to reveal, or if others believe that the illness is an actual illness.
- Use touch only after a thorough assessment and as appropriate.
- ▲ Have all team members approach the client in a consistent manner.
- Provide time for one-on-one interactions to establish a therapeutic relationship.
- Encourage the client to verbalize feelings about self and body image. Have the client make a list of strengths.
- Hold the client responsible for age-appropriate behavior. Involve the client in the planning of self-care.
- Give positive feedback when appropriate self-control is used.
- ▲ Encourage participation in group therapy for building relationship skills and getting feedback from others with regard to behavior.
- Encourage the client to use a daily diary to set achievable and realistic goals and to monitor successes.
- ▲ Refer for rational emotive therapy to help dispel underlying irrational thinking.

## Geriatric

- ▲ Monitor for signs of depression, grief, and withdrawal and make an appropriate referral.
- Address the client by his or her full name preceded by

• = Independent          ▲ = Collaborative

the proper title (Mr., Mrs., Ms., Miss); use a nickname or first name only if suggested by the client, and do not use terms of endearment (e.g., "honey").
- Practice reality-orientation principles; ask specifically how the client feels about events that are happening.
- Ask the client about important past experiences.
▲ If the client's symptoms are associated with a stroke, refer the client for longer rehabilitation that includes physical programs addressing psychological as well as neuromuscular issues.

## Multicultural
- Assess for the influence of cultural beliefs, norms, and values on the family's perceptions of infant/child behavior.
- Use a neutral, indirect style when addressing areas in which improvement is needed (such as a need for verbal or oral stimulation) when working with Native-American clients.
- Acknowledge and praise parenting strengths noted.
- Use therapeutic communication techniques that emphasize acceptance, offer the self, validate the client's concerns, and convey respect.

## Home Care
- The interventions described previously may be adapted for home care use.
- Assess the client's immediate support system and family for relationship patterns and content of communication.
- Encourage the family to provide support and feedback regarding the client's identity and ego boundaries.
▲ If the client is involved in counseling or self-help groups, monitor and encourage attendance. Help the client identify the value of group participation after each group encounter.
▲ If the client is taking prescribed psychotropic medications, assess for understanding of possible side effects

• = Independent        ▲ = Collaborative

and the reasons for taking medication. Teach as
necessary.
▲ Assess medications for effectiveness and side effects and
monitor for compliance.
▲ If the client is homebound, refer for psychiatric home
health care services for client reassurance and implementation of a therapeutic regimen.

## Client/Family Teaching

• Teach stress reduction and relaxation techniques.
▲ Refer to community resources or other self-help groups
appropriate for the client's underlying problem (e.g.,
Adult Children of Alcoholics, parent effectiveness
group).
▲ Refer to appropriate treatment as soon as signs of depression are noted.
• Be a role model for family members: talk to, not around,
the client; give choices to the client when family members may be listening; always address the client by name;
and do not interrupt when the client is attempting to
communicate.

# Functional urinary Incontinence

## NANDA Definition

Impairment or loss of continence due to functional deficits,
including altered mobility, dexterity, or cognition, or environmental barriers

## Defining Characteristics

The relationship between functional limitations and urinary
incontinence remains controversial. While functional impairment clearly exacerbates the severity of urinary incontinence, the
underlying factors that contribute to these functional limitations
themselves contribute to abnormal lower urinary tract function
and impaired continence.

        • = Independent          ▲ = Collaborative

## Related Factors (r/t)

Cognitive disorders (delirium, dementia, severe or profound retardation); neuromuscular limitations impairing mobility or dexterity; environmental barriers to toileting

## Client Outcomes

### Client Will (Specify Time Frame):

- Eliminate or reduce incontinent episodes
- Eliminate or overcome environmental barriers to toileting
- Use adaptive equipment to reduce or eliminate incontinence related to impaired mobility or dexterity
- Use portable urinary collection devices or urine containment devices when access to the toilet is not feasible

## Nursing Interventions

- Perform a history taking and physical assessment focusing on bothersome lower urinary tract symptoms, cognitive status, functional status (particularly physical mobility and dexterity), frequency and severity of leakage episodes, and alleviating and aggravating factors.
- ▲ Consult with the client and family, the client's physician, and other health care professionals concerning treatment of incontinence in the elderly client undergoing detailed geriatric evaluation.
- ▲ Teach the client, the client's care providers, or the client's family to complete a voiding diary (bladder log) by recording voiding frequency, the frequency of urinary incontinent episodes, and their association with urgency (a sudden and strong desire to urinate that is difficult to defer) over a 3- to 7-day period. An electronic voiding diary may be kept whenever feasible. In addition to these parameters, the patient may be asked to record voided volume and fluid intake.
- ▲ Assess the patient for potentially reversible or modifiable causes of acute/transient urinary incontinence (e.g., urinary tract infection; atrophic urethritis; constipation or impaction; use of sedatives or narcotics interfering with the ability to reach the toilet in a timely fashion, anti-

• = Independent          ▲ = Collaborative

depressants or psychotropic medications interfering with efficient detrusor contractions, parasympatholytics, or alpha-adrenergic antagonists; polyuria caused by uncontrolled diabetes mellitus or insipidus).

- Assess the client in an acute care or rehabilitation facility for risk factors for functional incontinence.
- Assess the client for coexisting or premorbid urinary incontinence.
- Assess the home, acute care, or long-term care environment for accessibility to toileting facilities, paying particular attention to the following:
  - Distance of the toilet from the bed, chair, and living quarters
  - Characteristics of the bed, including presence of side rails and distance of the bed from the floor
  - Characteristics of the pathway to the toilet, including barriers such as stairs, loose rugs on the floor, and inadequate lighting
  - Characteristics of the bathroom, including patterns of use, lighting, height of the toilet from the floor, presence of handrails to assist transfers to the toilet, and breadth of the door and its accessibility for a wheelchair, walker, or other assistive device
- Assess the client for mobility, including the ability to rise from chair and bed, transfer to the toilet, and ambulate, and the need for physical assistive devices such as a cane, walker, or wheelchair.
- ▲ Assess the client for dexterity, including the ability to manipulate buttons, hooks, snaps, Velcro, and zippers as needed to remove clothing. Consult a physical or occupational therapist to promote optimal toilet access as indicated.
- Evaluate cognitive status with a Neecham Confusion Scale in cases of acute cognitive change or with a Folstein Mini-Mental State Examination or other tool as indicated.
- Remove environmental barriers to toileting in the acute care, long-term care, or home setting. Assist the client in

● = Independent          ▲ = Collaborative

removing loose rugs from the floor and improving lighting in hallways and bathrooms.

- Provide an appropriate, safe urinary receptacle such as
  a three-in-one commode, female or male handheld urinal, no-spill urinal, or containment device when toileting access is limited by immobility or environmental
  barriers.

▲ Help the client with limited mobility to obtain evaluation
  by a physical therapist and to obtain assistive devices as
  indicated; assist the client in selecting shoes with a
  nonskid sole to maximize traction when arising from a
  chair and transferring to the toilet.

- Assist the client in altering the wardrobe to maximize
  toileting access. Select loose-fitting clothing with stretch
  waistbands rather than buttoned or zippered waist;
  minimize buttons, snaps, and multilayered clothing; and
  substitute Velcro or other easily loosened systems for
  buttons, hooks, and zippers in existing clothing.

- Begin a prompted voiding program or patterned urge response toileting program for the elderly client in the
  home or a long-term care facility who has functional in-
  continence and dementia:
  - Determine the frequency of current urination using an
    alarm system or check-and-change device.
  - Record urinary elimination and incontinent patterns
    in a bladder log to use as a baseline for assessment and
    evaluation of treatment efficacy.
  - Begin a prompted toileting program based on the re-
    sults of this program; toileting frequency may vary
    from every 1.5 to 2 hours to every 4 hours.
  - Praise the client when toileting occurs with
    prompting.
  - Refrain from any socialization when incontinent epi-
    sodes occur; change the client and make her or him
    comfortable.

## Geriatric
- Institute aggressive continence management programs

• = Independent          ▲ = Collaborative

for the cognitively intact, community-dwelling client in consultation with the client and family.
- Monitor the elderly client in a long-term care facility, acute care facility, or home for dehydration.

## Home Care
- The interventions described previously may be adapted for home care use.
- Assess current strategies used to reduce urinary incontinence, including limitation of fluid intake, restriction of bladder irritants, prompted or scheduled toileting, and use of containment devices.
- Encourage a mind-set and program of self-care management.
- Implement a bladder training program, including self-monitoring activities (reducing caffeine intake, adjusting amount and timing of fluid intake, decreasing long voiding intervals while awake, instituting dietary changes to promote bowel regularity), bladder training, and pelvic muscle exercise.
- For a memory-impaired elderly client, implement an individualized scheduled toileting program (on a schedule developed in consultation with the caregiver, approximately every 2 hours, with toileting reminders provided and existing patterns incorporated, such toileting before or after meals).
- Teach the family the general principles of bladder health, including avoidance of bladder irritants, adequate fluid intake, and a routine schedule of toileting (refer to the care plan for **Impaired Urinary elimination**).
- Teach prompted voiding to the family and client for the client with mild to moderate dementia (refer to previous description).
- Teach the principles of perineal skin care to the client or care provider, including routine cleansing following incontinent episodes, daily cleaning and drying of perineal skin, and the use of moisture barriers as indicated.
- Advise the client about the advantages of using dispos-

able or reusable insert pads, pad-pant systems, or replacement briefs specifically designed for urinary incontinence (or double urinary and fecal incontinence) as indicated.

- Assist the family with arranging care in a way that allows the client to participate in family or favorite activities without embarrassment. Elicit discussion of the client's concerns about the social or emotional burden of incontinence.
- ▲ Refer to occupational therapy for help in obtaining assistive devices and adapting the home for optimal toilet accessibility.
- ▲ Consider the use of an indwelling catheter for continuous drainage in the client who is both homebound, bed-bound, or receiving palliative or end-of-life care (requires a physician's order).
- ▲ When an indwelling catheter is in place, follow prescribed maintenance protocols for managing the catheter, drainage bag, perineal skin, and urethral meatus. Teach infection control measures adapted to the home care setting.
- Assist the client in adapting to the catheter. Encourage discussion of the client's response to the catheter.

## Client/Family Teaching

- Work with the client, family, and their extended support systems to assist with needed changes in the environment and wardrobe, and other alterations required to maximize toileting access.
- Work with the client and family to establish a reasonable, manageable, prompted voiding program using environmental and verbal cues to remind caregivers of voiding intervals, such as television programs, meals, and bedtime.
- Teach the family to use an alarm system for toileting or to carry out a check-and-change program and to maintain an accurate log of voiding and incontinence episodes.

• = Independent          ▲ = Collaborative

# Reflex urinary Incontinence

## NANDA Definition

Involuntary loss of urine at somewhat predictable intervals when a specific bladder volume is reached; involuntary loss of urine caused by a defect in the spinal cord between the nerve roots at or below the first cervical segment and those above the second sacral segment; urine elimination occurs at unpredictable intervals; micturition may be elicited by tactile stimuli, including stroking of inner thigh or perineum

## Defining Characteristics

Urinary incontinence caused by neurogenic detrusor overactivity, in which disruption of spinal pathways leads to absent or diminished awareness of the desire to void or the occurrence of an overactive detrusor contraction; incomplete bladder emptying caused by dyssynergia of striated sphincter mechanism, which produces functional outlet obstruction of bladder; reflex urinary incontinence may be associated with sweating and acute elevation in blood pressure and pulse rate in clients with spinal cord injury (see the care plan for **Autonomic dysreflexia**)

## Related Factors (r/t)

Paralyzing spinal disorder affecting spinal segments C1 to S2

## Client Outcomes

### Client Will (Specify Time Frame):

- Follow prescribed schedule for bladder evacuation
- Demonstrate successful use of triggering techniques to stimulate voiding
- Have intact perineal skin
- Remain clear of symptomatic urinary tract infection
- Demonstrate how to apply containment device or insert indwelling catheter or be able to provide caregiver with instructions for performing these procedures
- Demonstrate awareness of risk of autonomic dysreflexia, its prevention and management

• = Independent          ▲ = Collaborative

## Nursing Interventions

- Assess the client's neurological status, including the type of neurological disorder, the functional level of neurological impairment, its completeness (effect on motor and sensory function), and the ability to perform bladder management tasks, including intermittent catheterization, application of a condom catheter, etc.
- Knowledge of functional impairments related to a spinal cord injury (including upper extremity function) is essential because it determines the client's ability to manage the bladder by self-catheterization.
- Perform a focused assessment of the urinary system, including perineal skin integrity.
- Complete a bladder log to determine the pattern of urine elimination, incontinence episodes, and current bladder management program.
- ▲ Consult with the physician concerning current bladder function and the potential of the bladder to produce upper urinary tract distress (hydronephrosis, vesicoureteral reflux, febrile urinary tract infection, or compromised renal function).
- ▲ Determine a bladder management program in consultation with the client, family, and rehabilitation team.
- ▲ In consultation with the rehabilitation team, counsel the client and family concerning the merits and potential risks associated with each possible bladder management program, including spontaneous voiding, intermittent self-catheterization, reflex voiding with condom catheter containment, and indwelling catheterization.
- Teach the client with reflex incontinence to consume an adequate amount of fluids on a daily basis (approximately 30 ml/kg of body weight).
- Advise clients that while consumption of cranberry products or cranberry tablets is in no way harmful or contraindicated, it does not reduce the risk for urinary tract infection.
- Teach the client with reflex urinary incontinence that is managed by spontaneous voiding to self-administer an

• = Independent            ▲ = Collaborative

alpha-adrenergic blocking medication as directed and to recognize and manage potential side effects.

▲ Begin intermittent catheterization using a modified clean or sterile technique based on facility policies.

▲ Teach intermittent catheterization as the client approaches discharge as directed. Instruct the client and at least one family member, spouse, or partner in the performance of catheterization using clean technique. Teach the client with quadriplegia how to instruct others to perform this procedure.

▲ Teach the client managed by intermittent catheterization to self-administer antispasmodic (parasympatholytic) medications as directed, and to recognize and manage potential side effects.

▲ Consult with the physician and occupational therapist concerning the use of a neuroprosthesis or other device designed to improve hand use for the quadriplegic client with partial hand function.

▲ For a male client with reflex incontinence who cannot manage the condition effectively with spontaneous voiding, does not choose to perform intermittent catheterization, or cannot perform catheterization, teach the client and his family to obtain, select, and apply a condom catheter with drainage bag. Assist them in choosing a product that adheres to the penile shaft without allowing seepage of urine onto surrounding skin or clothing, contains a material and adhesive that does not produce hypersensitivity reactions on the skin, and includes a leg bag that is easily concealed under the clothing and does not cause irritation to the skin of the thigh.

• Teach the client who uses a condom catheter to remove the condom device, inspect the skin, cleanse the penis thoroughly, and reapply a new catheter every day.

• Teach the client whose incontinence is managed by a condom catheter to routinely inspect the skin with each catheter change for evidence of lesions caused by pressure from the containment device or by exposure to urine.

• Teach the client managed by intermittent or indwelling

• = Independent        ▲ = Collaborative

catheter to recognize signs of significant urinary tract infection and to seek care promptly when these signs occur. The signs of significant infection are the following:

- Discomfort over the bladder or during urination
- Acute onset of urinary incontinence
- Fever
- Markedly increased spasticity of muscles below the level of the spinal lesion
- Malaise, lethargy
- Hematuria
- Autonomic dysreflexia (hyperreflexia)

## Geriatric

▲ If difficulties are encountered in client teaching, refer the elderly client to a nurse who specializes in care of the aging client with urinary incontinence.

## Home Care

- The interventions described previously may be adapted for home care use.
- Teach the client what the complications of reflex incontinence are and when to report changes to a physician or primary nurse.
- ▲ If the client is taught intermittent self-catheterization, arrange for contingency care in the event that the client is unable to perform self-catheterization.
- Assess and instruct the client and family in care of the catheter and supplies in the home.
- Encourage a mind-set and program of self-care management.
- Assist the family with arranging care in a way that allows the client to participate in family or favorite activities without embarrassment. Elicit discussion of the client's concerns about the social or emotional burden of incontinence.
- ▲ If medications are ordered, instruct the family or caregivers and the client in medication administration, use, and side effects.

• = Independent          ▲ = Collaborative

## Client/Family Teaching

- Teach the client with a spinal injury the signs of autonomic dysreflexia, its relationship to bladder fullness, and management of the condition. (Refer to the care plan for **Autonomic dysreflexia.**)
- Teach the client and several significant others the techniques of intermittent catheterization, indwelling catheter care and removal, or condom catheter management as appropriate.
- Teach the client and family techniques to clean catheters used for intermittent catheterization, including washing with soap and water and allowing to air dry, and using microwave cleaning techniques.

I

# Stress urinary Incontinence

## NANDA Definition

State in which the individual experiences urine loss of less than 50 mL accompanied by increased intra-abdominal pressure
NOTE: The value of less than 50 mL for the volume of urine loss may be exceeded by women and men with severe stress incontinence caused by incompetence of the urethral sphincter mechanism. This is sometimes classified as "total incontinence." In this book, however, "total incontinence" will be used to refer exclusively to incontinence due to extraurethral causes, and all forms of stress incontinence are reviewed under this diagnosis, regardless of severity.

## Defining Characteristics

Observed urine loss with physical exertion (sign of stress incontinence); reported loss of urine associated with physical exertion or activity (symptom of stress incontinence); urine loss associated with increased abdominal pressure (urodynamic stress urinary incontinence)

• = Independent        ▲ = Collaborative

## Related Factors (r/t)

Urethral hypermobility/pelvic organ prolapse (familial predisposition, multiple vaginal deliveries, delivery of infant large for gestational age, forceps-assisted or breech delivery, obesity, changes in estrogen levels at climacteric, extensive abdominopelvic or pelvic surgery)

Urethral sphincter mechanism incompetence (multiple urethral suspensions in women, radical prostatectomy in men, uncommon complication of transurethral prostatectomy or cryosurgery of prostate, spinal lesion affecting sacral segments 2 to 4 or cauda equina, pelvic fracture)

## Client Outcomes

### Client Will (Specify Time Frame):

- Report fewer stress incontinence episodes and/or a decrease in the severity of urine loss
- Experience reduction in grams of urine loss measured objectively by a pad test
- Experience reduction in frequency of urinary incontinence episodes as recorded on voiding diary (bladder log)
- Identify containment devices that assist in management of stress incontinence

## Nursing Interventions

- Take a focused history addressing duration of urinary leakage and related lower urinary tract symptoms, including daytime voiding frequency, urgency, frequency of nocturia, frequency of urinary leakage, and factors provoking urine loss.
- Perform a focused physical assessment, beginning with perineal skin assessment.
- Attempt to reproduce the sign of stress urinary incontinence by asking the client to perform a Valsalva maneuver or to cough while observing the urethral meatus for urine loss.
- Perform a focused pelvic examination including visual in-

spection of the vaginal mucosa, observation of urethral hypermobility and related pelvic floor descent (prolapse), and digital assessment of pelvic floor muscle strength.

- Determine the client's current use of containment devices; evaluate the devices for their ability to adequately contain urine loss, protect clothing, and control odor. Assist the client in identifying containment devices specifically designed to contain urinary leakage.

▲ Teach the client to complete a voiding diary (bladder log) by recording voiding frequency, the frequency of urinary incontinent episodes, and their association with urgency (a sudden and strong desire to urinate that is difficult to defer) over a 3- to 7-day period. An electronic voiding diary may be kept whenever feasible. In addition to these parameters, the client may be asked to record voided volume and fluid intake.

▲ With the client and in close consultation with the physician, review treatment options, including behavioral management; drug therapy; use of a pessary, vaginal device, or urethral insert; and surgery. Outline their potential benefits, efficacy, and side effects.

▲ Assess the client's pelvic muscle strength immediately prior to initiating a pelvic floor muscle rehabilitation using pressure manometry, a digital evaluation technique, or urine stop test.

- Begin a pelvic floor muscle rehabilitation program.

- Teach the client undergoing pelvic muscle rehabilitation to identify, contract, and relax the pelvic floor muscles without contracting distant muscle groups (such as the abdominal muscles) using tactile, audible, or visual biofeedback techniques.

ʼ Incorporate principles of exercise physiology into a pelvic muscle rehabilitation program using the following strategies:

■ Begin a graded exercise program, usually starting with 5 to 10 repetitions and advancing gradually to no more than 35 to 50 repetitions every day or every

• = Independent          ▲ = Collaborative

other day based on baseline and ongoing evaluation of maximal strength and endurance.

- Continue exercise sessions over a period of 3 to 6 months.
- Integrate muscle training into activities of daily living.
- Assess progress every 2 weeks during the first month and every 4 to 6 weeks thereafter.

• Alternatively, the female client may be taught to achieve pelvic muscle rehabilitation using weighted vaginal cones.

▲ Begin transvaginal or transrectal electrical stimulation therapy in selected persons with stress incontinence in consultation with the client and physician.

• Teach the principles of bladder training to women with stress urinary incontinence:

- Assist the client in completing a voiding diary over a period of a minimum of 3 days or up to 7 days.
- Review the results with the client, determining typical voiding frequency and establishing goals for voiding frequency.
- Using baseline voiding frequency, as determined by the diary, teach the client to urinate by the clock when awake, typically every 30 to 120 minutes.
- Encourage adherence to the program with timing devices and verbal encouragement and support, and address individual reasons for schedule interruption.
- Gradually increase the time between urinations to the negotiated goal. Time intervals between voiding are typically increased in increments of 15 to 30 minutes for clients with a baseline frequency of less than every 60 minutes and increments of 25 to 30 minutes for clients with a baseline frequency of more than every 60 minutes.

▲ Teach the client to self-administer alpha-adrenergic agonist medications, imipramine, and topical estrogens as directed.

▲ Refer the female client with stress urinary incontinence

• = Independent          ▲ = Collaborative

and pelvic organ prolapse who wishes to employ a pessary, vaginal device, or urethral insert to manage stress incontinence to a nurse specialist or gynecologist with expertise in the placement and maintenance of these devices.

- Discuss potentially reversible or controllable risk factors with the client with stress incontinence and assist the client to formulate a strategy to alleviate or eliminate these conditions.
▲ Provide information about support resources such as the Simon Foundation for Continence or the National Foundation for Continence.
▲ Refer the client with persistent stress incontinence to a continence service, physician, or nurse who specializes in the management of this condition.

### Geriatric
- Evaluate the elderly client's functional and cognitive status to determine the impact of functional limitations on the frequency and severity of urine loss and on plans for management.

### Home Care
- The interventions described previously may be adapted for home care use.
- Elicit discussion of the client's concerns about the social or emotional burden of stress incontinence.
- Encourage a mind-set and program of self-care management.
- Implement a bladder training program, including self-monitoring activities (reducing caffeine intake, adjusting amount and timing of fluid intake, decreasing long voiding intervals while awake, making dietary changes to promote bowel regularity), bladder training, and pelvic muscle exercise.
▲ Consider the use of an indwelling catheter for continuous drainage in the client with severe stress urinary incontinence who is homebound, bed-bound, or receiv-

• = Independent          ▲ = Collaborative

ing palliative or end-of-life care (requires a physician's order).

▲ When an indwelling catheter is in place, follow the prescribed maintenance protocols for managing the catheter, drainage bag, and perineal skin and urethral meatus. Teach infection control measures adapted to the home care setting.

• Assist the client in adapting to the catheter. Encourage discussion of the client's response to the catheter.

• Begin a program of pelvic muscle rehabilitation in the homebound elderly client who is motivated to adhere to the program and has adequate cognitive function to understand and follow instructions.

## Client/Family Teaching

• Teach the client to perform pelvic muscle exercise using an audiotape or videotape if indicated.

• Teach the client the importance of avoiding dehydration and instruct the client to consume fluid at the rate of 30 mL/kg of body weight daily ($1/2$ ounce per pound per day).

• Teach the client the importance of avoiding constipation by a combination of adequate fluid intake, adequate intake of dietary fiber, and exercise.

• Teach the client to apply and remove support devices such as a urethral insert.

• Teach the client to select and apply urine containment devices.

# Total urinary Incontinence

## NANDA Definition

State in which the individual experiences continuous and unpredictable loss of urine

NOTE: In this book, the diagnosis **Total urinary Incontinence**

• = Independent          ▲ = Collaborative

will be used to refer to continuous urine loss due to an extraurethral cause, and the diagnosis **Stress urinary Incontinence** will be used to refer to leakage caused by urethral sphincter incompetence, regardless of severity.

## Defining Characteristics

Continuous urine flow varying from dribbling incontinence superimposed on an otherwise identifiable pattern of voiding to severe urine loss without identifiable micturition episodes

## Related Factors (r/t)

Ectopia (ectopic ureter opens into vaginal vault or cutaneously; bladder ectopia with exstrophy/epispadias complex); fistula (opening from bladder or urethra to vagina or skin that bypasses urethral sphincter mechanism, allowing continuous urine loss)

## Client Outcomes

**Client Will (Specify Time Frame):**

- Experience urine loss that is adequately contained, with clothing remaining unsoiled and odor controlled
- Maintain intact perineal skin
- Maintain dignity, hide urine containment device in clothing, and minimize bulk and noise related to device

## Nursing Interventions

- Obtain a history of the duration and severity of urine loss, prior management, and aggravating or alleviating features.
- ▲ Perform a focused physical assessment, including inspection of the perineal skin, examination of the vaginal vault, reproduction of the sign of stress incontinence (refer to the care plan for **Stress urinary Incontinence**), and testing of bulbocavernosus reflex and perineal sensations.
- ▲ Consult a physician concerning the results of colposcopy, cystourethroscopy, intravenous urogram, cystogram, Pyridium pad test, or pelvic examination.
- Assist the client in selecting and applying a urine con-

• = Independent          ▲ = Collaborative

tainment device(s). Review types of containment products with the client, including advantages and potential complications associated with each type of product.

- Evaluate disposable vs. reusable products for urine containment, considering the setting (home care vs. acute care vs. long-term care), preferences of the client and care-giver(s), and immediate vs. long-term costs.

- Cleanse the perineal skin regularly using a cleanser capable of removing irritants (including urine, stool, and materials). Select a product with a slightly acidic pH close to that of normal skin, with a water base and surfactant designed to remove irritants from the skin with minimal physical force. Avoid vigorous scrubbing with water, soap and a washcloth. Consider selection of a product with a moisturizer.

- Apply a moisture barrier containing dimethicone or zinc oxide to clients with severe urinary incontinence or those with double urinary and fecal incontinence.

- When cleansing a client with a moisture barrier containing zinc oxide, avoid vigorous scrubbing or use of a traditional washcloth to remove the paste. Instead, cleanse fecal materials away from the skin, leaving a clean layer of zinc oxide paste when cleansing after a single episode or gently removing the paste with mineral oil.

▲ Consult the physician concerning use of a moisture barrier with active healing ingredients when perineal dermatitis exists. In addition, an antifungal powder may be applied underneath the ointment when perineal dermatitis is complicated by monilial infection. Teach the client to use the product sparingly when applying to affected areas.

▲ Consult the physician concerning placement of an indwelling catheter when severe urine loss is complicated by urinary retention, when careful fluid monitoring is indicated, when perineal dryness is required to promote healing of a stage 3 or 4 pressure ulcer, during periods of critical illness, or in the terminally ill client when use of absorbent products produces pain or distress.

▲ Refer the client with "intractable" or extraurethral incon-

I

• = Independent          ▲ = Collaborative

tinence to a continence service or specialist for further
evaluation and management of urine loss.

### Geriatric

- Provide privacy and support when changing incontinent
  devices in elderly clients.
- Avoid brisk scrubbing and use of a washcloth when
  cleansing the skin of an aging client.
- Employ meticulous infection control procedures when
  using an indwelling catheter.

### Home Care

- The interventions described previously may be adapted
  for home care use.
- Encourage a mind-set and program of self-care
  management.
- Assist the family with arranging care in a way that allows
  the client to participate in family or favorite activities
  without embarrassment. Elicit discussion of the client's
  concerns about the social or emotional burden of
  incontinence.
- ▲ Consider the use of an indwelling catheter for continuous drainage in the client with severe urinary incontinence who is homebound, bed-bound, or receiving palliative or end-of-life care (requires a physician's order).
- ▲ When an indwelling catheter is in place, follow the prescribed maintenance protocols for managing the catheter,
  drainage bag, and perineal skin and urethral meatus.
  Teach infection control measures adapted to the home
  care setting.
- Assist the client in adapting to the catheter. Encourage
  discussion of the client's response to the catheter.

### Client/Family Teaching

- Teach the family to obtain, apply, and dispose of or clean
  and reuse urine containment devices.
- Teach the family a routine perineal skin care regimen,
  including daily or every other day hygiene and cleansing
  with containment product changes.

• = Independent          ▲ = Collaborative

- Teach the client and family to recognize and manage perineal dermatitis, ammonia contact dermatitis, and monilial rash.
- Teach the client to maintain adequate fluid intake (30 mL/kg of body weight per day).
- Teach the client and family to recognize and manage urinary tract infection.

# Urge urinary Incontinence

## NANDA Definition

State in which the individual experiences involuntary passage of urine occurring with precipitous desire to urinate; urge incontinence is defined within the context of overactive bladder syndrome; the overactive bladder is characterized by bothersome urgency (a sudden and strong desire to urinate that is not easily deferred); overactive bladder is typically associated with frequent daytime voiding and nocturia, and approximately 37% will experience urge incontinence

### Defining Characteristics

Diurnal urinary frequency (voiding more than once every 2 hours while awake); nocturia (awakening 3 or more times per night to urinate; voiding more than 8 times within a 24-hour period as recorded on a voiding diary (bladder log); bothersome urgency (a sudden and strong desire to urinate that is not easily deferred); symptom of urge incontinence (urine loss associated with desire to urinate); enuresis (involuntary passage of urine while asleep)

### Related Factors

- Neurological disorders (brain disorders, including cerebrovascular accident, brain tumor, normal pressure hydrocephalus, traumatic brain injury)
- Inflammation of bladder (calculi; tumor, including transitional cell carcinoma and carcinoma in situ; inflammatory lesions of the bladder; urinary tract infection)

• = Independent          ▲ = Collaborative

- Bladder outlet obstruction (see **Urinary retention**)
- Stress urinary incontinence (mixed urinary incontinence; these conditions often coexist but relationship between them remains unclear)
- Idiopathic causes (implicated factors include depression, sleep apnea/hypoxia)

## Client Outcomes

### Client Will (Specify Time Frame):

- Report relief from urge urinary incontinence or a decrease in the incidence or severity of incontinent episodes
- Identify containment devices that assist in the management of urge urinary incontinence

## Nursing Interventions

- Take a nursing history focusing on duration of urinary incontinence, diurnal frequency, nocturia, severity of symptoms, and alleviating and aggravating factors.
- Perform a focused physical assessment, beginning with perineal skin assessment.
- ▲ Perform a focused pelvic examination including visual inspection of the vaginal mucosa, observation of urethral hypermobility and related pelvic floor descent (prolapse) and digital assessment of pelvic floor muscle strength. Assist the woman with moderately severe to severe vaginal wall prolapse (descent to or beyond the introitus) to a female urologist or urogynecologist.
- ▲ Complete a urinalysis, examining for the presence of nitrites, leukocytes, glucose, or hemoglobin (red blood cells).
- ▲ Teach the client to complete a voiding diary (bladder log) by recording voiding frequency, the frequency of urinary incontinent episodes, and their association with urgency (a sudden and strong desire to urinate that is difficult to defer) over a 3- to 7-day period. An electronic voiding diary may be kept whenever feasible. In addition to these parameters, the client may be asked to record voided volume and fluid intake.

• = Independent          ▲ = Collaborative

▲ Review all medications the client is receiving, paying particular attention to sedatives, narcotics, diuretics, antidepressants, psychotropic drugs, and cholinergics. Consult the physician or nurse practitioner about altering or eliminating these medications if they are suspected of affecting incontinence.

• Assess the client for urinary retention (see the care plan for **Urinary retention**).

• Assess the client for functional limitations (environmental barriers, limited mobility or dexterity, impaired cognitive function (see the care plan for **Functional urinary Incontinence**).

▲ Consult the physician concerning diabetic management and pharmacotherapy for urinary tract infection when indicated.

▲ Assess for signs and symptoms of atrophic vaginal changes in the perimenopausal or postmenopausal woman, including vaginal dryness, tenderness to touch, mucosal dryness, friability, and discomfort with gentle palpation. Specifically query the woman with atrophic vaginitis concerning associated lower urinary tract symptoms (usually voiding frequency, urgency, and dysuria). Refer the woman with atrophic vaginal changes and bothersome lower urinary tract symptoms to a gynecologist, urologist, or women's health nurse-practitioner for further evaluation and management.

• Teach the principles of bladder training to women with urge urinary incontinence.

   ■ Assist the client in completing a voiding diary over a period of a minimum of 3 days or up to 7 days.

   ■ Review the results with the client, determining typical voiding frequency and establishing goals for voiding frequency.

   ■ Using baseline voiding frequency, as determined by the diary, teach the client to urinate by the clock when awake, typically every 30 to 120 minutes.

   ■ Encourage adherence to the program with timing devices and verbal encouragement and support, and address individual reasons for schedule interruption.

• = Independent          ▲ = Collaborative

■ Gradually increase the time between urinations to the negotiated goal. Time intervals between voiding are typically increased in increments of 15 to 30 minutes for clients with a baseline frequency of less than every 60 minutes and increments of 25 to 30 minutes for clients with a baseline frequency of more than every 60 minutes.

- Review with the client the types of beverages consumed, focusing on the intake of bladder irritants, including caffeine and alcohol.

- Review with the client the volume of fluids consumed and gradually adjust the fluid intake to meet the Adequate Intake recommendation of 3 liters for the 19- to 30-year-old male and 2.2 liters for the 19- to 30-year-old female. Water balance studies suggest that adult men require 2.5 liters per day.

- Instruct in techniques of urge suppression. Teach the client to identify, isolate, contract, and relax the pelvic floor muscles. When a strong or precipitous urge to urinate is perceived, teach the client to avoid running to the toilet. Instead, she or he should perform repeated, rapid pelvic muscle contractions until the urge is relieved. Relief is followed by micturition within 5 to 15 minutes, using nonhurried movements when locating a toilet and voiding.

▲ Begin transvaginal or transrectal electrical stimulation using a low-frequency current (5 to 20 Hz) in consultation with the physician.

▲ Teach the client to self-administer antimuscarinic (anticholinergic) drugs as directed. Teach dosage and administration of the medication and the importance of combining pharmacotherapy with scheduled voiding, adequate fluid intake, restriction of bladder irritants, and urge suppression techniques.

▲ Assist the client in selecting, obtaining, and applying a containment device for urine loss as indicated (see the care plan for **Total urinary Incontinence**).

▲ Provide the client with information about incontinence

● = Independent          ▲ = Collaborative

support groups such as the National Association for
Continence and the Simon Foundation for Continence.

## Geriatric

- Assess the functional and cognitive status of the elderly
  client with urge incontinence.
- Plan care in long-term or acute care facilities based on
  knowledge of the elderly client's established voiding patterns, paying particular attention to patterns of nocturia.
- ▲ Carefully monitor the elderly client for potential adverse
  effects of antispasmodic medications, including a severely dry mouth interfering with the use of dentures,
  eating, or speaking, or confusion, nightmares, constipation, mydriasis, or heat intolerance.

## Home Care

- The interventions described previously may be adapted
  for home care use.
- Teach the importance of avoiding dehydration or excessive fluid consumption and the paradoxical relationship between dehydration and symptoms of urgency.
- Teach the family and client to identify and correct environmental barriers to toileting within the home.
- Encourage a mind-set and program of self-care
  management.
- Implement a bladder training program as appropriate,
  including self-monitoring activities (reducing caffeine intake, adjusting amount and timing of fluid intake, decreasing long voiding intervals while awake, making dietary changes to promote bowel regularity), bladder
  training, and pelvic muscle exercise.
- Help the client and family to identify and correct environmental barriers to toileting within the home.

## Client/Family Teaching

- Teach the client and family to recognize foods and beverages that are likely to irritate the bladder.
- Teach the family and client to recognize and manage side

• = Independent          ▲ = Collaborative

effects of antispasmodic medications used to treat urge incontinence.

- Help the client and family to recognize and manage side effect of anticholinergic medications used to manage irritative lower urinary tract symptoms.

# Risk for urge urinary Incontinence

## NANDA Definition

At risk for involuntary loss of urine associated with a sudden, strong sensation of urinary urgency

## Risk Factors

Overactive bladder dysfunction with associated detrusor overactivity; inflammation from urinary tract infection; inflammatory lesion; bladder to lower ureteral stone; bladder outlet obstruction; dietary risk factors; consumption of caffeine
NOTE: Overactive bladder is a symptom syndrome characterized by bothersome urgency (a sudden and strong desire to urinate that is not easily deferred) that is typically associated with day and nighttime voiding frequency (more than 8 urinations per day). While urge urinary incontinence affects approximately 37% of clients with overactive bladder, 63% have an identifiable condition that is not adequately described by this diagnosis. It is hoped that "risk for urge urinary incontinence" will evolve in a manner that more clearly describes the underlying syndrome, overactive bladder.

## Client Outcomes

### Client Will (Specify Time Frame):

- Report relief from urge urinary incontinence or a decrease in the incidence or severity of incontinent episodes
- Identify containment devices that assist in the management of urge urinary incontinence

• = Independent          ▲ = Collaborative

## Nursing Interventions

- Take a nursing history focusing on the following lower urinary tract symptoms: daytime voiding frequency, nocturia, presence of bothersome urgency (precipitous desire to urinate that interferes with activities of daily living), and presence of urine loss.
- Query the client about specific risk factors for urge urinary incontinence, such as childhood enuresis, depression, prostate enlargement with bladder outlet obstruction, and neurological disorders, including stroke or parkinsonism.
- Assess the client's functional status, focusing on mobility, dexterity, and cognitive status.
- ▲ Complete a urinalysis, focusing on the presence of nitrites, leukocytes, glucose, or hemoglobin (red blood cells).
- ▲ Teach the client to complete a voiding diary (bladder log) by recording voiding frequency, the frequency of urgency episodes over a 3- to 7-day period. An electronic voiding diary may be kept whenever feasible. In addition to these parameters, the client may be asked to record voided volume and fluid intake.
- Advise all clients to reduce or eliminate intake of caffeinated beverages or over-the-counter medications of dietary aids containing caffeine.
- Advise community-dwelling men that moderate consumption of beer may reduce the risk of developing overactive bladder dysfunction and the associated risk for urge urinary incontinence.
- Advise community-dwelling women that intake of a balanced diet, and supplementation of vitamin D to ensure meeting daily recommended allowances may reduce the risk of developing overactive bladder dysfunction and the associated risk for urge urinary incontinence.
- Additional bladder irritants, including aspartame, carbonated drinks, decaffeinated coffee or tea, citrus juices, highly spiced foods, chocolates, and vinegar-containing foods, may be eliminated from the diet and

• = Independent ▲ = Collaborative

added back singly to determine their impact on lower
urinary tract symptoms and urgency.

- Review with the client the volume of fluids consumed
and gradually adjust the fluid intake to meet the Adequate Intake recommendation of 3 liters for the 19-
to 30-year-old male and 2.2 liters for the 19- to 30-year-
old female. Water balance studies suggest that adult
men require 2.5 liters per day.

▲ Review all medications the client is receiving, paying particular attention to sedatives, narcotics, diuretics, antidepressants, psychotropic drugs, and cholinergics. Consult the physician about altering or eliminating these
medications if they are suspected of affecting
incontinence.

▲ Consult the physician concerning diabetic management
and pharmacotherapy for urinary tract infection when
indicated.

▲ Assess for signs and symptoms of atrophic vaginal
changes in the perimenopausal or postmenopausal
woman, including vaginal dryness, tenderness to touch,
dryness of mucosa on touch with friability, and discomfort with gentle palpation. Specifically query the client with atrophic vaginitis concerning associated lower
urinary tract symptoms (voiding frequency, urgency or
dysuria). Refer the client with atrophic vaginal
changes and bothersome lower urinary tract symptoms to
a gynecologist, urologist, or women's health nurse-
practitioner for further evaluation and management.

- Teach clients techniques of bladder training and pelvic
muscle rehabilitation focusing on urge suppression.

- Provide the client with information about incontinence
support groups such as the National Association for
Continence and the Simon Foundation for Continence

## Geriatric

- Assess the functional and cognitive status of an elderly
client with irritative lower urinary tract symptoms or urge
incontinence.

▲ Advise a male client with bothersome lower urinary tract

• = Independent          ▲ = Collaborative

symptoms to see his physician or nurse-practitioner, since these symptoms may be related to prostate enlargement.

▲ Carefully monitor the elderly client for potential adverse effects of anticholinergic medications, including severe dry mouth interfering with the use of dentures, eating, or speaking, or the occurrence of confusion, nightmares, constipation, mydriasis, or heat intolerance.

## Home Care

- The interventions described previously may be adapted for home care use.
- Encourage a mind-set and program of self-care management.
- Implement a bladder training program, including self-monitoring activities (reducing caffeine intake, adjusting amount and timing of fluid intake, decreasing long voiding intervals while awake, making dietary changes to promote bowel regularity), bladder training, and pelvic muscle exercise.
- Teach the client and family to recognize foods and beverages that are likely to irritate the bladder.
- Teach the importance of avoiding dehydration or excessive fluid consumption and the paradoxical relationship between dehydration and symptoms of urgency.
▲ Teach the family and client to recognize and manage side effects of anticholinergic medications used to treat irritative lower urinary tract symptoms.
- Teach the family and client to identify and correct environmental barriers to toileting within the home.
- Assist the family with arranging care in a way that allows the client to participate in family or favorite activities without embarrassment. Elicit discussion of the client's concerns about the social or emotional burden of incontinence.

## Client/Family Teaching

- Teach the client and family to recognize foods and beverages that are likely to irritate the bladder.

• = Independent          ▲ = Collaborative

- Teach the importance of avoiding dehydration or excessive fluid consumption and the paradoxical relationship between dehydration and symptoms of urgency.

## Disorganized Infant behavior

### NANDA Definition

Disintegrated physiological and neurobehavioral responses to the environment; A state of being of the infant/child displaying altered regulation, and modulation of the physiological and behavior subsystems of functioning (i.e., autonomic, motor, state, self-regulatory, and attention-interaction systems) that impairs the infant's ability of achieving homeostasis and interacting with the environment in an organized, adaptive way

### Defining Characteristics

#### Physiological/Autonomic

*Cardiorespiratory:* Bradycardia <100, tachycardia >180, tachypnea >60, dysrhythmias; irregular respirations, pauses, apnea, nasal flaring, chest retractions; skin color—rapid change, pale, mottled, dusky, perioral/periorbital duskiness, cyanotic; stress cues—gaze averting, hiccoughing, coughing, sneezing, sighing, drawn face, slack jaw, open mouth, tongue thrust; oxygen desaturation

*Visceral:* feeding intolerances; coughing; gagging; emesis; vomiting; hiccoughing; bowel straining; bowel movement with stress

*Neuromotor:* tremors; tremulous, excessive startles; twitches; jitteriness; seizures; coughing; sneezing

#### Motor System

*Hyper/increased tone:* frantic/disorganized movements; arching; finger splays; rapid extensions and flexions of arms/legs; facial grimaces

*Hypo/decreased tone:* flaccid/limp; drawn face; body squirming; uncoordinated and purposeless movements

• = Independent            ▲ = Collaborative

## State-Organization System

*Diffuse/disorganized sleep:* difficulty falling asleep, maintaining quiet/deep sleep; frequent awakening; frequent body movements; irregular respirations; whimpering

*Diffuse/disorganized arousal and awake state:* hyper-aroused, irritable, fussy, restless; infrequent quiet awake state; dull facial expression, glassy eyes, floating eyes, worried-panic look

*Rapid state oscillations:* difficulty transitioning between states; jumps from sleep to cry and cry to sleep

## Self-Regulation System

*Deficient and/or ineffective self-regulatory capabilities:* common behaviors include: hands to mouth, hand grasping/clasping, foot/leg bracing, sucking efforts, tucking body, hyperattending to visual and/or auditory stimuli used effectively to regain or maintain control

## Attention-Interaction System

*Attention:* difficulty achieving and maintaining focus attention to orient to visual and auditory sensory stimuli

*Interactional:* difficulty engaging in social interactions; easily stressed communicating avoidance/stress behaviors (e.g., gaze aversion, arching, fussing, irritable, turning away, finger splays leading to physiologic/autonomic indices); easily stressed with more than one type of sensory stimuli (visual, auditory, tactile, movement)

## Related Factors (r/t)

### Prenatal

Congenital or genetic disorders; congenital infections; perinatal asphyxia; central nervous system insult; maternal illness (uncontrolled diabetes, mental illness); maternal substance exposure (drugs, alcohol); poor maternal nutrition, excessive maternal smoking

### Postnatal

Immature central nervous system; prematurity; small for gestational age (SGA); malnutrition; neurological and/or neuromotor problems; oral motor problems resulting in feeding problems/

• = Independent          ▲ = Collaborative

intolerances; internal stress (pain, gastrointestinal, respiratory problems, etc.); external stress (invasive and painful procedures, inadequately pain medicated, medical illness, environmental stressors, etc.)

## Individual
Medical illness; immature physiological and/or neurological systems; prematurity; unclear cues communicating "hunger," "satiety," attention and consoling needs; sensory integration problems resulting in over- and/or underreactions to sensations (sights/visual, sounds/auditory, touch/tactile, and vestibular/movement); separated from parents; isolation during quiet awake times; imbalance between nurturing touch and task/procedure touch

## Environmental
Transition to extrauterine life creates challenges for preterm infants struggling to maintain previously organized patterns of functioning and experiencing non-contingent, non-reciprocal stimulation within the environment; imbalance between sensory overstimulation and sensory deprivation; hospitalization, care practices non-contingent with infant's state and behavior cues, frequent sleep interruptions

## Caregiver
Misreading or insensitive to infant's cues; cue deficient knowledge; mismatch between infant/child cues and contingent responding; lack of warmth and pleasure in caregiver's voice; negative mood; unable to successfully console and relieve the infant's distress; does not engage with and display interest in the infant; environmental stimulation contribution

## Client Outcomes

**Client Will (Specify Time Frame):**

### Infant/Child
- Display clear behavior cues that communicate approach/engagement and stress/avoidance engagement needs

        • = Independent          ▲ = Collaborative

- Display organized and physiologic/autonomic stability: cardiorespiratory, visceral, and neuromotor
- Display organized motor system: balance between flexion and extension, smooth, synchronous, and purposeful movements
- Display state organizational stability: robust sleep and awake states, ability to maintain organized sleep and awake states, smooth transition between sleep and awake states
- Demonstrate progress to and effective self-regulation: displays range of self-regulatory behaviors that facilitate regulation
- Demonstrate ability to effectively orally feed
- Demonstrate ability to process, organize and respond to sensory information sights/vision, sounds/auditory, touch/tactile), movement/vestibular in an adaptive way
- Demonstrate ability to engage in pleasurable parent/caregiver-infant/child interactions

## Parents/Significant Other
- Recognize infant/child behaviors as a unique way of communicating needs and goals
- Recognize infant behaviors used to communicate stress/avoidance and disengagement and approach/engagement.
- Recognize and support infant's/child's drive and coping behaviors used to self-regulate
- Demonstrate ways to facilitate state modulation and organization
- Read and sensitively respond to infant/child behavior cues and needs
- Recognize how their style of interactions can positively or negatively affect the infant's/child's responses and allow the infant/child to take the lead and by following his or her lead will foster adaptive communication patterns
- Structure and modify the environment in response to infant/child's behaviors, personal, nurturing, medical and sensory needs
- Identify appropriate positioning and handling techniques that enhance motor organization, comfort, normal development and prevent positioning-acquired abnormalities

• = Independent            ▲ = Collaborative

- Promote infant's/child's attention capabilities to orient and process sensory information (visual, auditory, tactile, vestibular/movement)
- Engage in pleasurable parent-infant/child interactions that encourage bonding and attachment
- Identify available community resources that provide early intervention services, community health nursing, parenting information and parent-to-parent support

## Nursing Interventions

- Identify infant's/child's behavioral organization as his or her unique way of communicating in five subsystems of functioning (i.e., physiological/autonomic, motor, state, self-regulation, attention-interactional).
- Provide individualized developmental care for low-birthweight, preterm infants that positively influences neurodevelopmental functioning, parenting competence, and reduces the severity of medical illnesses.
- Recognize behavior used to communicate stress/avoidance/disengagement and approach/engagement.
- Identify and support the infant's/child's use of self-regulatory/consoling and habituation behaviors needed for mastering the environment.
- Demonstrate ways to facilitate state organization and control.
- Cluster care whenever possible allowing for longer periods of uninterrupted sleep.
- Correlate stress/disorganization behaviors to internal factors (e.g., pain, hunger, discomfort) and/or external factors (e.g., lights, noise, handling).
- Structure and organize the environment.
- Identify appropriate position and handling techniques that enhance motor organization, comfort, and normal development and prevent positioning-acquired abnormalities.
- Provide lots of opportunities for physical closeness, loving touch, massaging, cuddling, skin to-skin (Kangaroo Care) and rocking.

• = Independent          ▲ = Collaborative

- Encourage parents' competence by praising their parenting strengths and capabilities when caring for their infants.
- Identify and support infant's/child's attention capabilities.
- Provide opportunities for parent/caregiver to engage in pleasurable parent-infant interactions contingent with infant cue responses; begin slowly and introduce one sensory stimulus at a time—looking, then slowly begin talking softly, adding gentle touch; if infant remains stable, swaddle and slowly pick up. Assess and respond contingently to infant cues.
- Provide pleasurable sensory motor experiences (i.e., visual, auditory, tactile, vestibular/movement, proprioceptive) that enhance development of sensory pathways.
- Knowledge of community-based follow-up programs for preterm and infants at risk and their families discharged from the NICU.

## Multicultural

- Assess for the influence of cultural beliefs, norms, and values on the family's perceptions of infant/child behavior.
- Use a neutral, indirect style when addressing areas where improvement is needed (such as a need for verbal or oral stimulation) when working with Native-American clients.
- Acknowledge and praise parenting strengths noted.
- Use therapeutic communication techniques that emphasize acceptance, offer the self, validate the client's concerns, and convey respect when discussing the infant/child behavior.

## Home Care

- Above interventions may be adapted for home care use.
- Educate families in preparing home environment.
- Prepare families for realistic challenges of caring for preterm and at risk infants prior to discharge. Differences include: understanding "corrected" age, feeding

• = Independent          ▲ = Collaborative

skills, poor endurance/tires easily, shorter sleep-wake cycles, less alert and more fussy when awake, fussy before returning to sleep, overstimulation, etc.

- Encourage families to teach friends/visitors to recognize and respond to infant's unique behavioral cues.
- Provide information of community resources, developmental follow-up services, and parent-to-parent support programs.

## Family Teaching

- Assist families/support systems in recognizing and responding to infant's unique behavioral cues.
- Give anticipatory guidance to parents about what infant/child behaviors are possible in given situations.
- Model calming interventions to provide parents with tools for positive interactions with their infant/child
- Nurture parents so that they in turn can nurture their infant/child.
- Establish a nurturing environment in which parents can interact with their infant/child
- Have knowledge of community early intervention services and follow-up programs for preterm and at risk infants and families.

# Risk for disorganized Infant behavior

## NANDA Definition

Disintegrated physiological and neurobehavioral responses to the environment, a state of being of the infant/child displaying altered regulation, and modulation of the physiological and behavior subsystems of functioning (i.e., autonomic, motor, state, self–regulatory, and attention-interaction systems) that impairs the infant's ability of achieving homeostasis and interacting with the environment in an organized, adaptive way

• = Independent          ▲ = Collaborative

## Defining Characteristics

### Physiological/Autonomic

*Cardiorespiratory:* bradycardia <100, tachycardia >180, tachypnea >60, dysrhythmias; irregular respirations, pauses, apnea, nasal flaring, chest retractions; skin color—rapid change, pale, mottled, dusky, perioral/periorbital duskiness, cyanotic; stress cues—gaze averting, hiccoughing, coughing, sneezing, sighing, drawn face, slack jaw, open mouth, tongue thrust); oxygen desaturation

*Visceral:* feeding intolerances; coughing; gagging; emesis; vomiting; hiccoughing; bowel straining; bowel movement with stress

*Neuromotor:* tremors; tremulous, excessive startles; twitches; jitteriness; seizures; coughing; sneezing

### Motor System

*Hyper/increased tone:* frantic/disorganized movements; arching; finger splays; rapid extensions and flexions of arms/legs; facial grimaces

*Hypo/decreased tone:* flaccid/limp; drawn face; body squirming; uncoordinated and purposeless movements

### State-Organization System

*Diffuse/disorganized sleep:* difficulty falling asleep, maintaining quiet/deep sleep; frequent awakening; frequent body movements; irregular respirations; whimpering

*Diffuse/disorganized arousal and awake state:* hyper-aroused, irritable, fussy, restless; infrequent quiet awake state; dull facial expression, glassy eyes, floating eyes, worried-panic look

*Rapid state oscillations:* difficulty transitioning between states; jumps from sleep to cry and cry to sleep

### Self-Regulation System

*Deficient and/or ineffective self-regulatory capabilities:* common behaviors include: hands to mouth, hand grasping/clasping, foot/leg bracing, sucking efforts, tucking body, hyper-attending to visual and/or auditory stimuli used effectively to regain or maintain control

● = Independent          ▲ = Collaborative

## Attention-Interaction System

*Attention:* difficulty achieving and maintaining focus attention to orient to visual and auditory sensory stimuli

*Interaction:* difficulty engaging in social interactions; easily stressed communicating avoidance/stress behaviors (e.g., gaze aversion, arching, fussing, irritable, turning away), finger splays leading to physiologic/autonomic indices, easily stressed with more than one type of sensory stimuli (visual, auditory, tactile, movement)

## Related Factors (r/t)

### Prenatal

Congenital or genetic disorders; congenital infections; perinatal asphyxia; central nervous system insult; maternal illness (uncontrolled diabetes, mental illness); maternal substance exposure (drugs, alcohol); poor maternal nutrition, excessive maternal smoking

### Postnatal

Immature central nervous system; prematurity; small for gestational age (SGA); malnutrition; neurological and/or neuromotor problems; oral motor problems resulting in feeding problems/intolerances; internal stress (pain, gastrointestional, respiratory problems, etc.); external stress (invasive and painful procedures, inadequately pain medicated, medical illness, environmental stressors, etc.)

### Individual

Medical illness; immature physiological and/or neurological systems; prematurity; unclear cues communicating "hunger," "satiety," attention and consoling needs; sensory integration problems resulting in over- and/or underreactions to sensations (sights/visual, sounds/auditory, touch/tactile, and vestibular/movement); separated from parents; isolation during quiet awake times; imbalance between nurturing touch and task/procedure touch

### Environmental

Transition to extrauterine life creates challenges for preterm

• = Independent          ▲ = Collaborative

infants struggling to maintain previously organized patterns of functioning and experiencing non-contingent, non-reciprocal stimulation within the environment; imbalance between sensory overstimulation and sensory deprivation; hospitalization, care practices non-contingent with infant's state and behavior cues, frequent sleep interruptions

## Caregiver

Misreading or insensitive to infant's cues; cue deficient knowledge; mismatch between infant/child cues and contingent responding; lack of warmth and pleasure in caregiver's voice; negative mood; unable to successfully console and relieve the infant's distress; does not engage with and display interest in the infant; environmental stimulation contribution

## Client Outcomes

### Client Will (Specify Time Frame):

### Infant/Child

- Display clear behavior cues that communicate approach/engagement and stress/avoidance engagement needs
- Display organized and physiologic/autonomic stability: cardiorespiratory, visceral, and neuromotor
- Display organized motor system: balance between flexion and extension, smooth, synchronous, and purposeful movements
- Display state organizational stability: robust sleep and awake states, ability to maintain organized sleep and awake states, smooth transition between sleep and awake states
- Demonstrate progress to and effective self-regulation: displays range of self-regulatory behaviors that facilitate regulation
- Demonstrate ability to effectively orally feed
- Demonstrate ability to process, organize, and respond to sensory information sights/vision, sounds/auditory, touch/tactile), movement/vestibular in an adaptive way
- Demonstrate ability to engage in pleasurable parent/caregiver-infant/child interactions

• = Independent          ▲ = Collaborative

## Parents/Significant Other

- Recognize infant/child behaviors as a unique way of communicating needs and goals
- Recognize infant behaviors used to communicate stress/avoidance and disengagement and approach/engagement
- Recognize and support infant's/child's drive and coping behaviors used to self-regulate
- Demonstrate ways to facilitate state modulation and organization
- Read and sensitively respond to infant/child behavior cues and needs
- Recognize how their style of interactions can positively or negatively affect the infant's/child's responses and allow the infant/child to take the lead and by following his or her lead will foster adaptive communication patterns
- Structure and modify the environment in response to infant's/child's behaviors, personal, nurturing, medical and sensory needs
- Identify appropriate positioning and handling techniques that enhance motor organization, comfort, normal development and prevent positioning-acquired abnormalities
- Promote infant's/child's attention capabilities to orient and process sensory information (visual, auditory, tactile, vestibular/movement)
- Engage in pleasurable parent-infant/child interactions that encourage bonding and attachment
- Identify available community resources that provide early intervention services, community health nursing, parenting information and parent-to-parent support

## Nursing Interventions

- Identify infant's/child's behavioral organization as his or her unique way of communicating in five subsystems of functioning (i.e., physiological/autonomic, motor, state, self-regulation, attention-interactional).
- Provide individualized developmental care for low-birthweight, preterm infants that positively influences neurodevelopmental functioning and parenting competence and reduces the severity of medical illnesses.

• = Independent          ▲ = Collaborative

- Recognize behavior used to communicate stress/avoidance/disengagement and approach/engagement.
- Identify and support the infant's/child's use of self-regulatory/consoling and habituation behaviors needed for mastering the environment.
- Demonstrate ways to facilitate state organization and control.
- Cluster care whenever possible allowing for longer periods of uninterrupted sleep.
- Correlate stress/disorganization behaviors to internal factors (e.g., pain, hunger, discomfort) and/or external factors (e.g., lights, noise, handling).
- Structure and organize the environment.
- Identify appropriate position and handling techniques that enhance motor organization, comfort, and normal development and prevent positioning-acquired abnormalities.
- Provide lots of opportunities for physical closeness, loving touch, massaging, cuddling, skin-to-skin (Kangaroo Care) and rocking.
- Encourage parents' competence by praising their parenting strengths and capabilities when caring for their infants.
- Identify and support infant's/child's attention capabilities.
- Provide opportunities for parent/caregiver to engage in pleasurable parent-infant interactions contingent with infant cue responses; begin slowly and introduce one sensory stimulus at a time—looking, then slowly begin talking softly, adding gentle touch, if infant remains stable, swaddle and slowly pick up. Assess and respond contingently to infant cues.
- Provide pleasurable sensory motor experiences (i.e., visual, auditory, tactile, vestibular/movement, proprioceptive) that enhance development of sensory pathways.
- Knowledge of community based follow-up programs for preterm and infants at risk and their families discharged from the NICU.

● = Independent          ▲ = Collaborative

## Multicultural

- Assess for the influence of cultural beliefs, norms, and values on the family's perceptions of infant/child behavior.
- Use a neutral, indirect style when addressing areas where improvement is needed (such as a need for verbal or oral stimulation) when working with Native-American clients.
- Acknowledge and praise parenting strengths noted.
- Use therapeutic communication techniques that emphasize acceptance, offer the self, validate the client's concerns, and convey respect when discussing infant/child behavior.

I

## Home Care

- Above interventions may be adapted for home care use.
- Educate families in preparing home environment.
- Prepare families for realistic challenges of caring for pre-term and at risk infants prior to discharge. Differences include: understanding "corrected" age, feeding skills, poor endurance/tires easily, shorter sleep-wake cycles, less alert and more fussy when awake, fussy before returning to sleep, overstimulation, etc.
- Encourage families to teach friends/visitors to recognize and respond to infant's unique behavioral cues.
- Provide information on community resources, developmental follow-up services, and parent-to-parent support programs.

## Family Teaching

- Assist families/support systems in recognizing and responding to infant's unique behavioral cues.
- Give anticipatory guidance to parents about what infant/child behaviors are possible in given situations.
- Model calming interventions to provide parents with tools for positive interactions with their infant/child.
- Nurture parents so that they in turn can nurture their infant/child.

● = Independent          ▲ = Collaborative

- Establish a nurturing environment in which parents can interact with their infant/child.
- Have knowledge of community early intervention services and follow-up programs for preterm and at risk infants and families.

# Readiness for enhanced organized Infant behavior

## NANDA Definition

A pattern of regulation and modulation of the physiological and behavioral subsystems of functioning (i.e., autonomic, motor, state-organizational, self-regulation, and attentional-interactional systems) that is satisfactory but that can be improved, resulting in higher levels of integration in response to environmental stimuli; a pattern of stable regulation and modulation of the physiological and behavioral subsystems (i.e., autonomic, motor, state-organization, self-regulation and attentional-interactional) to function harmoniously that allows the infant/child to interact with the environment in an organized way; the organized infant/child is able to process external sensory stimuli without disrupting his/her physiological and behavioral functioning; if their balance is disrupted, they are more adaptable by being able to regain system balance through self-regulatory behaviors

## Defining Characteristics

Definite sleep-wake states; use of some self-regulatory behaviors; response to visual/auditory stimuli; stable physiological measures

### Physiological/Autonomic

*Cardiorespiratory:* stable heart rate, respiratory rate, and skin color
*Visceral:* digestion stable; absence of feeding intolerances/problems; regular elimination patterns

• = Independent        ▲ = Collaborative

*Neuromotor:* absence/minimal startles, tremors, twitches, jitteriness

## Motor System

*Posture and tone:* balanced of flexion, extension, and rotation; able to lie in safe tucked position; does not stiffen or become rigid or stiff

*Movements:* smooth, symmetrical, and purposeful movements; no extensions

## State-Organization System

*State:* displays full range of states from deep sleep (State I) to robust crying (State VI)

*Clarity:* ability to maintain a state for period of time from deep sleep to quiet, alert state (ideal state for learning and interacting with caregivers)

*Modulation:* smooth transition/oscillation between states (awakens gradually, falls asleep easily)

*Habituation:* ability to decrease motor activity resulting in a sleep state with the presence of repetitive stimuli

## Self-Regulation System

*Range:* exhibits repertoire of self-regulatory/coping behaviors (postural change, hand clasp/grasp, hand holding, foot bracing, sucking, visual and auditory attending, habituation, etc.)

*Effective:* adequately uses self-regulatory behaviors to maintain a balance between physiologic and behavior function when exposed to environmental stimuli; if balance state is disrupted is able to return to state of balance with assistance from the caregiver; continually learning and adding new behaviors to repertoire

## Attention-Interaction System

*Attention:* ability to *focus* attention and *orient* to visual and auditory sensory stimuli; ability to *sustain and increase attention* periods; ability to *shift* attention from one stimulus to another; ability to *inhibit* distractions

• = Independent          ▲ = Collaborative

*Interaction:* ability to engage in reciprocal interactions (mutual gazing, eye contact, turning to voice, smiling, vocalizing); elicits attention behaviors, enjoys social play; is able to smoothly engage and disengage easily without becoming overstimulated

## Related Factors (r/t)

Refer to **Disorganized Infant behavior** as appropriate, although with potential for enhanced organized behavior, related factors will be minimal

## Client Outcomes

### Client Will (Specify Time Frame):

### Infant/Child
- Display stable vital signs and skin color
- Display smooth, synchronous, and purposeful body movements
- Display range of clear sleep and awake states
- Display smooth transitions between sleep and awake states
- Demonstrate range of effective self-consoling behaviors
- Demonstrate smooth visceral/digestive functioning without feeding intolerances
- Effectively attend and interact with the environment with minimal stress
- Enjoy engaging in reciprocal social play experiences
- Display pleasure with sensory-motor experiences
- Not be "over" or "under" reactive to sensory-motor experiences (visual, auditory, tactile, movement, body awareness)
- Continue to demonstrate progressive growth and development

### Parents/Significant Other
- Demonstrate ways to structure and modify the environment that enhances the infant's/child's own adaptive capacity for achieving optimal physiologic and neurobehavioral functioning

● = Independent          ▲ = Collaborative

- Identify their infant's/child's behaviors which signal "stress/ avoidance" or "approach"
- Demonstrate ways to facilitate motor organization and development by appropriate handling and positioning techniques
- Demonstrate care that is contingent with the state of the infant/child
- Demonstrate additional ways to facilitate state organization/ development
- Support and expand infant's/child's self-regulatory skills
- Demonstrate ways to help infant/child achieve an attentive state that allows them to orient to visual and auditory sensory stimuli
- Support and expand infant's/child's calm alert periods, the ideal state for learning and interacting
- Demonstrate ways to engage the infant/child in social interactions and allow the infant/child to lead the interaction and respond contingently to his or her approach/engagement and avoidance/disengagement cues
- Demonstrate ways to provide pleasurable and developmentally appropriate sensory-motor experiences (visual, auditory, tactile, movement, body awareness)

## Nursing Interventions

Refer to **Disorganized Infant behavior** and **Risk for disorganized Infant behavior** Nursing Interventions.

NOTE: The interventions should be based on individual response of the infant/child to each intervention. Interventions appropriate for one infant/child may not be appropriate for another. In addition, a particular intervention that seems appropriate for one infant/child at a particular time may not be as effective with the same infant/child at another time. Carefully observe for the desired adaptive response or expected outcomes and continually reevaluate. Nursing care that is responsive and contingent with the state of the infant is ideal; however, if stressful events occur provide appropriate interventions to minimize stress and facilitate self-regulation.

• = Independent      ▲ = Collaborative

# Ineffective Infant feeding pattern

## NANDA Definition

Impaired ability to suck or coordinate the suck-swallow response

## Defining Characteristics

Inability to coordinate sucking, swallowing, and breathing; inability to initiate or sustain an effective suck

## Related Factors (r/t)

Prolonged NPO; anatomic abnormality; neurological impairment/delay; coordination of suck-swallow-breathe; tongue thrusting; biting; gagging; abnormal muscle tone-increased and/or decreased; depressed oral reflexes; inappropriate positioning; altered parent/caregiver interaction; prolonged tube feedings; oral hypersensitivity/oral aversion; jaw instability; disorganized tongue and/or jaw movements; pre-term birth; hypersensitivity (tactile defensiveness); poor lip closure; altered sensory processing—over- or underreaction to sensory stimuli (i.e., sights, sounds, tactile, movement, body awareness); negative environmental stimuli; sensory overload; swallowing difficulties; cardiorespiratory problems; poor sleep-wake regulation; poor endurance; gastrointestinal problems; gastroesophageal reflux disease (GERD); unclear cues for "hunger" and "satiety"

## Client Outcomes

### Client Will (Specify Time Frame):

### Infant

- Consume adequate calories to sustain temperature, to provide "catch-up" growth for preterm infants and to facilitate optimal growth and development
- Have opportunity for skin-to-skin (Kangaroo Care) experience
- Have opportunity for "trophic" enteral feedings prior to oral feedings
- Progress to safe, self-regulated oral feedings
- Progress to and maintain stable neurobehavioral organization

• = Independent          ▲ = Collaborative

(i.e., motor, state, self-regulation, attention-interaction) behavior subsystems of functioning
- Coordinate suck-swallow with breathing with/without minimal stress behaviors
- Able to demonstrate self-regulated feeding behaviors
- Display clear behavior cues related to "hunger," "satiety,"
approach/engagement, avoidance/disengagement
- Display alertness and evidence of pleasure with feedings
- Progress to and ability to engage in mutually positive
parent/caregiver–infant/child interactions during
feedings

## Parent/Family

- Recognize necessity of consuming adequate calories for optimal growth and development
- Learn to read and respond contingently to infant's behavior
cues (e.g., "hunger," "satiety," approach/engagement,
stress/avoidance/disengagement)
- Learn strategies that promote organized infant behavior
(e.g., physiologic/autonomic, motor, state)
- Learn appropriate positioning and handling techniques
- Learn effective ways to relieve stress behaviors during
nippling
- Learn ways to help infant coordinate suck-swallow with
breathing
- Engage in mutually positive interactions with infant during
feeding experiences
- Recognize ways to facilitate effective feedings including: feed
in quiet alert state; appropriate length of feeding; burping;
prepare/structure environment; signs of sensory overload; self-regulation using semi-demand protocols, allow
pauses between sucking bursts; avoid pulling and twisting
nipple during pauses; allow infant to resume sucking when
ready; provide oral support (cheek and/or jaw) as needed; use
appropriate nipple hole size and flow rate

## Nursing Interventions

- Refer to care plans for **Readiness for enhanced orga-**

• = Independent        ▲ = Collaborative

**nized Infant behavior, Disorganized Infant behavior, and Risk for disorganized Infant behavior.**

- Interventions follow sequential pattern of implementation that can be adapted as appropriate.
- Provide developmentally supportive neonatal intensive care for preterm infants that facilitates self-regulation of the physiological/autonomic, motor, state organizational, attention-interaction systems).
- Provide opportunities for skin-to-skin (Kangaroo Care) care.
- ▲ Discuss using "trophic" feedings for high-risk hospitalized infants as appropriate.
- ▲ Implement gavage feedings (or another alternative feeding method) using breast milk whenever possible, before infant's readiness for feedings by mouth.
- ▲ Provide naturalistic environment for tube feedings (naso-oral, gastric gavage, or other alternative tube feedings) similar to oral feeding experience; include: pleasurable tactile experiences, hold in semi-upright/flexed position, offer nonnutritive sucking (NNS), quiet environment, pace feeding, semi-demand method contingent on infant behavior cues, rest breaks, burp, as appropriate.
- Assess infant's oral reflexes (i.e., root, gag, suck, and swallow).
- Prepare and structure the environment minimizing unnecessary sensory stimuli.
- Modify stimulation based on infant's physiological and behavioral state organization/disorganization.
- Feed infant in quiet alert state, the optimal state for feeding.
- Position pre-term infant in semi-upright flexed feeding posture, head neutral alignment, slight chin tuck, back straight with shoulders/arms forward, hands midline, keeping hips flexed 90 degrees.
- Before feeding, assess the infant's baseline parameters of vital signs, state, and activity level.
- Provide 10 minutes nonnutritive sucking (NNS) prior to oral feeding.

• = Independent         ▲ = Collaborative

- Determine the appropriate flow rate of nipple for pre-term infants that facilitates a 1:1:1 ratio of coordinated suck-swallow-breathe.
- Assess infant's ability to sustain coordinated suck, swallow, breathe pattern for 2 minutes.
- Assess infant's suck, swallow, and breathing coordination 1:1:1 ratio pattern during active sucking.
- Use techniques that support the infant's suck-swallow-breathe coordination and prevent development of abnormal compensatory patterns used to protect the airway.
- Provide oral support measures for preterm infants by giving jaw and/or cheek support as appropriate.
▲ Collaborate with other health care providers (e.g., physician, neonatal nutritionist, physical and occupational therapists, lactation specialists) to develop a feeding plan.
- Allow appropriate time for nipple feeding to ensure infant's safety without exceeding calorie expenditure.
- Monitor the length of the feeding not to exceed 30 minutes.
- Encourage transitioning from standard care, scheduled feeding method to a semi-demand feeding method contingent on infant behavior cues.
- Assess quality of parent-infant interactions.
- Assess for attachment behaviors that can positively or negatively impact a feeding.
- Encourage family to participate in the feeding process.
▲ Refer to a neonatal nutritionist, physical or occupational therapist, or lactation specialist as needed.

**Home Care**
- Above appropriate interventions may be adapted for home care use.
▲ Infants with risk factors and clinical indicators of feeding problems present prior to hospital discharge should be referred to appropriate community early intervention service providers (e.g., community health nursing, Early-On, OT, Speech Pathologists, Feeding Specialists, etc.) to ensure effective feeding outcomes that facili-

• = Independent          ▲ = Collaborative

tate adequate weight gain for optimal growth and development.

## Family Teaching

- Provide anticipatory guidance for infant's expected feeding course.
- Teach various effective feeding methods/strategies to parent(s).
- Teach parents how to read, interpret and respond contingently to infant cues.
- Provide a family-focused caring environment that supports parents in their role as their infant's primary caregiver—strengths are supported while vulnerabilities are partnered.
- Help parents identify their support system including immediate and extended family members and friends prior to hospital discharge; if necessary, include these persons in family teaching sessions.
- Provide anticipatory guidance for the infant's discharge.

# Risk for Infection

## NANDA Definition

At increased risk for being invaded by pathogenic organisms

## Risk Factors

Invasive procedures; insufficient knowledge regarding avoidance of exposure to pathogens; trauma; tissue destruction and increased environmental exposure; rupture of amniotic membranes; pharmaceutical agents (e.g., immunosuppressants); malnutrition; increased environmental exposure to pathogens; immunosuppression; inadequate acquired immunity; inadequate secondary defenses (e.g., decreased hemoglobin, leukopenia, suppressed inflammatory response); inadequate primary defenses (e.g., broken skin, traumatized tissue, decrease in ciliary action, stasis of

• = Independent          ▲ = Collaborative

body fluids, change in pH secretions, altered peristalsis); chronic disease

### Related Factors (r/t)

See Risk Factors

### Client Outcomes

### Client Will (Specify Time Frame):

- Remain free from symptoms of infection
- State symptoms of infection of which to be aware
- Demonstrate appropriate care of infection-prone site
- Maintain white blood cell (WBC) count and differential within normal limits
- Demonstrate appropriate hygienic measures such as hand washing, oral care, and perineal care

### Nursing Interventions

- ▲ Observe and report signs of infection such as redness, warmth, discharge, and increased body temperature.
- ▲ Assess temperature of neutropenic clients every 4 hours; report a single temperature of greater than 38.5° C or three temperatures of greater than 38° C in 24 hours.
- • Oral or tympanic thermometers may be used to assess temperature in adults and infants.
- • Use oral thermometers for critically ill adults.
- ▲ Note and report laboratory values (e.g., WBC count and differential, serum protein, serum albumin, and cultures).
- • Remove the granulocytopenic client from areas exposed to construction dust so that the client will not inhale fungal spores. Remove all plants and flowers from the client's room.
- • Assess skin for color, moisture, texture, and turgor (elasticity). Keep accurate, ongoing documentation of changes. Preventive skin assessment protocol, including documentation, assists in the prevention of skin breakdown.
- • Carefully wash and pat dry skin, including skinfold areas. Use hydration and moisturization on all at-risk surfaces.

• = Independent          ▲ = Collaborative

▲ Encourage a balanced diet, emphasizing proteins, fatty acids, and the following vitamins: essential amino acids, linoleic acid, vitamin A, folic acid, vitamins $B_6$ and $B_{12}$, vitamin C, zinc, iron, and selenium.

• Monitor weight loss, leaving 25% or more of food uneaten at most meals.

• Use strategies to prevent nosocomial pneumonia (NP): assess lung sounds, sputum, and redness or drainage around stoma sites; use sterile water rather than tap water for mouth care of immunosuppressed clients; provide a clean manual resuscitation bag for each client; use sterile technique when suctioning; suction secretions above tracheal tube before suctioning; drain accumulated condensation in ventilator tubing into a fluid trap or other collection device before repositioning the client; assess patency and placement of nasogastric tubes; elevate the client's head to 30 degrees or higher to prevent gastric reflux of organisms in the lung; institute feeding as soon as possible; assess for signs of feeding intolerance—no bowel sounds, abdominal distension, increased residual, emesis.

• Encourage fluid intake

• Use appropriate "hand hygiene" (i.e., hand washing or use of alcohol-based hand rubs).

• When using an alcohol-based hand rub, apply product to palm of one hand and rub hands together, covering all surfaces of hands and fingers, until hands are dry. Note that the volume needed to reduce the number of bacteria on hands varies by product.

• Follow Standard Precautions and wear gloves during any contact with blood, mucous membranes, nonintact skin, or any body substance except sweat. Use goggles, gloves, and gowns when appropriate.

• Follow Transmission-Based Precautions for airborne-, droplet-, and contact-transmitted microorganisms:

  ■ **Airborne:** Isolate the client in a room with monitored negative air pressure, with the room door closed, and the client remaining in the room. Always wear appropriate respiratory protection when you enter the

• = Independent          ▲ = Collaborative

room. For tuberculosis, you should wear an approved particulate respirator mask. Limit the movement and transport of the client from the room to essential purposes only. If at all possible, have the client wear a surgical mask during transport.

- **Droplet:** Keep the client in a private room, if possible. If not possible, maintain a spatial separation of 3 feet from other beds or visitors. The door may remain open. You should wear a mask when you must come within 3 feet of the client. Some hospitals may choose to implement a mask requirement for droplet precautions for anyone entering the room. Limit transport to essential purposes and have the client wear a mask if possible.

- **Contact:** Place the client in a private room if possible or with someone who has an active infection from the same microorganism. Wear clean, nonsterile gloves when entering the room. When providing care, change gloves after contact with any infective material such as wound drainage. Remove the gloves and wash your hands before leaving the room and take care not to touch any potentially infectious items or surfaces on the way out. Wear a gown if you anticipate your clothing may have substantial contact with the client or other potentially infectious items. Remove the gown before leaving the room. Limit transport of the client to essential purposes and take care that the client does not contact other environmental surfaces along the way. Dedicate the use of noncritical client care equipment to a single client. If use of common equipment is unavoidable, adequately clean and disinfect equipment before use with other clients.

Standard Precautions are based on the likely routes of transmission of pathogens. The second tier of the new CDC guidelines is Transmission-Based Precautions. This replaces many old categories of isolation precautions and disease-specific precautions with three simpler sets of precautions.

• = Independent        ▲ = Collaborative

- Sterile technique must be used when inserting urinary catheters. Catheters must be cared for at least every shift.
- Use careful technique when changing and emptying urinary catheter bags; avoid cross-contamination.
- ▲ Use alternatives to indwelling catheters whenever possible (external catheters, incontinence pads, bladder control techniques).
- ▲ Provide well-designed site care for all peripheral, central venous, and arterial catheters: standardize insertion technique; select catheters with as few lumens as necessary; avoid use of femoral catheters in clients with fecal or urinary incontinence; use aseptic technique for insertion and care; stabilize cannula and tubing; maintain a sterile occlusive dressing (change every 72 hours per hospital policy); label insertion sites and all tubing with date and time of insertion, inspect every 8 hours for signs of infection, record and report; replace peripheral catheters per hospital policy (usually every 48 to 72 hours); when fever of unknown origin develops, obtain culture.
- Use careful sterile technique wherever there is a loss of skin integrity.
- Ensure the client's appropriate hygienic care with hand washing; bathing; and hair, nail, and perineal care performed by either the nurse or the client.
- ▲ Recommend responsible use of antibiotics; use antibiotics sparingly.
- ▲ Carefully screen and treat women with infertility who may have female genital tuberculosis

## Pediatric

NOTE: Many of the above interventions are appropriate for the pediatric client.

- Follow meticulous hand hygiene when working with premature infants.
- Cluster nursing procedures to decrease number of contacts with infants allowing time for appropriate hand hygiene.

• = Independent          ▲ = Collaborative

- Assess child's temperature with a rectal thermometer after other vital signs have been obtained.
▲ Avoid the prophylactic use of topical cream in premature infants.

## Geriatric

- Recognize that geriatric clients may be seriously infected but have less obvious symptoms. The immune system declines with aging.
▲ Suspect pneumonia when the client has symptoms of lethargy or confusion. Most clients develop NP by either aspirating contaminated substances or inhaling airborne particles. Refer to care plan for **Risk for Aspiration.**
▲ Carefully screen elderly women with symptoms of urinary tract infections for salmonella.
▲ Foot care other than simple toenail cutting should be performed by a podiatrist.
▲ Observe and report if the client has a low-grade temperature or new onset of confusion.
- During the peak of the influenza epidemic, limit visits by relatives and friends.
▲ Recommend that the geriatric client receive an annual influenza immunization and one-time pneumococcal vaccine.
- Recognize that chronically ill geriatric clients, particularly those with depression, have an increased susceptibility to infection; practice meticulous care of all invasive sites.
- Recognize that older adults are at risk for HIV/AIDS; institute Universal Precautions and appropriate instruction for all age groups.

## Home Care

- Some of the above interventions may be adapted for home care use.
- Review standards for surveillance of infections in home care.
- Maintain strong infection control policies.

● = Independent          ▲ = Collaborative

- Assess home environment for general cleanliness, storage of food items, and appropriate waste disposal. Instruct as necessary in proper disposal and use of disinfecting agents.
▲ Assess home care environment for appropriate disposal of used dressing materials.
▲ Role-model all preventive behaviors in care of the client (e.g., Universal Precautions).
- Do not visit the client when you are ill.
- Maintain the cleanliness of all irrigation and cleansing solutions. Change solutions when cleanliness has not been maintained—do not wait to finish bottle.
- Assess and teach clients about current medications and therapies that promote susceptibility to infection: corticosteroids, immunosuppressants, chemotherapeutic agents, and radiation therapy.
- Assess the client for knowledge of infections that have been drug resistant.
▲ Instruct the client to complete any course of prophylactic antibiotic therapy unless experiencing adverse side effects.
- Monitor recurrent antibiotic use in infants. Instruct parents on appropriate indicators for medical visits, and on the influence of breastfeeding and day care at home for avoiding increased need for antibiotics.
▲ Monitor for the occurrence of infectious exacerbation of chronic obstructive pulmonary disease (COPD); refer to physician for treatment.
▲ Refer for nutritional evaluation; implement dietary changes to support recovery and address antibiotic side effects.

## Client/Family Teaching

- Teach the client risk factors contributing to surgical wound infection, smoking, and higher body mass index.
▲ Teach the client and family the symptoms of infection that should be promptly reported to a primary medical caregiver (e.g., redness; warmth; swelling; tenderness or pain; new onset of drainage or change in drainage from wound; increase in body temperature).
▲ Teach signs of hepatitis B virus (HBV)/AIDS symp-

• = Independent          ▲ = Collaborative

toms: malaise, abdominal pain, vomiting or diarrhea, enlarged glands, rash; tuberculosis symptoms: cough, night sweats, dyspnea, changes in sputum, changes in breath sounds; insulin-dependent diabetes mellitus (IDDM) symptoms: sores or wounds that do not heal).

▲ Encourage high-risk persons, including health care workers, to have influenza vaccinations.

• Assess whether the client and family know how to read a thermometer; provide instructions if necessary. Chemical dot thermometers are easy to use and decrease risk of infection. Clients need to know that the instructions should be followed carefully and that electronic thermometers may be the best choice for accuracy.

• Instruct the client and family about the need for good nutrition (especially protein) and proper rest to prevent infection.

• If the client has AIDS, discuss the continued need to practice safe sex, avoid nonsterile needle use, and maintain a healthy lifestyle to prevent infection.

▲ Refer the client and family to social services and community resources to obtain support in maintaining a lifestyle that increases immune function (e.g., adequate nutrition and rest, freedom from excessive stress).

# Risk for Injury

## NANDA Definition

At risk of injury as a result of the interaction of environmental conditions interacting with the individual's adaptive and defensive resources

NOTE: This nursing diagnosis overlaps with other diagnoses such as **Risk for Falls, Risk for Trauma, Risk for Poisoning, Risk for Suffocation, Risk for Aspiration,** and if the client is at risk of bleeding, **Ineffective Protection.** See care plans for these diagnoses if appropriate.

• = Independent          ▲ = Collaborative

## Risk Factors

### External

Mode of transport or transportation; people or provider (e.g., nosocomial agents; staffing patterns; cognitive, affective, and psychomotor factors); physical (e.g., design, structure, and arrangement of community, building, and/or equipment); nutrients (e.g., vitamins, food types); biological (e.g., immunization level of community, microorganism); chemical (e.g., pollutants, poisons, drugs, pharmaceutical agents, alcohol, caffeine, nicotine, preservatives, cosmetics, dyes)

### Internal

Psychological (affective orientation); malnutrition; abnormal blood profile (e.g., leukocytosis/leukopenia); altered clotting factors; thrombocytopenia; sickle cell; thalassemia; decreased hemoglobin; immune-autoimmune dysfunction; biochemical, regulatory function (e.g., sensory dysfunction, integrative dysfunction, effector dysfunction, tissue hypoxia); developmental age (physiological, psychosocial); physical (e.g., broken skin, altered mobility)

## Related Factors (r/t)

See Risk Factors.

## Client Outcomes

### Client Will (Specify Time Frame):

• Remain free of injuries
• Explain methods to prevent injury

## Nursing Interventions

▲ Prevent iatrogenic harm to the hospitalized client by following these guidelines for giving care:
  ■ Use at least two methods to identify the client before administering medications or blood products, such as the client's name and medical record number or birth date.
  ■ Prior to beginning any invasive or surgical procedure,

• = Independent    ▲ = Collaborative

have a final verification to confirm the correct client, the correct procedure, and the correct site for the procedure using active or passive communication techniques.

■ When taking verbal or telephone orders, the orders should be written down, and then read back for verification to the individual giving the order.
■ Standardize use of abbreviations and eliminate abbreviations that are prone to cause errors.
■ Take high alert medications off the nursing unit, such as potassium chloride. Standardize concentrations of medications such as morphine in PCA pumps.
■ Use only intravenous pumps that prevent free flow of intravenous solution when the tubing is taken out of the pump.
■ Improve the effectiveness of alarm systems in the clinical area.
■ Reduce the risk of infections by following CDC hand hygiene guidelines.
■ Identify all of the client's current medications upon admission to a health care facility, and ensure that all health care staff have access to the information.
■ Evaluate all clients for fall risk and take appropriate actions to prevent falls.

• Thoroughly orient the client to environment.
• Place call light within reach and show how to call for assistance; answer call light promptly.
• Screen clients using a fall risk factor assessment tool to identify those at risk for falls.
▲ Avoid use of restraints if at all possible. Obtain a physician's order if restraints are necessary.
• In place of restraints, use the following:
  ■ Well staffed and educated nursing personnel with frequent client contact
  ■ Nursing units designed to care for clients with cognitive or functional impairments
  ■ Nonskid footwear
  ■ Alarm systems with ankle, above the knee, or wrist sensors

• = Independent        ▲ = Collaborative

- Bed or wheelchair alarms
- Increased observation of the client
- Locked doors to unit
- Low or very low height beds
- Border-defining pillow/mattress to remind the client to stay in bed

- For an agitated client, consider providing individualized music of the client's choice.
- Review drug profile for potential side effects that may increase risk of injury.
- Use $1/4$- to $1/2$-length side rails only, and maintain bed in a low position. Ensure that wheels are locked on bed and commode. Keep dim light in room at night.
▲ If the client has a new onset of confusion (delirium), recognize this is a medical emergency and refer for evaluation and treatment. Also provide reality orientation when interacting with him or her. Have family bring in familiar items, clocks, and watches from home to maintain orientation. If the client has chronic confusion with dementia, use validation therapy that reinforces feelings but does not confront reality.
- Ask family to stay with the client to prevent the client from accidentally falling or pulling out tubes.
- Remove all possible hazards in environment such as razors, medications, and matches.
- Place an injury-prone client in a room that is near the nurses' station.
- Help clients sit in a stable chair with armrests. Avoid use of wheelchairs and geri-chairs except for transportation as needed.
▲ Refer to physical therapy for strengthening exercises and gait training to increase mobility.
▲ For the agitated psychotic client, use nonphysical forms of behavior management, such as verbal intervention or show of force. If medication is required, use oral medications if at all possible.

**Pediatric**

- Teach parents the need for close supervision of all young

• = Independent          ▲ = Collaborative

children playing near water, including washing machines.
- If child has epilepsy, recommend showers instead of tub baths, and no unsupervised swimming is ever allowed.
- Assess the client's socioeconomic status.
- Never leave young children unsupervised around cooking areas.
- Teach parents and children the need to maintain safety for the exercising child, including wearing helmets when biking, using breakaway bases for baseball, and having the needed conditioning for the activity.
- Teach both parents and children the need for gun safety.

## Geriatric
- Encourage the client to wear glasses and hearing aids and to use walking aids when ambulating.
- If the client experiences dizziness because of orthostatic hypotension when getting up, teach methods to decrease dizziness, such as rising slowly, remaining seated several minutes before standing, flexing feet upward several times while sitting, sitting down immediately if feeling dizzy, and trying to have someone present when standing.
- Discourage driving at night.

## Multicultural
- Acknowledge racial/ethnic differences at the onset of care.
- Assess for the influence of cultural beliefs, norms, and values on the client's perceptions of risk for injury.
- Assess whether exposure to community violence is contributing to risk for injury.
- Use culturally relevant injury prevention programs whenever possible.
- Validate the client's feelings and concerns related to environmental risks.

## Home Care
- Some of the above interventions may be adapted for home care use.

• = Independent          ▲ = Collaborative

- Assess home environment for threats to safety: clutter, inappropriate storage of chemicals, slippery floors, scatter rugs, unsafe stairs and stairwells, blocked entries, dim lighting, extension cords across pathways, unsafe electrical or gas connections, unsafe heating devices, unsafe oxygen placement, high beds without rails, excessively hot water, pets, and pet excrement.
▲ Instruct the client and family or caregivers in correcting identified hazards. Refer to occupational therapy services for assistance if needed. Notify landlord or code enforcement office of any structural building hazards.
- Provide assistive devices in bathrooms (e.g., hand rails, nonslip decals on the floor of the shower and bathtub).
▲ Refer to physical therapy services for the client and family education in safe transfers and ambulation and for strengthening exercises for ambulation and transfers.
- Avoid extreme hot and cold around clients at risk for injury (e.g., heating pads, hot water for baths/showers).
▲ Monitor blood glucose patterns for indicators of need for client instruction or referral to physician for treatment changes.
▲ Provide a signaling device for clients who wander or are at risk for falls. If the client lives alone, provide a Lifeline or similar call device.
▲ Provide medical identification bracelet for clients at risk for injury from dementia, seizures, or other medical disorders.

## Client/Family Teaching

- Teach how to safely ambulate at home, including using safety measures such as handrails in bathroom.
- Recommend client use a night light after dark.
- If the client has visual impairment, teach the client and caregiver to label with bright colors such as yellow or red significant places in environment that must be easily located (e.g., stair edges, stove controls, light switches).
- Encourage the use of proper car seats and safety belts.
- Instruct the client not to drive under the influence of alcohol or drugs. Assess for a substance abuse problem

• = Independent          ▲ = Collaborative

and refer to appropriate resources for drug and alcohol education.

- Counsel the client not to use alcohol to protect from injury.
- Teach the client to avoid excessive noise at work or at home, wearing hearing protection when necessary. Any noise that hurts the ears or is above 90 decibels is excessive.

# Risk for perioperative positioning Injury

## NANDA Definition

At risk for injury as a result of the environmental conditions found in the perioperative setting

## Risk Factors

Disorientation; edema; emaciation; immobilization; muscle weakness; obesity; sensory/perceptual disturbances resulting from anesthesia; high pressure for short periods of time and low pressure for extended periods of time are risk factors for tissue injury

NOTE: The following systems are most frequently affected by surgical positioning: neurological, musculoskeletal, integumentary, respiratory, and cardiovascular. Risk factors contributing to the incidence of injury related to surgical positioning include but are not limited to the client's age; height; weight; nutritional status; skin condition; the presence of preexisting conditions such as diabetes, vascular disease, and/or respiratory disease; immuno-compromise; impaired nerve function; physical mobility limitations such as arthritis, limited range of motion (ROM), presence of implants/prosthesis or malignancy; effects of anesthesia; staff's knowledge of the equipment; required position for the procedure; and the duration of the procedure. As a result of these factors, there is the potential for impaired tissue perfusion, impaired skin integrity, or neuromuscular or joint injury related to surgical positioning. The anesthetized client is at increased risk of injury

• = Independent        ▲ = Collaborative

due to positioning because anesthesia prevents the body's defense mechanism from warning the client of exaggerated stretching, twisting, or compression of his or her body.

## Complications of Surgical Positioning

Complications of positioning include, but are not limited to, mechanical restriction of the rib cage, vasodilatation, hyper/hypotension, decreased cardiac output, inhibition of normal compensatory mechanisms, redistribution and congestion of the blood supply, and nerve and muscle trauma due to stretching and compression.

Transient physiological reactions to surgical positioning include skin redness and/or bruising, lumbar backache, stiffness in the limbs and neck, numbness, and generalized muscle aches that usually resolve within 24 to 48 hours without treatment. Lumbar back pain, previously considered a transient physiological reaction to positioning, may be an indication of rhabdomyolysis.

More serious complications of surgical positioning include pressure ulcers, peripheral nerve injury, deep venous thrombosis, joint dislocation, compartment syndrome (impairment of micro-circulation in soft tissue), rhabdomyolysis, and joint injury.

## Nursing Interventions

### General Interventions for Any Surgical Patient

- The nurse must demonstrate knowledge of not only the equipment, but also anatomy and the application of physiological principles in order to properly position the client.
- A preoperative assessment should be completed prior to the surgical procedure to "identify physical alterations that may require additional precautions for procedure-specific positioning."
- Clients with limited mobility/ROM should be asked to position themselves under the nurse's guidance before induction of anesthesia so that the client can verify that a position of comfort has been obtained.
- Appropriate numbers of personnel should be present to assist in positioning the client.

• = Independent          ▲ = Collaborative

- Monitor pressure being applied to the client intraoperatively by staff, equipment, and/or instruments.
- Keep linens on the OR table free of wrinkles.
- Equipment should be checked to verify it is in good working order and it should be used according to manufacturer's instructions: verify that the equipment is clean, operating properly, free of sharp edges, able to maintain normal capillary interface pressure, and nonallergenic to the client.
- Reassess the client after positioning and periodically during the procedure for maintenance of proper alignment and skin integrity.
- Do not allow extremities to extend beyond/off the OR table.
- Avoid contact with metal when positioning the client.
- Avoid hyperextension of joints.
- Move and position client slowly and smoothly.
- Lock the OR table, cart, or bed and stabilize the mattress before transfer/positioning of the client
- Pad the operating room table well. Use a static air overlay or full-length silicone gel pad to prevent pressure injuries.
- Prevent pooling of preparative solutions, blood, irrigation, urine, and feces.
- Ensure privacy and dignity for the client during positioning, by reducing unnecessary exposure.
- Implement measures to prevent inadvertent hypothermia.
- If the client is positioned in Trendelenburg/reverse Trendelenburg or with the head of the bed raised/lowered every attempt should be made to lift the patient for several seconds, prior to prepping and draping, to allow the skin to realign itself.
- Lift rather than pull or slide the client when positioning.
- Position the client's legs parallel and uncrossed.
- Maintain alignment of head with cervical, thoracic, and lumbar spine.
- Body supports and restraint straps (safety belt) should be loose and secured over waist or mid-thigh at least 2

I

● = Independent        ▲ = Collaborative

inches above knees, avoiding bony prominences by placing a blanket between the strap and the client's skin.
- Recognize that the longer the surgery, the more the
chance of the client developing pressure ulcers.

## Supine Position (Dorsal Recumbent)
- Pad all bony prominences and positioning devices.
- Place a safety strap 2 inches above the knees, with a
sheet or blanket between the strap and the client's
skin.
- Support lumbar and popliteal areas.
- Use a pillow, padded footboard, or donut under the
heels.
- Arms positioned on padded armboards should be in the
palms-up position, with the armboards at less than a
90-degree angle (some sources recommend less than
60 degrees) to the body and the armboard pad level with
the OR table pad.
- Arms positioned at the sides of the body should have the
palms against the sides of the body and fingers extended along the length of the body. The sheet flaps
should be brought down over the arms and tucked under
the client's sides.
- When placing a pregnant client in the supine position,
place a small roll under her right flank.

## Prone Position (Modification: Kneeling, Jackknife, or Kraske Position)
- Provide an adequate number of personnel to accomplish
"logroll" turning of the anesthetized client.
- Pad all bony prominences and positioning devices.
- Arms and heels should not be in contact with hard surfaces or hanging over the edge of the OR table.
- Arms secured at the patient's sides should be in an
elbow-up position to decrease mattress pressure on the
ulnar nerve.
- When placing the client's arms on armboards, they
should be brought down slowly and then forward with
minimal abduction.

• = Independent          ▲ = Collaborative

- Place chest rolls from the acromioclavicular joint to the iliac crests.
- Male genitalia and female breasts should be checked and positioned to eliminate pressure. Male genitalia should be allowed to hang loosely and without pressure. Female breasts should be angled toward the sternum to reduce compression on them.
- Place a bolster or pillow under the pelvis.
- Place padding under the knees to prevent undue pressure on the patellas.
- Shoulders should be kept in a neutral position with the elbows bent at 90 degrees and the hands resting alongside the head.
- Place the head, turned to one side, on a padded headrest, maintain neck in alignment with the spine, and protect the client's ears and eyes. Pad the head and eyeballs to avoid pressure from the operating table.
- Care must be taken when positioning obese clients in the Kraske position (a modified form of the prone position).
- Clients placed in the Kraske position should be observed for respiratory and circulatory changes.

## Lateral Position (Lateral Chest or Kidney)

- Pad all bony prominences and positioning devices.
- Provide adequate personnel to properly position the client.
- Use a lift sheet to facilitate the turn.
- Place a support under the head.
- Keep the top leg straight or slightly flexed and flex the bottom leg at the hip and knee.
- Place padded beanbags, sandbags, or bolsters against the back and abdomen.
- Pad the lateral aspect of the bottom knee.
- Place a pillow between the client's legs lengthwise so that the pillow also supports the foot.
- Pad the lower shoulder and bring it forward slightly; the lower arm is extended on a padded armboard.
- Place the upper arm on a padded raised armboard or over the lower arm with padding between the two arms.

• = Independent          ▲ = Collaborative

- Place an axillary roll at the apex of the scapula in the axillary space of the dependent arm.
- When using positioning straps or tape to hold the client in the lateral position, place a towel or blanket between the client's skin and the strap/tape.

## Lithotomy Position

- Pad all bony prominences and positioning devices.
- Check the stirrups to ensure they are fastened securely to the OR table before placing the client in the lithotomy position.
- Position the client's arms loosely secured across the abdomen, extended on padded armboards, or at the client's sides.
- Pad the sacral area and provide a small lumbar roll. The client's buttocks should be even with the table edge once the lower portion of the OR table has been lowered.
- Stirrups should be positioned at equal height and adjusted according to the length of the client's legs and at the level of the client's upper thighs.
- Place the client's legs in the stirrups simultaneously, using one hand to hold the foot and the other to hold the calf at the knee.
- Lower the client's legs simultaneously and slowly, extending the legs fully.
- Minimize the height of the legs.
- Avoid hyperabduction of the thighs, and excessive external rotation and flexion of the hips.
- Select lithotomy leg holders with optimal body alignment and weight bearing in mind (e.g., combination knee-crutch-and-boot).
- Pad all bony prominences and surfaces that may contact the leg support system.

NOTE: The hemilithotomy position (one leg in the lithotomy position) is often used when operating to repair a fractured hip or femur.

- Arms should be positioned on armboards or loosely cra-

• = Independent          ▲ = Collaborative

dled over the lower abdomen and secured with the blanket.

- Assess the need for sequential compression stockings
- Monitor the length of time the client remains in the lithotomy position. Clients who have been in the lithotomy position for 4 hours should be repositioned supine for 20–30 minutes in an attempt to avert peroneal nerve injury and/or development of compartment syndrome.

NOTE: If assessment reveals conditions that place the client at increased risk for injury in this position, attempting this position while the client is awake and can report any discomfort may help prevent positioning complications.

- To decrease the length of time the client is in the lithotomy position, evaluate the procedure to determine if any portion can be done in the supine position.

### Trendelenburg/Reverse Trendelenburg Position

- Either of these positions can have adverse effects on both the circulatory system (i.e., increased blood pressure and intracranial pressure) and the respiratory system (i.e., diaphragm movement is impeded), which in most circumstances are monitored and controlled by anesthesia personnel.
- Modifications of both positions may be suggested and implemented by the nurse in collaboration with the surgeon and anesthesiologist.
- Padded shoulder braces may be used in the Trendelenburg position. They should be placed at an equal distance from the head of the table and lateral on the acromioclavicular joint, with a 1/2-inch space allowed between the brace and the shoulder and without medial deviation towards the neck.
- Knees should be positioned at the break in the operating table.
- Length of time in this position should be as short as possible.

● = Independent        ▲ = Collaborative

# Decreased Intracranial adaptive capacity

## NANDA Definition

Intracranial fluid dynamic mechanisms that normally compensate for increases in intracranial volumes are compromised, resulting in repeated disproportionate increases in intracranial pressure (ICP) in response to a variety of noxious and non-noxious stimuli

## Defining Characteristics

Repeated increases in ICP of greater than 10 mm Hg for more than 5 minutes following a variety of external stimuli; disproportionate increases in ICP following a single environmental or nursing maneuver stimulus; baseline ICP greater than 10 mm Hg; elevated P2 component of ICP waveform; wide-amplitude ICP waveform; volume-pressure response test variation (volume-pressure ratio of 2, pressure-volume index of less than 10)

## Related Factors (r/t)

Decreased cerebral perfusion less than 50 to 60 mm Hg; sustained increase in ICP greater than 10 to 15 mm Hg; systemic hypotension with intracranial hypertension; brain injuries

## Client Outcomes

### Client Will (Specify Time Frame):

- Experience fewer than five episodes of disproportionate increases in ICP (DIICP) in 24 hours
- Have neurological status changes that are not triggered by episodes of DIICP
- Have CPP remain greater than 60 to 70 mm Hg in adults

## Nursing Interventions

- For episodes of DIICP, do the following:
  - Reverse stimulus if readily apparent.
  - Evaluate position of the client. Head should be in midline without neck flexion to prevent intracranial trapping of jugular venous outflow.

• = Independent          ▲ = Collaborative

- ■ Return the client to original position if a position change has triggered DIICP.
- ■ Stop suctioning if routine suctioning is triggering DIICP. Follow preventive protocol if future suctioning is indicated.
- ■ Have clients who can follow directions exhale through their mouth if they are doing a Valsalva maneuver.
- ■ Reduce environmental noise and painful or unexpected touching of the client.
- • Elevate head of bed if the client maintains CPP.
- ▲ For DIICP, if baseline ICP rises above 15 mm Hg or CPP (mean arterial blood pressure minus mean ICP) is less than 60 mm Hg in adults for 5 minutes or more, do the following:
  - ■ Initiate protocols for lowering ICP according to a collaborative plan with attending physician if ICP remains elevated or CPP decreases outside parameters—usually ICP greater than 15 to 20 mm Hg or CPP less than 60 mm Hg for 10 or more minutes (less than 40–65 mm Hg in children).
  - ■ Use cerebrospinal fluid (CSF) drainage via ventriculostomy intermittently to maintain a given ICP level.
  - ■ Add sedation (e.g., morphine, midazolam, propofol) and analgesia with or without paralysis (e.g., atracurium, pancuronium [Pavulon]) if body movements or fighting respirator continuously stimulate a CPP decrease.
  - ■ Bolus administration of osmotic diuretic or other hyperosmotic agent (e.g., mannitol, mannitol plus furosemide) may be followed with continuous administration if CPP is not maintained with bolus administration. Note that it is essential to keep serum osmolality less than 320 mOsm/L to prevent hyperosmolality-related seizures.
  - ■ In adults, control hyperventilation, maintaining $Pco_2$ of 30 to 35 mm Hg unless ICP continues to be refractory, in which case $Pco_2$ may be briefly decreased below 30 mm Hg if ICP is responsive. Mild or pro-

• = Independent          ▲ = Collaborative

phylactic hyperventilation should be avoided in
children, unless ICP is refractory.

▲ To prevent DIICP in clients at risk (clients with elevated
P2 waveforms and ICP of less than 10 mm Hg; clients
previously responsive to general stimuli), do the
following:

- Maintain 15- to 30-degree head elevation if CPP is
  maintained at greater than 70 mm Hg.
- Maintain systemic blood pressure adequate to keep
  CPP greater than 70 mm Hg by body positioning and
  use of vasoactive protocols.
- Maintain adequate respiratory status; suction if
  needed but not prophylactically.
- Use gentle touching and talking or family visitations.
- Use mechanical turning beds if manual repositioning
  is a stimulus to DIICP.
- Avoid 90-degree hip flexion and use of the knee gatch
  of the bed.
- Sequence nursing care to allow for recovery of base-
  line ICP between noxious activities, such as suctioning, and position changes that involve neck flexion.

▲ With regard to general ICP monitoring:

- Monitor ICP and CPP continuously with alarm settings on.
- Notify physician if nursing interventions and collaborative protocols do not maintain a CPP of greater
  than 60 mm Hg and an ICP of less than 20 mm Hg
  for adults; 40–65 mm Hg for infants and children.
- Monitor neurological status and CPP, including level
  of arousal, ability to follow commands, response to
  painful stimuli if arousal is decreased, and brainstem
  signs (pupil response, respiratory pattern, symmetry of
  motor response, and vital signs).
- Notify physician of signs of neurological deterioration
  regardless of levels of ICP and CPP.

## Home Care

NOTE: Clients experiencing potentially rapid changes in
ICP are not candidates for home care. However, clients

• = Independent          ▲ = Collaborative

experiencing potentially gradual changes in ICP (i.e., clients with developmental delays resulting from genetic dysfunction), or clients with post ICP changes secondary to brain trauma, may be served by home care with the following considerations:

- Some of the above interventions may be adapted for home care use.
- Identify baseline neurological data before discharge from institutional care.
- Evaluate neurological functioning at regular intervals.
- Instruct the caregiver about client-specific changes that will indicate increased ICP. Examples include changes in speech articulation and eye coordination, decreased ability to focus, increased seizure activity, and decreased coping ability. The nurse is cautioned that changes will be specific to the disability of the client. Early reporting of status changes allows for early intervention in neurologically impaired clients.
- Instruct the client/family in appropriate expectations of cognitive recovery following minor brain injury.
- ▲ For clients with a history of traumatic brain injury, assess for mood, thought process, or personality disturbances and refer for appropriate mental health follow-up.
- Assist clients to identify resources/situations they can attend or in which they can participate to enhance a sense of valued fit. Identify and problem solve around issues of stress.
- ▲ Institute case management of frail elderly to support continued independent living.

# Deficient Knowledge (specify)

## NANDA Definition

Absence or deficiency of cognitive information related to a specific topic

• = Independent        ▲ = Collaborative

## Defining Characteristics

Verbalization of the problem; inaccurate follow-through of instruction; inaccurate performance of test; inappropriate or exaggerated behaviors (e.g., hysterical, hostile, agitated, apathetic)

## Related Factors (r/t)

Lack of exposure; lack of recall; information misinterpretation; cognitive limitation; lack of interest in learning; unfamiliarity with information resources

## Client Outcomes

### Client Will (Specify Time Frame):

- Explain disease state, recognize need for medications, and understand treatments.
- Explain how to incorporate new health regimen into lifestyle.
- State an ability to deal with health situation and remain in control of life.
- Demonstrate how to perform health related procedure(s) satisfactorily.
- List resources that can be used for more information or support after discharge.

## Nursing Interventions

- Observe the client's ability and readiness to learn (e.g., mental acuity, ability to see or hear, no existing pain, emotional readiness, absence of language or cultural barriers) and previous knowledge.
- Assess barriers to learning (e.g., perceived change in lifestyle, financial concerns, cultural patterns, lack of acceptance by peers or coworkers).
- Involve clients in writing specific outcomes for the teaching session, such as identifying what is most important to learn from their viewpoint and lifestyle.
- When teaching, build on the client's literacy skills.
- Present material that is most significant to the client first, such as how to give injections or change dressings;

• = Independent          ▲ = Collaborative

present additional material once the client's most pressing educational needs have been met.

- Use easy-to-understand language when giving information to clients. Encourage clients to ask the following questions: What is my main problem? What do I need to do? Why is it important for me to do this? Have clients repeat back information.
- ▲ Carefully evaluate information that is given to client regarding "disease state"; focus on wellness.
- Evaluate the readability of the material in pamphlets or written instructions.
- Use visual aids such as diagrams, pictures, videotapes, audiotapes, and interactive Internet websites.
- Provide clients with appropriate preoperative information.
- Assess willingness of family to incorporate new information, immunizations, medical/dental care, and diet/behavior modifications in support of the client.
- ▲ Help the client identify community resources for continuing information and support.
- ▲ Consider an experience-based group educational program for clients with type 2 diabetes.
- Evaluate the client's learning through return demonstrations, verbalizations, or the application of skills to new situations.

## Pediatric

- Consider the developmental needs of teens when designing programs related to pregnancy.
- ▲ Consider a pregnancy prevention intervention program for teens using Baby Think It Over infant simulator.

## Geriatric

- Adapt the teaching process for the physical constraints of the aging process (e.g., speak clearly, use a variety of audio-visual-psychomotor methods, provide examples, and allow time for the client to repeat and review).
- Ensure that the client uses necessary reading aids (e.g.,

● = Independent          ▲ = Collaborative

eyeglasses, magnifying lenses, large-print text) or hearing aids.
- Use printed material, videotapes, lists, diagrams, and Internet addresses that the client can refer to at another time.
- Repeat and reinforce information during several brief sessions.
- Discuss healthy lifestyle changes that promote wellness for the older adult.
- Evaluate readability of the material.
- ▲ Consider health education programs using television and newspapers.

## Multicultural
- Acknowledge racial/ethnic differences at the onset of care.
- Assess for the influence of cultural beliefs, norms, and values on the client's knowledge base.
- Use a neutral indirect style when addressing areas where improvement is needed when working with Native-American clients.
- Validate the client's feelings and concerns related to previous learning experiences.
- Approach individuals of color with respect, warmth, and professional courtesy.
- Provide health care information to mothers and grandmothers in African-American families.
- Provide written health care information in their native language to patients with limited English proficiency.

## Home Care
NOTE: Because home care is an intermittent model of care having a goal of safety and optimal wellness of the client between visits, the importance of teaching (by the nurse) and learning (by the client) should not be understated. All of the previously mentioned interventions are applicable to the home setting.
- ▲ Select a space and time for teaching in which the client and/or caregiver can focus on information to be learned.

• = Independent          ▲ = Collaborative

▲ Consider the complexity of material or behaviors to be learned. Adjust care plan and respective teaching and learning experiences accordingly to build client confidence in ability to learn (and change).

- Assess the client for low or absent literacy. Use illustrations for instruction that are as closely equivalent as possible to written instructions.

- Assess the client/family learning needs and current level of knowledge.

- Assess for specific areas of learning that have the potential for strong emotional responses by the client or family/caregiver. Allow time for expression of feelings and encourage acceptance of need for learning.

- Use visual aids and other available media that engage multiple senses to maximize learning. Leave visually-oriented/written materials in home.

- Document the client's and caregivers' responses to learning. Clear documentation supports continuity in the learning experience.

- Explore resources for teaching relative to specific illnesses.

- Encourage self-care management of illness. Refer to care plan for **Powerlessness.**

- Consider high tech options for delivery of home-based instruction.

# Readiness for enhanced Knowledge (specify)

## NANDA Definition

The presence or acquisition of cognitive information related to a specific topic is sufficient for meeting health-related goals and can be strengthened

## Defining Characteristics

Expresses an interest in learning; explains knowledge of the topic;

• = Independent          ▲ = Collaborative

behaviors congruent with expressed knowledge; describes previous experiences pertaining to the topic

## Related Factors (r/t)

To be developed

## Client Outcomes

### Client Will (Specify Time Frame):

- Demonstrate knowledge of new information.
- Meet personal health-related goals.
- Explain how to incorporate new health regimen into lifestyle.
- List sources to obtain information.

## Nursing Interventions

- Include clients as members of the health care team when providing education.
- Use open-ended questions and encourage two-way communication.
- Provide appropriate individualized health education when clients visit health care providers.
- Ensure that clients receive appropriate health-oriented education during hospitalization.
- When developing written information, assess and provide information that is important to clients.
- Carefully develop written materials to ensure that the client's literacy levels, including English as a second language, are addressed.
- Assist clients to find access to the Internet, libraries, and schools to find health information.
- Assist clients with questions about health information to find quality sites on the Internet.
- ▲ Provide a previsit questionnaire to facilitate individualized proactive planning before the visit to health care provider.
- ▲ Provide information about the prognosis, the alternatives of treatment, and the effects of treatment when the diagnosis is cancer. Consider providing informational leaflets.

• = Independent          ▲ = Collaborative

- Provide appropriate health care information and screening for clients with physical disabilities.
▲ Prior to the initiation of a mood stabilizer, the potential benefits, risks, and adverse effects should be communicated to the patient. Provide information on potential severe and life-threatening adverse cutaneous drug reactions (ACDRs) to all clients on mood-stabilizing agents such as carbamazepine, lithium carbonate, valproic acid, topiramate, lamotrigine, gabapentin, and oxcarbazepine. Patients should be advised to seek medical attention if they suspect a drug-induced skin reaction.
▲ Refer to nurse practitioners for client education. Use the HOPE model (health-oriented patient education) instead of the DOPE model (disease-oriented patient education).
- Refer to care plan for **Deficient Knowledge.**

### Pediatric
▲ Provide adolescents with cancer with developmentally appropriate information.

### Geriatric
▲ Consider using an interactive multimedia computer software program to disburse education.

### Multicultural
- Refer to **Deficient Knowledge** care plan.
- Provide health care information to mothers and grandmothers in African-American families.

### Home Care
NOTE: Because home care is an intermittent model of care having a goal of safety and optimal wellness of the client between visits, the importance of teaching (by the nurse) and learning (by the client) should not be understated. All of the previously mentioned interventions are applicable to the home setting.
▲ Consider high-tech options for delivery of home-based instruction.

• = Independent        ▲ = Collaborative

# Sedentary Lifestyle

## NANDA Definition

Reports a habit of life that is characterized by a low physical activity level

## Defining Characteristics

Chooses a daily routine lacking physical exercise; demonstrates physical deconditioning; verbalizes preference for activities low in physical activity

## Related Factors

Deficient knowledge of health benefits of physical exercise; lack of training for accomplishment of physical exercise; lack of resources (time, money, companionship, facilities); lack of motivation; lack of interest

## Client Outcomes

**Client Will (Specify Time Frame):**

- Increase physical activity to minimum of 10,000 steps per day.
- Meet mutually defined goals of increased exercise.
- Verbalize feeling of increased strength and ability to move.

## Nursing Interventions

- Observe the client for cause of sedentary lifestyle. Determine whether cause is physical or psychological.
- ▲ Assess for reasons why the client would be unable to participate in an exercise program—refer for evaluation by a primary care practitioner as needed.
- Use the Outcome Expectation for Exercise Scale to determine client's self-efficacy expectations and outcomes expectations toward exercise.
- Recommend the client enter an exercise program with a friend.
- Recommend the client begin a walking program utilizing the following criteria:
  - Buy a pedometer.

• = Independent          ▲ = Collaborative

- Determine common times when walking can be incorporated into usual lifestyle.
- Set goal of walking 10,000 steps per day, which equals 5 miles per day.
- If when client comes home from work, he or she does not have required number of steps, go for a walk until reaching designated goal of 10,000 steps per day.

### Pediatric

- Encourage child to increase the amount of walking done per day—if child is willing, ask him or her to wear a pedometer to measure number of steps.
- Encourage the adolescent to increase exercise to help themselves feel better.

### Geriatric

- Assess ability to move using the "Up & Go" test. Ask the client to rise from a sitting position, walk 10 feet, turn, and return to the chair to sit.
- Recommend the client begin a regular exercise program, even if generally active.
- ▲ Refer the client to physical therapy for resistance exercise training as able including abdominal crunch, leg press, leg extension, leg curl, calf press, and more.
- Use the WALC Intervention (Walk; Address pain, fear, fatigue during exercise; Learn about exercise; Cue by self-modeling) to improve exercise adherence in the older adult.
- Recommend the client begin a tai chi practice.
- If client is frail, ensure good nutrition, appropriate medications, attention to vision and hearing deficits, and increase social support along with exercise.
- If client is scheduled for an elective surgery that will result in admission into ICU and immobility, or recovery from a knee replacement, initiate a prehabilitation program that includes a warm-up, aerobic strength, flexibility, and functional task work.
- ▲ Evaluate the client for signs of depression (flat affect, in-

• = Independent      ▲ = Collaborative

somnia, anorexia, frequent somatic complaints) or cognitive impairment (use Mini-Mental State Exam [MMSE]). Refer for treatment or counseling as needed.

## Home Care

- Above interventions may be adapted for home care use.
- ▲ Assess home environment for factors that create barriers to mobility. Refer to occupational therapy services if needed to assist the client in restructuring home and daily living patterns.

## Client/Family Teaching

- Work with the client using the Transtheoretical Model of behavior change and determine if the client is in the precontemplation, contemplation, preparation, action, or maintenance state of behavior change about exercise. Provide appropriate strategies to support change to exercising based on determined state of change.
- Develop a series of contracts with mutually agreed-on goals of increased activity. Include measurable landmarks of progress, consequences for meeting or not meeting goals, and evaluation dates. Sign the contracts with the client.

# Risk for Loneliness

## NANDA Definition

At risk for experiencing vague dysphoria

## Risk Factors

Affectional deprivation; social isolation; cathectic deprivation; physical isolation

## Related Factors (r/t)

See Risk Factors

• = Independent          ▲ = Collaborative

## Client Outcomes

### Client Will (Specify Time Frame):

- Maintain one or more meaningful relationships (growth enhancing versus codependent or abusive in nature)—relationships allowing self-disclosure—and demonstrate a balance between emotional dependence and independence.
- Participate in ongoing positive and relevant social activities and interactions that are personally meaningful.
- Demonstrate positive use of time alone when socialization is not possible.

## Nursing Interventions

- Assess the client's perception of loneliness (is the person alone by choice, or do others impose the aloneness?). See care plan for **Social isolation.**
- Assess the client's ability and/or inability to meet physical, psychosocial, spiritual, and financial needs and how unmet needs further challenge the ability to be socially integrated (e.g., loss of job leading to inability to afford usual and familiar social interaction, fatigue; lack of energy necessary for social interaction and personal engagement; impaired skin integument and its relationship to real and/or perceived social isolation). NOTE: See care plan for **Disturbed Body image** if loneliness is associated with impaired skin integument.
- Use active listening skills. Establish therapeutic relationship and spend time with the client.
- Assist the client with identifying loneliness as a feeling and the causes related to loneliness.
- Evaluate the client's desire for social interaction in relation to actual social interaction.
- Explore ways to increase the client's support system and participation in groups and organizations.
- Encourage the client to be involved in meaningful social relationships that are characteristic of both giving and receiving support.
- Encourage social support for patients with visual impairments.

• = Independent          ▲ = Collaborative

- Encourage the client to develop closeness in at least one relationship.

## Adolescents

- Assess the client's social support system.
- Evaluate the depth and level of character traits, shyness, and self-esteem, particularly of younger and middle adolescent clients.
- Evaluate the family stability of younger and middle adolescent clients and advocate and encourage healthy, growth-producing relationships with family and support systems.
- For older adolescents, encourage close relationships with peers and involvement with groups and organizations.
- Consider use of pets to cope with loneliness.

## Geriatric

- Assess the client's adaptive sensory functions or any other health deviations that may limit or decrease his or her ability to interact with others.
- ▲ Assess the client's potential or actual hearing loss or hearing impairment and make appropriate referrals if a problem is identified.
- Assess caregivers for Alzheimer's clients for depression related to loneliness.
- ▲ Identify community support systems specific to elderly populations.
- Ask the client to consider living in a retirement community.
- Encourage support by friends and family when the decision to stop driving must be made.
- Encourage physical activity such as aerobics or stretching and toning in a group.
- Provide opportunities for indoor gardening.
- Provide reading materials for clients who are able to read.

## Multicultural

- Acknowledge racial/ethnic differences at the onset of care.

• = Independent        ▲ = Collaborative

- Assess for the influence of cultural beliefs, norms, and values on the client's perception of social activity and relationships.
- Approach individuals of color with respect, warmth, and professional courtesy.
- Assess the use of personal space needs, communication styles, acceptable body language, eye contact, perception of touch, and use of paraverbals when communicating with the client.
- Use a family-centered approach when working with Latino, Asian-American, African-American, and Native-American clients.
- Promote a sense of ethnic attachment.
- Validate the client's feelings regarding isolation and loneliness.
- Support spirituality as a source of support.

## Home Care

- Above interventions may be adapted for home care use.
- ▲ Assess for depression with lonely elderly client and make appropriate referrals.
- ▲ If the client is experiencing somatic complaints, evaluate client complaints to ensure physical needs are being met, and then identify relationship between somatic complaints and loneliness.
- Assist clients to identify resources/situations they can attend or in which they can participate to enhance a sense of valued fit.
- ▲ Help the client to identify periods when loneliness is greatest (e.g., certain times of day, anniversaries of past special events). With the client's permission, refer for services of visiting volunteers.
- To keep older people independent, interventions to prevent loneliness should be explored. Consider using art as an intervention.
- Identify alternatives to eating alone. Clients are often susceptible to loneliness at mealtimes. Loneliness may contribute to nutritional deficiencies or excesses.

• = Independent    ▲ = Collaborative

- Identify alternatives to being alone (e.g., telephone contact).
- Consider using computers and the Internet to alleviate or reduce loneliness and social isolation.
- Support religious beliefs.
- Discuss the meaning of death and fears associated with dying alone. Explore the possibility of significant others being with the client at the time of death.

## Client/Family Teaching

- Encourage positive use of solitude to prevent loneliness (e.g., reading, listening to music, enjoying nature and art).
- Include the family in all client-teaching activities, and give them accurate information regarding the illness severity.
- Give family members something to do such as holding a hand, applying lotion, or assisting with feeding.
- Encourage family members to express caring by telling the client where they will be and sending messages when they cannot be present.

M

# Impaired Memory

## NANDA Definition

Inability to remember or recall bits of information or behavioral skills; impaired memory may be attributed to pathophysiological or situational causes that are either temporary or permanent

## Defining Characteristics

Inability to recall factual information; inability to recall recent or past events; inability to learn or retain new skills or information; inability to determine whether a behavior was performed; observed or reported experiences of forgetting; inability to perform

• = Independent          ▲ = Collaborative

a previously learned skill; forgets to perform a behavior at a scheduled time

## Related Factors (r/t)

Fluid and electrolyte imbalance; neurological disturbances; excessive environmental disturbances; anemia; acute or chronic hypoxia; decreased cardiac output

## Client Outcomes

### Client Will (Specify Time Frame):

* Demonstrate use of techniques to help with memory loss.
* State has improved memory for everyday concerns.

## Nursing Interventions

* Assess cognitive function and memory. The emphasis of the assessment is everyday memory, the day-to-day operations of memory in real-world ordinary situations. Use an assessment tool such as the Mini-Mental State Examination (MMSE) and/or the Metamemory in Adulthood (MIA) questionnaire.
* ▲ Determine whether onset of memory loss is gradual or sudden. If memory loss is sudden, refer the client to a physician or neuropsychologist for evaluation.
* Determine amount and pattern of alcohol intake.
* Note the client's current medications and intake of any mind-altering substances such as benzodiazepines, ecstasy, marijuana, cocaine, or glucocorticoids.
* Note the client's current level of stress. Ask if there has been a recent traumatic event.
* If stress is associated with memory loss, refer to a stress reduction clinic. If not available, suggest that the client meditate, receive massages, participate in moderate physical activity, all of which may promote stress reduction and reduce anxiety and depression. Encourage the client to develop an aerobic exercise program.
* Determine the client's sleep patterns. If insufficient, refer to care plan for **Disturbed Sleep pattern.**
* ▲ Determine the client's blood sugar levels. If they are ele-

• = Independent          ▲ = Collaborative

vated, refer to physician for treatment and encourage
healthy diet and exercise to improve memory.

▲ If signs of depression such as weight loss, insomnia, or
sad affect are evident, refer the client for psychotherapy.

▲ Perform a nutritional assessment. If nutritional status is
marginal, confer with a dietitian and primary care practitioner to evaluate whether the client needs supplementation with foods or vitamins. Teach the client the
need to eat a healthy diet with adequate intake of whole
grains, fruits, and vegetables to decrease cerebrovascular infarcts.

▲ Question the client about cholesterol level. If it is high,
refer to physician or dietitian for help in lowering.
Encourage the client to eat a healthy diet, avoiding saturated fats and *trans*-fatty acids.

• Suggest the client use cues, including alarm watches,
electronic organizers, calendars, lists, or pocket computers, to trigger certain actions at designated times.

• Encourage the client to use external memory devices,
such as a calendar for appointments, keep reminder lists,
place a string around finger or rubber band around wrist
as reminders, or enlist someone else to remind him or
her of important events.

• Help the client set up a medication box that reminds the
client to take medication at needed times; assist the client with refilling the box at intervals if necessary.

• If safety is an issue with certain activities (e.g., the client
forgets to turn off stove after use or forgets emergency
telephone numbers), suggest alternatives such as using a
microwave or whistling teakettle for heating water and
programming emergency numbers in telephone so
that they are readily available.

▲ Refer the client to a memory clinic (if available), a neuropsychologist, or an occupational therapist.

• For clients with memory impairments associated with
dementia, see care plan for **Chronic Confusion.**

### Geriatric

• Assess for signs of depression.

• = Independent          ▲ = Collaborative

- Evaluate all medications that the client is taking to determine whether they are causing the memory loss.
- Recommend that elderly clients maintain a positive attitude and active involvement with the world around them and that they maintain good nutrition.
- Encourage the elderly to believe in themselves and to work to improve their memory. Negative attitudes and belief may decrease motivation and impair everyday memory function.
▲ Refer the client to a memory class that focuses on helping older adults learn memory strategies.
- Help family develop a memory aid booklet or wallet that contains pictures and labels from the client's life, or develop a video movie that includes familiar pictures with narration.
- Help family label items such as the bathroom or sock drawer to increase recall.

## Multicultural

- Assess for the influence of cultural beliefs, norms, and values on the family or caregivers' understanding of impaired memory.
- Use bias-free instruments when assessing memory in the culturally diverse client.
- Inform the client's family or caregiver of meaning of and reasons for common behavior observed in the client with impaired memory.
- Validate family members' feelings regarding the impact of the client's behavior on family lifestyle.

## Home Care

- Above interventions may be adapted for home care use.
- Arrange cues for medication taking that are focused around daily events (e.g., meals and bedtimes).
- Assess the client's need for outside assistance with recall of treatment, medications, and willingness/ability of family to provide needed support.

• = Independent        ▲ = Collaborative

- Identify a checking-in support system (e.g., Lifeline or significant others).
- Keep furniture placement and household patterns consistent.
▲ In the presence of a medical disorder, institute case management of frail elderly to support continued independent living.

## Client/Family Teaching

- When teaching the client, determine what the client knows about memory techniques and then build on that knowledge.
- When teaching a skill to the client, set up a series of practice attempts. Begin with simple tasks so that the client can be positively reinforced and progress to more difficult concepts.
- Teach clients to use memory techniques such as repeating information they want to remember, making mental associations to remember information, and placing items in strategic places so that they will not be forgotten.

M

# Impaired bed Mobility

## NANDA Definition

Limitation of independent movement from one bed position to another

## Defining Characteristics

Impaired ability to turn from side to side; impaired ability to move from supine to sitting or sitting to supine; impaired ability to "scoot" or reposition self in bed; impaired ability to move from supine to prone or prone to supine; impaired ability to move from supine to long sitting or long sitting to supine

• = Independent        ▲ = Collaborative

## Related Factors (r/t)

Intolerance to activity; decreased strength and endurance; pain or discomfort; perceptual or cognitive impairment; neuromuscular impairment; musculoskeletal impairment; depression; severe anxiety

Suggested functional level classifications may include the following:

0—Completely independent
1—Requires use of equipment or device
2—Requires help from another person
3—Requires help from another person and equipment device
4—Dependent (does not participate in activity)

## Client Outcomes

### Client Will (Specify Time Frame):

- Demonstrate optimal independence in positioning, exercising, and performing functional activities in bed.
- Demonstrate ability to direct others on how to do bed positioning, exercising, and functional activities.

## Nursing Interventions

- Perform physical assessment to determine the client's risk for ICP, respiratory, and cardiovascular abnormalities, increased muscle tone, aspiration, pressure ulcer and pain.
- Use critical thinking and priority setting to decide most therapeutic bed positions and frequency of turns; base this on client's history, risk profile, and preventive needs.
- Raise the head of the bed to 30 degrees if the client has increased intracranial pressure (ICP). Refer to care plan for **Decreased Intracranial adaptive capacity.**
- Assist client to sit upright during and after feedings or ingestion of pills if dysphagia presents. Refer to care plan for **Impaired Swallowing.**
- Periodically position the client in an upright sitting posi-

• = Independent          ▲ = Collaborative

tion as tolerated. If vital signs and oxygen saturation levels are stable, dangle patient's legs if applicable.

- Maintain the head of the bed at the lowest degree of elevation possible, depending on medical condition to prevent pressure ulcer.
- Position the bed flat at intervals, unless contraindicated for a medical reason.
- Tilt patients 30 degrees or less while side lying.
- Place a pillow under heels of immobile, supine lying patients unless contraindicated (e.g., postoperatively after total knee replacement).
- Prevent complications of immobility.
- If high risk for pressure ulcer development exists, place the client on a static or dynamic surface in bed. Routinely place palm of hand under the overlay and susceptible bony areas to check for "bottoming out" (body sinks into mattress, thus the recommended one inch between the surface and client is absent). Refer to care plan for **Risk for impaired Skin integrity.**
- ▲ Place the client with stage III or IV pressure ulcer on low-air-loss surface or air-fluidized bed. Consult enterostomal therapy nurse to determine appropriate surface for complex clients.
- Encourage the client to take deep breaths, cough, reposition self, drink adequate fluids, and use incentive spirometer.
- Ensure the client receives adequate fiber, fluid, and a stool softener and/or bulking agent to prevent constipation. Refer to care plan for **Constipation.**
- Recognize clients at risk for venous thromboembolism (VTE) and implement prophylactic measures such as antiembolic stockings, elastic wraps, sequential compression devices; joint ROM and leg exercises; adequate fluid intake and anticoagulant medications. Refer to care plan for **Ineffective Tissue perfusion.**
- Encourage fluid intake of 2000 to 3000 mL/day as tolerated by medical condition.

**M**

• = Independent          ▲ = Collaborative

- Take scrupulous care of indwelling Foley catheter; detect and report signs of urinary tract infection as early as possible.
- Implement the following interventions during bed mobility activities:
  - Place positioning devices such as pillows or foam wedges between bony prominences.
  - Use lifting or lateral transferring devices such as: trapeze, bed linen, mechanical lateral transfer aid, ceiling mounted lift, or transfer chair, and bed scale to move (rather than drag) for dependent or obese individuals.
- Use large beds and special equipment to reposition the bariatric (very obese) client, such as air mattress overlay with rotation function, trapeze, and stirrup and pulley attached to an overhead traction system (to place one leg in thus raising it during pericare). Logroll and tilt dependent bariatric client (avoid full side-lying position) until familiar with his or her ability to help turn in bed.

M

▲ Apply elbow pads to comatose clients, to those with arm restraints, and to clients who use their elbows to prop or scoot themselves up in bed. Apply nocturnal elbow splint to promote extension if an ulnar nerve palsy exists or if there is pain at the elbow and paresthesia in the ulnar side of the 4th and 5th fingers.
- Teach proper ROM, self-care activities, and apply extremity splints/boots on a rotating schedule to prevent joint contracture and disuse syndrome.
- Explain the importance of exhaling when pulling self up or rolling in bed and during any activity that precipitates breath holding or straining.
▲ If movement intensifies pain level, then preventively administer analgesics before bed repositioning, exercising, or self-cares.
- Assist clients to splint an incision, wound, or other painful abdominal area with a pillow as they change positions, cough, or perform functional activities.
▲ Administer oral antispasmodic medications as pre-

● = Independent             ▲ = Collaborative

scribed to control muscle spasms that interfere with movement.

▲ Apply ice as ordered by physician to sites after nerve and motor point blocks and assess for side effects of pain, sensory deficits, or vascular problems.

▲ Recognize that intractable chronic spasticity and pain can interrupt function, bed/chair positioning, hygiene, and quality of life. If conservative treatment fails, some clients benefit from continuous intrathecal baclofen infusion (CITB) via an implanted pump in the spinal canal.

▲ Refer clients to a dietitian, or provide dietary information to promote normal body weight.

## Exercising

• Perform passive ROM at least twice a day to immobile body parts. Support limb above and below the joint being ranged (e.g., hold the forearm and hand while ranging the wrist).

• Range hemiplegic client's affected upper extremity with the shoulder in slight external rotation.

• Perform ROM slowly and rhythmically. Do not range beyond the point of pain in those with sensation; range only to the point of resistance in those with poor sensation and mental awareness.

• Reinforce client's self-initiated practice of exercise programs, developed by therapists including muscle setting, active strengthening, contraction of muscles against resistance, and weight lifting.

• Intervene for misalignment, flaccidity and spasticity, inability to shift weight, reduced sensation, and excessive effort while moving.

• Use manual guidance and verbal cueing during bed mobility to facilitate more normal tone, posture, and movement. Allow clients to do as much of the activity as they can.

## Positioning

• Incorporate the following measures to promote normal tone and prevent complications.

• = Independent        ▲ = Collaborative

- Position head and neck in midline.
- Use a flat pillow when clients are supine if neck flexion occurs. Use a small pillow behind the head and/or between the shoulder blades if extension occurs.
- If lateral head flexion occurs, place a sandbag under the pillow along one or both sides of the head when the client is supine, and place one or two pillows under the head in the side-lying position.
- Change the position of client's shoulders and arms frequently. Abduct the shoulders of persons with high paraplegia or quadriplegia horizontally to 90 degrees briefly twice a day.
- Do not position hemiplegics' shoulders in abduction.
- Apply resting forearm, wrist, and hand splints as ordered. Routinely check underlying skin for pressure and poor circulation. Strictly adhere to on/off orders.
- Use hard cone or splint in hands as ordered to help prevent hand contractures.
- Elevate the affected arm of persons with hemiplegia and apply an isotoner glove.
- Place a thin pillow under the weak pelvic girdle, hip and upper thigh of persons with hemiplegia. Place a trochanter roll along the outside of the legs of persons with hemiplegia or leg paralysis.
- Strictly maintain leg abduction in persons with a surgical hip pinning or hip replacement by placing an abductor splint or pillow between the legs.
- Apply foot splints, boots, or high top tennis shoes as recommended by the physical therapist. Routinely assess underlying skin for signs of pressure.

- Assist clients to lie prone or semiprone routinely (may be contraindicated in those with cardiopulmonary disturbances or increased intracranial pressure).
- Position hemiplegics on the unaffected and affected sides. Position the affected shoulder slightly forward by moving the shoulder, not the arm.

M

• = Independent          ▲ = Collaborative

- Components of normal bed mobility include rolling, bridging, scooting, long sitting, and sitting upright. Most movements start with the client supine, flat in bed.

## Bed Mobility—Rolling
- Assist the client into the set position for rolling. For hemiplegics, this includes:
  - Moving the shoulder and arm on the side to which the client will turn outward with palm facing up
  - Flexing the knees with the feet flat on the bed
- For persons with bilateral leg paralysis, this includes:
  - Crossing the outside leg over the other leg or manually flexing the outside leg
  - Placing the arms in front of the chest with the hands clasped together
- Instruct and guide the client to roll over segmentally (e.g., start by turning the head toward the direction of the turn, then move the shoulders/arms/trunk, as the hips and flexed knees follow). Staff should be prepared to assist the affected side of hemiplegics, and the legs of paraplegics and quadriplegics.

NOTE: For safety, always logroll a client with spinal cord injury and persons with severe back pain or recent back surgery.

## Bed Mobility—Bridging
- Teach clients to use bridging (lifting hips off the bed) during functional activities such as using the bedpan or pulling up pants.
- Reinforce the set position (e.g., knees flexed and feet flat on the bed close to the buttocks). Assist by preventing external rotation of the legs.
- Have the client rest his or her arms and hands on the bed alongside the trunk.
- Instruct the client to push down on the bed with the feet thus lifting his/her buttocks. Assistance may be needed to lift the pelvis upward or to hold a weak foot down.

M

• = Independent          ▲ = Collaborative

## Bed Mobility—Scooting Laterally

- Communicate which direction the client is to move towards and help the client bridge.
- Support the client's pelvis to the extent needed as he or she pushes down on the bed with the feet, and lifts the hips up and over onto the side of the bed.
- Instruct the client to lift head and shoulders up off the bed and move them and the trunk sideways. If the client has hemiplegia, support the affected shoulder from the scapula and help move the trunk as needed.

## Bed Mobility—Side-Lying to Sitting Upright

- Assess whether the client is over to one side of the bed far enough; if not, help the client to move over.
- Assist or cue the client to turn on his/her side (to the affected side if hemiplegic) if possible.
- Instruct the client to lower the legs slowly over the edge of the bed with knees flexed and close to chest unless the client has recently had back or neck surgery, or has back pain. If so, the legs should be lowered slowly off the bed by staff at the same time the client lifts his/her head and pushes up with the arms, keeping the spine straight.
- Ask the client to lift his or her head off the bed.
- Ensure that the bottom shoulder is positioned slightly forward before sitting up (move it forward from the shoulder).
- Instruct the client to bear weight on the bottom arm and elbow while at the same time pushing against the mattress with the palm of other hand to sit up.
- Help the client sit up by placing one of your hands under the bottom shoulder blade to keep it well forward and pushing down on the opposite with your other hand. Shift the client's weight; do not lift it. Encourage the client to complete as much of the movement as possible.
- Assist clients to sit on the edge of the bed with weight on

• = Independent           ▲ = Collaborative

both buttocks. Hips and knees should flex to 90 degrees, and if possible feet should be flat on the floor.

## Bed Mobility—Long Sitting (for Clients with Paretic or Immobile Legs)

- Assess the client's ability for 100-degree straight leg raises; if absent, avoid this position.
- Cue the client to start from the flat and supine position and to grasp the side rails.
- Instruct client to pull self up to a sitting position. If hand function is poor, teach the client to raise the head/trunk and then push against the mattress with flexed forearms, until sitting upright. The legs remain in extension as the client sits up.

## Geriatric

- Discriminately raise elders' side rails. Try alternatives such as body pillows, height-adjustable beds, bed alarms, and antislip floor mats next to the bed instead.
- Develop strategies for bed positioning and mobility based on the client's multiple chronic and disabling conditions.
- Assess caregivers' strength, health history, and cognitive status, to predict ability and risk for helping clients with bed mobility at home. Explore alternative options if risk is too high.
- Assess the client's stamina and energy level during bed mobility activities; rest breaks may be needed.
- Spread out bed activities and exercise programs rather than clumping them together.
- Incorporate memory aids and strategies (e.g., written schedules, directions, sketches, or notes), timers, etc, so that clients with cognitive decline can function as independently as possible.

## Home Care

- ▲ Utilize nurse case managers, care coordinators or social workers to assess support systems and identify need for

M

• = Independent        ▲ = Collaborative

assistive technology devices and community or home health services.

- Encourage use of the client's regular bed in the home unless contraindicated for medical reasons. Foam wedges or blocks can raise the head of bed if necessary. Place indented or grooved-out areas in wood pieces under each leg of the bed and set bed against the walls in a corner of the room.
- Suggest rearranging furniture at home to make it accessible and to meet sleeping, toileting, and living needs.
- Discuss the psychological and physical benefits of allowing clients to be as self-sufficient as possible with bed mobility even though it may be time consuming.
- Prepare family members for potential regression in client's self-care during the transition from hospital to home.
- Offer emotional support and suggest community social supports to help with adjustment and independence issues.
- Provide information about options for durable medical equipment and assistive technology and help families creatively problem-solve ways to access funding sources to pay for such devices.
- In the presence of medical disorder, institute case management of the frail elderly to support continued independent living.
- See the Home Care Interventions section of the care plan for **Impaired physical Mobility.**

## Client/Family Teaching

- Use various sensory modalities to teach the client, family, and caregivers correct techniques for ROM, exercising, repositioning, and bed mobility activities.
- Give visual information (e.g., demonstrations, sketches, instructional videos, written instructions).
- Give tactile stimulation (e.g., manual guidance, hand-on-hand technique, return demonstrations, note taking).
- Give auditory information (e.g., verbal instructions, instructional audiotapes, verbal repetition of instruc-

• = Independent         ▲ = Collaborative

tions, self-talk during a motor activity, reading aloud written instructions).
- Schedule time with family and caregivers for education and practice. Suggest that family members come prepared with questions and wear comfortable and safe clothing and shoes for practice.
- Teach caregivers proper body mechanics and use of assistive devices (if applicable) while assisting clients with bed mobility activities.

# Impaired physical Mobility

## NANDA Definition

A limitation in independent, purposeful physical movement of the body or of one or more extremities

## Defining Characteristics

M

Postural instability during performance of routine ADLs; limited ability to perform gross motor skills; limited ability to perform fine motor skills; uncoordinated or jerky movements; limited range of motion; difficulty turning; decreased reaction time; movement-induced shortness of breath; gait changes (e.g., decreased walking speed, difficulty initiating gait, small steps, shuffles feet, exaggerated lateral postural sway); engages in substitutions for movement (e.g., increased attention to other's activity, controlling behavior, focus on preillness/predisability); slowed movement; movement-induced tremor; medications; prescribed movement restrictions; discomfort; lack of knowledge regarding value of physical activity; body mass index greater than 30; sensoriperceptual impairments; neuromuscular impairment; pain; musculoskeletal impairment; intolerance to activity/ decreased strength and endurance; depressive mood state or anxiety; cognitive impairment; decreased muscle strength, control, and/or mass; reluctance to initiate movement; sedentary lifestyle or disuse or deconditioning; selective or generalized malnutrition; loss of integrity of bone structures; developmental

• = Independent          ▲ = Collaborative

delay; joint stiffness or contractures; limited cardiovascular endurance; altered cellular metabolism; lack of physical or social environmental supports; cultural beliefs regarding age-appropriate activity

Suggested functional level classifications may include the following:

0—Completely independent
1—Requires use of equipment or device
2—Requires help from another person for assistance, supervision, or teaching
3—Requires help from another person and equipment device
4—Dependent (does not participate in activity)

## Client Outcomes

### Client Will (Specify Time Frame):

- Increase physical activity.
- Meet mutually defined goals of increased mobility.
- Verbalize feeling of increased strength and ability to move.
- Demonstrate use of adaptive equipment (e.g., wheelchairs, walkers) to increase mobility.

## Nursing Interventions

- Screen for mobility skills in the following order: (1) bed mobility; (2) supported and unsupported sitting; (3) transition movements such as sit to stand, sitting down, and transfers; and (4) standing and walking activities. Use a tool such as the Assessment Tool for Safe Patient Handling and Movement.
- Observe the client for cause of impaired mobility. Determine whether cause is physical or psychological. See interventions for **Ineffective Coping** or **Hopelessness.**
- Monitor and record the client's ability to tolerate activity and use all four extremities; note pulse rate, blood pressure, dyspnea, and skin color before and after activity. See care plan for **Activity intolerance.**
- ▲ Before activity, observe for and, if possible, treat pain. Ensure that the client is not oversedated.

• = Independent          ▲ = Collaborative

▲ Consult with physical therapist for further evaluation, strength training, gait training, and development of a mobility plan.

▲ Obtain any assistive devices needed for activity, such as gait belt, walker, cane, crutches, or wheelchair, before the activity begins.

• If the client is immobile, perform passive ROM exercises at least twice a day unless contraindicated; repeat each maneuver three times.

▲ If the client is immobile, consult with physician for a safety evaluation before beginning an exercise program; if program is approved, begin with the following exercises:

 ■ Active ROM exercises using both upper and lower extremities (e.g., flexing and extending at ankles, knees, hips)

 ■ Chin-ups and pull-ups using a trapeze in bed (may be contraindicated in clients with cardiac conditions)

 ■ Strengthening exercises such as gluteal or quadriceps sitting exercises

• If client is immobile, consider use of a transfer chair, a chair that becomes a stretcher.

• Help the client achieve mobility and start walking as soon as possible if not contraindicated.

• Use a gait walking belt when ambulating the client.

• Apply any ordered brace before mobilizing the client.

• Initiate a "No Lift" policy where appropriate assistive devices are utilized for manual lifting.

• Increase independence in ADLs, encouraging self-efficacy and discouraging helplessness as the client gets stronger.

▲ If client has had a CVA with hemiparesis, consider use of constraint-induced movement therapy (CIMT), where the functional extremity is purposely constrained and the client is forced to use the involved extremity.

• If the client does not feed or groom self, sit side-by-side with the client, put your hand over the client's hand, support the client's elbow with your other hand, and help the client feed self; use the same technique to help the client comb hair.

M

• = Independent          ▲ = Collaborative

## Geriatric

- Assess ability to move using the "Up & Go" test. Ask the client to rise from a sitting position, walk 10 feet, turn, and return to the chair to sit.
- Help the mostly immobile client achieve mobility as soon as possible, depending on physical condition.
- If client is frail, ensure good nutrition, appropriate medications, attention to vision and hearing deficits, and increase social support along with exercise.
- Use the Outcome Expectation for Exercise Scale to determine client's self-efficacy expectations and outcomes expectations toward exercise.
- For a client who is mostly immobile, minimize cardiovascular deconditioning by positioning the client in the upright position several times daily.
- If the client is mostly immobile, encourage him or her to attend a low-intensity aerobic chair exercise class that includes stretching and strengthening chair exercises.
- Initiate a walking program in which the client walks with or without help every day as part of daily routine.
- ▲ Refer the client to physical therapy for resistance exercise training as able including abdominal crunch, leg press, leg extension, leg curl, calf press, and more.
- Use the WALC Intervention (Walk; Address pain, fear, fatigue during exercise; Learn about exercise; Cue by self-modeling) to improve exercise adherence in the older adult.
- If client is scheduled for an elective surgery that will result in admission into ICU and immobility, or recovery from a knee replacement, initiate a prehabilitation program that includes a warm-up, aerobic strength, flexibility, and functional task work.
- ▲ Evaluate the client for signs of depression (flat affect, insomnia, anorexia, frequent somatic complaints) or cognitive impairment (use Mini-Mental State Exam [MMSE]). Refer for treatment or counseling as needed.
- Watch for orthostatic hypotension when mobilizing elderly clients. Have the client dangle at the side of the bed with legs hanging over the edge of the bed, flex and ex-

• = Independent          ▲ = Collaborative

tend feet several times after sitting up, then stand up slowly with someone holding the client. If client becomes light-headed or dizzy, return him or her to bed immediately.

- Be very careful when getting a mostly immobile client up. Be sure to lock the bed and wheelchair and have sufficient personnel to protect the client from falls.
- Do not routinely assist with transfers or bathing activities unless necessary.
- Use gestures and nonverbal cues when helping clients move if they are anxious or have difficulty understanding and following verbal instructions.
- Recognize that wheelchairs are not a good mobility device and often serve as a mobility restraint.
- Ensure that chairs fit clients. Chair seat should be 3 inches above the height of the knee. Provide a raised toilet seat if needed.
- If the client is mainly immobile, provide opportunities for socialization and sensory stimulation (e.g., television and visits). See **Deficient Diversional activity, Acute Confusion** or **Hopelessness** as appropriate.

## Home Care

- Above interventions may be adapted for home care use.
- ▲ Begin discharge planning as soon as possible with case manager or social worker to assess need for home support systems, assistive devices, and community or home health services.
- ▲ Assess home environment for factors that create barriers to physical mobility. Refer to occupational therapy services if needed to assist the client in restructuring home and daily living patterns.
- ▲ Refer to home health aide services to support the client and family through changing levels of mobility. Reinforce need to promote independence in mobility as tolerated.
- ▲ Refer to physical therapy for gait training, strengthening, and balance training.
- Assess skin condition at every visit. Establish a skin care

M

• = Independent          ▲ = Collaborative

program that enhances circulation and maximizes position changes.

- Once the client is able to walk independently, and needs an exercise program, suggest the client enter an exercise program with a friend.
- Provide support to the client and family/caregivers during long-term impaired mobility.
- ▲ Institute case management of frail elderly to support continued independent living.

## Client/Family Teaching

- Teach the client to get out of bed slowly when transferring from the bed to the chair.
- Teach the client relaxation techniques to use during activity.
- Teach the client to use assistive devices such as a cane, a walker, or crutches to increase mobility.
- Teach family members and caregivers to work with clients during self-care activities such as eating, bathing, grooming, dressing, and transferring rather than having the client be a passive recipient of care.
- Work with the client using the Transtheoretical Model of behavior change and determine if the client is in the precontemplation, contemplation, preparation, action, or maintenance state of behavior change about exercise. Provide appropriate strategies to support change to exercising based on determined state of change.
- Develop a series of contracts with mutually agreed-on goals of increased activity. Include measurable landmarks of progress, consequences for meeting or not meeting goals, and evaluation dates. Sign the contracts with the client.

M

# Impaired wheelchair Mobility

## NANDA Definition

Limitation of independent movement within the environment using a device equipped with wheels

• = Independent          ▲ = Collaborative

## Defining Characteristics

Impaired ability to operate a manual or power wheelchair on even or uneven surface; impaired ability to operate manual or power wheelchair on an incline or decline; impaired ability to operate wheelchair on curbs

## Related Factors (r/t)

Intolerance to activity; decreased strength and endurance; pain or discomfort; perceptual or cognitive impairment; neuromuscular impairment; musculoskeletal impairment; depression; severe anxiety

Suggested functional level classifications may include the following:

0—Completely independent
1—Requires use of equipment or device
2—Requires help from another person for assistance, supervision, or teaching
3—Requires help from another person and equipment or device
4—Dependent—does not participate in activity

M

## Client Outcomes

### Client Will (Specify Time Frame):

- Demonstrate optimal independence in operating and moving a wheelchair or other device equipped with wheels.
- Demonstrate the ability to direct others in operating and moving a wheelchair or other device equipped with wheels.
- Demonstrate therapeutic positioning, pressure relief, and safety principles while operating and moving wheelchair or other device equipped with wheels.

## Nursing Interventions

- Assist client to don and doff equipment (e.g., braces, corsets, orthoses, immobilizers, and abdominal binders) in bed.
- ▲ Obtain referrals for physical therapy (PT), occupational therapy (OT), or a wheelchair seating clinic.
- Realize the seating system allows the client to propel the

• = Independent          ▲ = Collaborative

chair safely and ably use the hands, reach the foot rests and floor with the feet, and stand up from the chair without falling. In the disabled, the chair is part of their identity.

- Keep the right cushion and wheelchair with the right patient.
- Use of contoured surfaces/cushions/cutouts/supports, strict continence management, adequate nutrition and hydration, and repositioning are key strategies to prevent sitting-acquired pressure ulcers. Never use doughnut-type cushions or sheepskin.
- ▲ Obtain a PT, OT or wheelchair seating clinic referral for cushion re-evaluation if signs of pressure exist after chair sitting.
- Emphasize importance of weight shifts every 15 minutes with safety belts in place, including: lateral leans (leaning toward one side of chair), forward leans (leaning forward as arms lie alongside thighs), and pushups if balance and trunk control are present (pushing up with hands on armrests to lift buttocks off the seat).
- Manually tilt the wheelchair backward 45 to 65 degrees for 3-5 minutes, hourly. Client may also sit with the back of the wheelchair reclined (150 degrees) with legs on leg/foot rests.
- Activate passive standing position in wheel chair if applicable, or if client has partial weight bearing, stand him/her briefly.
- Inspect skin under orthoses, braces, etc. once removed and check bony prominences after client returns to bed.
- Place feet level with both feet on footrests or on the floor when passively sitting in the wheelchair.
- Routinely assess the client's sitting posture and help reposition him/her into sound alignment as needed.
- Place client's feet securely on footrests and fasten seat belts across the top of the thighs before propelling the wheelchair.
- Remove leg and foot rests from wheelchairs of clients who can "walk" it by taking short steps with their legs while seated to move the chair.

● = Independent          ▲ = Collaborative

- Implement precautionary measures including use of friction-coated projection hand rims and leather gloves as clients propel manual wheelchairs.
- Guide client's hands onto wheelchair rims and explain how to push forward on both wheel rims to move ahead, to push the right rim to turn left and vice versa, and to pull backward on both wheel rims to back up.
- Use a wheelchair low enough so both feet touch flat on the floor.
- Guide and instruct clients with unilateral arm and leg function to propel the wheelchair by: (1) raising that foot plate then putting foot flat on the floor, (2) placing sound hand on the wheel rim, (3) pushing forward with the sound hand while (4) "walking" the chair forward by extending the knee, putting the heel then the entire foot on the floor, flexing the knee and pulling the chair forward. NOTE: A hemi, one-arm drive wheelchair is recommended for persons with hemiplegia.
- Recommend clients back their wheelchairs (wheeled devices) into an elevator. If entering face first, instruct them to turn chair around to face the elevator doors.
- Reinforce principle of descending a curb backward ("popping a wheelie") if balance, trunk control, strength, and timing are adequate. Client needs to lean slightly forward and guide both wheels off curb at the same time.
- Recommend ascending curbs in a forward position by popping a wheelie or having an assistant tilt the chair back, place the front wheels over the curb, and roll the back wheels up it. If surface is soft (muddy, sandy) go up curb backward via a wheelie.
- During assisted wheelies, the helper must hold the wheelchair until all four wheels are back on the ground and the client has balance and control of the wheelchair.
- When client has unilateral neglect, agnosia, or proprioception deficits, nurses should reinforce the team's compensatory strategies as clients propel the wheelchair, enter doorways, and detect and avoid obstacles. Strategies may include: visual scanning, self-talk, self-questioning about what could be wrong, and manual guiding.

**M**

• = Independent          ▲ = Collaborative

- • Use an individualized wheelchair with clients sitting as upright as possible versus a geri-chair when feeding dysphagic elders.
- ▲ Implement and teach the following measures:
  - ■ Consult therapists for ROM, exercises, strengthening, and gentle stretching; and for wheelchair setup, seat height and "pushing" evaluations.
  - ■ Encourage doing more leans and chair tilts versus push-ups as weight shifts.
  - ■ Ensure transfer surfaces are as even in height as possible.
  - ■ Advocate for ultralightweight manual; or pushrim activated power assisted or electric powered wheelchairs (therapists and physicians will need to document evaluations and write letters of necessity to justify/request funding from payors).
  - ■ Stress that clients maintain normal versus extra body weight.
  - ■ Reinforce these principles as clients propel their wheelchairs, "Use long and smooth strokes that limit high forces and rate of loading on the pushrim" and "Allow the hand to naturally drift down when letting go of the pushrim; make an effort to keep the hand below the pushrim when not in contact with the pushrim."
  - ■ Remind clients to avoid putting pressure on their elbows and remind them to distribute pressure the length of the arm during repositioning and weight shifts. Splints (especially nocturnal), elbow pads, assistance with transfers, and temporary use of an electric wheelchair may relieve tendonitis.
  - ■ Recognize the value systems of clients and nurses regarding use of a wheelchair may create tension. Need for a wheelchair may symbolize weakness and loss of autonomy to clients; it may symbolize increased independence and functioning to professionals.
- ▲ Offer support and referrals to help clients cope with

• = Independent          ▲ = Collaborative

issues related to physical disability and loss of
independence.

- Suggest and help clients transition from a manual to a
powered wheelchair if progressive physical disability
occurs.
- Request and receive client's permission before moving
client's unoccupied wheelchair within the room or out to
the hall or another room.

## Geriatric

- Alternate wheelchair mobility with rest periods.
▲ Avoid using restraints on elderly, fidgeting clients because they slide down in a wheelchair or try to reposition
themselves. Rather, assess for deformities, spinal curva-
tures, abnormal tone, discomfort, and limited joint range.
If present, obtain a consult for a proper wheelchair seating system.
- Ensure proper lower extremity positioning when clients
are sitting up. Do not use elevating leg rests to prevent them from sliding down in the wheelchair, instead
use custom foot rests. Place both feet either on foot
rests or on the floor when the wheelchair is stationary.
▲ Assess for side effects of medications and potential need
for dosage readjustments to increase wheelchair mobility tolerance.
- Allow the client to propel the wheelchair independently
at his or her own speed. Avoid rushing client.

## Home Care

- Assess the home environment for barriers to wheelchair
accessibility and for a support system for emergency
and contingency care (e.g., Lifeline).
- Arrange traffic patterns so they are wide enough for a
wheelchair or wheeled device to get around in.
- Explain a 5-foot turning space is necessary to maneuver
wheelchairs in (e.g., in a bathroom), doorways need to be
32 to 36 inches wide, entrance ramps or paths should
slope 1 inch per foot, and one outside entrance should

M

have space enough to open the door and accommodate the wheelchair or wheeled device in.

- Suggest simple and economic changes such as replacing door hardware with fold-back hinges, removing doorway encasements if doorways are too narrow and removing or replacing thresholds if existing ones are too high.
- Suggest rearranging room functions, furniture, and storage so that toileting, sleeping, bathing, and preparing and eating meals can safely take place on one level of the home.
- ▲ Request PT and OT referrals to evaluate wheelchair skills and safety; teach client how to improve endurance, propel wheelchair on carpet and irregular surfaces, how to get back into wheelchair if he or she falls (or intentionally moves) onto the floor; and to make home modifications for safety.
- Reinforce clients or caregiver assess for skin breakdown daily and establish programs to enhance circulation and decrease risk of sitting-acquired pressure ulcers.
- ▲ Supply home health aide services as appropriate for assistance with ADLs, bathing, and skin care.
- ▲ Provide support to clients and make referrals to medical social services or mental health/support group services.
- ▲ Provide client with information about advocacy, accessibility, assistive technology, potential funding, and issues under the Americans with Disabilities Act.
- ▲ Investigate community resources and written information for locating wheelchair parts and services for repair and tune up if the client is unable to do it (an annual tune-up is wise).

## Client/Family Teaching

- Suggest that the client test-drive wheelchairs and try out cushions and postural supports before purchasing them.
- Discuss advantages, disadvantages, and long-term care involved with various cushions that distribute pressure. (1) Air cushions evenly distribute pressure, can be changed to optimize flotation, wash easily in case of incontinence, and are lightweight but they leak air and

• = Independent        ▲ = Collaborative

need reinflation. As flotation increases, a lightweight client's sense of stability may decrease. (2) Gel cushions are durable and give support because they contour to the buttock; however, they may be hot, heavy, and create a moist environment. The gel must be pushed back in place to provide pressure relief. (3) Foam cushions are light, inexpensive, and can be cut to fit client contour but they compress and break down. They may need to be replaced and are not waterproof.

- Instruct and have the client demonstrate reinflation of pneumatic tires; encourage the client to monitor tire pressure every 2 to 3 weeks.
- Instruct client and family to remove as many wheelchair parts as possible when lifting wheelchair into the car. Check that armrests and all parts of chair are fastened securely before picking them or the chair up. Check temperature of wheelchair or wheeled device before sitting in it.
- ▲ Teach or secure social service referrals to educate clients on financial coverage/regulations of third-party payers and HCFA for durable medical equipment. Realize that light and ultralight wheelchairs are easier to propel and are more comfortable and adjustable than heavier models. They are expensive, but over time cost less to operate than heavier chairs.
- Teach the client the importance of using seatbelts or chair tie-downs when riding in motor vehicles. If unavailable, clients in wheelchairs should be transported in large, heavy vehicles.

# Nausea

## NANDA Definition

An unpleasant wavelike sensation in the back of the throat, epigastrium, or throughout the abdomen that may or may not lead to vomiting

• = Independent          ▲ = Collaborative

## Defining Characteristics

Usually precedes vomiting, but may be experienced after vomiting or when vomiting does not occur; accompanied by pallor, cold and clammy skin, increased salivation, tachycardia, gastric stasis, and diarrhea; accompanied by swallowing movements affected by skeletal muscles; reports "nausea" or "sick to stomach"

## Related Factors (r/t)

### Treatment related

Gastric irritation: pharmaceuticals (e.g., aspirin, nonsteroidal anti-inflammatory drugs, steroids, antibiotics), alcohol, iron, and blood, gastric distention: delayed gastric emptying caused by pharmacological interventions (e.g., narcotics administration, anesthesia agents), pharmaceuticals (e.g., analgesics, antivirals for HIV, aspirin, opioids, chemotherapeutic agents), toxins (e.g., radiotherapy)

### Biophysical

Biochemical disorders (e.g., uremia, diabetic ketoacidosis, pregnancy), cardiac pain, cancer of stomach or intraabdominal tumors (e.g., pelvic or colorectal cancers), esophageal or pancreatic disease, gastric distention due to delayed gastric emptying, pyloric intestinal obstruction, genitourinary and biliary distention, upper bowel stasis, compression of the stomach (liver, spleen, or other organ enlargement that slows the stomach functioning [squashed stomach syndrome]), excess food intake, gastric irritation due to pharyngeal and/or peritoneal inflammation, liver or splenetic capsule stretch, local tumors (e.g., acoustic neuroma, primary or secondary brain tumors, bone metastases at base of skull), motion sickness, Menière's disease, or labyrinthitis

### Physical Factors

Examples include increased intracranial pressure, meningitis, and toxins (e.g., tumor-produced peptides, abnormal metabolites due to cancer)

### Situational

Psychological factors (e.g., pain, fear, anxiety, noxious odors, taste, unpleasant visual stimulation)

• = Independent            ▲ = Collaborative

## Client Outcomes

### Client Will (Specify Time Frame):

- State relief of nausea.
- Explain methods he or she can use to decrease nausea and vomiting (N&V).

## Nursing Interventions

- Determine cause of N&V (e.g., medication effects, viral illness, food poisoning, extreme anxiety, anesthetic agents, pregnancy).
- Provide distraction from sensation of nausea using soft music, television, and videos per the client preference.
- Apply a cold washcloth to the forehead of a nauseated client.
- ▲ Apply supplemental oxygen if ordered.
- Maintain a quiet, well-ventilated environment free of strong odors from food, perfume, or cleaning solutions.
- Avoid sudden movement of the client; allow the client to lie still.
- If nausea is associated with frequent vomiting, assess client for fluid and electrolyte imbalances.
- Keep a clean emesis basin and tissues within the client's reach.
- ▲ Administer ordered antiemetic medications as needed.
- Provide oral care after the client vomits.
- Stay with the client to give support, place hand on shoulder, and hold the emesis basin.
- After vomiting is controlled and nausea abates, begin feeding the client small amounts of clear fluids such as clear soda or preferably ginger ale, and then bland foods such as crackers or dry toast; progress to a soft diet.
- Remove cover of food tray before bringing it into the client's room.
- ▲ Refer HIV-positive clients for management of antiretroviral-related nausea.

## Nausea in Pregnancy

- Recommend that the woman eat dry crackers or dry toast in bed before arising and then get up slowly. Also ad-

**N**

•  = Independent          ▲ = Collaborative

vise to chew gum or suck hard candies, eat small frequent meals, avoid foods with offensive odors, and avoid preparing food or shopping when nauseated.
- ▲ Discuss with the primary care practitioner the possibility of using transcutaneous electrical stimulation in the form of Relief Band Device (Woodside Biomedical) to help relieve nausea.
- • Consider the use of continuous acupressure at P6 applied by Sea-Bands with acupressure buttons to both wrists or P6 acupressure.
- ▲ Refer for acupuncture.

## Nausea Following Surgery

- • Medicate the client for nausea as ordered.
- ▲ Alleviate postoperative pain using ordered analgesic agents (refer to care plan for **Acute Pain**).
- • Ensure that the nauseated client is not hypotensive. Check blood pressure and note signs of postural hypotension.
- • Consider use of a recliner chair postoperatively if not contraindicated.
- • Recommend that client sit down when experiencing nausea.
- ▲ Refer for possible use of isopropyl alcohol (IPA) inhalation for treatment of postoperative N&V for patients who have general anesthesia for a surgical procedure.
- ▲ Consult with primary care practitioner for use of nonpharmacological techniques such as acupuncture, electroacupuncture, acupoint stimulation, or transcutaneous electrical nerve stimulation as an adjunct for controlling postoperative N&V.
- ▲ Teach the use of acupressure on two acupressure points on the wrist.
- • Use relaxation, imagery, and distraction techniques for nausea: encourage the client to take slow, deep breaths.

## Nausea Following Chemotherapy

- ▲ Consult with physician regarding need for antiemetic medications either prophylactic or when N&V occurs.

• = Independent          ▲ = Collaborative

▲ Use antiemetics and nursing interventions of increased access to support and increase information.

▲ If nausea is associated with the use of opioids, consult with primary care practitioner for possible use of alternative pain medication and consider the possible use of olanzapine as an antiemetic for advanced cancer patients.

▲ Consult with primary care provider on the use of transcutaneous electrical nerve stimulation as an adjunct for controlling chemotherapy-induced N&V.

• Help the client learn how to use acupressure for nausea, applying pressure bilaterally at P6 and ST36 acupressure points on the back of the wrist and by the knee.

▲ For clients who continue to experience nausea after antiemetic drugs or other treatments, consult with the primary care practitioner regarding the possibility of using acupuncture or transcutaneous nerve stimulation wristband to control N&V.

• Offer the nauseated client a 10-minute foot massage.

• If client has anticipatory nausea, utilize interventions such as education, relaxation therapy, and imagery to help client decrease nausea associated with event.

**N**

## Geriatrics

▲ Administer antiemetic drugs carefully; watch for side effects.

▲ Evaluate NSAIDs as a possible cause of nausea.

## Home Care

• Above interventions may be adapted for home care use.

• Assess for causes of nausea in the hospice care client such as constipation, bowel obstruction, adverse effects of medications and onset of increased intracranial pressure; refer to primary care practitioner if needed.

• Assist the client and family with identifying and avoiding irritants in the home setting that exacerbate nausea (e.g., strong odors from food, plants, perfume, and room deodorizers).

• = Independent          ▲ = Collaborative

## Client/Family Teaching

- Teach the client techniques to use when uncomfortable, including relaxation techniques, guided imagery, hypnosis, and music therapy.

# Unilateral Neglect

## NANDA Definition

Lack of awareness and attention to one side of the body

## Defining Characteristics

Consistent inattention to stimuli on an affected side; does not look toward affected side; inadequate positioning and/or safety precautions with regard to the affected side; inadequate self-care; leaves food on plate on the affected side

## Related Factors (r/t)

Effects of disturbed perceptual abilities (e.g., hemianopsia [one-sided blindness], neurological illnesses, trauma)
NOTE: Because the right hemisphere is dominant in directing attention, unilateral neglect is more common if neurological pathology occurs in the right hemisphere of the brain, which results in left-sided neglect. Also, unilateral neglect frequently occurs with damage to the right parietal lobe, the right frontal lobe, the thalamus, and basal ganglia

## Client Outcomes

### Client Will (Specify Time Frame):

- Demonstrate techniques that can be used to minimize unilateral neglect.
- Care for both sides of the body appropriately and keep affected side free from harm.
- Return to the highest functioning level possible based on personal goals and abilities.

• = Independent          ▲ = Collaborative

## Nursing Interventions

- Monitor the client for signs of unilateral neglect (e.g., not washing, shaving, or dressing one side of the body; sitting or lying inappropriately on affected arm or leg; failing to respond to stimuli on the contralateral side of lesion; eating food on only one side of plate; or failing to look to one side of the body).
- If available, use the "star cancellation test" to evaluate presence of unilateral neglect. The star cancellation test consists of a series of big and little stars and words scattered on a page. When directed to cross out all the little stars, clients with unilateral neglect will miss stars on one side of the paper.
- Use the Draw-A-Man test as a means of verifying the presence of unilateral neglect.
- Use the wheelchair collision test for screening for behavior assessment of unilateral neglect; set up four round chairs in two rows and ask the client in a wheelchair to propel the wheelchair around the chairs. NOTE: There are 62 assessment tools for evaluation of the presence of unilateral neglect; of these 28 are standardized.
- Provide a safe, well-lighted, and clutter-free environment. Place call light on unaffected side. Cue the client to environmental hazards when mobile.
- Nursing interventions for clients with unilateral neglect should be implemented in the following stages as the client progresses:
  - **Stage I:** Focus attention mainly on non-neglected side.
    - ❑ Set up environment so that most activity is on unaffected side.
    - ❑ Keep the client's personal items within view and on unaffected side.
    - ❑ Position the client's bed so that activity is on unaffected side.
  - **Stage II**: Help the client develop an awareness of neglected side.

• = Independent          ▲ = Collaborative

        ❑ Gradually focus the client's attention on affected side.

        ❑ Gradually move personal items and activity to affected side.

        ❑ Stand on the client's affected side when assisting with ambulation or ADLs.

- **Stage III**: Help the client develop ability to compensate for neglect.

        ❑ Encourage the client to bathe and groom affected side first.

        ❑ Focus touch and talking on affected side; use a positive approach (e.g., "Mary, turn your head to the left and you'll see your daughter").

        ❑ Use constant and positive reminders to keep the client scanning the entire environment.

        ❑ Use bright yellow or red stickers on outer margins in reading or writing exercises. Have the client look for the sticker before reading or writing.

        ❑ Help the client do ordinary tasks, compensating for their neglect situation. Use cues and anchors to promote attention to the neglected side and help the client develop compensatory mechanisms to deal with the neglect syndrome.

- Recognize that unilateral neglect can improve following a stroke, and it is practical to postpone evaluation until two weeks after a stroke.

▲ Refer to a rehabilitation team including a nurse rehabilitation specialist, a neuropsychologist, an occupational therapist, and physical therapist for continued help in dealing with unilateral neglect.

▲ Refer client to an ophthalmologist who specializes in low vision rehabilitation. By use of specialized glasses with built-in prisms, more normal vision may be restored.

## Home Care

- Many of the listed interventions may be adapted for use in the home care setting.

    • = Independent         ▲ = Collaborative

- Position bed at home so that client gets out of bed on unaffected side.

## Client/Family Teaching

- Explain pathology and symptoms of unilateral neglect to both the client and family.
- Teach the client how to scan regularly to check the position of body parts and to regularly turn head from side to side for safety when ambulating, using a wheelchair, or doing other tasks. Recommend the client think of self like a horizon-illuminating lighthouse.
- Teach caregivers positive cueing (reminders to help the client remember to interact with entire environment).

# Noncompliance

## NANDA Definition

Behavior of person and/or caregiver that fails to coincide with a health-promoting or therapeutic plan agreed on by the person (and/or family and/or community) and health care professional; in the presence of an agreed-on, health-promoting, or therapeutic plan, person's or caregiver's behavior is fully or partially nonadherent and may lead to clinically ineffective or partially ineffective outcomes

## Defining Characteristics

Behavior indicative of failure to adhere (directly observed or verbalized by patient or significant others) (critical); objective tests (e.g., physiological measures, detection of markers); evidence of development of complications; evidence of exacerbation of symptoms; failure to keep appointments; failure to progress

## Related Factors (r/t)

### Health Care Plan

Duration; significant others; cost; intensity; complexity

• = Independent        ▲ = Collaborative

## Individual Factors
Personal and developmental abilities; health beliefs, cultural influences, spiritual values; individual's value system; knowledge and skill relevant to the regimen behavior; motivational forces

## Health System
Satisfaction with care; credibility of provider; access and convenience of care; financial flexibility of plan; client-provider relationships; provider reimbursement of teaching and follow-up; provider continuity and regular follow-up; individual health coverage; communication and teaching skills of the provider

## Network
Involvement of members in health plan; social value regarding plan; perceived beliefs of significant others
NOTE: The nursing diagnosis **Noncompliance** is judgmental and places blame on the client. The authors recommend use of the diagnosis **Ineffective Therapeutic regimen management** in place of the diagnosis **Noncompliance**. The diagnosis **Ineffective Therapeutic regimen management** has interventions that are developed by both the health care providers and the client. It is a more respectful and efficacious nursing diagnosis than **Noncompliance**.

## Client Outcomes

### Client Will (Specify Time Frame):

- Describe consequence of continued noncompliance with treatment regimen.
- State goals for health and the means by which to obtain them.
- Communicate an understanding of disease and treatment.
- List treatment regimens and expectations and agree to follow through.
- List alternative ways to meet goals.
- Describe the importance of family participation to help achieve goals.

● = Independent          ▲ = Collaborative

# Nursing Interventions

- Ask the client why he or she has not complied with the prescribed treatment. Have the client "tell his or her story." Listen nonjudgmentally.
- Make the client an active partner in his or her own health care management. Recognize that the client has absolute control over whether he or she follows the health care regimen. Always treat the client with respect, and develop mutual outcomes for treatment.
- Work with the client to problem-solve how to handle the illness and need for medications or prescribed care.
- If the client is in denial: provide information, communicate unconditional positive regard, avoid distancing yourself, and look for opportunities for authentic contact with your client, being present psychologically and physically.
- Observe for cause of noncompliance (see Related Factors). Recognize that noncompliance is very common.
- Recognize that behavioral change comes slowly, and often in stages:
  - Precontemplation—change is not contemplated; unaware of problem or risk
  - Contemplation—aware that problem exists; no specific plans or commitment to change
  - Preparation—plan to take action within the next 30 days
  - Action—now taking action to improve health; often behavior not consistently carried out
  - Maintenance—consistently engages in healthful behavior for more than 6 months
- Determine the client's and family's knowledge of illness and treatment. Teach them about the illness and purpose of the treatment regimen if necessary.
- Observe whether locus of control is internal or external for the client. Recognize that people with external locus of control are more likely to be noncompliant because they do not believe they can help themselves. They believe that it is a matter of luck or destiny that they are ill.

N

• = Independent          ▲ = Collaborative

- ▲ Monitor the client for signs of depression that may cause noncompliance. Refer for treatment if appropriate.
- • Monitor the client's ability to follow directions, solve problems, concentrate, and read.
- • Avoid using threats, pressure, and inappropriate fear arousal to increase compliance.
- • Determine whether the client's support system helps or hinders therapy. Bring family members and significant others into the educational process as desired by the client.
- • Listen to the client's descriptions of abilities; encourage the client to use these abilities in self-care. When dealing with complex health care regimens, start the client with small behavioral changes (e.g., have chemotherapy client rinse mouth with a saliva substitute twice daily). When one step has been accomplished, add another step.
- • Work with the client to develop cues that trigger needed health care behaviors (e.g., checking blood sugar level before putting on makeup each morning), including weekends, holidays, and vacations.
- • Work with the client to develop an instruction and reminder sheet that fits medications and treatments into the client's lifestyle.
- • Observe the noncompliant client for possibility of secondary gain such as increased attention if the client continues to be ill and noncompliant.
- ▲ Consider allowing the client to take his or her own medications while in the hospital if appropriate.
- • Develop a mutually agreed-on written contract with the client regarding needed health care behaviors; give reinforcement as the client meets defined goals.
- ▲ Consult with primary care practitioner regarding the possibility of simplifying the health care regimen so that it more easily fits into the client's lifestyle (e.g., taking medications one time per day versus four times per day).
- ▲ Refer for compliance therapy (motivational interviewing and cognitive behavioral therapy) for medication management for clients with schizophrenia.

• = Independent          ▲ = Collaborative

# Geriatric

- Make the client an explicit medication instruction sheet using bulleted lists and simple icons.
- ▲ If the client has sensory and coordination deficits, use a medication organizer and have the home health nurse or family place the client's medications in daily compartments.
- Help the client feel like a partner in managing health care condition; use caring, encouragement, written goals, and a "power with" relationship with nurse.
- ▲ Ask clients if they can afford medications. Refer for financial help from social worker or case manager if needed.
- ▲ Monitor the client for signs of depression associated with noncompliance (e.g., refusing to eat or take medications). Refer the client for treatment of depression as needed.
- Use repetition, verbal cues, and memory aids such as pictures, schedule, or reminder sheet when teaching the health care regimen. Use events such as meals, bedtime, etc., as reminders when to take medications.
- Consider assistive medication technology: talking reminders, pill dispensers, etc.

**N**

# Multicultural

- Assess for the influence of cultural beliefs, norms, and values on the client's ability to modify health behavior.
- Discuss with the client those aspects of their health behavior/lifestyle that will remain unchanged by their health status.
- Negotiate with the client regarding the aspects of health behavior that will need to be modified.
- Assess the role of fatalism on the client's ability to modify health behavior.
- Validate the client's feelings regarding the impact of health status on current lifestyle.
- Use mechanical reminders to cue patients as a means to improve adherence.

● = Independent          ▲ = Collaborative

## Home Care

NOTE: Because the home care nurse enters the client's home as a guest, the ability of the nurse to establish a supportive, therapeutic relationship is especially important. A paradigm shift in nurses' view of noncompliance has been proposed, to include the recognition of clients as experts on their own lives, and the assessment of client social context to determine possible rationales for not following professional advice.

- Above interventions may be adapted for home care use.
- Before providing any care, review the Home Health Care Bill of Rights with the client, including the right to refuse treatment.
- If included in agency policies and procedures, also review patient responsibilities with the client (which is often part of a printed Bill of Rights).
- When the client is noncompliant, redefine personal and health priorities (contract for services) with the client to determine alternative motivational strategies or health actions to meet health goals.
- Institute self-care management to maximize client responsibility for own care. Refer to care plan for **Powerlessness.**
- Elicit and answer questions respectfully regarding illness and treatment, correcting any misconceptions and highlighting the importance of assisting the client to incorporate treatment plan into daily lifestyle. Do not use medical jargon in explanations.
- Explore barriers to medical regimen adherence. Review medications and treatment regularly for needed modifications. Take complaints of side effects seriously and serve as the client advocate to address changes as indicated.
- ▲ If noncompliance compromises the client's health status, refer for psychiatric home health care services to assess the client's motivation and implement therapeutic regimen.
- ▲ If noncompliant behavior continues and the client

• = Independent          ▲ = Collaborative

chooses not to cooperate with medical regimen, the
home health care agency cannot continue to provide
services.

- If care is to be terminated, identify all possible alternatives for the client, and assist with making an informed choice about future health actions.

- Respect the wishes of terminally ill clients to refuse selected aspects of medical regimen. With terminally ill clients, do not terminate care. Provide those aspects of care
that the client and family or caregivers will accept. The
goal of hospice care is to provide comfort and dignity
in the dying process.

## Client/Family Teaching

▲ Teach clients about medication side effects (e.g., mental
changes, sexual dysfunction) so that they understand
them and feel comfortable discussing them.

- Teach clients to control their "self-talk" by giving themselves positive messages that will be used to promote
desired behaviors, such as taking medications and controlling food intake.

N

# Readiness for enhanced Nutrition

## NANDA Definition

A pattern of nutrient intake that is sufficient for meeting
metabolic needs and can be strengthened

## Defining Characteristics

Expresses willingness to enhance nutrition; eats regularly; consumes adequate food and fluid; expresses knowledge of healthy
food and fluid choices; follows an appropriate standard for intake
(e.g., the food pyramid, U.S. Dietary Guidelines or America
Diabetic Association guidelines); safe preparation and storage for
food and fluids; attitude toward eating and drinking is congruent
with health goals

• = Independent          ▲ = Collaborative

## Related Factors (r/t)

Motivation to improve health through diet

## Client Outcomes

### Client Will (Specify Time Frame):

- Explain how to eat according to the U.S. Dietary Guidelines.
- Design dietary modifications to meet individual long-term goal of health, using principles of variety, balance, and moderation.
- Weigh within normal range for height and age.

## Nursing Interventions

- Ask the client to keep a one-day to three-day food diary where everything eaten or drunk is recorded. Analyze the quality, quantity, and pattern of food intake.
- Advise the client to measure food periodically. Help the client learn usual portion sizes.
- Help the client determine their body mass index (BMI). Use a chart or one of the formulas below:
  - Weight in kilograms divided by height (in meters) squared ($kg/m^2$)
  - Weight in pounds multiplied by 705, divided by height in inches, divided again by height in inches
- Recommend the client use the interactive Food Pyramid site at www.MyPyramid.gov to determine the number of calories to eat, and gain more information on how to eat in a healthy fashion.
- Recommend the client follow the Dietary Guidelines for Americans, which can be found at this website: www.healthierus.gov/dietaryguidelines/. Use the Food Pyramid to analyze the quality of the diet.
- Recommend the client eat a healthy breakfast every morning.
- Recommend the client avoid eating in fast food restaurants.
- Review the client's current exercise level. With the client and primary health care provider, design a long-term exercise program. Encourage the client to adopt an exer-

• = Independent        ▲ = Collaborative

cise program that involves 45 minutes of exercise five times/week.

- Demonstrate the use of food labels to make healthful choices. Alert the client/family to focus on serving size, total fat, and simple carbohydrates.
- Determine the client's knowledge of the need for supplements. Discourage the client from taking excessive amounts of vitamins unless prescribed by a physician.

## Carbohydrates

- Encourage the client to *decrease* intake of sugars including intake of soft drinks, desserts, and candy. Limit sugar intake to 12 teaspoons of added sugar daily.
- Recommend the client eat whole grains whenever possible, and explain how to find whole grains using the food label.
- Evaluate the client's usual intake of fiber.
- Recommend the client eat five to nine fruits and vegetables per day, with a minimum of two servings of fruit and three servings of vegetables. Encourage client to eat a rainbow of fruits and vegetables because bright colors are associated with increased nutrients.

## Fats

- Recommend the client limit intake of saturated fats and *trans*-fatty acids; instead increase intake of vegetable oils such as canola oil and olive oil. Limit fat intake to around 30% of total calories per day.
- Recommend client use low fat choices when selecting and cooking meat, also when selecting dairy products
- Recommend that the client eat cold water fish such as salmon, tuna, or mackerel at least two times per week to ensure adequate intake of omega-3 fatty acids. If unwilling to eat fish suggest sources such as flaxseed, soy, or walnuts. NOTE: Fish oil capsules should be taken cautiously; some brands can be contaminated with mercury or pesticides. Intake of excessive omega-3 fatty acids can result in bleeding.

• = Independent        ▲ = Collaborative

## Protein

- Recommend the client decrease intake of red meat and processed meats, instead eat more poultry, fish, and dairy sources of protein.
- Recommend the client eat meatless meals at intervals and try alternative sources of protein including nuts, especially almonds (one handful), and nut butters.
- Recommend the client eat beans and especially soy as an alternative to animal proteins at intervals. Introduce the client to soy products such as flavored soymilk. NOTE: women with diagnosed estrogen-dependent cancer of the breast should generally avoid eating soy foods.

## Fluid and Electrolytes

- Recommend the client choose and prepare foods with less salt, aim for a maximum of 2300 mg per day, which is approximately 1 teaspoon of salt.
- If the client drinks alcohol, encourage to drink in moderation, no more than one drink per day for women, and two drinks per day for men.
- Recommend client increase intake of water, to at least 2000 mL or 2 quarts per day. A guideline is 1 to 1.5 mL of fluid per each calorie needed, so an average intake would be between 2000 and 3000 mL/day, or at least 8 cups of fluid.

## Geriatric

- Assess changes in lifestyle and eating patterns.
- ▲ Recommend the client discuss the need for a low-dose balanced multiple vitamin and mineral supplement with physician.
- Assess fluid intake. Recommend routine drinks of water whether thirsty or not.
- Observe for socioeconomic factors that influence food choices (e.g., funds, cooking facilities).
- Suggest a variety of seasonings.

## Multicultural

- Assess for dietary intake of essential nutrients.

• = Independent          ▲ = Collaborative

- Assess for the influence of cultural beliefs, norms, and values on the client's nutritional knowledge.
- Discuss with the client those aspects of his or her diet that will remain unchanged.
- Determine the motivational factors operating within the client at the present time.
- Negotiate with the client regarding the aspects of his or her diet that will need to be modified.
- Explore strategies that appeal to the client.
- Validate the client's feelings regarding the impact of current lifestyle, finances, and transportation on ability to obtain nutritious food.
- Encourage family meals.

## Client/Family Teaching

- The majority of interventions above involve teaching.
- Work with the family members regarding information on how to improve nutritional status.
- Teach the importance of exercise in a weight control program.

N

# Imbalanced Nutrition: less than body requirements

## NANDA Definition

Intake of nutrients insufficient to meet metabolic needs

## Defining Characteristics

Body weight less than 20% under ideal weight; pale conjunctival and mucous membranes; weakness of muscles required for swallowing or mastication; sore, inflamed buccal cavity; satiety immediately after ingesting food; reported or evidence of lack of food; reported inadequate food intake less than RDA (Recommended Dietary Allowance); reported altered taste sensation; perceived inability to ingest food; misconceptions; loss of weight with adequate food intake; aversion to eating; abdominal cramp-

• = Independent          ▲ = Collaborative

ing; poor muscle tone; abdominal pain with or without pathology; lack of interest in food; capillary fragility; diarrhea and/or steatorrhea; excessive loss of hair; hyperactive bowel sounds; lack of information; misinformation

### Related Factors (r/t)

Inability to ingest or digest food or absorb nutrients because of biological, psychological, or economic factors

### Client Outcomes

### Client Will (Specify Time Frame):

- Progressively gain weight toward desired goal.
- Weigh within normal range for height and age.
- Recognize factors contributing to underweight.
- Identify nutritional requirements.
- Consume adequate nourishment.
- Be free of signs of malnutrition.

### Nursing Interventions

- Monitor for signs of malnutrition including: brittle hair that is easily plucked, bruises, dry skin, pale skin and conjunctiva, muscle wasting, smooth red tongue, cheilosis, "flaky paint" rash over lower extremities, and disorientation.
- ▲ Note laboratory test results as available: serum albumin, serum total protein, serum ferritin, transferrin, hemoglobin, hematocrit, and electrolytes.
- Weigh the client daily in acute care, weekly in extended care under same conditions.
- Determine healthy body weight for age and height. Refer to dietitian for complete nutrition assessment if 10% under healthy body weight or if rapidly losing weight.
- ▲ Monitor food intake; record percentages of served food that is eaten (25%, 50%); consult with dietitian for actual calorie count if needed.
- Observe the client's relationship to food. Attempt to separate physical from psychological causes for eating difficulty.

• = Independent        ▲ = Collaborative

- Compare usual food intake with the Food Pyramid, noting slighted or omitted food groups.
- If the client is a vegetarian, evaluate vitamin $B_{12}$ and iron intake.
- Observe the client's ability to eat (time involved, motor skills, visual acuity, and ability to swallow various textures).

NOTE: If the client is unable to feed self, refer to Nursing Interventions for **Feeding Self-care deficit.** If the client has difficulty swallowing, refer to Nursing Interventions for **Impaired Swallowing.**

▲ If the client is recovering from a gastrointestinal disorder such as gastroenteritis, surgery, or previous obstruction and is malnourished, consult with dietitian regarding use of a clear liquid product that contains increased amounts of protein and calories such as citrotein, Boost Breeze, or Resource Fruit Beverage.
- For the client with anorexia, who will not eat foods, consider offering 30 cc of a nutritional supplement in a medication cup every hour.
- For the client who is malnourished, and can eat, offer small quantities of food, served in an appetizing fashion, at frequent intervals.
- If the client lacks endurance, schedule rest periods before meals and open packages and cut up food for the client.
- When the client is malnourished, watch carefully for signs of infection and maintain every action possible to protect the client from infection.
- Assess for recent changes in physiological status that may interfere with nutrition.
- If the client is pregnant, ensure that she is receiving adequate amounts of folic acid by eating a balanced diet and taking prenatal vitamins as ordered.
- Provide companionship at mealtime to encourage nutritional intake.
- Monitor state of oral cavity (gums, tongue, mucosa, teeth). Provide good oral hygiene before and after meals.
- If a client has anorexia and dry mouth from medication

N

• = Independent          ▲ = Collaborative

side effects, offer sips of fluids throughout the day, along with sugarless hard candy and chewing gum to stimulate saliva formation.

- Determine relationship of eating and other events to onset of nausea, vomiting, diarrhea, or abdominal pain.
- Determine time of day when the client's appetite is the greatest. Offer highest calorie meal at that time.
▲ Administer antiemetics and pain medications as ordered and needed before meals.
- Prepare the client for meals. Clear unsightly supplies and excretions. Avoid invasive procedures before meals.
- If client is nauseated, remove cover of food tray before bringing it into the client's room.
- If vomiting is a problem, discourage consumption of favorite foods.
- Work with the client to develop a plan for increased activity.
- If the client is anemic, offer foods rich in iron and vitamins $B_{12}$, C, and folic acid.
- For the agitated client, offer finger foods (sandwiches, fresh fruit) and fluids.
▲ If client has been malnourished for a significant length of time, consult with dietitian and refeed carefully after correcting electrolyte balance. Watch for heart and respiratory failure.

### Geriatric
- Assess for protein-energy malnutrition in elderly clients regardless of setting. Utilize a screening tool such as the Mini Nutritional Assessment.
- Assess for factors contributing to a current acute illness.
- Implement strategies to ensure good nutrition to prevent recurrence of illness.
- Interpret laboratory findings cautiously. Compromised kidney function makes reliance on urine samples for nutrient analyses less reliable in the elderly than in younger persons.
- Offer high protein supplements based on individual needs and capabilities.

• = Independent        ▲ = Collaborative

- Give the client a choice of supplements to increase personal control. If the client is unwilling to drink a glass of liquid supplement, offer 30 mL/hr in a medication cup.
- Offer liquid energy supplements. When given liquid preloads 60 minutes before the next meal, older persons consistently ate a greater total energy load.
- Unless medically contraindicated, permit self-selected seasonings and foods.
- Serve food in a restaurant style manner if possible.
- Play relaxing dinner music during mealtime.
- Assess components of bone health: calcium intake, the elderly adult needs 1200 mg and adequate amounts of Vitamin D.
- Consider social factors that may interfere with nutrition (e.g., lack of transportation, inadequate income, lack of social support).
- Assess for psychological and mental factors that impact nutrition. Watch for signs of depression.
- Consider the effects of medications on food intake. Appetite-stimulating drugs may have a role in some cases.
- ▲ Provide appropriate food textures for chewing ease. Insert dentures (if needed) before meals. Assess fit of dentures. Refer for dental consultation if needed.

NOTE: If the client is unable to feed self, refer to Nursing Interventions for **Feeding Self-care deficit.** If client has impaired physical function, malnutrition, depression, and cognitive impairment, please refer to care plan on **Adult Failure to thrive.**

## Multicultural
- Assess for dietary intake of essential nutrients.
- Assess for the influence of cultural beliefs, norms, and values on the client's nutritional knowledge.
- Discuss with the client those aspects of his or her diet that will remain unchanged.
- Negotiate with the client regarding the aspects of his or her diet that will need to be modified.

• = Independent          ▲ = Collaborative

- Validate the client's feelings regarding the impact of current lifestyle, finances, and transportation on ability to obtain nutritious food.
- Encourage family meals.

## Home Care

- Above interventions may be adapted for home care use.
- Monitor food intake. Instruct the client in intake of small frequent meals and liquid supplements (e.g., Ensure, Instant Breakfast).
- Assess client's willingness to eat; fashion interventions accordingly.
- ▲ Assess the client for depression. Refer for mental health services as indicated.
- Recognize that older women may continue their younger preoccupation with weight and recurrent dieting, despite being at normal weight. Assess source of low weight or weight loss with this in mind.
- ▲ Administer and monitor total parenteral nutrition (TPN) as ordered by physician. TPN requires monitoring for potential complications and client/caregiver education.
- ▲ In the presence of depression diagnosis, refer for psychiatric home health care services for client reassurance and implementation of therapeutic regimen.

## Client/Family Teaching

- Help the client/family identify the area to change that will make the greatest contribution to improved nutrition.
- Build on the strengths in the client's/family's food habits. Adapt changes to their current practices.
- Select appropriate teaching aids for the client's/family's background.
- Implement instructional follow-up to answer the client's/family's questions.
- ▲ Suggest community resources as suitable (food sources, counseling, Meals on Wheels, Senior Centers).
- Teach the client and family how to manage tube feedings or parenteral therapy at home.

• = Independent          ▲ = Collaborative

# Imbalanced Nutrition: more than body requirements

## NANDA Definition

Intake of nutrients that exceeds metabolic needs

## Defining Characteristics

Triceps skin fold of more than 25 mm in women; triceps skin fold of more than 15 mm in men; body weight more than 20% over ideal for height and frame; eating in response to external cues (e.g., time of day, social situation); eating in response to internal cues other than hunger (e.g., anxiety); reported or observed dysfunctional eating pattern pairing food with other activities; sedentary activity level; concentration of food intake at the end of the day

## Related Factors (r/t)

Excessive intake in relation to metabolic need; deficient knowledge related to desirability of nutritional supplements

## Client Outcomes

### Client Will (Specify Time Frame):

- State pertinent factors contributing to weight gain.
- Identify behaviors that remain under client's control.
- Claim ownership for current eating patterns.
- Design dietary modifications to meet individual long-term goal of weight control, using principles of variety, balance, and moderation.
- Accomplish desired weight loss in a reasonable period (1 to 2 lb/wk).
- Incorporate appropriate activities requiring energy expenditure into daily life.

## Nursing Interventions

- Ask the client to keep a one-day to three-day food diary where everything eaten or drunk is recorded.
- Advise the client to measure food periodically. Help the client learn usual portion sizes.

• = Independent          ▲ = Collaborative

- Help the client determine his or her body mass index (BMI). Use a chart or one of the formulas below:
  - Weight in kilograms divided by height (in meters) squared ($kg/m^2$)
  - Weight in pounds multiplied by 705, divided by height in inches, divided again by height in inches
- Recommend the client follow the U.S. Dietary Guidelines, which can be found at this website: www.healthierus.gov/dietaryguidelines.
- Recommend the client use the interactive Food Pyramid site at www.MyPyramid.gov to determine the number of calories to eat, and gain more information on how to eat in a healthy fashion.
- Establish a reasonable goal for the client's body weight and for weight loss (e.g., 1 to 2 lb/wk).
- Recommend that client lose weight slowly, based on a healthy eating pattern and increased exercise. The number of calories consumed should be at least 1600 for men, and 1300 for women.
- Demonstrate the use of food labels to make healthful choices. Alert the client/family to focus on serving size, total fat, and simple carbohydrates.
- Initiate a client contract that involves rewarding and reinforcing progressive goal attainment.
- Weigh the client twice a week under the same conditions.
- Watch the client for signs of depression: flat affect, poor sleeping habits, lack of interest in life.
- Determine the client's knowledge of the need for supplements. Discourage the client from taking excessive amounts of vitamins unless prescribed by a physician.

## Pattern of Dietary Intake

- Recommend the client eat a healthy breakfast every morning.
- Recommend the client avoid eating in fast-food restaurants.
- ▲ Obtain a thorough history. Refer to a dietitian if the client has a medical condition.

• = Independent          ▲ = Collaborative

## Recommended Foods/Fluids

- Encourage the client to increase intake of vegetables and fruits to at least five servings per day, preferably 9 servings per day.
- Encourage the client to eat at least 3 whole grain servings per day, preferably more.
- Evaluate the client's usual intake of fiber.
- Encourage the client to *decrease* intake of sugars including intake of soft drinks, desserts, and candy.
- Recommend client increase intake of water, to at least 2000 mL or 2 quarts per day. A guideline is 1 to 1.5 mL of fluid per each calorie needed, so an average intake would be between 2000 and 3000 mL/day, or at least 8 cups of fluid.
- For more information on healthy eating, please see interventions for **Readiness for enhanced Nutrition.**

## Behavioral Methods for Weight Loss

- Familiarize the client with the following behavior modification techniques:
  - Self-monitoring of food intake, including keeping a food and exercise diary
  - Graphing weight weekly
  - Controlling stimuli that causes overeating such as watching TV with frequent food-related commercials
  - Limiting food intake to one site in the home
  - Sitting down at the table to eat
  - Planning food intake for each day
  - Rearranging the schedule to avoid inappropriate eating
  - Saving or rescheduling everyday activities for times when one is hungry
  - Avoiding boredom; keeping a list of activities on the refrigerator
  - For a party, eating before arriving, sitting away from the snack foods, and substituting lower-calorie beverages for alcoholic ones
  - Deciding beforehand what to order in a restaurant

N

• = Independent      ▲ = Collaborative

- Bringing only healthy foods into the house to decrease temptation
- Slowing mealtime by swallowing food before putting more food on the utensil, pausing for a minute during the meal and attempting to increase the number of pauses, and trying to be the last one to finish eating
- Drinking a glass of water before each meal; taking sips of water between bites of food
- Charting one's progress
- Making an agreement with oneself or a significant other for a meaningful reward, and not rewarding oneself with food
- Changing one's mind-set, as in control of eating behavior
- Viewing exercise as a means of controlling hunger
- Practicing relaxation techniques
- Imagining oneself ordering a side salad, diet dressing, low-fat milk, and a small hamburger at a fast-food restaurant
- Visualizing oneself enjoying a fresh apple in preference to apple pie

**N**

## Physical Activity
- ▲ Assess for reasons why the client would be unable to participate in an exercise program; refer for evaluation by a primary care practitioner as needed. Encourage activity to help with weight loss.
- • Use the Outcome Expectation for Exercise Scale to determine client's self-efficacy expectations and outcomes expectations toward exercise.
- • Recommend the client enter an exercise program with a friend.
- • Recommend the client begin a walking program utilizing the following guidelines:
  - Buy a pedometer.
  - Determine times when walking can be incorporated into usual lifestyle.
  - Set a goal of walking 10,000 steps per day, which equals 5 miles per day.

• = Independent          ▲ = Collaborative

- ■ If when the client comes home from work, he or she does not have required number of steps, go for a walk until reaching designated goal of 10,000 steps per day.

## Pediatric

- Work with parents of the overweight child by encouraging the following behaviors:
  - ■ Emphasize providing good food, not depriving children of food.
  - ■ Accept the child's natural size and shape; the child needs the parents' unconditional love.
  - ■ Make family meals a priority.
  - ■ Involve the child in helping plan menus, doing cooking, and preparation as appropriate for the child's age.
  - ■ Be active with children.
  - ■ Encourage children to love their bodies.
- Determine the child's BMI after the child is 3 years of age. The Centers for Disease Control and Prevention's BMI chart for children and teens is available at this website: www.cdc.gov/nccdphp/dnpa/bmi/bmi-for-age.htm
- Work with the child and parent to develop an appropriate weight maintenance plan, including behavior methods of weight loss, as well as increased activity.
- Encourage child to increase the amount of walking done per day, if the child is willing, ask them to wear a pedometer to measure number of steps.
- Do not use food as a reward for good behavior, especially not foods that are concentrated sources of sugar or fat.
- Recommend to the child decrease television viewing, watching movies, and playing video games. Ask parents to limit television to 1–2 hours per day maximum.

## Geriatric

- Assess changes in lifestyle and eating patterns. Energy needs decrease an estimated 5% per decade after the age

• = Independent          ▲ = Collaborative

of 40 years, but often eating patterns remain unchanged from youth.

- Assess fluid intake. Recommend routine drinks of water whether thirsty or not.
- Observe for socioeconomic factors that influence food choices (e.g., inadequate funds or cooking facilities).
- Suggest a variety of seasonings.

## Multicultural

- Assess for the influence of cultural beliefs, norms, acculturation, and values on the client's nutritional knowledge and practices.
- Encourage parental efforts at increasing physical activity and decreasing dietary fat for their children.
- Assess for the influence of cultural beliefs, norms, and values on the client's ideal of acceptable body weight and body size.
- Discuss with the client those aspects of his or her diet that will remain unchanged, and work with the client to adapt cultural core foods.
- Negotiate with the client regarding the aspects of his or her diet that will need to be modified.
- Validate the client's feelings regarding the impact of current lifestyle, finances, and transportation on the ability to obtain and prepare nutritious food.
- Limit television viewing and consumption of soft drinks.
- Encourage family meals.

## Client/Family Teaching

- Provide the client and family with information regarding the treatment plan options.
- Inform the client about the health risks associated with obesity, which include cancer, diabetes, heart disease, strokes, hypertension, gastroesophageal reflux, gallstones, osteoarthritis, and venous thrombosis.
- Inform the client and family of the disadvantages of trying to lose weight by dieting alone.
- Teach the importance of exercise in a weight control program.

• = Independent          ▲ = Collaborative

- Recommend the client receive adequate amounts of sleep.
- Teach stress reduction techniques as alternatives to eating.

# Risk for imbalanced Nutrition: more than body requirements

## NANDA Definition

At risk for intake of nutrients that exceeds metabolic needs

### Risk Factors

Reported use of solid food as major food source before 5 months of age; concentration of food intake at end of day; reported or observed obesity in one or both parents; reported or observed higher baseline weight at beginning of each pregnancy; rapid transition across growth percentiles in infants or children; pairing of food with other activities; observed use of food as reward or comfort measure; eating in response to internal cues other than hunger (e.g., anxiety); eating in response to external cues (e.g., time of day, social situation); dysfunctional eating patterns

### Client Outcomes

**Client Will (Specify Time Frame):**

- Explain concept of a balanced diet.
- Compare current eating pattern with recommended healthy one.
- Design dietary modifications to meet individual long-term goal of weight control, using principles of variety, balance, and moderation.
- Identify role of exercise in weight control.

### Nursing Interventions

Please refer to care plan for **Imbalanced Nutrition: more than body requirements.**

• = Independent          ▲ = Collaborative

# Impaired Oral mucous membrane

## NANDA Definition

Disruptions of lips and soft tissues of oral cavity

## Defining Characteristics

Purulent drainage or exudates; gingival recession, pockets deeper than 4 mm; tonsils enlarged beyond what is developmentally appropriate; smooth, atrophic, sensitive tongue; geographic tongue; mucosal denudation; presence of pathogens; difficulty in speech; self-report of bad taste; gingival or mucosal pallor; oral pain/discomfort; xerostomia (dry mouth); vesicles, nodules, or papules; white patches/plaques, spongy patches, or white curdlike exudate; oral lesions or ulcers; halitosis; edema; hyperemia; desquamation; coated tongue; stomatitis; self-report of difficult eating or swallowing; self-report of diminished or absent taste; bleeding; macroplasia; gingival hyperplasia; fissures; cheilitis; red or bluish masses (e.g., hemangiomas)

## Related Factors (r/t)

Chemotherapy; chemical exposure (e.g., alcohol, tobacco, acidic foods, regular use of inhalers); depression; immunosuppression; aging-related loss of connective, adipose, or bone tissue; barriers to professional care; cleft lip or palate; medication side effects; lack of or decreased salivation; chemical trauma (e.g., acidic foods, drugs, noxious agents, alcohol); pathological conditions—oral cavity (radiation to head or neck); nothing-by-mouth status for more than 24 hours; mouth breathing; malnutrition or vitamin deficiency; dehydration; infection; ineffective oral hygiene; mechanical factors (e.g., ill-fitting dentures, braces, tubes [endotracheal/nasogastric], surgery in oral cavity); decreased platelet count; immunocompromise; radiation therapy; barriers to oral self-care; diminished hormone levels (women); stress; loss of supportive structures

## Client Outcomes

### Client Will (Specify Time Frame):

- Maintain intact, moist oral mucous membranes that are free of ulceration and debris.

● = Independent          ▲ = Collaborative

• Demonstrate measures to regain or maintain intact oral mucous membranes.

## Nursing Interventions

▲ Inspect the oral cavity at least once daily and note any discoloration, lesions, edema, bleeding, exudate, or dryness. Refer to a physician or specialist as appropriate.

• Assess for mechanical agents such as ill-fitting dentures and chemical agents such as frequent exposure to tobacco that could cause or increase trauma to oral mucous membranes.

• Monitor the client's nutritional and fluid status to determine if it is adequate. Refer to the care plan for **Deficient Fluid volume** or **Imbalanced Nutrition: less than body requirements** if applicable.

• Encourage fluid intake of up to 3000 mL/day if not contraindicated by the client's medical condition.

• Determine the client's mental status. If the client is unable to care for himself or herself, oral hygiene must be provided by nursing personnel. The nursing diagnosis **Bathing/Hygiene Self-care deficit** is then also applicable.

• Determine the client's usual method of oral care and address any concerns regarding oral hygiene.

• If the client does not have a bleeding disorder and is able to swallow, encourage the client to brush the teeth with a soft toothbrush using a fluoride-containing toothpaste at least twice per day.

• Encourage the client to brush the tongue with the toothbrush, or use a tongue scraper twice a day.

• If the client does not have a bleeding disorder, encourage the client to floss once per day or use an interdental cleaner.

## Client Receiving Chemotherapy/Radiation

▲ Ensure that the client receives a comprehensive oral examination before initiation of chemotherapy or radiation, with aggressive preventative dental care given as needed.

• Provide instructions about the need for and method of

• = Independent          ▲ = Collaborative

providing frequent oral care to the patient one week before radiotherapy.

- For measurement of presence or severity of mucositis, use the Oral Mucositis Assessment Scale (OMAS).
- For the client receiving bolus fluorouracil, use cryotherapy with ice chips dissolving in client's mouth for 5 minutes before and 25 minutes after bolus administration of fluorouracil to reduce the severity of mucositis.
- Give the client frequent sips of water, and ask client to rinse the mouth with water regularly.
- Provide ice chips frequently to keep the mouth moist.
- ▲ If radiation induced mucositis, request an order for benzydamine hydrochloride as a mouthwash for prevention or treatment of radiation induced mucositis.
- Help client use a mouth rinse of salt and soda every 1 to 2 hours for prevention and treatment of stomatitis.
- ▲ If the mouth is severely inflamed and it is painful to swallow, contact the physician for a topical anesthetic or analgesic order. Modification of oral intake (e.g., soft or liquid diet) may also be necessary to prevent friction trauma. The nursing diagnosis **Imbalanced Nutrition: less than body requirements** may apply.
- If the client's platelet count is lower than $50,000/mm^3$ or the client has a bleeding disorder, use a specially made toothbrush designed for sensitive or diseased tissue, or a toothette that is not soaked in glycerin or flavorings; if the client cannot tolerate a toothbrush or a toothette, a piece of gauze wrapped around a finger can be used to remove plaque and debris.
- Use tap water or normal saline to provide oral care; do not use commercial mouthwashes containing alcohol or hydrogen peroxide. Also, do not use lemon-glycerin swabs.
- Use foam sticks to moisten the oral mucous membranes, clean out debris, and swab out the mouth of the edentulous client. Do not use foam sticks to clean the teeth unless the platelet count is very low and the client is prone to bleeding gums.

• = Independent        ▲ = Collaborative

- Keep the lips well lubricated using a lip balm that is water or aloe-based.

## Client on a Ventilator

- Use a pediatric sized toothbrush to brush teeth, use suction to remove secretions.
- Use water as a rinsing agent and mouthwash.
- ▲ Apply chlorhexidine gluconate in the oral cavity by swab or spray early after intubation if ordered.
- Provide scrupulous oral care to a critically ill client.
- ▲ If whitish plaques are present in the mouth or on the tongue and can be rubbed off readily with gauze, leaving a red base that bleeds, suspect a fungal infection and contact the physician for follow-up.
- Refer to the care plan for **Impaired Dentition** if the client has problems with the teeth.

## Geriatric

- Determine the functional ability of the client to provide his or her own oral care. Refer to **Bathing/hygiene Self-care deficit.**
- Provide appropriate oral care to the elderly with a self-care deficit, brushing the teeth after every meal.
- Carefully observe the oral cavity and lips for abnormal lesions such as white or red patches, masses, ulcerations with an indurated margin, or a raised granular lesion.
- Ensure that dentures are removed and scrubbed at least once daily, removed and rinsed thoroughly after every meal, and removed and kept in an appropriate solution at night.
- ▲ If the client has xerostomia, evaluate medications to see if they could be the cause, provide synthetic saliva products to moisten the oral cavity, and offer frequent sips of water and sugarless gum or candy to provide lubrication.

## Home Care

- The interventions described previously may be adapted for home care use.

O

• = Independent          ▲ = Collaborative

▲ If dryness is a side effect of the client's medication(s), instruct the client in the use of artificial saliva. Monitor sodium intake in hypertensive clients. Use alternatives to sodium chloride rinses.

• Instruct the client to avoid alcohol-based or hydrogen peroxide–based commercial products for mouth care and to avoid other irritants to the oral cavity (e.g., tobacco, spicy foods).

▲ Instruct the client in ways to soothe the oral cavity (e.g., cool beverages, Popsicles, viscous lidocaine).

• If the client often breathes by mouth, add humidity to the room unless contraindicated.

▲ If necessary, refer for home health aide services to support the family in oral care and observation of the oral cavity.

## Client/Family Teaching

• Teach the client how to inspect the oral cavity and monitor for signs and symptoms of infection or complications, and when to call the health care practitioner.

• Teach the client and family if necessary how to perform appropriate mouth care.

P

# Acute Pain

## NANDA Definition

Pain is whatever the experiencing person says it is, existing whenever the person says it does; unpleasant sensory and emotional experience arising from actual or potential tissue damage or described in terms of such damage; sudden or slow onset of pain of any intensity from mild to severe with anticipated or predictable end

## Defining Characteristics

### Subjective

Pain is always subjective and cannot be proved or disproved. A client's report of pain is the most reliable indicator of pain. A

• = Independent          ▲ = Collaborative

client with cognitive ability who can speak or point should use a pain rating scale (e.g., 0 to 10) to identify the current level of pain intensity (self-report) and determine a comfort-function goal. Establishment of a comfort-function goal involves helping the client to select a pain rating level that will allow the client to easily perform identified functional goals (e.g., a pain rating of 3 on a scale of 0 to 10 to cough, deep breathe, and ambulate).

## Objective

Expressions of pain are extremely variable and cannot be used in lieu of self-report. Neither behavior nor vital signs can substitute for the client's self-report. However, observable responses to pain may be helpful in assessing clients who cannot or will not use a self-report pain rating scale. Observable responses may be loss of appetite and inability to deep breathe, ambulate, sleep, or perform activities of daily living. Clients may show guarding, self-protective behavior, self-focusing or narrowed focus, distraction behavior ranging from crying to laughing, and muscle tension or rigidity. In sudden and severe pain, autonomic responses such as diaphoresis, blood pressure and pulse changes, pupillary dilation, or increases or decreases in respiratory rate and depth may be present.

## Related Factors (r/t)

Actual or potential tissue damage (mechanical [e.g., incision or tumor growth], thermal [e.g., burn], or chemical [e.g., toxic substance])

## Client Outcomes

### Client Will (Specify Time Frame):

- Use pain rating scale to identify current pain intensity and determine comfort/function goal (if client has cognitive abilities).
- Describe how unrelieved pain will be managed.
- Report that pain management regimen relieves pain to satisfactory level with acceptable and manageable side effects.
- Perform activities of recovery with reported acceptable level of pain (if pain is above comfort-function goal, take ac-

• = Independent        ▲ = Collaborative

tion that decreases pain or notify a member of health care team).
- If cognitively impaired, demonstrate a reduction in pain behaviors, have manageable and tolerable side effects, and perform recovery activities satisfactorily.
- State ability to obtain sufficient amounts of rest and sleep.
- Describe nonpharmacological methods that can be used to help control pain.

## Nursing Interventions

▲ Determine whether the client is experiencing pain at the time of the initial interview. If so, intervene at that time to provide pain relief. Assess and document the intensity, character, onset, duration, and aggravating and relieving factors of pain during the initial evaluation of the client.
- Assess pain in a client using a self-report 0 to 10 numerical pain rating scale or the Faces Pain Scale.
- Question the client regarding pain at frequent intervals, often at the same time as doing vital signs.
- Ask the client to describe past experiences with pain and the effectiveness of methods used to manage pain, including experiences with side effects, typical coping responses, and the way the client expresses pain.
- Question the client regarding the level of pain that they think is appropriate to achieve a state of comfort and appropriate function. Attempt to keep below that level, preferably much lower.
- Describe the adverse effects of unrelieved pain.
- Assess and document the intensity of the pain and discomfort after any known pain-producing procedure, with each new report of pain, and at regular intervals.
- If the client is cognitively impaired and unable to report pain and use a pain rating scale, assess and document behaviors that might be indicative of pain (e.g., change in activity, loss of appetite, guarding, grimacing, moaning).
- Assume that pain is present and treat accordingly in a

• = Independent          ▲ = Collaborative

client who has a pathological condition or who is undergoing a procedure thought to be painful.

▲ Prevent pain when possible during procedures such as venipuncture. Utilize a topical local anesthetic such as EMLA cream, or LMX-4.

· Determine the client's current medication use.

▲ Explore the need for both opioid (narcotic) and nonopioid analgesics.

▲ Obtain a prescription to administer a nonopioid, such as acetaminophen, a nonselective nonsteroidal anti-inflammatory drug (NSAID), or a COX-2 (cyclooxygenase-2) selective NSAID ATC, unless contraindicated.

▲ Obtain a prescription to administer an opioid analgesic if indicated, especially for severe pain.

▲ Administer opioids orally or intravenously (IV), not intramuscularly (IM). Use a preventive approach to keep pain at or below an acceptable level. Provide PCA and intraspinal routes of administration when appropriate and available.

· Explain to the client the pain management approach that has been ordered, including therapies, medication administration, side effects, and complications.

· Discuss the client's fears of undertreated pain, overdose, and addiction.

▲ When opioids are administered, assess pain intensity, sedation, and respiratory status at regular intervals. Assess sedation and respiratory status at least every 2 hours in opioid-naïve clients (those who have not been taking regular daily doses of opioids) during the first 24 hours of opioid therapy. Decrease the opioid dose if the client is excessively sedated.

▲ Review the client's flow sheet and medication records to determine overall degree of pain relief, side effects, and analgesic requirements during the previous 24 hours.

▲ Administer supplemental opioid doses as needed to keep pain ratings at or below the comfort-function goal.

▲ Obtain prescriptions to increase or decrease opioid doses

P

· = Independent          ▲ = Collaborative

as needed; base prescriptions on the client's report of pain severity and response to the previous dose in terms of relief, side effects, and ability to perform the activities of recovery. Increase or decrease the dosage of opioid based on assessment of the client's response.

▲ When the client is able to tolerate oral analgesics, obtain a prescription to change to the oral route; use an equianalgesic chart to determine initial dose.

• In addition to administering analgesics, support the client's use of nonpharmacological methods to help control pain, such as distraction, imagery, relaxation, and application of heat and cold.

• Teach and implement nonpharmacological interventions when pain is relatively well controlled with pharmacological interventions.

• Plan care activities around periods of greatest comfort whenever possible.

▲ Ask the client to describe appetite, bowel elimination, and ability to rest and sleep. Administer medications and treatments to improve these functions. Obtain a prescription for a peristaltic stimulant to prevent opioid-induced constipation.

## Pediatric

• For the neonate, utilize oral sucrose for pain of short duration such as heel stick or venipuncture.

▲ Utilize a topical local anesthetic such as EMLA cream, or LMX-4 before performing venipuncture in an infant or child.

▲ For the neonate experiencing moderate to severe pain, utilize opioid analgesics and anesthetics in appropriate dosages.

• For the young child (1–4 years of age) utilize a Faces Pain Scale to determine the level of pain present.

## Geriatric

▲ Always take the older client's reports of pain seriously and ensure that the pain is relieved.

• = Independent        ▲ = Collaborative

- When assessing pain, speak clearly, slowly, and loudly enough for the client to hear, and if the client uses a hearing aid, be sure it is in place; repeat information as needed. Be sure the client can see well enough to read the pain scale (use an enlarged scale) and written materials.
- Handle the client's body gently. Allow the client to move at his or her own speed.
▲ Use acetaminophen and NSAIDs with low gastrointestinal side-effect profiles, such as the selective COX-2 NSAIDs (celecoxib) and watch for side effects, such as gastrointestinal disturbances and renal dysfunction.
▲ Avoid or use with caution drugs with a long half-life, such as the NSAID piroxicam (Feldene), and the opioids methadone (Dolophine) and levorphanol (LevoDromoran).
▲ Use opioids with caution in the older client.
▲ Avoid the use of opioids with toxic metabolites, such as meperidine (Demerol) and propoxyphene (Darvon, Darvocet), in older clients.

## Multicultural

- Assess for the influence of cultural beliefs, norms, and values on the client's perception and experience of pain.
- Assess for the effect of fatalism on the client's beliefs regarding the current state of comfort.
- Assess for pain disparities among racial and ethnic minorities.
- Incorporate safe and effective folk health care practices and beliefs into care whenever possible. It is the responsibility of the caregiver to ensure that safe and effective pain management is provided. Although support of an individual's health care beliefs is recommended, when research does not support the safety or effectiveness of a method or when research does not exist, this should be explained fully to the client.
- Use a family-centered approach to care.
- Teach information about pain medications and their side effects, how to work with health care providers to man-

P

• = Independent          ▲ = Collaborative

age pain, and encouragement to use religious faith to cope with pain.

- Use culturally relevant pain scales (e.g., the Oucher Scale), if available, to assess pain in the client.
- Ensure that directions for medication use are available in the client's language of choice and are understood by the client and caregiver.

## Home Care

- Develop the treatment plan with the client and caregivers.
- ▲ Develop a full medication profile, including medications prescribed by all physicians and all over-the-counter medications. Assess for drug interactions. Instruct the client to refrain from mixing medications without physician approval.
- Assess the client's and family's knowledge of side effects and safety precautions associated with pain medications (e.g., use caution in operating machinery when opioids are first taken or dosage has been increased significantly).
- If medication is administered using highly technological methods, assess the home for the necessary resources (e.g., electricity) and ensure that there will be responsible caregivers available to assist the client with administration.
- ▲ Assess the knowledge base of the client and family with regard to highly technological medication administration. Teach as necessary. Be sure the client knows when, how, and whom to contact if analgesia is unsatisfactory.

## Client/Family Teaching

NOTE: To avoid the negative connotations associated with the words *drugs* and *narcotics*, use the term *pain medicine* when teaching clients.

- Provide written materials on pain control.
- Discuss the various discomforts encompassed by the word *pain* and ask the client to give examples of previ-

---

ously experienced pain. Explain the pain assessment process and the purpose of the pain rating scale.

▲ Teach the client to use the pain rating scale to rate the intensity of past or current pain. Ask the client to set a comfort-function goal by selecting a pain level on the rating scale that makes it easy to perform recovery activities (e.g., turn, cough, deep breathe). If pain is above this level, the client should take action that decreases pain or notify a member of the health care team.

▲ Demonstrate medication administration and the use of supplies and equipment. If PCA is ordered, determine the client's ability to press the appropriate button. Remind the client and staff that the PCA button is for client use only.

• Reinforce the importance of taking pain medications to keep pain under control.

• Reinforce that taking opioids for pain relief is not addiction and that addiction is very unlikely to occur.

• Demonstrate the use of appropriate nonpharmacological approaches in addition to pharmacological approaches for helping to control pain, such as application of heat and/or cold, distraction techniques, relaxation breathing, visualization, rocking, stroking, music listening, and television watching.

P

# Chronic Pain

## NANDA Definition

Pain is whatever the experiencing person says it is, existing whenever the person says it does; unpleasant sensory and emotional experience arising from actual or potential tissue damage or described in terms of such damage; sudden or slow onset of pain of any intensity from mild to severe, constant or recurring, without anticipated or predictable end; state in which the individual experiences pain that persists for a period of time beyond the usual course of acute illness or a reasonable duration

• = Independent          ▲ = Collaborative

for the injury to heal, is associated with a chronic pathological process, or recurs at intervals for months or years

## Defining Characteristics

### Subjective

Pain is always subjective and cannot be proved or disproved. The client's report of pain is the most reliable indicator of pain. Clients with cognitive abilities who can speak or point should use a pain rating scale (e.g., 0 to 10) to identify their current level of pain intensity (self-report) and determine a comfort-function goal. Establishment of a comfort-function goal involves assisting clients in selecting a pain rating that will allow them to easily perform identified functional goals, e.g., a pain rating of 3 on a scale of 0 to 10 to work or walk the dog.

### Objective

Expressions of pain are extremely variable and cannot be used in lieu of self-report. Neither behavior nor vital signs can substitute for the client's self-report. However, observable responses to pain may be helpful in pain assessment, especially in clients who cannot or will not use a self-report pain rating scale. Observable responses may be loss of appetite or the inability to ambulate, perform activities of daily living (ADLs), work, or sleep. Clients may show guarding, self-protective behavior, self-focusing or narrowed focus, distraction behavior ranging from crying to laughing, and muscle tension or rigidity. In sudden severe pain, autonomic responses such as diaphoresis, blood pressure and pulse changes, pupillary dilation, and increase or decrease in respiratory rate and depth may be present but are usually not seen with chronic pain that is relatively stable. Clients with chronic or persistent cancer or nonmalignant pain may experience threats to self-image, a perceived lack of options for coping, and worsening helplessness, anxiety, and depression. Chronic pain may affect almost every aspect of the client's daily life, including concentration, work, and relationships.

## Related Factors (r/t)

Actual or potential tissue damage; tumor progression and related

• = Independent        ▲ = Collaborative

pathology; diagnostic and therapeutic procedures; central or
peripheral nerve injury (neuropathic pain)

NOTE: The cause of chronic nonmalignant pain may not be
known because pain study is a new science and an area encom-
passing diverse types of problems.

## Client Outcomes

### Client Will (Specify Time Frame):

- Use pain rating scale to identify current level of pain intensity, determine comfort/function goal, and maintain a pain
  diary (if client has cognitive abilities).
- Describe total plan for pharmacological and nonpharmacological pain relief, including how to safely and effectively take
  medicines and integrate nondrug therapies.
- Demonstrate ability to pace self, taking rest breaks before
  they are needed.
- Function on acceptable ability level with minimal interference from pain and medication side effects (if pain is
  above comfort-function goal, take action that decreases pain
  or notify a member of health care team).
- If cognitively impaired, demonstrate a reduction in pain behaviors, have manageable and tolerable side effects, and
  perform ADLs satisfactorily.

## Nursing Interventions

P

- ▲ Determine whether the client is experiencing pain at the
  time of the initial interview. If so, intervene at that time
  to provide pain relief. Assess and document the intensity,
  character, onset, duration, and aggravating and relieving factors of pain during the initial evaluation of the
  client.
- • Assess pain in a client using a self-report 0 to 10 numerical pain rating scale or a Faces Pain Scale.
- • Question the client regarding pain at frequent intervals,
  often at the same time as doing vital signs.
- • Tell the client to report pain location, intensity, and
  quality when experiencing pain. Assess and document

• = Independent          ▲ = Collaborative

the intensity of pain and discomfort after any known pain-producing procedure, with each new report of pain, and at regular intervals.

- Question the client regarding the level of pain that they think is appropriate to achieve a state of comfort and appropriate function. Attempt to keep pain level no higher than that level, preferably much lower.
- Ask the client to describe past and current experiences with pain and the effectiveness of the methods used to manage the pain, including experiences with side effects, typical coping responses, and the way the client expresses pain.
- Describe the adverse effects of unrelieved pain.
- Ask the client to maintain a diary of pain ratings, timing, precipitating events, medications, treatments, and steps that work best to relieve pain.
- If the client is cognitively impaired and unable to report pain and use a pain rating scale, assess and document behaviors that might be indicative of pain (e.g., change in activity, loss of appetite, guarding, grimacing, moaning).
- ▲ Assume that pain is present and treat accordingly in clients who have a pathological condition or are undergoing a procedure thought to be painful.
- Determine the client's current medication use. To aid in planning pain treatment, obtain a medication history.
- ▲ Explore the need for medications from the three classes of analgesic: opioids (narcotics), nonopioids (acetaminophen, nonselective nonsteroidal anti-inflammatory drugs [NSAIDs], and COX-2 [cyclo-oxygenase-2] selective NSAIDs), and adjuvant medications. For chronic neuropathic pain, consider adjuvant medications that are analgesic, such as anticonvulsants and antidepressants.
- ▲ For persistent cancer pain, obtain a prescription to administer opioid analgesics. When pain persists or increases, an opioid such as oxycodone should be added to the nonopioid. If this is not effective, switch to morphine or other single-entity opioids.

• = Independent        ▲ = Collaborative

▲ For persistent chronic nonmalignant pain, discuss the use of opioid analgesics with the health care team and obtain a prescription to administer if appropriate.

▲ The oral route for pain medication administration is preferred. If the client is receiving parenteral analgesia, use an equianalgesic chart to convert to a controlled release, long acting oral medication as soon as possible.

▲ Establish ATC dosing and administer supplemental opioid doses for breakthrough pain as needed to keep pain ratings at or below the comfort-function goal.

▲ Ask the client to describe appetite, bowel elimination, and ability to rest and sleep. Administer medications and treatments to improve these functions. Always obtain a prescription for a stool softener and a peristaltic stimulant daily to prevent opioid-induced constipation in clients taking regular daily doses of opioids.

• Explain to the client the pain management approach that has been ordered, including therapies, medication administration, side effects, and complications.

• Discuss the client's fears of undertreated pain, addiction, and overdose.

▲ Review the client's pain diary, flow sheet, and medication records to determine the overall degree of pain relief, side effects, and analgesic requirements for an appropriate period (e.g., 1 week).

▲ Obtain prescriptions to increase or decrease analgesic doses when indicated. Base prescriptions on the client's report of pain severity and the comfort-function goal and response to previous dose in terms of relief, side effects, and ability to perform ADLs and comply with the prescribed therapeutic regimen.

▲ If opioid dose is increased, monitor sedation and respiratory status for a brief time.

▲ In addition to the use of analgesics, support the client's use of nonpharmacological methods to help control pain, such as physical therapy, group therapy, distraction, imagery, relaxation, massage, and application of heat and cold.

P

• = Independent          ▲ = Collaborative

- Teach and implement nonpharmacological interventions when pain is relatively well controlled with pharmacological means.
- Encourage the client to plan activities around periods of greatest comfort whenever possible.
- Explore appropriate resources for management of pain on a long-term basis (e.g., hospice, pain care center).
- If the client has progressive cancer pain, assist the client and family with handling issues related to death and dying.
- Assist the client and family in minimizing the effects of pain on interpersonal relationships and daily activities such as work and recreation.

## Pediatric

- For the young child (1–4 years of age) utilize a Faces Pain Scale to determine the level of pain present.
- Help children and adolescents learn and utilize techniques such as relaxation and cognitive behavioral techniques to handle pain.

## Geriatric

- ▲ Always take an older client's reports of pain seriously and ensure that the pain is relieved.
- When assessing pain, speak clearly, slowly, and loudly enough for the client to hear, and if the client uses a hearing aid, be sure it is in place; repeat information as needed. Be sure the client can see well enough to read the pain scale (use an enlarged scale) and written materials.
- Handle the client's body gently. Allow the client to move at his or her own speed.
- ▲ Use acetaminophen and NSAIDs with low gastrointestinal side-effect profiles, such as a COX-2 selective NSAID, choline and magnesium salicylates (Trilisate), and diflunisal (Dolobid), and watch for side effects, such as gastrointestinal disturbances and bleeding problems.
- ▲ Avoid or use with caution drugs with a long half-life, such as the NSAID piroxicam (Feldene), and the opioids

P

• = Independent          ▲ = Collaborative

methadone (Dolophine) and levorphanol (LevoDromoran).

▲ Use opioids cautiously in the older client with moderate to severe pain unrelieved by NSAIDS. Reduce initial doses by 25 to 50%. After titrating to comfort with a short-acting opioid, switch to an extended-release opioid.

▲ Avoid the use of opioids with toxic metabolites, such as meperidine (Demerol) and propoxyphene (Darvon, Darvocet), in older clients.

• Monitor for signs of depression in the elders, refer for treatment if needed.

## Multicultural

• Assess for the influence of cultural beliefs, norms, and values on the client's perception and experience of pain.

• Assess for the effect of fatalism on the client's beliefs regarding the current state of comfort.

• Assess for pain disparities among racial and ethnic minorities.

• Incorporate safe and effective folk health care practices and beliefs into care whenever possible. It is the responsibility of the caregiver to ensure that safe and effective pain management is provided. Although support of an individual's health care beliefs is recommended, when research does not support the safety or effectiveness of a method or when research does not exist, this should be explained fully to the client.

• Use a family-centered approach to care.

• Teach information about pain medications and their side effects, how to work with health care providers to manage pain, and encouragement to use religious faith to cope with pain.

• Use culturally relevant pain scales (e.g., the Oucher Scale), if available, to assess pain in the client.

• Ensure that directions for medication use are available in the client's language of choice and are understood by the client and caregiver.

P

• = Independent          ▲ = Collaborative

## Home Care

- • Develop the treatment plan with the client and care-givers.
- ▲ Develop a full medication profile, including medications prescribed by all physicians and all over-the-counter medications. Assess for drug interactions. Instruct the client to refrain from mixing medications without physician approval.
- • Assess the client's and family's knowledge of side effects and safety precautions associated with pain medications (e.g., use caution if operating machinery when opioids are first taken or dosage has been increased significantly).
- ▲ Collaborate with the health care team (including the client and family) on an ongoing basis to determine an optimal pain control profile. Identify the most effective interventions and the medication administration routes most acceptable to the client and family.
- ▲ If medication is administered using highly technological methods, assess the home for necessary resources (e.g., electricity) and ensure that responsible caregivers will be available to assist the client with administration.
- ▲ Assess the knowledge base of the client and family for highly technological medication administration. Teach as necessary. Be sure the client knows when, how, and whom to contact if analgesia is unsatisfactory.
- • Support the client and family in the use of opioid analgesics.

## Client/Family Teaching

NOTE: To avoid the negative connotations associated with the words *drugs* and *narcotics,* use the term *pain medicine* when teaching clients.

- • Provide written materials on pain control.
- • Discuss the various discomforts encompassed by the word *pain* and ask the client to give examples of previously experienced pain. Explain the pain assessment process and the purpose of the pain rating scale.

• = Independent          ▲ = Collaborative

▲ Ask the client to set a comfort-function goal by selecting a pain level on the rating scale that takes it easy to perform recovery activities (e.g., turn, cough, deep breathe). If pain is above this level, the client should take action that decreases pain or notify a member of the health care team.

▲ Discuss the total plan for pharmacological and nonpharmacological treatment, including the medication plan for ATC administration and supplemental doses, the maintenance of a pain diary, and the use of supplies and equipment.

• Reinforce the importance of taking pain medications to keep pain under control.

• Reinforce that taking opioids for pain relief is not addiction and that addiction is very unlikely to occur.

▲ Explain to a client with chronic neuropathic pain the process of taking adjuvant analgesics (e.g., tricyclic antidepressants).

• Suggest the client with cancer try having a massage, with aromatherapy if desired.

• Emphasize to the client the importance of pacing himself or herself and taking rest breaks before they are needed.

▲ Demonstrate the use of appropriate nonpharmacological approaches in addition to pharmacological approaches for helping to control pain (e.g., physical therapy, group therapy, distraction, imagery, and application of heat and cold).

• Teach and implement nonpharmacological interventions when pain is relatively well controlled with pharmacological means.

# Readiness for enhanced Parenting

## NANDA Definition

Pattern of providing an environment for children or other dependent person(s) that is sufficient to nurture growth and development and can be strengthened

• = Independent          ▲ = Collaborative

## Defining Characteristics

Expresses willingness to enhance parenting; children or other dependent person(s) express satisfaction with home environment; emotional and tacit support of children or dependent person(s) is evident; bonding or attachment is evident; physical and emotional needs of children or other dependent person(s) are met; realistic expectations of children or other dependent person(s) are exhibited

## Client Outcomes

### Client/Family Will (Specify Time Frame):

- Affirm desire to improve parenting skills to further support growth and development of children.
- Demonstrate loving relationship with children.
- Provide a safe, nurturing environment.
- Assess risks in home/environment and takes steps to prevent possibility of harm to children.
- Meet physical, psychosocial, and spiritual needs or seek appropriate assistance.

## Nursing Interventions

- Use family-centered care and role modeling for holistic care of families.
- Assess parents' feelings when dealing with a child who has a chronic illness.
- Encourage positive parenting: respect for children, understanding of normal development, and use of creative and loving approaches to meet parenting challenges.
- Promote low-tech interventions, such as massage and multisensory interventions (maternal voice, eye-to-eye contact, and rocking) to reduce maternal and infant stress and improve mother-infant relationship.
- Provide opportunities for mother-infant skin-to-skin contact (kangaroo care [KC]) for preterm infants.
- Provide the parent with the opportunity to assist in the newborn's first bath, allowing a flexible bath time.
- When the person who is ill is the parent, use family-centered assessment skills to determine the impact of an

• = Independent          ▲ = Collaborative

adult's illness on the child and then guide the parent through those topics that are most likely to be of concern, including (a) the name of the illness, (b) the cause of the illness, (c) the potential contagion or spread of the illness, and (d) the ultimate impact of the illness on the life of the child.
- Have family members participate in client conferences that involve all members of the health care team.
- Help parents develop realistic expectations of their child's development.
- Provide practical and psychologic assistance for parents of patients with psychiatric diagnoses, such as schizophrenia.

## Multicultural
- Assess for the influence of cultural beliefs, norms, and values on the client's perception of parenting.
- Acknowledge racial/ethnic differences at the onset of care.
- Acknowledge that value conflicts from acculturation stresses may contribute to increased anxiety and significant conflict with children.
- Acknowledge and praise parenting strengths noted.

## Home Care
- The nursing interventions described previously should be used in the home environment with adaptations as necessary.
- ▲ Refer to a parenting program to facilitate learning of parenting skills.

## Client/Family Teaching
- ▲ Refer to Client/Family Teaching for **Impaired Parenting** and **Risk for impaired Parenting** for suggestions that may be used with minor adaptations.
- Teach parents home safety: reduction of hot water temperature, proper poison storage, use of smoke alarms, installation of safety gates for stairs, and use of ipecac syrup.

• = Independent          ▲ = Collaborative

- Teach parents and young teens conflict resolution using a hypothetical conflict solution with and without a structured conflict resolution guide.
▲ Refer mothers of children with type 1 diabetes for community support in baby-sitting, child care, or respite.
- Support empowerment of parents of children with asthma.
- Teach families the importance of monitoring television viewing and limiting exposure to violence.
- Consider individual and/or group-based parenting programs for teenage mothers.
- Consider group-based parenting programs for parents for children under the age of three years with emotional and behavioral problems.
- Consider group-based parenting programs for parents with anxiety, depression, and/or low self-esteem.
▲ Refer adolescent parents for comprehensive psychoeducational parenting classes.

# Impaired Parenting

P **NANDA Definition**

Inability of primary caretaker to create, maintain, or regain an environment that promotes optimum growth and development of the child

## Defining Characteristics

### Infant/Child

Poor academic performance; frequent illness; running away; physical and psychological trauma or abuse; frequent accidents; lack of attachment; failure to thrive; behavioral disorders; poor social competence; lack of separation anxiety; poor cognitive development

### Parental

Inappropriate child care arrangements; rejection of or hostility toward child; statements of inability to meet child's needs;

• = Independent         ▲ = Collaborative

inflexibility in meeting needs of child or situation; poor or inappropriate caretaking skills; regular punitive behavior; inconsistent care; child abuse; inadequate child health maintenance; unsafe home environment; verbalization of inability to control child; negative statements about child; verbalization of role inadequacy or frustration; inappropriate visual, tactile, or auditory stimulation of child; abandonment; insecure attachment or lack of attachment to infant; inconsistent behavior management; child neglect; little cuddling; maternal-child interaction deficit; poor parent-child interaction

## Related Factors (r/t)

### Social

Lack of access to resources; social isolation; lack of resources; poor home environment; lack of family cohesiveness; inadequate child care arrangements; lack of transportation; unemployment or job problems; role strain or overload; marital conflict, declining satisfaction; lack of value of parenthood; change in family unit; low socioeconomic class; unplanned or unwanted pregnancy; presence of stress (e.g., financial or legal difficulties, recent crisis, cultural move); lack of or poor parental role model; single parenthood; lack of social support network; lack of involvement of father of child; history of being abusive; history of being abused; financial difficulties; maladaptive coping strategies; poverty; poor problem-solving skills; inability to put child's needs before own; low self-esteem; relocation; legal difficulties

### Knowledge

Lack of knowledge about child health maintenance; lack of knowledge about parenting skills; unrealistic expectations for self, infant, partner; limited cognitive functioning; lack of knowledge about child development; inability to recognize and act on infant cues; low educational level or attainment; poor communication skills; lack of cognitive readiness for parenthood; preference for physical punishment

### Physiological

Physical illness

### Infant/Child
Premature birth; illness; prolonged separation from parent; not desired gender; attention deficit/hyperactivity disorder; difficult temperament; separation from parent at birth; lack of goodness of fit (temperament) with parental expectations; unplanned or unwanted child; handicapping condition or developmental delay; multiple births; altered perceptual abilities

### Psychological
History of substance abuse or dependencies; disability; depression; difficult labor and/or delivery; young age, especially adolescence; history of mental illness; high number of or closely spaced pregnancies; sleep derivation or disruption; lack of or late prenatal care; separation from infant/child

NOTE: It is important to reaffirm that adjustment to parenting in general is a normal maturational process that elicits nursing behaviors to prevent potential problems and to promote health.

### Client Outcomes

### Client Will (Specify Time Frame):

- Affirm desire to develop constructive parenting skills to support infant/child growth and development.
- Initiate appropriate measures to develop a safe, nurturing environment.
- Acquire and display attentive, supportive parenting behaviors.
- Identify strategies to protect child from harm and/or neglect and initiate action when indicated.

### Nursing Interventions

- Use the Parenting Risk Scale to assess parenting.
- Examine the characteristics of parenting style and behaviors, including the following:
  - Emotional climate at home
  - Attribution of negative traits to the child
  - Failure to support the child's increases in autonomy
  - Type of interaction with the infant/child

• = Independent          ▲ = Collaborative

- Competition with the child for attention of spouse/ significant other
- Lack of knowledge/concern about health maintenance or behavioral problems
- Other behaviors or concerns

▲ Institute abuse/neglect protection measures if there is evidence of an inability to cope with family stressors or crisis, signs of parental substance abuse are observed, or a significant level of social isolation is apparent.

▲ For a mother with a toddler, assess maternal depression, perceptions of difficult temperament in the toddler, and low maternal self-efficacy. Make appropriate referral.

• Appraise the parent's resources and the availability of social support systems. Determine the single mother's particular sources of support, especially the availability of her own mother and partner. Encourage the use of healthy, strong support systems.

• Provide education to at-risk parents on behavioral management techniques such as looking ahead, giving good instructions, providing positive reinforcement, redirecting, planned ignoring, and instituting time-outs.

• Support parents' competence in appraising their infant's behavior and responses.

• Promote low-tech interventions, such as massage and multisensory interventions (maternal voice, eye-to-eye contact, and rocking) to reduce maternal and infant stress and improve mother-infant relationship.

• Encourage skin-to-skin care by parents of preterm infants.

• Model age-appropriate and cognitively appropriate caregiver skills by doing the following:
  - Communicating with the child at an appropriate cognitive level of development
  - Giving the child tasks and responsibilities appropriate to age or functional age/level
  - Instituting safety considerations such as the use of assistive equipment
  - Encouraging the child to perform activities of daily living as appropriate

P

• = Independent                    ▲ = Collaborative

- Encourage mothers to understand and capitalize on their infants' capacity to interact, particularly in the very early months of life.
- Provide practical and psychologic assistance for parents of patients with psychiatric diagnoses, such as schizophrenia.
▲ Provide programs for homeless mothers with severe mental illness who have lost physical custody of their children.
▲ Provide a recovery program that includes instruction in parenting skills and child development for mothers who are addicted to cocaine.

## Multicultural

- Assess for the influence of cultural beliefs, norms, and values on the client's perception of parenting.
- Acknowledge racial/ethnic differences at the onset of care.
- Approach individuals of color with respect, warmth, and professional courtesy.
- Give a rationale when assessing African-American individuals about sensitive issues.
- Acknowledge that value conflicts from acculturation stresses may contribute to increased anxiety and significant conflict with children.
- Use a neutral, indirect style when addressing areas in which improvement is needed (such as a need for verbal stimulation) when working with Native-American clients.
- Provide support for Chinese families caring for children with disabilities.
- Acknowledge and praise parenting strengths noted.
- Validate the client's feelings regarding parenting.
- Facilitate modeling and role playing to help the family improve parenting skills.

## Home Care

- The interventions described previously may be adapted for home care use.

● = Independent          ▲ = Collaborative

- Assess parenting stress at each home visit to provide appropriate support and anticipatory guidance to families of children with chronic disease.
▲ Assess the single mother's history regarding childhood and partner abuse, and current status regarding depressive symptoms, abusive parenting attitudes (lack of empathy, favorable opinion of corporal punishment, parent-child role-reversal, inappropriate expectations). Refer for mental health services as indicated.
▲ Implement behavioral parent training (BPT), including enhancement of skills in child-directed play, effective use of commands, use of discipline measures such as imposing time-outs and providing immediate and natural consequences, problem solving, and communication strategies.

## Client/Family Teaching

- Consider individual and/or group-based parenting programs for teenage mothers.
- Consider group-based parenting programs for parents for children under the age of three years with emotional and behavioral problems.
- Consider group-based parenting programs for parents with anxiety, depression, and/or low self-esteem.
▲ Refer adolescent parents for comprehensive psychoeducational parenting classes.
- Explain individual differences in children's temperaments and compare and contrast with the parents' expectations. Help parents determine and understand the implications of their child's temperament.
- Discuss sound disciplinary techniques, which include catching children being good, listening actively, conveying positive regard, ignoring minor transgressions, giving good directions, using praise, and imposing time-outs.
- Encourage positive parenting: respect for children, understanding of normal development, and creative and loving approaches to meet parenting challenges.

P

• = Independent          ▲ = Collaborative

- Plan parental education directed toward the following age-related parental concerns:
  - Birth to 2 years—transition, sleep, aggression
  - 3 to 5 years—transition, parent-child relationship, sleep
  - 6 to 10 years—school, parent-child relationship, divorce
  - 11 to 18 years—parent-child relationship, divorce, school
- ▲ Initiate referrals to community agencies, parent education programs, stress management training, and social support groups.
- ▲ Provide information regarding available telephone counseling services.
- Refer to the care plan for **Delayed Growth and development** for additional teaching interventions.

# Risk for impaired Parenting

## NANDA Definition

Risk for inability of the primary caretaker to create, maintain, or regain an environment that promotes the optimum growth and development of the child

## Risk Factors

### Social

Marital conflict, declining satisfaction; history of being abused; poor problem-solving skills; role strain/overload; social isolation; legal difficulties; lack of access to resources; lack of value of parenthood; relocation; poverty; poor home environment; lack of family cohesiveness; lack of or poor parental role model; lack of involvement of father of child; history of being abusive; financial difficulties; low self-esteem; lack of resources; unplanned or unwanted pregnancy; inadequate child care arrangements; maladaptive coping strategies; low socioeconomic class; lack of transportation; change in family unit; unemployment or job

• = Independent    ▲ = Collaborative

problems; single parenthood; lack of social support network; inability to put child's needs before own; stress

## Knowledge

Low educational level or attainment; unrealistic expectations of child; lack of knowledge about parenting skills; poor communication skills; preference for physical punishment; in ability to recognize and act on infant cues; low cognitive functioning; lack of knowledge about child health maintenance; lack of knowledge about child development; lack of cognitive readiness for parenthood

## Physiological

Physical illness

## Infant/Child

Multiple births; handicapping condition or developmental delay; illness; altered perceptual abilities; lack of goodness of fit (temperament) with parental expectations; unplanned or unwanted child; premature birth; not desired gender; difficult temperament; attention deficit/hyperactivity disorder; prolonged separation from parent; separation from parent at birth

## Psychological

Separation from infant/child; large number of closely spaced children; disability; sleep deprivation or disruption; difficult labor and/or delivery; young age (especially adolescence); depression; history of mental illness; lack of or late prenatal care; history of substance abuse or dependence

NOTE: It is important to reaffirm that adjustment to parenting in general is a normal maturational process that elicits nursing behaviors to prevent potential problems and to promote health.

## Client Outcomes

### Client Will (Specify Time Frame):

- Successfully establish a nurturing parenting role.
- Affirm desire to acquire and maintain constructive parenting skills to support infant/child growth and development.

• = Independent          ▲ = Collaborative

- Maintain appropriate measures to develop a safe, nurturing environment.
- Display attentive, supportive parenting behaviors.
- Have knowledge of strategies to protect child from harm and/or neglect.

## Nursing Interventions

NOTE: Management of a risk diagnosis necessitates approaches using primary and secondary prevention. Primary prevention interventions include activities such as safety instruction and focus on forestalling the development of a disease or condition. Early detection through screening, monitoring, and surveillance is secondary prevention.

- Conduct risk identification, noting the presence of a history of abuse, parental/family stressors, strength and adequacy of social support systems, established coping styles, and other related factors (see Related Factors).
- Screen for maternal psychiatric-mental health symptoms and negative experiences in the mother's family of origin.
- Support parents' competence in appraising their infant's behavior and responses.
- Promote low-tech interventions, such as massage and multisensory interventions (maternal voice, eye-to-eye contact, and rocking) to reduce maternal and infant stress and improve mother-infant relationship.
- Encourage skin-to-skin care by parents of preterm infants.
- Provide education to at-risk parents on behavioral management techniques such as looking ahead, giving good instructions, providing positive reinforcement, redirecting, planned ignoring, and using time-outs.
- Monitor parent-infant interactions that may signal interrupted or inadequate attachment or other parenting issues.
- Encourage mothers to understand and capitalize on their infants' capacity to interact, particularly in the very early months of life.
- Provide practical and psychologic assistance for parents

of patients with psychiatric diagnoses, such as schizophrenia.
- Refer to the care plan for **Impaired Parenting** for other interventions as appropriate to the situation.

## Multicultural

- Assess for the influence of cultural beliefs, norms, and values on the client's perception of parenting.
- Acknowledge racial/ethnic differences at the onset of care.
- Approach individuals of color with respect, warmth, and professional courtesy.
- Give a rationale when assessing African-American individuals about sensitive issues.
- Acknowledge that value conflicts from acculturation stresses may contribute to increased anxiety and significant conflict with children.
- Use a neutral, indirect style when addressing areas in which improvement is needed (such as a need for verbal stimulation) when working with Native-American clients.
- Acknowledge and praise parenting strengths noted.
- Validate the client's feelings regarding parenting.
- Facilitate modeling and role playing to help the family improve parenting skills.

P

## Home Care

- The interventions described previously may be adapted for home care use.
- Assess parenting stress at each home visit to provide appropriate support and anticipatory guidance to families of children with chronic disease.

## Client/Family Teaching

- Consider individual and/or group based parenting programs for teenage mothers.
- Consider group based parenting programs for parents for children under the age of three years with emotional and behavioral problems.

• = Independent     ▲ = Collaborative

- Consider group-based parenting programs for parents with anxiety, depression, and/or low self-esteem.
▲ Refer adolescent parents for comprehensive psychoeducational parenting classes.
▲ Initiate referrals to an appropriate community agency for early follow-up if an actual problem is identified.
- Refer to the care plan for **Impaired Parenting** for additional teaching interventions.


# Risk for Peripheral neurovascular dysfunction

## NANDA Definition

At risk for disruption in circulation, sensation, or motion of an extremity

## Risk Factors

Trauma; fractures; mechanical compression (e.g., tourniquet, cast, brace, dressing, restraints); orthopedic surgery; immobilization; burns; vascular obstruction

## Client Outcomes

### Client Will (Specify Time Frame):

- Maintain circulation, sensation, and movement of an extremity within client's own normal limits.
- Explain signs of neurovascular compromise and ways to prevent venous stasis.

## Nursing Interventions and Rationales

- Perform neurovascular assessment every 1 to 4 hours or every 15 minutes as ordered.
- Use the six *P*s of assessment:
  - **Pain**—Assess severity (on a scale of 1 to 10), quality, radiation, and relief by medications. Diffuse pain that is aggravated by passive movement and is unre-

• = Independent          ▲ = Collaborative

lieved by medication can be an early symptom of compartment syndrome or a symptom of limb ischemia.

- **Pulses**—Check the pulses distal to the injury. Check the uninjured side first to establish a baseline for a bilateral comparison.
- **Pallor/Poikilothermia**—Check color and temperature changes below the injury site. Check capillary refill. If pallor is present, record the level of coldness carefully.
- **Paresthesia** (change in sensation)—Check by lightly touching the skin proximal and distal to the injury. Ask if the client has any unusual sensations such as hypersensitivity, tingling, prickling, decreased feeling, or numbness.
- **Paralysis**—Ask the client to perform appropriate range-of-motion exercises in the unaffected and then the affected extremity.
- **Pressure**—Check by feeling the extremity; note new onset of firmness of the extremity.
- Monitor the client for symptoms of compartment syndrome evidenced by pain greater than expected, pain with passive movement, decreased sensation, weakness, loss of movement, absence of pulse, and tension in the skin that surrounds the muscle compartment. These symptoms are not always present and can be difficult to assess.
- Monitor appropriate application and function of corrective device (e.g., cast, splint, traction) every 1 to 4 hours as needed.
- Position the extremity in correct alignment with each position change; check every hour to ensure appropriate alignment.
- ▲ Get the client out of bed and mobilize the client as soon as possible, after consultation with the physician.
- ▲ Monitor for signs of DVT, especially in high-risk populations, including persons older than 40 years of age; persons with immobility or obesity; persons taking estrogen or oral contraceptives; persons with a history of trauma, surgery, or previous DVT; and persons with a

P

• = Independent          ▲ = Collaborative

cerebrovascular accident, varicose veins, malignancy, or cardiovascular disease.
▲ Apply graduated compression stockings if ordered; measure carefully to ensure proper fit, removing at least daily to assess circulation and skin condition.
▲ Watch for and report signs of DVT as evidenced by pain, deep tenderness, swelling in the calf and thigh, and redness in the involved extremity. Take serial leg measurements of the thigh and leg circumferences. In some clients a tender venous cord can be felt in the popliteal fossa. Do not rely on Homans' sign.
▲ Help the client perform prescribed exercises every 4 hours as ordered.
• Provide a nutritious diet and adequate fluid replacement.

## Geriatric
• Use heat and cold therapies cautiously.

## Home Care
• Assess the knowledge base of the client and family following any institutional care.
• Teach about the disease process and care as necessary.
• If risk is related to fractures and cast care, teach the family to complete a neurovascular assessment; it may be performed as often as every 4 hours but is more commonly done two to three times per day.
• If the fracture is peripheral, position the limb for comfort and change position frequently, avoiding dependent positions for extended periods.
▲ Refer to physical therapy services as necessary to establish an exercise program and safety in transfers or mobility within limitations of physical status.
• Establish an emergency plan.

## Client/Family Teaching
• Teach the client and family to recognize signs of neurovascular dysfunction and to report signs immediately to the appropriate person.
• Emphasize proper nutrition to promote healing.

• = Independent          ▲ = Collaborative

▲ If necessary, refer the client to a rehabilitation facility for instruction in proper use of assistive devices and measures to improve mobility without compromising neurovascular function.

## Risk for Poisoning

### NANDA Definition

Accentuated risk of accidental exposure to, or ingestion of, drugs or dangerous products in doses sufficient to cause poisoning

### Risk Factors
### External

Unprotected contact with heavy metals or chemicals; storage of medicines in unlocked cabinets accessible to children or confused persons; presence of poisonous vegetation; presence of atmospheric pollutants, paint, lacquer, etc., in poorly ventilated areas or without effective protection; flaking, peeling paint or plaster in presence of young children; chemical contamination of food and water; availability of illicit drugs potentially contaminated by poisonous additives; presence of large supplies of drugs in home; placement or storage of dangerous products within reach of children or confused persons

### Internal

Verbalization that occupational setting is without adequate safeguards; reduced vision; lack of safety or drug education; lack of proper precautions; insufficient finances; cognitive or emotional difficulties

### Related Factors (r/t)

See Risk Factors.

### Client Outcomes
### Client Will (Specify Time Frame):

- Prevent inadvertent ingestion of or exposure to toxins or poisonous substances.

● = Independent          ▲ = Collaborative

- Explain and undertake appropriate safety measures to prevent ingestion of or exposure to toxins or poisonous substances.

## Nursing Interventions

- When a client comes to the hospital with possible poisoning, begin care following the "ABCs," and administer oxygen if needed.
- Obtain a thorough history of what was ingested, how much, when, and ask to look at the container. Note the client's age, weight, medications, and any medical conditions.
- Inspect carefully for signs of ingestion of poisons including an odor on the breath, a trace of the substance on the clothing, burns or redness around the mouth and lips, as well as signs of confusion, vomiting, or dyspnea.
- ▲ Note results of toxicology screens, arterial blood gasses, blood glucose levels, and any other ordered laboratory tests.
- ▲ Initiate any ordered treatment for poisoning quickly.
- Prevent iatrogenic harm to the hospitalized client by following these guidelines for administering medications:
  - Use at least two methods to identify the client before administering medications or blood products, such as the client's name and medical record number or birth date.
  - When taking verbal or telephone orders, the orders should be written down, and then read back for verification to the individual giving the order.
  - Standardize use of abbreviations and eliminate abbreviations that are prone to cause errors.
  - Take high alert medications off the nursing unit, such as potassium chloride. Standardize concentrations of medications such as morphine in PCA pumps.
  - Use only intravenous pumps that prevent free flow of intravenous solution when the tubing is taken out of the pump.
  - Identify all of the client's current medications upon

P

• = Independent          ▲ = Collaborative

admission to a health care facility, and ensure that all health care staff have access to the information.
- Detect possible interactions and cumulative or other adverse effects among prescribed medications, self-administered over-the-counter products, culturally based home treatments, herbal remedies and foods.

## Pediatrics

▲ Evaluate lead exposure risk and consult the health care provider regarding lead screening measures as indicated (public/ambulatory health).
- Supply "Mr. Yuk" labels for families with children.
- Provide guidance for parents/caregivers regarding age-related safety measures, including the following:
  - Store potentially harmful substances in the original containers with safety closures intact.
  - Recognize that no container is completely "child proof."
  - Avoid storage of medications or toxic substances in food containers.
  - Place poisonous houseplants out of the reach of infants and children; preferably remove from the home. Teach children not to put leaves or berries into their mouths.
  - Keep cleaning agents, disinfectants, and other hazardous materials out of sight and out of children's reach; keep them locked up.
  - Do not take medications in front of children; children mimic parents' behaviors.
  - Do not suggest that medications such as aspirin and children's vitamins are candy.
  - If interrupted when using a harmful product, take it with you; children can get into it within seconds.
  - Use extreme caution with pesticides and gardening materials close to children's play areas.
  - Keep perfume and makeup out of reach of children.
- Teach the family to keep the home safe for children by keeping harmful cleaning products and all liquids

P

• = Independent          ▲ = Collaborative

containing hydrocarbons away from children and using child-resistant packaging as available.

- Advise families that syrup of ipecac is generally no longer recommended to be kept and used in the home.

## Geriatric

- Caution the client and family to avoid storing medications with similar appearances close to one another (e.g., nitroglycerin ointment near toothpaste or denture creams).
- Place medications in a medication box that indicates when medications are to be taken.
- Remind the older client to store medications out of reach when young children come to visit.

## Home Care

- The interventions described previously may be adapted for home care use.
- Provide the client and/or family with a poison control diagram to be kept on the refrigerator or a bulletin board. Ensure that the telephone number for local poison control information is readily available.
- Prepour medications for a client who is at risk of ingesting too much of a given medication because of mistakes in preparation. Delegate this task to the family or caregivers if possible.
- Identify poisonous substances in the immediate surroundings of the home, such as a garage or barn, including paints and thinners, fertilizers, rodent and bug control substances, animal medications, gasoline, and oil. Label with the name, a poison warning sign, and a poison control center number. Lock out of the reach of children.
- Identify the risk of toxicity from environmental activities such as spraying trees or roadside shrubs. Contact local departments of agriculture or transportation to obtain material substance data sheets or to prevent the activity in desired areas.
- Avoid carbon monoxide poisoning. Instruct the client

• = Independent          ▲ = Collaborative

and family in the importance of using a carbon monoxide detector in the home, having the chimney professionally cleaned each year, having the furnace professionally inspected each year, ensuring that all combustion equipment is properly vented, and installing a chimney screen and cap to prevent small animals from moving into the chimney.

## Multicultural

- Assess housing for pathways of lead poisoning.
- Prompt caregivers to take action to prevent lead poisoning.
- Inform minority parents of children who present for treatment of a poisoning episode of poisoning prevention education as part of the medical encounter.
- Poison control centers (PCCs) should offer information in bilingual and bicultural manner.

## Client/Family Teaching

- Counsel the client and family members regarding medication safety:
  - Avoid sharing prescriptions.
  - Read and follow labeling instructions on all products; adjust dosage for age.
  - Avoid excessive amounts and/or frequency of doses ("If a little does some good, a lot should do more").
- Advise the family to post first aid charts and poison center instructions in an accessible location. Poison control center telephone numbers should be posted close to each telephone, and the number programmed into cell phones.
- Advise family when calling the poison control center to:
  - Give as much information as possible, including your name, location, and telephone number, so that the poison control operator can call back in case you are disconnected or summon help if needed.
  - Give the name of the potential poison ingested and, if possible, the amount and time of ingestion. If the bottle or package is available, give the trade name and ingredients if they are listed.

P

• = Independent          ▲ = Collaborative

- Be prepared to tell the person the child's height and weight.
- Describe the state of the poisoning victim. Is the victim conscious? Are there any symptoms? What is the person's general appearance, skin color, respiration, breathing difficulties, mental status (alert, sleepy, unusual behavior)? Is the person vomiting? Having convulsions?

- Encourage the client and family to take first aid and other types of safety-related programs.
▲ Initiate referrals to peer group interventions, peer counseling, and other types of substance abuse prevention/rehabilitation programs when substance abuse is identified as a risk factor.

## Post-trauma syndrome

### NANDA Definition

Sustained maladaptive response to a traumatic, overwhelming event

### P Defining Characteristics

Avoidance; repression; difficulty in concentrating; grief; intrusive thoughts; neurosensory irritability; palpitations; enuresis (in children); anger and/or rage; intrusive dreams; nightmares; aggression; hypervigilance; exaggerated startle response; hopelessness; altered mood state; shame; panic attack; alienation; denial; horror; substance abuse; depression; anxiety; guilt; fear; gastric irritability; detachment; psychogenic amnesia; irritability; numbing; compulsive behavior; flashbacks; headaches

### Related Factors (r/t)

Events outside range of usual human experience; physical and psychosocial abuse; tragic occurrence involving multiple deaths; epidemic; sudden destruction of one's home or community; confinement as prisoner of war or criminal victimization (tor-

• = Independent          ▲ = Collaborative

ture); war; rape; natural and/or manmade disaster; serious accident; witnessing of mutilation, violent death, or other horror; serious threat or injury to self or loved ones; industrial or motor vehicle accident; military combat

## Client Outcomes

### Client Will (Specify Time Frame):

- Return to pretrauma level of functioning as quickly as possible.
- Acknowledge traumatic event and begin to work with the trauma by talking about the experience and expressing feelings of fear, anger, anxiety, guilt, and helplessness.
- Identify support systems and available resources and be able to connect with them.
- Return to and strengthen coping mechanisms used in previous traumatic event.
- Acknowledge event and perceive it without distortions.
- Assimilate event and move forward to set and pursue life goals.

## Nursing Interventions

- Observe for a reaction to a traumatic event in all clients regardless of age.
- Provide a safe and therapeutic environment.
- Remain with the client and provide support during periods of overwhelming emotions.
- Assist the individual to try to comprehend the trauma if possible.
- Use touch with the client's permission (e.g., a hand on the shoulder, holding a hand).
- Explore and enhance available support systems.
- Assist the client in regaining previous sleeping and eating habits.
- ▲ Provide the client with pain medication if they are experiencing physical pain.
- ▲ Consider the use of medication to ease symptoms associated with post-traumatic stress disorder.

• = Independent        ▲ = Collaborative

- Help the client use positive cognitive restructuring to re-establish feelings of self-worth.
- Provide the means for the client to express feelings through therapeutic drawing.
- Encourage the client to return to the normal routine as quickly as possible.
- Talk to and assess the client's social support after a traumatic event.

## Geriatric

- Use environmental assessment skills to identify elderly clients who are traumatized by disaster, loss, or both.
- Observe the client for concurrent losses that may affect coping skills.
- Allow the client more time to establish trust and express anger, guilt, and shame about the trauma. Review past coping skills and give the client positive reinforcement for successfully dealing with other life crises.
- ▲ Monitor the client for clinical signs of depression and anxiety; refer to a physician for medication if appropriate.
- Instill hope.

## Multicultural

- Assess for the influence of cultural beliefs, norms, and values on the client's ability to cope with a traumatic experience.
- Acknowledge racial/ethnic differences at the onset of care.
- Use a family-centered approach when working with Latino, Asian, African-American, and Native-American clients.
- When working with an Asian American client, provide opportunities by which the family can save face.
- Validate the client's feelings regarding the trauma.
- Incorporate cultural traditions as appropriate.

## Home Care

- ▲ Assess family support and the response to the client's

**P**

• = Independent          ▲ = Collaborative

coping mechanisms. Refer the family for medical social services or other counseling as necessary.

• Provide a stable routine of day-to-day activities consistent with pretrauma experience. Do not force a new routine on the client.

▲ If the client is receiving medications, assess the client's self-medicating ability. Assign a responsible person to administer medications if necessary.

▲ Assess the impact of the trauma on significant others (e.g., a father may have to take over his partner's parenting responsibility after she has been raped and injured). Provide empathy and caring to significant others. Refer for additional services as necessary.

## Client/Family Teaching

• Explain to the client and family what to expect the first few days after the traumatic event and in the future.

• Teach positive coping skills and avoidance of negative coping skills.

• Teach stress reduction methods such as deep breathing, visualization, meditation, and physical exercise. Encourage their use especially when intrusive thoughts or flashbacks occur.

• Encourage other healthy living habits of proper diet, adequate sleep, regular exercise, family activities, and spiritual pursuits.

▲ Refer the client to peer support groups.

• Instruct the family in ways to be helpful to and supportive of the traumatized person. Emphasize the importance of listening and being there. Also emphasize that there are no magic phrases capable of easing the person's emotional suffering.

▲ Consider the use of complementary and alternative therapies.

**P**

• = Independent          ▲ = Collaborative

## Risk for Post-trauma syndrome

### NANDA Definition

At risk for sustained maladaptive response to a traumatic, overwhelming event

### Risk Factors

Exaggerated sense of responsibility; perception of event; survivor's role in the event; occupation (e.g., police, fire, rescue, corrections, emergency department, mental health worker); displacement from home; inadequate social support; non-supportive environment; diminished ego strength; duration of event

### Client Outcomes

#### Client Will (Specify Time Frame):

- Identify symptoms associated with post-traumatic stress disorder (PTSD) and seek help.
- Identify the event in realistic, cognitive terms.
- State that he or she is not to blame for the event.

### Nursing Interventions

- Assess for PTSD in a client who has chronic illness, anxiety, or personality disorder; was a witness to serious injury or death; or experienced sexual molestation.
- Consider the use of the Stanford Acute Stress Reaction Questionnaire to evaluate anxiety and dissociation symptoms after traumatic events.
- Assess for ongoing symptoms of dissociation, avoidant behavior, hypervigilance, and re-experiencing.
- Assess for past experiences with traumatic events.
- Consider screening for PTSD in a client who is a high utilizer of medical care.
- Provide peer support to contact co-workers experiencing trauma to remind them that others in the organization are concerned about their welfare; provide an opportunity to discuss the traumatic incident and assess for the need for further post-trauma services.

• = Independent          ▲ = Collaborative

- Provide post-trauma debriefings. Effective post-trauma coping skills are taught, and each participant creates a plan for his or her recovery. During the debriefing, the facilitators assess participants to determine their needs for further services in the form of post-trauma counseling. For maximum effectiveness, the debriefing should occur within 2 to 5 days of the incident.
- Provide post-trauma counseling. Counseling sessions are extensions of debriefings and include continued discussion of the traumatic event and post-trauma consequences, and the further development of coping skills.
- Instruct the client to use the following critical incident stress management techniques:
  - Within the first 24 to 48 hours, engaging in periods of appropriate physical exercise alternated with relaxation will alleviate some of the physical reactions.
  - Structure your time—keep busy.
  - You're normal and are having normal reactions—don't label yourself as crazy.
  - Talk to people—talk is the most healing medicine.
  - Be aware of numbing the pain with overuse of drugs or alcohol; you don't need to complicate the stress with a substance abuse problem.
  - Reach out—people do care.
  - Maintain as normal a schedule as possible.
  - Spend time with others.
  - Help your co-workers as much as possible by sharing feelings and checking out how they are doing.
  - Give yourself permission to feel rotten and share your feelings with others.
  - Keep a journal—write your way through those sleepless hours.
  - Do things that feel good to you.
  - Realize that those around you are under stress.
  - Don't make any big life changes.
  - Do make as many daily decisions as possible to give you a feeling of control over your life (i.e., if someone asks you what you want to eat, answer them even if you're not sure).

P

• = Independent          ▲ = Collaborative

- Get plenty of rest.
- Reoccurring thoughts, dreams, or flashbacks are normal—don't try to fight them; they'll decrease over time and become less painful.
- Eat well-balanced and regular meals (even if you don't feel like it).
- Assess for a history of life-threatening illness such as cancer and provide appropriate counseling.

## Pediatric

- Children with cancer should continue to be assessed for PTSD into adulthood.
- Provide protection for a child who has witnessed violence or who has had traumatic injuries. Help the child to acknowledge the event and to express grief over the event.
- Consider implementation of a school-based program for children to decrease PTSD after catastrophic events.

## Multicultural

- Assess for the influence of cultural beliefs, norms, and values on the client's ability to cope with a traumatic experience.
- Use a family-centered approach when working with Latino, Asian, African-American, and Native-American clients.
- Acknowledge racial/ethnic differences at the onset of care.
- Assure the client of confidentiality.
- Validate the client's feelings regarding the trauma and allow the client to tell the trauma story.
- Incorporate cultural traditions as appropriate.

## Home Care

- ▲ Assess the client's ability to meet primary needs of shelter, nourishment, and safety. Refer to medical social services, state departments of human services, or other organizations as appropriate.
- Identify other losses or stressors that may affect coping ability (e.g., role or relationship changes, deaths).

● = Independent          ▲ = Collaborative

▲ Assess the family's response to the client's risk. Refer the family to medical social services or mental health services or support groups as necessary. Provide nursing support.

▲ If the client is on medication, assess its effectiveness and the client's compliance with the regimen. Identify who administers the medication.

• Assist the client in the home in identifying and establishing daily patterns that have meaning for the client.

▲ For a client who is displaced from the home, identify internal values that can be maintained while the client is displaced, such as respite, contact with specific persons, and honesty.

▲ Encourage the client to verbalize feelings of risk and trauma to therapeutic staff or other supportive persons. Refer to medical social services or mental health/support group services as appropriate.

▲ Evaluate the client's response to a traumatic or critical event. If screening warrants, refer to a therapist for counseling/treatment.

• See the care plan for **Post-trauma syndrome.**

## Client/Family Teaching

• Instruct the family and friends to use the following critical incident stress management techniques:
  ▪ Listen carefully.
  ▪ Spend time with the traumatized person.
  ▪ Offer your assistance and a listening ear, even if the person has not asked for help.
  ▪ Help the person with everyday tasks like cleaning, cooking, caring for the family, and minding children.
  ▪ Give the person some private time.
  ▪ Don't take the individual's anger or other feelings personally.
  ▪ Don't tell the person that he or she is "lucky it wasn't worse"; such statements do not console traumatized people. Instead, tell the person that you are sorry such an event has occurred and you want to understand and assist him or her.

• = Independent          ▲ = Collaborative

- Teach the client and family to recognize symptoms of PTSD and to seek treatment when the client does the following:
  - Relives the traumatic event by thinking or dreaming about it frequently
  - Is unsettled or distressed in other areas of his or her life such as in school, at work, or in personal relationships
  - Avoids any situation that might cause him or her to relive the trauma
  - Demonstrates a certain amount of generalized emotional numbness
  - Shows a heightened sense of being on guard
- Instruct the parents to monitor a child who sustained minor injuries for symptoms of PTSD.
- Provide education to explain that acute stress disorder symptoms are normal reactions that are likely to resolve. Instruct to seek help if the symptoms persist.

# Powerlessness

## P  NANDA Definition

Perception that one's own actions will not significantly affect an outcome; perceived lack of control over current situation or immediate happening

### Defining Characteristics

#### Low

Expressions of uncertainty about fluctuating energy levels; passivity

#### Moderate

Nonparticipation in care or decision making when opportunities are provided; resentment, anger, and guilt; reluctance to express true feelings; passivity; dependence on others that may result in irritability; fearing alienation from caregivers; expressions of

• = Independent          ▲ = Collaborative

dissatisfaction and frustration because of inability to perform previous tasks/activities; expression of doubt regarding role performance; failure to monitor progress; failure to defend self-care practices when challenged; inability to seek information regarding care

## Severe

Verbal expressions of having no control over self-care, or influence over situation, or influence over outcome; apathy; depression regarding physical deterioration that occurs despite client's compliance with regimens

## Related Factors (r/t)

Health care environment; interpersonal interactions; lifestyle of helplessness; illness-related regimen

## Client Outcomes

### Client Will (Specify Time Frame):

- State feelings of powerlessness and other feelings related to powerlessness (e.g., anger, sadness, hopelessness).
- Identify factors that are uncontrollable.
- Participate in planning and implementing care; make decisions regarding care and treatment when possible.
- Ask questions about care and treatment.
- Verbalize hope for the future and sense of participation in planning and implementing care.

## Nursing Interventions

NOTE: Prior to implementation of interventions in the face of client powerlessness, nurses should examine their own philosophies of care to ensure that control issues or lack of faith in client capabilities will not bias the ability to intervene sincerely and effectively.

- Observe for factors contributing to powerlessness (e.g., immobility, hospitalization, unfavorable prognosis, lack of support system, misinformation about situation, inflexible routine, chronic illness).

• = Independent          ▲ = Collaborative

- Be alert to client behaviors that attempt to assert power, even if they seem confrontational. Assist clients to channel their behaviors in an effective manner.
- Assess for ineffective therapeutic regimen management or noncompliance.
- Assess the client's locus of control related to his or her health.
- Assess for signs/symptoms of hopelessness depression and pay particular attention to the availability of social support. Hopelessness depression is characterized by a negative cognitive style (i.e., a tendency to perceive negative events as stable and global).
- Establish a therapeutic relationship with the client by spending one-on-one time with him or her, assigning the same caregiver, keeping commitments (e.g., saying, "I will be back to answer your questions in the next hour"), providing encouragement, and being empathetic.
- Allow the client to express hope, which may range from "I hope my coffee will be hot" to "I hope I will die with my significant other here." Listen to the client's priorities and incorporate those priorities in the therapeutic regimen wherever possible.
- Allow the client to share feelings. Evaluate the influence those feelings could have on the client's decision making and actions. Help the client to focus on objective elements of his or her situation, rather than on the emotionally threatening aspects of the experience. The experience of feeling overwhelmed by a medical situation can increase feelings of powerlessness.
- Support clients' efforts to regain control of their lives by learning everything they can about their illnesses.
- Encourage the client to participate in self-regulation and self-care management of the client's illness. Have the client assist in planning care whenever possible (e.g., determining what time to bathe, taking pain medication before uncomfortable procedures, expressing food and fluid preferences). Document specifics in the care plan.
- Encourage the client to share his or her beliefs, thoughts, and expectations about his or her illness.

• = Independent ▲ = Collaborative

- Make the time to learn the client's needs and be sure that nurse and client are operating with mutual understanding.
- Assist the client in specifying the health goals he or she would like to achieve, prioritizing those goals with regard to immediate concerns, and identifying actions that will achieve the goals. Offer feedback and education to ensure that goals and the expected time frame for meeting them are realistic. Goals may need to be small to be attainable (e.g., dangle legs at bedside for 2 days, then sit in chair 10 minutes for 2 days, then walk to window).
- Help the client identify factors not under his or her control.
- Assist the client in identifying a repertoire of strategies to implement in managing his or her symptoms.
- Encourage the client in goal-directed activities that promote a sense of accomplishment, especially regular exercise.
- Discuss with the client areas in which he or she feels the need to protect himself or herself or others, and the strategies used. Support appropriate protective measures while assisting the client in identifying more effective and stress-reducing measures.
- Recognize the client's need to experience a sense of reciprocity in dealing with others. Negotiate actions that the client can contribute to the caregiving partnership with both family and nurse; e.g., have the client prepare a cup of tea for the nurse during visits if the client is able.
- Help the client to identify and persist with self-care strategies that are effective; extinguish strategies that are ineffective.
- Allow time for questions (15 to 20 minutes each shift); have the client write down questions; encourage the client to record a summary of answers received if desired or practicable, or provide written material that reinforces answers.
- Keep items the client uses and needs, such as a urinal, tissues, telephone, and television controls, within reach.
- Give realistic and sincere praise for accomplishments.

P

• = Independent                  ▲ = Collaborative

- Keep interactions with the client focused on the client, not on the family or physician. Actively listen to the client.
- Acknowledge subjective concerns or fears.
- Encourage the client to take control of as many ADLs as possible; keep the client informed of all care that will be given.
- Develop a contract with the client that states the client's and nurse's responsibilities and privileges.
- See the care plans for **Hopelessness** and **Spiritual distress.**

## Geriatric

- ▲ Initiate focused assessment questioning and education regarding syndromes common in the elderly.
- Explore feelings of powerlessness—the feeling that the client's behavior will not affect outcomes.
- Explore personality resources and inner strengths that the client has used in the past. Incorporate these into the treatment plan.
- Establish therapeutic relationships by listening; participate with the client in generating choices and incorporate his or her statement of limitations.
- Emphasize client control in all possible ADLs.
- Encourage the positive use of solitude—reading, listening to music, enjoying nature—to prevent loneliness. Encourage socialization with others when possible; advocate for the client regarding family visitation if relationships are viewed positively by the client.
- ▲ Monitor the use of alternative therapies but do not intervene unless the therapy interacts negatively with the existing therapeutic regimen. Ensure that all health care providers involved with the client are aware of the alternative therapies being used.

## Multicultural

- Assess for the influence of cultural beliefs, norms, and values on the client's feelings of powerlessness. The cli-

P

• = Independent          ▲ = Collaborative

ent's expressions of powerlessness may be based on cultural perceptions or expectations.

- Assess the effect of fatalism on the client's expression of powerlessness.
- Encourage spirituality as a source of support to decrease powerlessness.
- Validate the client's feelings regarding the impact of health status on current lifestyle.
- For inner-city clients, help the client to redefine behaviors as ways of coping with a hostile environment and to reconnect with community supports.
- Utilize an empowerment approach when working with African-American women.

## Home Care

- ▲ Include an initial and ongoing assessment and evaluation of potential abuse and neglect. Photograph evidence of abuse or neglect when possible.
- ▲ If neglect or abuse is suspected, identify an emergency plan that addresses the problem immediately, ensures client safety, and includes a report to the appropriate authorities.
- Develop a therapeutic relationship in the home setting that respects the client's domain.
- Develop a written contract with the client that designates what care will be given and who has responsibility for care elements. Focus should be on care that is controlled by the client. Enable the client to develop his or her own resources actively.
- ▲ Empower the client by encouraging the client to guide specifics of care such as wound care procedures and dressing and grooming details. Confirm the client's knowledge and document in the chart that the client is able to guide procedures. Document in the home and in the chart the preferred approach to procedures. Orient the family and caregivers to the client's role.
- Identify the client's concerns and implement interven-

• = Independent          ▲ = Collaborative

tions to address the consequences of disability in clients with medical illness.

- Enhance self-efficacy by creating an environment that supports physical activities; provide support in the form of encouragement, anticipatory guidance, sharing of how others perform, and realistic assessment of the client's abilities.
- Respect the client's choices regarding desired assistance. Identify knowledge deficits and provide education to address them to ensure that the client's choice is accurately informed.
- Assess the affective climate within the family and family support system (including other caregivers). Instruct the family in appropriate expectations of the client and in the specifics of the client's illness. Encourage the family and client in efforts toward educating friends and co-workers regarding appropriate expectations for the client. Serve as the client's advocate.
- Evaluate the powerlessness of caregivers, to insure they continue their ability to care for the client. Provide assistance using interventions from this care plan.
- Be aware of and assist clients with potential needs for help in negotiating the health care system.
▲ Refer for homemaker or psychiatric home health care services for respite, client reassurance, and implementation of a therapeutic regimen.
▲ Explain all relevant symptoms, procedures, treatments, and expected outcomes.
▲ Provide written instructions for treatments and procedures for which the client will be responsible.
▲ Continually assess the client for signs of inappropriate exercise of self-care. Confront such applications of self-care; instruct the client in the dangers that inappropriate care may present and in alternatives for care that would be more effective.
- Teach stress reduction, relaxation, and imagery. Many cassette tapes are available on relaxation and meditation. Assist the client with relaxation based on the client's preference indicated in the initial assessment.

•  = Independent          ▲ = Collaborative

- Teach cognitive-behavioral activities, such as active problem solving, reframing (reappraising the situation from a different perspective), or thought stopping (in response to a negative thought, picturing a large stop sign and replacing the image with a prearranged positive alternative). Teach the client to confront his or her own negative thought patterns (or cognitive distortions), such as catastrophizing (expecting the very worst), dichotomous thinking (perceiving events as belonging in only one of two opposite categories), or magnification (placing distorted emphasis on a single event).
- Help the client practice assertive communication techniques.
- Role play (e.g., say, "Tell me what you are going to ask your doctor").
- Identify the strengths of the caregiver and efforts to gain control of unpredictable situations. Help the caregiver to stay connected with a client who may be behaving differently than usual, to make life as routine as possible, to help the client set goals and sustain hope, and to allow the client space to experience progress.
- ▲ Refer the client to support groups, pastoral care, or social services.

P

# Risk for Powerlessness

## NANDA Definition

At risk for perceived lack of control over a situation and/or one's ability to significantly affect an outcome

## Related Factors (r/t)

### Physiological

Chronic or acute illness (hospitalization, intubation, ventilator use, suctioning); acute injury or progressive debilitating disease process (e.g., multiple sclerosis); aging (e.g., decreased physical strength, decreased mobility); dying

• = Independent            ▲ = Collaborative

## Psychosocial

Lack of knowledge of illness or health care system; lifestyle of dependency with inadequate coping patterns; absence of integrality (e.g., essence of power); decreased self-esteem; low or unstable body image

## Client Outcomes

### Client Will (Specify Time Frame):

- State feelings of powerlessness and other feelings related to powerlessness (e.g., anger, sadness, hopelessness).
- Identify factors that are uncontrollable.
- Participate in planning and implementing care; make decisions regarding care and treatment when possible.
- Ask questions about care and treatment.
- Verbalize hope for the future and sense of participation in planning and implementing care.

## Nursing Interventions, Client/Family Teaching

See the care plan for **Powerlessness.**

# P | Ineffective Protection

## NANDA Definition

Decrease in ability to guard self from internal or external threats such as illness or injury

## Defining Characteristics

Maladaptive stress response; neurosensory alteration; impaired healing; deficient immunity; altered clotting; dyspnea; insomnia; weakness; restlessness; pressure ulcers; perspiring; itching; immobility; chilling; fatigue; disorientation; cough; anorexia

## Related Factors (r/t)

Abnormal blood profiles (e.g., leukopenia, thrombocytopenia, anemia, coagulation); extremes of age; inadequate nutrition;

alcohol abuse; drug therapies (e.g., antineoplastic, corticosteroid, immune, anticoagulant, thrombolytic); treatments (e.g., surgery, radiation); diseases such as cancer and immune disorders

## Client Outcomes

### Client Will (Specify Time Frame):

- Remain free of infection.
- Remain free of any evidence of new bleeding.
- Explain precautions to take to prevent infection.
- Explain precautions to take to prevent bleeding.

## Nursing Interventions

- Take temperature, pulse, and blood pressure (e.g., every 1 to 4 hours).
- ▲ Observe nutritional status (e.g., weight, serum protein and albumin levels, muscle mass, usual food intake). Work with the dietitian to improve nutritional status if needed. All clients diagnosed with HIV should have a dietary consult.
- Observe the client's sleep pattern; if altered, see Nursing Interventions for **Disturbed Sleep pattern**.
- Determine the amount of stress in the client's life. If stress is uncontrollable, see Nursing Interventions for **In-effective Coping**.

## Prevention of infection

- ▲ Monitor for and report any signs of infection (e.g., fever, chills, flushed skin, drainage, edema, redness, abnormal laboratory values, and pain) and notify the physician promptly.
- Use appropriate "hand hygiene" (i.e., hand washing or use of alcohol-based hand rubs).
- When using an alcohol-based hand rub, apply product to palm of one hand and rub hands together, covering all surfaces of hands and fingers, until hands are dry. Note that the volume needed to reduce the number of bacteria on hands varies by product.
- Consider warming the client before elective surgery.

• = Independent          ▲ = Collaborative

▲ If the client's immune system is depressed, notify the physician of elevated temperature, even in the absence of other symptoms of infection.

• If white blood cell count is severely decreased (absolute neutrophil count of <1000/mm$^3$), initiate the following precautions:

  ▪ Take vital signs every 4 hours.

  ▪ Complete a head-to-toe assessment twice daily, including inspection of oral mucosa, invasive sites, wounds, urine, and stool; monitor for onset of new complaints of pain.

  ▪ Avoid any invasive procedures, including catheterization, injections, or rectal or vaginal procedures.

▲ Administer granulocyte growth factor therapy as ordered.

• Take meticulous care of all invasive sites; use chlorhexidine gluconate for cleansing.

• Provide frequent oral care.

▲ Refer for prophylactic medication to prevent oral candidiasis.

▲ Refer for appropriate prophylactic antifungal treatment and avoid pathogen exposure (through air filtration, regular hand hygiene, avoidance of plants and flowers).

• Have the client wear a mask when leaving the room.

• Limit and screen visitors to minimize exposure to contagion.

• Help the client bathe daily.

• Serve the client well-cooked food only; avoid all raw foods, including salads. Avoid serving processed meats, cheeses, yogurt, and beer or wine. Have the client drink sterile or boiled water only, and make ice cubes out of sterile water.

• Ensure that the client is well nourished. Provide food with protein and consider vitamin supplements. If appetite is suppressed, institute a dietary referral. Keep track of serum albumin levels as well as transferrin and prealbumin levels.

• Help the client to cough and practice deep breathing regularly. Maintain an appropriate activity level.

• Obtain a private room for the client. Take ordered pre-

• = Independent          ▲ = Collaborative

cautions, including the use of a protective isolation or laminar airflow room, a Shinki bioclean room (SBCR), and/or high-energy particulate air (HEPA) filters if available and appropriate. Recognize that cotton cover gowns may not be effective in decreasing infection.

▲ Watch for signs of sepsis, including change in mental status, fever, shaking, chills, and hypotension. If present, notify the physician promptly.

## Pediatric

▲ Suggest Kangaroo care (KC) defined as skin-to-skin contact between a mother and her newborn, frequent and exclusive or nearly exclusive breastfeeding, and early discharge from hospital for low birth weight infants.

• For hand hygiene with low-birth-weight infants use alcohol hand rub and gloves.

• Avoid prophylactic application of topical ointment in preterm infants.

## Geriatric

• If not contraindicated, promote exercise to strengthen the immune system in the elderly.

• Give elderly clients with imbalanced nutrition a nutritional supplement to enhance immune function.

• See the care plan for **Risk for Infection** for more interventions related to the prevention of infection.

## Prevention of Bleeding

• Monitor the client's risk for bleeding; evaluate results of clotting studies and platelet counts.

• Watch for hematuria, melena, hematemesis, hemoptysis, epistaxis, bleeding from mucosa, petechiae, and ecchymoses.

▲ Give medications orally or intravenously only; avoid giving them intramuscularly, subcutaneously, or rectally. Apply pressure for a longer time than usual to invasive sites such as venipuncture or injection sites.

• = Independent          ▲ = Collaborative

- Take vital signs frequently; watch for changes associated with fluid volume loss.
- Monitor menstrual flow if relevant; have the client use pads instead of tampons.
- Have the client use a moistened toothette instead of a toothbrush, or a very soft child's toothbrush. Have the client use alcohol-free dental products and avoid flossing.
- Ask the client either not to shave or to use an electric razor only.
- To decrease risk of bleeding, avoid administering salicylates or nonsteroidal anti-inflammatory drugs (NSAIDs) if possible.

## Home Care
- Some of the interventions described previously may be adapted for home care use.
- Consider institution of a nurse-administered mobile care unit for monitoring anticoagulant therapy.
- ▲ For terminally ill clients, teach and institute all of the aforementioned noninvasive precautions that will maintain quality of life. Discuss with the client, family, and physician the consequences of contracting infection. Determine which precautions do not maintain quality of life and should not be used (e.g., physical assessment twice daily, multiple vital sign assessments).

## Client/Family Teaching
### Depressed Immune Function
- Teach precautions to take to decrease the chance of infection (e.g., avoiding uncooked fruits or vegetables, using appropriate self-care, ensuring a safe environment).
- Teach the client and family how to take a temperature. Encourage the family to take the client's temperature between 3 PM and 7 PM at least once daily.
- ▲ Teach the client and family to notify the physician of elevated temperature, even in the absence of other symptoms of infection.
- Teach the client to avoid crowds and contact with persons who have infections.

● = Independent          ▲ = Collaborative

## Bleeding Disorder

▲ Teach the client to wear a medical alert bracelet and notify all health care personnel of the bleeding disorder.

• Teach the client and family the signs of bleeding, precautions to take to prevent bleeding, and action to take if bleeding begins. Caution the client to avoid taking over-the-counter medications without the permission of the physician.

• Teach the client to wear loose-fitting clothes and avoid physical activity that might cause trauma.

# Rape-trauma syndrome

## NANDA Definition

Sustained maladaptive response to forced, violent sexual act (penetration may not actually occur) against victim's will and consent

## Defining Characteristics

Fear; disorganization; change in relationships; confusion; physical trauma (e.g., bruising, tissue irritation, injuries identified by use of new technology); suicide attempt; denial; guilt; paranoia; humiliation; embarrassment; aggression; muscle tension and/or spasms; mood swings; dependence; powerlessness; nightmares and sleep disturbances; sexual dysfunction; desire for revenge; phobias; loss of self-esteem; inability to make decisions; dissociative disorders; self-blame; hyperalertness; vulnerability; substance abuse; depression; helplessness; anger; anxiety; agitation; shame; shock

## Related Factors (r/t)

Rape; sexual assault; abuse

## Client Outcomes

### Client Will (Specify Time Frame):

• Share feelings, concerns, and fears.
• Recognize that the rape or attempt was not client's own fault.

• = Independent          ▲ = Collaborative

- State that, no matter what the situation, no one has the right to assault another.
- Describe medical/legal treatment procedures and reasons for treatment.
- Report absence of physical complications or pain.
- Identify support people and be able to ask them for help in dealing with this trauma.
- Function at same level as before crisis, including sexual functioning.
- Recognize that it is normal for full recovery to take a minimum of 1 year.

## Nursing Interventions

- Observe the client's responses, including anger, fear, self-blame, sleep pattern disturbances, and phobias.
- Monitor the client's verbal and nonverbal psychological state (e.g., crying, hand wringing, avoidance of interactions or eye contact with staff, silence, and denial).
- ▲ Stay with (or have a trusted person stay with) the client initially. If a law enforcement interview is permitted, provide support by staying with the client, but only at the client's request.
- Explain the entire medical/legal examination to the client before beginning any procedures.
- Obtain written permission to perform the examination but explain to the client that at any time during the examination the client may withdraw consent. Discuss with the client the importance of participating in the entire examination and the importance of the collection of evidence.
- Do not wait for the client to ask questions; explain everything you are doing, clarify why it must be done, and describe when and where you will touch.
- ▲ Observe for signs of physical injury as you are asking the client to undress and collecting the client's clothing for evidence. Ask the client where it hurts without asking leading questions. Do not ask specific questions but allow the client to give you a history of the sexual assault in the client's own words. If further clarification is

• = Independent        ▲ = Collaborative

needed by the examiner, ask the client to point to areas that were injured or touched. Inform the client that photographs of any injuries are necessary for forensic evidence. Obtain specific written permission for photographs to be taken and released to law enforcement personnel.

▲ Instruct the client to return for additional photographs either to the medical facility or to law enforcement personnel if bruises become more pronounced in a few days. It is recommended that all medical treatment be completed at the initial encounter due to the difficulty in getting clients to return for follow-up medical care.

• Documentation of a sexual assault examination is critical to evidentiary reports. It is important to document the client's exact description of the assault and then to collect evidence and photographs that validate the history the client reports.

• It is also very important for the examiner not to offer any opinions in the documentation about whether or not the assault occurred according to the physical findings.

▲ Document a one- or two-sentence summary of what happened. The chief complaint of the client reporting sexual assault should always be given as "reported sexual assault"; obtaining the details of the sequence of events is the police officer's job.

• Encourage the client to verbalize feelings.

• Escort the client to the treatment room immediately to remove the client from the general population; do not question the client in the triage area, close curtains and door, and avoid other interruptions during contact with the client (e.g., telephone calls, absence from the room, outside stimuli such as radios).

▲ Provide a sexual assault response team that includes a sexual assault nurse examiner (SANE), rape counseling advocate, and representative of law enforcement.

▲ The rape crisis center advocate should be part of the sexual assault response team (SART) and respond when the SANE responds. This person can encourage follow-up at the rape crisis center.

R

• = Independent          ▲ = Collaborative

- Provide items for self-care after examination (e.g., for cleansing the vaginal and rectal area).
▲ Most states provide sexual assault evidence collection kits that have been reviewed by the SART members to provide adequate evidence for analysis by the forensic laboratory. Explain to the client that all or some of the client's clothing may be kept for evidential purposes. Also explain that the client will receive replacement clothing or that the client can request that a friend or family member bring clothing from home to replace the clothing kept for evidence. Explain to the client that, if the clothing worn during the assault is still at the scene, the client should disclose this information to law enforcement officials so that law enforcement personnel can go to the scene and collect the evidence appropriately.
- An alternative light source will be used for direct inspection of the body for the presence of body fluids.
▲ Discuss the possibility of pregnancy and sexually transmitted diseases (STDs) and the treatments available.
▲ Encourage the client to report the rape to a law enforcement agency.
- Discuss the client's support system. Involve the support system if appropriate and if the client grants permission. Unsupportive and victim-blaming attitudes by significant others are common responses.
▲ Obtaining blood alcohol levels or levels of any drug should be discussed thoroughly with the medical director of your facility and the SART members.

### Geriatric
- Build a trusting relationship with the client.
▲ Explain reporting and encourage the client to report.
- Observe for psychosocial distress (e.g., memory impairment, sleep disturbances, regression, changes in bodily functions).
▲ All examinations should be done on the elderly as they would be done on any adult client after sexual assault. Evidence should be collected and consent for col-

• = Independent        ▲ = Collaborative

lection, photography, and law enforcement contact should be obtained as in all cases. Special attention should be given to the explanation of the genital examination, especially as it relates to the use of a speculum.

- Modify the rape protocol to promote comfort for the geriatric client. Consider positioning female clients with pillows rather than stirrups and consider using a smaller speculum.
- Assess for mobility limitations and cognitive impairment.
- Respect the client's need for privacy.
▲ Consider arrangements for temporary housing. Most sexual assaults of older clients occur in the home (or nursing home).

## Male Rape
- Reactions to male rape are often either disbelief or an assumption that the man who was raped is gay.

## Multicultural
- Assess for the influence of cultural beliefs, norms, and values on the client's ability to cope with the trauma of the rape experience.
- Acknowledge racial/ethnic differences at the onset of care.
- Use a family-centered approach when working with Latino, Asian, African-American, and Native-American clients.
- Provide opportunities by which the family and individual can save face when working with Asian-American clients.
- Assure the client of confidentiality.
- Validate the client's feelings regarding the rape and allow the client to tell his or her rape story.
- A culturally sensitive approach should be part of the training of all SARTs and members of the teams.

## Home Care
- Some of the interventions described previously may be adapted for home care use.

● = Independent        ▲ = Collaborative

- Interact with the client supportively and nonjudgmentally; this supports the client's self-worth.
- Assist the client with realistically assessing the home setting for safety and/or selecting a safe environment in which to live.
▲ Ensure that the client has a support system in place for long-term support. Instruct the family that recovery may take a long time. Refer for medical social work services to assist in setting up a support system if necessary. Refer for counseling if necessary.
▲ Make sure that physical symptoms from the rape or other physical conditions are followed up. Follow-up should include a visit to the primary care physician or the local health department in 3 to 4 weeks for repeat pregnancy testing and STD testing. Explain to the client that additional medication may be necessary for the treatment of STDs or pregnancy.
▲ If the client is homebound, refer for psychiatric home health care services for client reassurance and implementation of a therapeutic regimen.

## Client/Family Teaching

▲ Provide information on prophylactic antibiotic therapy, hepatitis B vaccination, and tetanus prophylaxis for nonimmunized clients with trauma.
- Discharge instructions should be written out for the client.
- Give instructions to significant others.
▲ Explain the potential for common side effects related to treatment with norgestrel, such as breast swelling or nausea and vomiting. (Call the emergency department if the client vomits within 1 hour of taking the pill because the pill may need to be taken again.) (Discuss any issues about prophylactic medications at the follow-up visit in 3 to 4 weeks.) It may take 3 to 30 days for the menstrual period to start; if menstruation has not begun in 30 days, contact a physician.
▲ Explain the potential for severe side effects related to treatment with norgestrel, such as severe leg or chest

R

• = Independent          ▲ = Collaborative

pain, trouble breathing, coughing up of blood, severe headache or dizziness, and trouble seeing or talking.

- Advise the client to call or return if new problems develop.
- Teach relaxation techniques.
- Discuss practical lifestyle changes within the client's control to reduce the risk of future attacks.
▲ Teach the client to use self-defense techniques to surprise an attacker and create an opportunity to run for help. Refer the client to a self-defense school.
- Teach the client appropriate outlets for anger.
- Emphasize the vulnerability of the client and ensure that reactions are appropriate for the victim of sexual assault.

NOTE: Post-traumatic stress disorder (PTSD) has a high probability of being a psychological sequela to rape. Research demonstrated two effective treatments for improvement of PTSD in rape victims—prolonged exposure and stress inoculation training. Prolonged exposure involves reliving the rape experience by imagining it as vividly as possible, describing it aloud in the present tense, taping this description, and listening to the tape at least once daily. Stress inoculation training uses breathing exercises to diminish anxiety and instruction in coping skills, thought stopping, cognitive restructuring, self-dialogue, and role playing. Research suggests that a combination of both treatments may provide the optimal effect.

R

# Rape-trauma syndrome: compound reaction

## NANDA Definition

Forced violent sexual act (penetration may not actually occur) against victim's will and consent resulting in a trauma syndrome that includes an acute phase of disorganization of victim's lifestyle and a long-term process or reorganization of lifestyle

• = Independent          ▲ = Collaborative

## Defining Characteristics

Change in lifestyle (e.g., changing residence, dealing with repetitive nightmares and phobias, seeking family support, seeking social network support in long-term phase); emotional reaction (e.g., anger, embarrassment, fear of physical violence and death, humiliation, desire for revenge, self-blame in acute phase); multiple physical symptoms (e.g., gastrointestinal irritability, genitourinary discomfort, muscle tension, sleep pattern disturbance in acute phase); reactivated symptoms of previous conditions (i.e., physical illness, psychiatric illness in acute phase); reliance on alcohol and/or drugs (acute phase)

## Related Factors (r/t)

Rape; sexual assault; abuse

## Client Outcomes

### Client Will (Specify Time Frame):

- Share feelings, concerns, and fears.
- Recognize that the rape or attempt was not client's own fault.
- State that, no matter what the situation, no one has the right to assault another.
- Describe medical/legal treatment procedures and reasons for treatment.
- Report absence of physical complications or pain.
- Identify support people and be able to ask them for help in dealing with this trauma.
- Function at same level as before crisis, including sexual functioning.
- Recognize that it is normal for full recovery to take a minimum of 1 year.

## Nursing Interventions

- See the care plans for **Rape-trauma syndrome, Powerlessness, Ineffective Coping, Dysfunctional Grieving, Anxiety, Fear, Risk for self-directed Violence,** and **Sexual dysfunction.**

• = Independent        ▲ = Collaborative

## Geriatric

▲ A new subgroup of rape victims resides in nursing homes. Treatment is necessary.

## Risk for Compound Reaction

• See the care plan for **Rape-trauma syndrome.**

## Multicultural

• Assess for the influence of cultural beliefs, norms, and values on the client's ability to cope with the trauma of the rape experience.

• Provide opportunities by which the family and individual can save face when working with Asian-American clients.

• Assure the client of confidentiality.

• Validate the client's feelings regarding the rape and allow the client to tell his or her rape story.

• A culturally sensitive approach should be part of the training of all sexual assault response teams and members of the teams.

## Home Care

▲ If the client has pursued psychiatric counseling, monitor and encourage attendance.

▲ If the client is receiving medication, assess the client's knowledge of its purpose, side effects, and interactions with medications for other diagnoses. Monitor for effectiveness, side effects, and interactions.

▲ Establish an emergency plan including use of hotlines. Contract with the client to use the emergency plan. Role play using the hotlines.

• For other home care and hospice considerations, see the care plan for **Rape-trauma syndrome.**

## Client/Family Teaching

• Teach the client what reactions to expect during the acute and long-term phases: acute phase—anger, fear, self-blame, embarrassment, vengeful feelings, physi-

R

• = Independent          ▲ = Collaborative

cal symptoms, muscle tension, sleeplessness, stomach upset, genitourinary discomfort; long-term phase—changes
in lifestyle or residence, nightmares, phobias, seeking of
family and social network support.
▲ Encourage psychiatric consultation if the client is suicidal, violent, or unable to continue activities of daily
living.
▲ Discuss any of the client's current stress-relieving medications that may result in substance abuse.

## Rape-trauma syndrome: silent reaction

### NANDA Definition

Forced violent sexual act (penetration may not actually occur)
against victim's will and consent resulting in a trauma syndrome
that includes an acute phase of disorganization of victim's
lifestyle and a long-term process of reorganization of lifestyle

### Defining Characteristics

Increased anxiety during interview (e.g., blocking of associations,
long periods of silence, minor stuttering, physical distress);
sudden onset of phobic reactions; lack of verbalization about the
rape; abrupt changes in relationships with males; increased
nightmares; pronounced changes in sexual behavior

### Related Factors (r/t)

Rape; sexual assault; abuse

### Client Outcomes

**Client Will (Specify Time Frame):**

- Resume previous level of relationships with significant
others.
- State improvement in sleep and fewer nightmares.
- Express feelings about and discusses the rape.

• = Independent          ▲ = Collaborative

- Return to usual pattern of sexual behavior.
- Remain free of phobic reactions.
- See the care plan for **Rape-trauma syndrome.**

## Nursing Interventions

- See the care plans for **Rape-trauma syndrome, Power-lessness, Ineffective Coping, Dysfunctional Griev-ing, Anxiety, Fear, Risk for self-directed Violence, Sex-ual dysfunction,** and **Impaired verbal Communication.**
- Observe for disruptions in relationships with significant others.
- Monitor for signs of increased anxiety (e.g., silence, stut-tering, physical distress, irritability, unexplained crying spells).
- Focus on the client's coping strengths.
- Observe for changes in sexual behavior.
- Identify phobic reactions to persons or objects in the en-vironment (e.g., strangers, doorbells, groups of people, knives).
- Provide support by listening when the client is ready to talk.
- Be nonjudgmental when feelings are expressed. Explain that anger is normal and needs to be verbalized. Reassure the client with phrases such as, "I'm sorry this hap-pened to you."
- Remain with an anxious client even if the client is silent. Use gentle speech and actions; move slowly.
- Evaluate somatic complaints.

## Geriatric

- A new subgroup of rape victims resides in nursing homes. Treatment is necessary.
- See the care plan for **Rape-trauma syndrome.**

## Multicultural

- Assess for the influence of cultural beliefs, norms, and values on the client's ability to cope with the trauma of the rape experience.

R

• = Independent        ▲ = Collaborative

- Provide opportunities by which the family and individual can save face when working with Asian-American clients.
- Assure the client of confidentiality.
- Allow the client to tell his or her rape story without probing.

## Home Care

- See the care plan for **Rape-trauma syndrome.**

## Client/Family Teaching

- Reassure the client that he or she is not bad and is not at fault. Avoid questions beginning with "why."
▲ Refer the client to a sexual assault counselor.
▲ Offer information about testing, treatment, and procedures related to pregnancy, hepatitis B, and sexually transmitted infection. Do not wait for the client to request information.
- See the care plan for **Rape-trauma syndrome.**

# Impaired Religiosity

## NANDA Definition

Impaired ability to exercise reliance on beliefs and/or participate in rituals of a particular faith tradition

## Defining Characteristics

Demonstrates or explains difficulty adhering to prescribed religious beliefs and rituals: religious ceremonies, dietary regulations, clothing, prayer, worship/religious services, private religious behaviors/reading religious materials/media, holiday observances, meetings with religious leaders; expresses emotional distress because of separation from faith community; expresses emotional distress regarding religious beliefs and/or religious social network; expresses a need to reconnect with previous belief patterns and customs; questions religious belief patterns and customs

• = Independent          ▲ = Collaborative

## Related Factors (r/t)

*Physical:* sickness/illness; *Psychological:* ineffective support/ coping, personal disaster/crisis, lack of security, anxiety, fear of death, ineffective coping with disease, use of religion to manipulate; *Sociocultural:* barriers to practicing religion, lack of social integration, lack of social/cultural interaction; *Spiritual:* spiritual crises, suffering; *Environmental:* barriers to practicing religion; *Developmental:* end-stage life crises, life transitions, aging

## Client Outcomes

### Client Will (Specify Time Frame):

- Express satisfaction with the ability to express religious practices.
- Express satisfaction with access to religious materials and rituals.
- Demonstrate balance between religious practices and healthy lifestyles.
- Avoid high-risk controlling religious relationships that inflict physical, sexual, or emotional harm and/or exploitation.

## Nursing Interventions

- Identify patient's concerns regarding religious expression.
- Encourage and/or coordinate the use of and participation in usual religious rituals or practices that are not detrimental to health.
- Coordinate or provide transportation to worship site, particularly for the elderly and in meeting the needs of the disabled or ill.
- Identify individuals at risk for an excessive dependence upon religion, religious leaders, or religious practices.
- ▲ Refer to religious leader, professional counseling, or support group as needed.

## Geriatric
- Promote established religious practices in the elderly.

## Multicultural
- Promote religious practices that are culturally appropriate.

● = Independent             ▲ = Collaborative

## Readiness for enhanced Religiosity

### NANDA Definition

Ability to exercise reliance on beliefs and/or participate in rituals of a particular faith tradition

### Defining Characteristics

Expresses desire to strengthen religious belief patterns and customs that had provided comfort/religion in the past; requests assistance to increase participation in prescribed religious beliefs through religious ceremonies, dietary regulations/rituals, clothing, prayer, worship/religious services, private religious behaviors, reading religious materials/media, holiday observances; requests assistance expanding religious options; expresses meeting with religious leaders/facilitators; requests forgiveness, reconciliation; questions or rejects belief patterns and customs that are harmful

### Related Factors (r/t)

Health-seeking behaviors to express one's chosen faith tradition or to reject harmful belief patterns and customs

### Client Outcomes

**Client Will (Specify Time Frame):**

- Express satisfaction with an enhanced ability to express religious practices.
- Express satisfaction with access to religious materials and rituals.
- Demonstrate balance between religious practices and healthy lifestyles.
- Avoid high-risk controlling religious relationships that inflict physical, sexual, or emotional harm and/or exploitation.

### Nursing Interventions

- Identify patient's desire regarding religious expression.
- Encourage and/or coordinate the use of and participation in usual religious rituals or practices that are not detrimental to health.

R

• = Independent          ▲ = Collaborative

- Coordinate or provide transportation to worship site, particularly for the elderly and in meeting the needs of the disabled or ill.
▲ Refer to religious leader, as appropriate.

## Pediatric
- Provide spiritual care for children based on developmental level.
  - **Infants:** Have the same nurse care for the child on a daily basis; hold, cuddle, rock, play with, and sing to the infant.
  - **Toddlers:** Provide consistency in care and familiar toys, music, stories, clothing blankets, pillows, and any other individual object of contentment. Schedule home religious routines into the plan of care and support home routines regarding good and bad behavior.
  - **School-age children and adolescents**: Encourage both groups to express their feelings regarding spirituality. Ask them, "Do you wish to pray and what do want to pray about?" Children of all ages can express feelings in storytelling. Offer age-appropriate complimentary therapies such as music, art, videos, and connectedness with peers through cards, letters, and visits.

## Geriatric
- Promote established religious practices in the elderly.

## Multicultural
- Promote religious practices that are culturally appropriate.

R

# Risk for impaired Religiosity

## NANDA Definition

Impaired ability to exercise reliance on beliefs and/or participate in rituals of a particular faith tradition

● = Independent        ▲ = Collaborative

## Risk Factors (r/t)

*Physical:* illness/hospitalization, pain; *Psychological:* ineffective support/coping/caregiving, depression, lack of security; *Sociocultural:* lack of social integration, cultural barriers to practicing religion, social isolation; *Spiritual:* suffering; *Environmental:* lack of transportation, barriers to practicing religion; *Developmental:* life transitions

## Client Outcomes

### Client Will (Specify Time Frame):

- Express satisfaction with the ability to express of religious practices.
- Express satisfaction with access to religious materials and rituals.
- Demonstrate balance between religious practices and healthy lifestyles.
- Avoid high-risk controlling religious relationships that inflict physical, sexual, or emotional harm and/or exploitation.

## Nursing Interventions

- Identify patient's concerns regarding religious expression.
- Encourage and/or coordinate the use of and participation in usual religious rituals or practices that are not detrimental to health.
- Coordinate or provide transportation to worship site, particularly for the elderly and in meeting the needs of the disabled or ill.
- Identify individuals at risk for an excessive dependence upon religion, religious leaders, or religious practices.
- ▲ Refer to religious leader, professional counseling, or support group as needed.

## Geriatric
- Promote established religious practices in the elderly.

## Multicultural
- Promote religious practices that are culturally appropriate.

• = Independent          ▲ = Collaborative

# Relocation stress syndrome

## NANDA Definition

Physiological and/or psychosocial disturbances that result from transfer from one environment to another

## Defining Characteristics

Temporary and/or permanent move; voluntary and/or involuntary move; aloneness, alienation, or loneliness; depression; anxiety (e.g., separation); sleep disturbance; withdrawal; anger; loss of identity, self-worth, or self-esteem; increased verbalization of needs, unwillingness to move or concern over relocation; increased physical symptoms/illness (e.g., gastrointestinal disturbance, weight change); dependency; insecurity; pessimism; frustration; worry; fear

## Related Factors (r/t)

Unpredictability of experience/isolation from family/friends; passive coping; language barrier; decreased health status; impaired psychosocial health; past, concurrent, and recent losses; feeling of powerlessness; lack of adequate support system/group; lack of predeparture counseling

## Client Outcomes

### Client Will (Specify Time Frame):

- Recognize and know the name of at least one staff member.
- Express concern about move when encouraged to do so during individual contacts.
- Carry out activities of daily living (ADLs) in usual manner.
- Maintain previous mental and physical health status (e.g., nutrition, elimination, sleep, social interaction).

## Nursing Interventions

- Obtain a history, including the reason for the move, the client's usual coping mechanisms, history of losses, and family support for the client.
- Consider the client's and family's cultural and ethnic val-

• = Independent          ▲ = Collaborative

ues as much as possible when choosing roommates, foods, and other aspects of care.

- Observe the following procedures if the client is being transferred to an extended care facility or assisted living facility:
  - Allow the client to have a choice of placement and arrange a preadmission visit if possible.
  - If the client cannot choose placement, arrange for a visit or telephone call by a member of the staff to welcome the client and show a videotape or at least provide pictures of the new care facility.
  - Have a familiar person accompany the client to the new facility.
  - Validate the caregiver's feelings of difficulty with putting a loved one in a different environment. This is a distressing experience, and caregivers feel responsible.
- Identify previous routines for ADLs. Try to maintain as much continuity with the previous schedule as possible.
- Bring in familiar items from home (e.g., pictures, clocks, afghans).
- Establish the way the client would like to be addressed (Mr., Mrs., Miss, first name, nickname).
- Thoroughly orient the client and the family to the new environment and routines; repeat directions as needed.
- Spend one-on-one time with the client. Allow the client to express feelings and convey acceptance of them; emphasize that the client's feelings are real and individual and that it is acceptable to be sad or angry about moving.
- Assign the same staff members to the client if compatible with client; maintain consistency in the personnel the client interacts with.
- Ask the client to state one positive aspect of the new living situation each day.
- Monitor the client's health status and provide appropriate interventions for problems with social interaction, nutrition, sleep, new onset of infection, or elimination problems.

● = Independent          ▲ = Collaborative

- If the client is being transferred within a facility, have staff members from the new unit visit the client before transfer.
- Work with the caregiver's family members by helping them deal with stages of "making the best of it," making the move, and "making it better."
- If a client is being transferred from the intensive care unit, have previous staff make occasional visits until the client is comfortable in the new surroundings. Ensure family are told relevant information.
- Watch for coping problems (e.g., withdrawal, regression, angry behavior, impaired sleeping, refusal to eat, flat affect) and intervene immediately.
- Allow the client to grieve for the loss of the old situation; explain that it is normal to feel sadness over change and loss.
- Encourage the client to participate in care as much as possible and make own decisions when possible (e.g., placement of the bed, choice of roommate, bathing routines). Make an effort to accommodate the client.

## Pediatric
- Provide support for a child and family who must relocate to be near a transplant center.
- If the client is an adolescent, try to avoid a move in the middle of the school year, find a newcomers' club for the adolescent to join, and refer for counseling if needed.

## Geriatric
- Monitor the need for transfer and transfer only when necessary.
- Protect the client from injuries such as falls.
- After the transfer, determine the client's mental status. Document and observe for any new onset of confusion.
▲ Refer for music therapy.
- Use reality orientation if needed (e.g., "Today is . . .," "The date is . . .," "You are at . . . facility"). Repeat the information as needed and provide a clock or calendar.

R

• = Independent            ▲ = Collaborative

## Client/Family Teaching

- Teach family members about relocation stress syndrome. Encourage them to monitor for signs of the syndrome.
- Help significant others learn how to support the client in the move by setting up a schedule of visits, arranging for holidays, bringing familiar items from home, and establishing a system for contact when the client needs support.

# Risk for Relocation stress syndrome

## NANDA Definition

At risk for physiological and/or psychosocial disturbances that result from transfer from one environment to another

### Risk Factors

Moderate to high degree of environmental change (e.g., physical, ethnic, cultural); temporary and/or permanent move; voluntary and/or involuntary move; lack of adequate support system/group; feelings of powerlessness; moderate mental competence (e.g., alert enough to experience changes); unpredictability of experiences; decreased psychosocial or physical health status; lack of predeparture counseling; passive coping; past, current, or recent losses

### Client Outcomes, Nursing Interventions, Client/Family Teaching

See care plan for **Relocation stress syndrome.**

# Ineffective Role performance

## NANDA Definition

Patterns of behavior and self-expression that do not match the environmental context, norms, and expectations

• = Independent      ▲ = Collaborative

## Defining Characteristics

Change in self-perception of role; role denial; inadequate external support for role enactment; inadequate adaptation to change or transition, system conflict; change in usual patterns of responsibility; discrimination; domestic violence; harassment uncertainty; altered role perceptions; role strain; inadequate self-management; role ambivalence; pessimistic attitude; inadequate motivation; inadequate confidence; inadequate role competency and skills; inadequate knowledge; inappropriate developmental expectations; role conflict; role confusion; powerlessness; inadequate coping; anxiety or depression; role overload; change in other's perception or role; role dissatisfaction; inadequate opportunities for role enactment

## Related Factors (r/t)

### Social

Inadequate or inappropriate linkage with the health care system; job schedule demands; young age; developmental level; lack of rewards; poverty; family conflict; inadequate support system; inadequate role socialization (e.g., role model, expectations responsibilities); low socioeconomic status; stress and conflict; domestic violence; lack of resources

### Knowledge

Inadequate role preparation (e.g., role transition, skill, rehearsal, validation); lack of knowledge about role, role skills; role transition; lack of opportunity for role rehearsal; developmental transitions; unrealistic role expectations; education attainment level; lack of or inadequate role model

### Physiological

Inadequate/inappropriate linkage with health care system; substance abuse; mental illness; body image alteration; physical illness; cognitive deficits; health alterations (e.g., physical health, body image, self-esteem, mental health, psychosocial health, cognitive, learning style, neurological health); depression; low self-esteem; pain; fatigue

NOTE: There is typology of roles: sociopersonal (friendship, family, marital, parenting, community), home management, inti-

● = Independent          ▲ = Collaborative

macy (sexuality, relationship building), leisure/exercise/recreation, self-management, socialization (developmental transitions), community contributor, and religious.

## Client Outcomes

### Client Will (Specify Time Frame):

- Identify realistic perception of role.
- State personal strengths.
- Acknowledge problems contributing to inability to carry out usual role.
- Accept physical limitations regarding role responsibility and consider ways to change lifestyle to accomplish goals associated with role performance.
- Demonstrate knowledge of appropriate behaviors associated with new or changed role.
- State knowledge of change in responsibility and new behaviors associated with new responsibility.
- Verbalize acceptance of new responsibility.

## Nursing Interventions

### Social

- Observe the client's knowledge of behaviors associated with role.
- Ask the client direct questions regarding new roles and how the health care system can help him or her continue in roles.
- Allow the client to express feelings regarding the role change.
- Reinforce the client's strengths, have the client identify past coping skills, and support the continued use of these skills.
- Have the client make a list of strengths that are needed for the new role. Acknowledge which strengths the client has and which strengths need to be developed. Work with the client to set goals for desired role.
- Have the client list problems associated with the new role and identify ways of overcoming them (e.g., if pain

• = Independent          ▲ = Collaborative

is worse late in day, have the client complete necessary role tasks early in day).
- Support the client's religious practices.

## Physiological
- ▲ Identify ways to compensate for physical disabilities (e.g., have a ramp built to provide access to house, put household objects within the client's reach from wheelchair) and provide technological assistance when available.
- See care plans for **Readiness for enhanced family Coping, Impaired Home maintenance, Impaired Parenting, Risk for Loneliness, Readiness for enhanced community Coping**, and **Ineffective Sexuality patterns.**

## Pediatric
- Assist new parents to adjust to changes in workload associated with childbirth.
- Assist parents in coping with infants with colic, a condition common in infants.
- ▲ Refer to home health agency for home visits when there is an infant who has excessive crying.
- Provide parents with coping skills when the role change is associated with a critically ill child.
- Assist families with life beyond the hospital when living with the illness of a child. Teach family members to value the small things children do, connect with other families, locate community resources, and understand the short- and long-term needs of the child.
- ▲ Consider the use of media-based behavioral treatments for children with behavioral disorders.

## Geriatric
- ▲ Provide support for grandparents raising grandchildren.
- ▲ Support the client's religious beliefs and activities and provide appropriate spiritual support persons.
- Encourage the use of humor by family caregivers to describe their role reversal.
- Explore community needs after assessing the client's

R

• = Independent          ▲ = Collaborative

strengths. Suggest functional activities (e.g., being a foster grandparent or a mentor for small businesses).
▲ Refer to appropriate support groups for adjustment to role changes.
▲ Refer to therapy to improve memory for patients with Alzheimer's disease.

## Multicultural

• Assess for the influence of cultural beliefs, norms, values, and expectations on the individual's role.
• Assess for conflicts between the caregiver's cultural role obligations and competing factors like employment.
• Negotiate with the client regarding the aspects of their role that can be modified and still honor cultural beliefs.
• Encourage family to use support groups or other service programs to assist with role changes.
• Validate the individual's feelings regarding the impact of role changes on family and personal lifestyle.

## Home Care

• Above interventions may be adapted for home care use.
• Determine the anticipated duration of role change.
• Assess family's ability to physically or psychologically assume responsibilities of decrease or change in the client's role function.
▲ Offer a referral to medical social services to assist with assessing the short- and long-term impacts of role change.

## Client/Family Teaching

• Provide educational materials to family members on patient behavior management plus caregiver stress-coping management.
• Help the client identify resources for assistance in caring for a disabled or aging parent (e.g., adult day care).
▲ Refer to appropriate community agencies to learn skills for functioning in the new or changed role (e.g., vocational rehabilitation, parenting classes, hospice, respite care).

• = Independent          ▲ = Collaborative

# Bathing/hygiene Self-care deficit

## NANDA Definition

Impaired ability to perform or complete bathing/hygiene activities for self

## Defining Characteristics

Inability to: wash body or body parts; obtain or get to water source; regulate temperature or flow of bath water; get bath supplies; dry body; get in and out of bathroom
Impaired physical mobility-functional level classification:

0—Completely independent
1—Requires use of equipment or device
2—Requires help from another person for assistance, supervision, or teaching
3—Requires help from another person and equipment or device
4—Dependent (does not participate in activity)

## Related Factors (r/t)

Decreased or lack of motivation; weakness or tiredness; severe anxiety; inability to perceive body part or spatial relationship; perceptual or cognitive impairment; pain; neuromuscular impairment; musculoskeletal impairment; environmental barriers

## Client Outcomes

### Client Will (Specify Time Frame):

S

- Remain free of body odor and maintain intact skin.
- Bathe with assistance of caregiver as needed and report sense of dignity is maintained.
- Bathe with assistance of caregiver as needed without exhibiting aggressive behaviors.
- State satisfaction with ability to use adaptive devices to bathe.
- Use methods to bathe safely with minimal difficulty.

• = Independent          ▲ = Collaborative

## Nursing Interventions

- If in a typical bathing setting for the client, assess the client's ability to bathe self via direct observation using physical performance tests for ADLs.
- Ask the client for input on bathing habits and cultural bathing preferences.
- Develop a bathing care plan based on the client's own history of bathing practices that addresses skin needs, self-care needs, client response to bathing, and equipment needs.
- Individualize bathing by identifying function of bath (e.g., odor or urine removal), frequency required to achieve function, and best bathing form (e.g., towel bathing, tub, or shower) to meet client preferences, preserve client dignity, make bathing a soothing experience, and reduce client aggression.
- ▲ Request referrals for occupational and physical therapy.
- Plan activities to prevent fatigue during bathing; seat the client with feet supported.
- ▲ Provide pain relief measures: ice packs, heat, and analgesics 45 minutes before bathing if needed.
- Consider environmental and human factors that may limit bathing ability, such as bending to get into tub, reaching required for bathing items, grasping force needed for faucets, and lifting of self. Adapt environment by placing items within easy reach, lowering faucets, and using a handheld shower.
- Teach use of adaptive bathing equipment (e.g., long-handled brushes, soap-on-a-rope, washcloth mitt, wall bars, tub bench, shower chair, commode chair without pan in shower) and follow up in the home.
- Ensure bathing assistance preserves client dignity through conveyance of honor, and recognition of the deservedness of respect and esteem of all persons regardless of their dependency or infirmity.
- Provide privacy: have only one caregiver providing bathing assistance, encourage a traffic-free bathing area, and post privacy signs.
- Keep the client warmly covered.

• = Independent        ▲ = Collaborative

- Enhance communication during bathing. Allow the client to participate as able in bathing. Smile and provide praise for accomplishments in a relaxed manner.
- Inspect skin condition during bathing.
- Use or encourage caregiver to use an unhurried, caring touch.
- If the client is bathing alone, place assistance call light within reach.
- Bathe cognitively impaired clients before bedtime.
- Nurture personal attributes such as humor, positive attitude, faith, and hope. Control stress for clients with multiple sclerosis.

## Geriatric

- Assess client's ability to perform ADLs independently with the Katz Index of Independence in Activities of Daily Living.
- Assess self-efficacy (The Self-Efficacy for Functional Activities scale); assess outcome expectations (Outcome Expectations for Functional Activities scale). Based on assessment promote motivation and self-efficacy for ADL functioning by: role modeling via videotape or partnering; verbal encouragement; individualizing care using humor, kindness, joy, and excitement with achievements; social supports; and decreasing unpleasant sensations with the ADL function.
- Assess for grieving resulting from loss of function.
- Develop client muscle strength building plan through exercise to build the client's physiological capacity and prevent decline in ADLs.
- Include exercise and walking program in plan of care.
- Provide same type of bathrobe and bathing articles, such as scented dusting powder and bath oil, that the client used previously.
- Emphasize how client experiences the bathing setting with secondary focus on ways environment can support caregiver.
- Design bathing environment for comfort: *Visual.* Reduce clutter and use partitions to hide equipment storage.

S

• = Independent          ▲ = Collaborative

Consider what bather looks at as he or she enters room, and bathes. Reduce institutional signs and blend into background. Laminate and put artwork or decorative objects in bather's view, or cue cards to bathing process (wall, ceiling, shower). Stand or sit in bather's position to experience what they see. Decrease glare from tiles, white walls, and artificial lights. Use contrasting colors and soft but adequate lighting on a dimming switch for adjustment.

- Arrange bathing environment to promote sensory comfort: *Auditory.* Reduce noise of voices and water. Do not allow traffic into bathing room. Add fabric to absorb sound (3–4 times the width of the opening for sound absorbing folds). Play soft music.
- Design bathing environment for comfort: *Tactile.* Use heat lamps or radiant heat panels to keep room warm. Use warmed towels. Use powder-coated grab bars in decorative colors with nonslip grip. Provide soft rug to stand on. Ensure flooring not slippery (a high coefficient of friction, ideally above 80 desired and obtained through flooring coatings).
- Teach caregivers to use behaviors that validate client's feelings, reassure, segment tasks, and explain the care process while bathing Alzheimer's clients.
- Advise caregivers to initiate shower spray or touch during bathing carefully with verbal prompts beforehand.
- Train caregivers bathing those with Alzheimer's disease, to avoid behaviors that can trigger assault: confrontational communication, invalidation of resident's feelings, failure to prepare a resident for a task, speaking disrespectfully to the client, and a hurried pace of the bath.
- When bathing a cognitively impaired client, have all bathing items ready for the client's needs before bathing begins.
- Teach caregiver to use massage for frail elderly clients during bathing. Massage is desired by clients to reduce pain or agitation.
- Bathe elderly clients before bedtime to improve sleep.

S

• = Independent        ▲ = Collaborative

- Limit bathing to once or twice a week; provide a partial bath at other times.
- Allow the client or caregiver adequate time to complete the bathing activity.
- Use a nondetergent, no-rinse cleanser for bed-bathing rather than soap and water.
- Avoid soap or use only mild soap on genital and axillary areas; rinse well.
- Use tepid water.
- Test water temperature before use with thermometer.
- Recommend use of water temperature-sensing shower valve to prevent scalding.
- Use a gentle touch when bathing; avoid vigorous scrubbing motions.
- Add hydrating bath oils to tub bath water 15 minutes after the client immerses in water.

## Home Care

- ▲ Based on functional assessment and rehabilitation capacity, refer for home health aide services to assist with bathing and hygiene.
- Turn down temperature of hot water heater.
- Show caregiver videotape of caregiver self-care activities (organizing day, talking when frustrated, self-time, and nonjudgmental person with whom to talk) followed by a discussion.
- Cue cognitively impaired clients in steps of hygiene.
- Respect the preference of terminally ill clients to refuse or limit hygiene care.
- If a terminally ill client requests hygiene care, make an extra effort to meet request and provide care when client and family will most benefit (e.g., before visitors, at bedtime, in the early morning).
- Maintain temperature of home at a comfortable level when providing hygiene care to terminally ill clients.

## Client/Family Teaching

- Teach the client and family how to use adaptive devices for bathing, and teach bathing techniques that promote

• = Independent                    ▲ = Collaborative

safety and prevent burns (e.g., getting into tub before filling it with water if temperature sensor valve used, testing water with thermometer, emptying water before getting out, using an antislip mat, wall-grab bars, tub bench).

- Teach the client and family an individualized bathing routine that includes a schedule, privacy, skin inspection, soap or lubricant, and chill prevention.

# Dressing/grooming Self-care deficit

## NANDA Definition

Impaired ability to perform or complete dressing and grooming activities for self

## Defining Characteristics

Impaired ability to put on or take off necessary items of clothing; impaired ability to fasten clothing; impaired ability to obtain or replace articles of clothing; inability to clothe upper body; inability to clothe lower body; inability to choose clothing; inability to use assistive devices; inability to use zippers; inability to remove clothes; inability to put on socks; inability to maintain appearance at a satisfactory level; inability to pick up clothing; inability to put on shoes

## Related Factors (r/t)

Decreased or lack of motivation; pain; severe anxiety; perceptual or cognitive impairment; weakness or tiredness; neuromuscular impairment; musculoskeletal impairment; discomfort; environmental barriers
NOTE: See suggested Functional Level Classification in the care plan for **Impaired physical Mobility.**

## Client Outcomes

**Client Will (Specify Time Frame):**

- Dress and groom self to optimal potential.

    • = Independent          ▲ = Collaborative

- Use adaptive devices to dress and groom.
- Explain and use methods to enhance strengths during dressing and grooming.
- Dress and groom with assistance of caregiver as needed.

## Nursing Interventions

- Observe the client's ability to dress and groom self through direct observation and from the client/caregiver report, noting specific deficits and their causes.
- Consider and remove environmental barriers and human factors that may limit dressing/grooming ability, such as reaching for clothes or grooming aids in closets or drawers. Help the client arrange clothing and grooming devices within easy reach. Installing turntables and closet rods or drawers between eye and hip level is helpful.
- Ask the client for input on clothing choices and how to increase the ease of dressing.
- ▲ Request referrals for occupational and physical therapy.
- ▲ Provide medication for pain 45 minutes before dressing and grooming if needed.
- Plan activities to prevent fatigue while dressing and grooming.
- Provide privacy and limit people/caregivers in room.
- Select larger-sized clothing, clothing with elastic waistbands, wide sleeves and pant legs, dresses that open down the back for wheelchair-bound women; and Velcro fasteners or larger buttons.
- Use adaptive dressing and grooming equipment as needed (e.g., long-handled brushes, grasping devices, Velcro closures, zipper pulls, button hooks, elastic shoelaces, large buttons, soap-on-a-rope, suction holders).
- Lay clothing out in the order that it will be put on by the client. Dress bottom half, then top half of body.
- Encourage the client to dress appropriately for time of day. Perform dressing and grooming activities in a consistent sequence each day.
- Teach CNAs to use graduated verbal prompting for clients with dementia to complete dressing task and provide

S

● = Independent        ▲ = Collaborative

positive reinforcement immediately for accomplished steps of task.
• Encourage participation; guide the client's hand through task if necessary.
• If the client does not groom self, sit side-by-side with the client, put your hand over the client's hand, support the client's elbow with your other hand, and help the client comb hair.
• Nurture personal attributes such as humor, positive attitude, faith, and hope and control of stress for clients with multiple sclerosis.
• Allow clients with a spinal cord injury to maximize control over activities and teach them how to direct their caregivers.
• Encourage family caregivers for clients with spinal cord injury.
▲ If client has had a CVA with hemi-paresis, consider use of constraint-induced movement therapy (CIMT), where the functional extremity is purposely constrained and the client is forced to use the involved extremity.

## Geriatric
• Assess for grieving resulting from loss of function.
▲ Provide medication for pain if needed and plan activities to prevent fatigue before dressing/grooming.
• Assess self-efficacy (The Self-Efficacy for Functional Activities scale); assess outcome expectations (Outcome Expectations for Functional Activities scale). Based on assessment, promote motivation and self-efficacy for ADL functioning by: role modeling via videotape or partnering; verbal encouragement; individualizing care using humor, kindness, joy, and excitement with achievements; social supports; and decreasing unpleasant sensations with the ADL function.
• Assess tasks the client can complete, noting areas of independence and difficulty to make adaptations
• Allow the client or caregiver adequate time to complete dressing (e.g., do not insist that the client is dressed at an early hour).

• = Independent          ▲ = Collaborative

- For clients with dementia, maintain a specific routine for dressing to prevent increase in dressing time required.
▲ Request referral for older women with cardiac disease to rehabilitation programs for strength training.
- Telehomecare can be an effective way to assess and monitor ADL performance for older adults.

## Home Care

- Involve the client in planning of informal care and provide access to health professionals and financial support for the care.
▲ Based on functional assessment and rehabilitation capacity, refer for home health aide services to assist with dressing and grooming.
- Have caregiver view videotape showing caregiver self-care activities (organizing day, talking when frustrated, self-time, and nonjudgmental person with whom to talk) followed by a discussion.
- Cue cognitively impaired clients in steps of dressing and grooming.
- Respect the preference of the terminally ill client to refuse dressing and limit grooming.
- If terminally ill clients request dressing and grooming, make an extra effort to meet the request and provide care when the client and family will most benefit (e.g., before visitors, in early morning).
- Maintain the temperature of the home at a comfortable level when dressing terminally ill client.

S

## Client/Family Teaching

- Teach the client to dress the affected side first, then the unaffected side.
- Teach the simplest step in a task until mastered, and then proceed to more complicated steps. Give praise.
- Teach the client how to use adaptive devices for dressing and grooming.
- Teach the client and family to select clothes appropriate for the season, temperature, and weather.

• = Independent        ▲ = Collaborative

# Feeding Self-care deficit

## NANDA Definition

Impaired ability to perform or complete feeding activities

### Defining Characteristics

Inability to swallow food; inability to prepare food for ingestion; inability to handle utensils; inability to chew food; inability to use assistive device; inability to get food onto utensils; inability to open containers; inability to ingest food safely; inability to manipulate food in mouth; inability to bring food from a receptacle to the mouth; inability to complete a meal; inability to ingest food in a socially acceptable manner; inability to pick up cup or glass; inability to ingest sufficient food

### Related Factors (r/t)

Weakness or tiredness; severe anxiety; neuromuscular impairment; pain; perceptual or cognitive impairment; discomfort; environmental barriers; decreased or lack of motivation; musculoskeletal impairment

NOTE: See suggested Functional Level Classification in the care plan for **Impaired physical Mobility.**

### Client Outcomes

**Client Will (Specify Time Frame):**

- Feed self safely.
- State satisfaction with ability to use adaptive devices for feeding.
- Utilize assistance with feeding when necessary (caregiver).

### Nursing Interventions

- Assess the client's ability to feed self and note specific deficits.
- Observe for cause of inability to feed self independently (see Related Factors).
- Ask the client for input on methods to facilitate eating and feeding (e.g., cultural foods, other food and fluid

• = Independent          ▲ = Collaborative

preferences), and provide four entrée choices, including ethnic choice.

▲ Consult speech-language pathologist for individualized feeding care plans.

▲ Request referral for occupational and physical therapy; request a dietician.

• Ensure that the client has dentures, hearing aids, and glasses in place.

• Use any necessary adaptive feeding equipment (e.g., rocker knives, plate guards, suction mats, built-up handles on utensils, scoop dishes, large-handled cups).

• Seat the client at table using name card and place mat with meal in visual range next to role model who can eat, if applicable.

• Prior to feeding the client with brain trauma or dementia: provide oral hygiene; for dry mouth give tart or sour foods/fluids before meals; give proteolytic enzymes before meals if thick oral secretions are a problem.

• Positioning the client with brain trauma or dementia for feeding: help client sit upright with hips and knees flexed, feet supported, trunk and head in midline position, and head slightly flexed with chin down; for immobilized client in bed, use high Fowler's position and support the head and neck with neck slightly flexed; with unilateral paralysis tilt head slightly to unaffected side and rotate the head towards the affected side.

• Prepare meal items before the client begins eating.

• Provide small portions of favorite foods, one entrée at a time, at proper serving temperature with unnecessary items, utensils removed.

• Provide consistency in caregiver and meal activities.

• To increase oral intake utilize feeding assistance intervention protocol: individual assistance, proper positioning, dining location preferences, and meal tray substitutions; use graduated prompting to enhance self-feeding ability as needed: (1) social stimulation and encouragement; (2) nonverbal cueing; (3) verbal cueing; (4) physical guidance; (5) full physical assistance.

• To increase oral intake utilize between-meal snacks

S

• = Independent          ▲ = Collaborative

3 times a day, alone or if intake is not increased 15% with the feeding assistance intervention protocol (above), delivered to the client on a movable cart with a variety of food/fluid choices.

- Caregiver should sit beside the client (on the client's unaffected side) at eye level.
- Caregiver can sit at a half circle table if interacting with a group of clients and should remain with clients until meal is completed.
- Allow the client to participate in feeding as able; provide verbal/visual cues with paced prompting; provide praise for all feeding attempts; increase tasks as able.
- Presentation of feeding: Provide 1/2 to 1 teaspoon of solid food or 10-15 mL of liquid at a time; wait until client has swallowed prior food/liquid.
- Provide the client with a pleasant, quiet meal environment with no distractions.
- Keep the environment free of toileting devices and odors, avoid painful procedures before meals, remove lids from tray, and provide clean utensils for separate courses.
- Do not mix different foods together when assisting the client with eating.
- Play slow-tempo, quiet music during meals.
- If client will not eat, provide 30 mL of nutritional supplement such as Ensure in a medication cup every hour while awake.
- Encourage the client to keep food on the unaffected side of mouth with a rocking motion to deposit the food, if applicable.
- Be prepared to intervene if choking occurs; have suction equipment readily available and know the Heimlich maneuver.
- ▲ For clients with conditions such as Parkinson's or myasthenia gravis ensure that their medications are given so that peak drug action occurs during meal times.
- ▲ Continue rehabilitation efforts with post stroke clients long term to achieve optimal functioning.
- ▲ If client has had a CVA with hemi-paresis, consider use of constraint-induced movement therapy (CIMT), where

• = Independent          ▲ = Collaborative

the functional extremity is purposely constrained and the client is forced to use the involved extremity.
- If the client does not feed self, sit side-by-side with the client, put your hand over the client's hand, support the client's elbow with your other hand, and help the client feed self.
- Provide oral hygiene after every meal eating and check for pocketing of food.

## Geriatric
- Provide nutrition care that honors the individual client and enhances, rather than detracts from, each client's quality of life.
- Develop client muscle strength building plan to build the client's physiological capacity.
- ▲ Implement Hospital Elder Life Program, a model of care to prevent functional and cognitive decline of older persons during hospitalization.
- ▲ Implement the Wellspring model, which advocates education and empowerment of CNAs to solve problems without direct administrative oversight.
- ▲ Ensure CNAs know the signs/symptoms of dysphagia such as choking, coughing, oral/chewing problems, throat clearing, wet voice, gurgly voice or pneumonia and if exhibited during feeding to report them promptly during feeding.
- ▲ Seek CNA input on feeding concerns to discussion possible actions and share techniques beneficial to specific clients.
- ▲ Ensure CNA feeding training includes the need to decrease command statements to clients being fed and instead offer encouraging statements.
- ▲ Suggest CNAs learn three to five personal details about client being fed during the feeding.
- ▲ Provide medication for pain before meals if needed and plan activities to prevent fatigue before meals.
- Assess and maintain documentation about poststroke client's eating and nutrition (include weight) upon admission to long-term care.

• = Independent            ▲ = Collaborative

- Serve meals "family-style" with food in serving bowls and an empty plate to be filled by patient.
- Obtain and value patient's view of agency's food selection and presentation. Present views to administration.
▲ Ensure adequate staffing at meal times.
- Choose soft foods rather than liquids, or use dietary thickeners.
- Assess for intolerance to food texture and, if found, reverse food texture pattern as tolerated, progressing finally to texture stage of thick liquids.
- Provide finger foods for clients with Alzheimer's disease and place in hands as needed to cue.
- Allow the client with dentures adequate time to chew.
- Provide emotionally neutral nonverbal cues to improve table-sitting behavior if patient rises from table early such as a firm hand on dominant shoulder indicating to re-sit.

## Home Care

▲ Based on functional assessment and rehabilitation capacity, refer for home health aide services to assist with feeding.
- Telehomecare can be an effective way to assess and monitor ADL performance for older adults.
- Cue cognitively impaired client when feeding.
- Respect the preference of terminally ill clients to refuse nutrition or assistance with eating. Refer to care plans for **Imbalanced Nutrition: less than body requirements** and **Impaired Swallowing.**
- If terminally ill client requests nutrition, take special care to provide foods and assistive devices that protect the client from aspiration, minimize energy requirements, and meet the client's taste preferences.

## Client/Family Teaching

- Teach the client how to use adaptive devices.
- Teach the client with hemianopsia to turn head so that the plate is in the line of vision.

• = Independent     ▲ = Collaborative

- Teach visually impaired client to locate foods according to numbers on a clock.

# Toileting Self-care deficit

## NANDA Definition

Impaired ability to perform or complete own toileting activities

## Defining Characteristics

Inability to get to toilet or commode; inability to sit on or rise from toilet or commode; inability to manipulate clothing for toileting; inability to carry out proper toilet hygiene; inability to flush toilet or commode

## Related Factors (r/t)

Environmental barriers; weakness or tiredness; decreased or lack of motivation; severe anxiety; impaired mobility status; impaired transfer ability; musculoskeletal impairment; neuromuscular impairment; pain; perceptual or cognitive impairment
NOTE: See suggested Functional Level Classification in the care plan for **Impaired physical Mobility.**

## Client Outcomes

**Client Will (Specify Time Frame):**

- Remain free of incontinence and impaction with no urine or stool on skin.
- State satisfaction with ability to use adaptive devices for toileting.
- Explain and use methods to be safe and independent in toileting.

## Nursing Interventions

- Observe cause of inability to toilet independently (see Related Factors).

● = Independent         ▲ = Collaborative

- Assess ability to toilet; note specific deficits.
- Ask the client for input on toileting methods and timing and how to better provide toileting activity assistance.
- Assess the client's usual bowel and bladder toileting patterns and the terminology used for toileting.
▲ Request referral for occupational and physical therapy for help in working with the client to transfer from bed to commode.
- Use any necessary assistive toileting equipment (e.g., raised toilet seat, suction mats, spill-proof urinals, support rails next to toilet, toilet safety frames, Sanifems [allows a woman to void standing], fracture bedpans, long-handled toilet paper holders).
- Provide privacy.
- Assess barriers to implementation of a toileting program.
- Assess client's voiding patterns and if consistent place on an individualized toileting schedule which is documented and allows the client to use the toilet/commode.
- Develop toileting schedule using clocks, written schedules, or verbal prompting as cues for the client and provide assistance at scheduled times.
- Schedule toileting to occur when defecation urge is strongest or voiding is likely (e.g., in the morning, every 2 hours, after meals, at bedtime). Assist the client until self-care ability increases.
- Allow the client to participate as able in toileting, and provide praise for accomplishments. Increase tasks as the client is able, and work with the client to aim toward independence in toileting.
- Obtain a bedside commode if necessary and adapt it for the client's needs; avoid bedpans if possible. If the client is acutely ill, provide bedpan at appropriate intervals.
- Make assistance call button readily available to the client and answer call light promptly.
- Assess and remove physical barriers to toilet, such as cluttered walkways.
▲ For clients with spinal cord injury select self-propelled commode-shower chair designed to enhance safety, ease

• = Independent          ▲ = Collaborative

of use and caregiver access marketed by Everest &
Jennings.
- Keep toilet paper and hand-washing items within easy
  reach of the client. Provide prompt skin care and
  linen changes after incontinence episodes.

## Geriatric

- Remove barriers to toileting, support client's cultural beliefs and preserve dignity.
- Develop client muscle strength building plan to build the
  client's physiological capacity.
- Include regular exercise and walking program in plan of
  care.
- Assist client (especially frail older clients) to exercise
  (walk 2 minutes, push wheelchair, sit-stand repetitions)
  for several minutes every time up to toilet.
- Provide equipment routinely that allows elevation of
  seat/head of bed to enhance bed/chair rising ability.
- Upper extremity use for disabled clients is an important
  consideration in equipment choice to facilitate use of
  hands in chair/bed rising abilities.
- ▲ Implement Hospital Elder Life Program, a model of care
  to prevent functional and cognitive decline of older persons during hospitalization.
- Assess self-efficacy (The Self-Efficacy for Functional
  Activities scale); assess outcome expectations (Outcome
  Expectations for Functional Activities scale). Based on
  assessment, promote motivation and self-efficacy for
  ADL functioning by: role modeling via videotape or
  partnering; verbal encouragement; individualizing care
  using humor, kindness, joy, and excitement with achievements; social supports; and decreasing unpleasant sensations with the ADL function.
- Assess self-efficacy of nursing assistants who provide restorative care activities (Self-Efficacy for Restorative
  Care Nursing Activities) and assess their outcome expectations (Outcome Expectancy for Restorative Care
  Activities).

• = Independent          ▲ = Collaborative

▲ Following hip fracture, focusing on hospital-based multi-disciplinary interventions and discharge planning.

• Monitor clients with dementia for behavioral toileting cues (e.g., pacing, restlessness, fidgeting) and assist with prompt toileting, or use an individualized scheduled toileting for memory-impaired elderly.

• Assess the client's mobility status and speed of movement.

• Reassure the client that call light will be answered promptly.

• Provide a small footstool in front of toilet or commode.

• Assess the client's functional ability to manipulate clothing for toileting. If necessary, modify clothing with Velcro fasteners and elastic waists.

▲ Avoid use of indwelling or condom catheters if possible.

## Home Care

• Have caregiver view videotape showing caregiver self-care activities (organizing day, talking when frustrated, self-time, and nonjudgmental person with whom to talk) followed by a discussion.

▲ Based on functional assessment and rehabilitation capacity, refer for home health aide services to assist with toileting.

• Cue cognitively impaired clients in steps of toileting.

▲ Avoid the use of medications that place undue toileting stress on the client who is terminally ill.

▲ Provide pain medication for terminally ill clients 20 to 45 minutes before toileting in anticipation of possible pain (e.g., in coordination with a bowel stimulation program). See care plan for **Constipation.**

▲ Consider use of an indwelling catheter for terminally ill clients in too much pain to move when hygiene and skin integrity are difficult to maintain.

## Client/Family Teaching

• Teach the client and family how to toilet the client with adaptive and safety devices.

• Have family install toilet seat of a contrasting color.

• = Independent          ▲ = Collaborative

- Prepare the client for toileting needs by teaching the action of medications such as diuretics.
- Help the visually impaired client to develop a plan for locating bathrooms in new environments.

# Readiness for enhanced Self-concept

## NANDA Definition

A pattern of perceptions or ideas about the self that is sufficient for well-being and can be strengthened

## Defining Characteristics

Expresses willingness to enhance self-concept; expresses satisfaction with thoughts about self, sense of worthiness, role performance, body image, and personal identity; actions are congruent with expressed feelings and thoughts; expresses confidence in abilities; accepts strengths and limitations

## Related Factors (r/t)

To be developed

## Client Outcomes

### Client Will (Specify Time Frame):

- State willingness to enhance self-concept.
- State satisfaction with thoughts about self, sense of worthiness, role performance, body image, and personal identity.
- Demonstrate actions that are congruent with expressed feelings and thoughts.
- State confidence in abilities.
- Accept strengths and limitations.

## Nursing Interventions

- Assess and support activities that promote self-concept developmentally.
- ▲ Support the client's choice of alternative therapies and

• = Independent        ▲ = Collaborative

provide information on appropriate therapies (e.g., using a certified massage therapist when massage is the treatment of choice).
▲ Clients with cancer often use massage therapy as an adjunct treatment.
▲ Support establishing a church-based community health promotion programs (CBHPPs) with the following key elements: partnerships, positive health values, availability of services, access to church facilities, community-focused interventions, health behavior change, and supportive social relationships.
▲ For clients who have had breast surgery and need prosthesis provide the appropriate prosthesis before the client leaves the health care facility.

## Pediatric

▲ Consider the development of a Healthy Kids mentoring program that has four components: (1) relationship building, (2) self-esteem enhancement, (3) goal setting, and (4) academic assistance (tutoring). Mentors met with students twice each week for $1^1/_2$ hours each session on school grounds. During each meeting, mentors devoted time to each program component.
▲ Assess and provide referrals to mental health professionals for clients with unresolved worries associated with terrorism.
▲ Provide an alternative school based program for pregnant and parenting teenagers.

## Geriatric

▲ Encourage clients to consider a web-based support program when they are in a caregiving situation.

## Multicultural

• Carefully assess each client and allow families to participate in providing care that is acceptable based on the client's cultural beliefs: silent presence, quiet prayers (Hasidic Jewish families), and telling stories and singing songs in their native language.

• = Independent          ▲ = Collaborative

- Provide support for health promoting behaviors and self-concept for clients from diverse cultures.
- Refer to care plans for **Disturbed Body image, Chronic low Self-esteem,** and **Readiness for enhanced Spiritual well-being.**

## Home Care

- Above interventions may be used in the home care setting.

# Chronic low Self-esteem

## NANDA Definition

Long-standing negative self-evaluations/feelings about self or self-capabilities

## Defining Characteristics

Rationalizes away/rejects positive feedback and exaggerates negative feedback about self (long-standing or chronic); self-negating verbalization (long-standing or chronic); hesitant to try new things/situations (long-standing or chronic); expressions of shame/guilt (long-standing or chronic); evaluates self as unable to deal with events (long-standing or chronic); lack of eye contact; nonassertive/passive; frequent lack of success in work or other life events; excessively seeks reassurance; overly conforming, dependent on others' opinions; indecisive

## Related Factors (r/t)

Chronic illness (specify); persistent mental illness (specify); ongoing relationship problems (specify); ongoing social problems (specify)

## Client Outcomes

- Demonstrates improved ability to interact with others (e.g., maintains eye contact, engages in conversation, expresses thoughts/feelings).
- Verbalizes increased self-acceptance through use of positive self-statements about self.

● = Independent          ▲ = Collaborative

- Identifies personal strengths, accomplishments, and values.
- Identifies and works on small, achievable goals.
- Improves independent decision-making and problem solving skills.

## Nursing Interventions

- Actively listen to and respect the client.
- Assess the client's environmental and every day stressors, including physical health concerns and the potential of abusive relationships.
- Assess existing strengths and coping abilities, and provide opportunities for their expression and recognition.
- Reinforce the personal strengths and positive self-perceptions that client identifies. Maintaining optimism may decrease anger and negative life events.
- Identify and limit client's negative self-assessments.
- Encourage realistic and achievable goal setting and evaluation of resources and impediments to achievement.
- Demonstrate and promote effective communication techniques; spend time with the client.
- Encourage independent decision-making by reviewing options and their possible consequences with client.
- Assist client to challenge negative perceptions of self and performance.
- Use failure as an opportunity to provide valuable feedback.
- Promote a positive environment and activities that enhance self-esteem.
- Assist client with evaluating the impact of family and peer group on feelings of self-worth.
- Support socialization and communication skills.
- Encourage journal/diary writing as a safe way of expressing emotions.
- Help client to increase sense of belonging.

● = Independent          ▲ = Collaborative

### Geriatric

- Support client in identifying and adapting to functional changes.
- Use reminiscence therapy to identify patterns of strength and accomplishment.
- Encourage participation in peer group activities.
- Encourage activities in which client can support/help others.

### Multicultural

- Assess for the influence of cultural beliefs, norms, and values on the client's sense of self-esteem.
- Validate the client's feelings regarding ethnic or racial identity.

### Home Care

- Assess client's immediate support system/family for relationship patterns and content of communication.
- Encourage family to provide support and feedback regarding client value or worth.
- ▲ Refer to medical social services to assist the family in pattern changes that could benefit the client.
- ▲ If client is involved in counseling or self-help groups, monitor and encourage attendance. Help client identify value of group participation after each group encounter.
- ▲ If client is taking prescribed psychotropic medications, assess for knowledge of medication side effects and reasons for taking medication. Teach as necessary.
- ▲ Assess medications for effectiveness and side effects and monitor client for compliance.

S

### Client/Family Teaching

- ▲ Refer to community agencies for psychotherapeutic counseling.
- ▲ Refer to psychoeducational groups on stress reduction and coping skills.
- ▲ Refer to self-help support groups specific to needs.

• = Independent         ▲ = Collaborative

## Situational low Self-esteem

### NANDA Definition

Development of a negative perception of self-worth in response to a current situation (specify)

### Defining Characteristics

Verbally reports current situational challenge to self-worth; self-negating verbalizations; indecisive, nonassertive behavior; evaluation of self as unable to deal with situations or events; expressions of helplessness and uselessness

### Related Factors (r/t)

Developmental changes (specify); disturbed body image; functional impairment (specify); loss (specify); social role changes (specify); history of learned helplessness; history of abuse, neglect, or abandonment; unrealistic self-expectations; lack of recognition/rewards; behavior inconsistent with values; failures/rejections; decreased power/control; change in health status

### Client Outcomes

**Client Will (Specify Time Frame):**
- State effect of life events on feelings about self.
- State personal strengths.
- Acknowledge presence of guilt and not blame self if an action was related to another person's appraisal.
- Seek help when necessary.
- Demonstrate self-perceptions are accurate given physical capabilities.
- Demonstrate separation of self-perceptions from societal stigmas.

### Nursing Interventions

▲ Assess the client for signs and symptoms of depression and potential for suicide and/or violence. If present, immediately notify the appropriate personnel of symptoms. See care plans for **Risk for other-directed Violence** and/or **Risk for Suicide.**

• = Independent          ▲ = Collaborative

- Actively listen to, demonstrate respect for, and accept client.
- Assist in the identification of problems and situational factors that contribute to problems, offering options for resolution.
- Mutually identify strengths, resources, and previously effective coping strategies.
- Have client list strengths.
- Accept client's own pace in working through grief or crisis situations.
- Accept the client's own defenses in dealing with the crisis.
- Assess for unhealthy coping mechanisms such as substance abuse.
- ▲ Provide information about support groups of people who have common experiences or interests.
- Teach the client mindfulness techniques to cope more effectively with strong emotional responses.
- Support problem-solving strategies but discourage decision-making when in crisis.
- Assess client's environmental and everyday stressors, including evidence of abusive relationships.
- Encourage objective appraisal of self and life events and challenge negative or perfectionist expectations of self.
- Provide psychoeducation to client and family.
- Validate confusion when feeling ill but looking well.
- Acknowledge the presence of societal stigma. Teach management tools.
- Validate the impact of past experiences on self-esteem and work on corrective measures.
- See care plan for **Chronic low Self-esteem.**

## Geriatric
- Support the client in identifying and adapting to functional changes associated with aging.
- Use reminiscence therapy to identify patterns of strength and accomplishment.
- Encourage participation in peer group activities.

• = Independent          ▲ = Collaborative

- Encourage activities in which the client can support/help others.

## Multicultural
- Assess for the influence of cultural beliefs, norms, and values on the client's sense of self-esteem.
- Validate the client's feelings regarding ethnic or racial identity.

## Home Care
- Establish an emergency plan and contract with the client for its use. Having an emergency plan is reassuring to the client. Establishing a contract validates the worth of the client and provides a caring link between the client and society.
- Access supplies that support client's success at independent living.
- See care plan for **Chronic low Self-esteem.**

## Client/Family Teaching
- Assess person's support system (family, friends, community) and involve if desired.
- Educate client and family regarding the grief process.
- Teach client and family that the crisis is temporary.
- ▲ Refer to appropriate community resources or crisis intervention centers.
- ▲ Refer to resources for handicap and/or disability services.
- ▲ Refer to illness-specific consumer support groups.
- ▲ Refer to self-help support groups specific to needs.

S

# Risk for situational low Self-esteem

## NANDA Definition

At risk for developing negative perception of self-worth in response to a current situation (specify)

• = Independent          ▲ = Collaborative

## Risk Factors

Developmental changes (specify); disturbed body image; functional impairment (specify); loss (specify); social role changes (specify); history of learned helplessness; history of abuse, neglect, or abandonment; unrealistic self-expectations; behavior inconsistent with values; lack of recognition/rewards; failures/rejections; decreased power/control over environment; physical illness (specify)

## Client Outcomes

### Client Will (Specify Time Frame)

- State accurate self-appraisal.
- Demonstrate the ability to self-validate.
- Demonstrate the ability to make decisions independent of primary peer group.
- Express effects of media on self-appraisal.
- Express influence of substances on self-esteem.
- Identify strengths and healthy coping skills.
- State life events and change as influencing self-esteem.

## Nursing Interventions

- Help client to identify environmental and/or developmental factors that increase risk for low self-esteem. Identification is early stage of problem solving process.
- Assess the client's previous experiences with health care and coping with illness to determine the level of education and support needed.
- Help client to identify current behaviors resulting from low self-esteem.
- Encourage creative problem solving through writing exercises.
- Encourage client to maintain highest level of functioning, including work schedule.
- Help the client to identify what has helped maintain positive self-esteem thus far.
- Help the client to identify the resources and social support network available to them at this time.

S

• = Independent        ▲ = Collaborative

- Assess for unhealthy coping mechanism such as substance abuse.
▲ Encourage the client to find a self-help or therapy group that focuses on self-esteem enhancement.
- Teach the client mindfulness techniques to cope with strong emotional responses and to prevent decreases in self-esteem.
- Encourage the client to create a sense of competence through short-term goal setting and goal achievement.
- Educate female clients about self-esteem differences between genders, and encourage exploration.
▲ Assess the client for symptoms of depression and anxiety. Refer to specialist as needed.
- Teach client a systematic problem-solving process. Crisis provides an opportunity for effective change in coping skills.
- See care plans for **Disturbed personal Identity** and **Situational low Self-esteem**.

### Geriatric
- Help the client to identify age-related and/or developmental factors that may be affecting self-esteem.
- Assist the client in life review and identifying positive accomplishments.
- Help client to establish a peer group and structured daily activities.

### Home Care
- Assess current environmental stresses and identify community resources.
- Encourage family members to acknowledge and validate the client's strengths.
- Assess the need for establishing an emergency plan.
- See care plans for **Situational low Self-esteem** and **Chronic low Self-esteem**.

### Client/Family Teaching
▲ Refer the client/family to community-based self-help and support groups.

• = Independent          ▲ = Collaborative

▲ Refer to educational classes on stress management, relaxation training, etc.
▲ Refer to community agencies that offer support and environmental resources.

# Self-mutilation

## NANDA Definition

Deliberate self-injurious behavior causing tissue damage with the intent of causing nonfatal injury to attain relief of tension

### Defining Characteristics

Cuts/scratches on body; picking at wounds; self-inflicted burns (e.g., eraser, cigarette); ingestion/inhalation of harmful substances/objects; biting; abrading; severing; insertion of object(s) into body orifice(s); hitting; constricting a body part

### Related Factors (r/t)

Psychotic state (command hallucinations); inability to express tension verbally; childhood sexual abuse; violence between parental figures; family divorce; family alcoholism; family history of self-destructive behaviors; adolescence; peers who self-mutilate; isolation from peers; perfectionism; substance abuse; eating disorders; sexual identity crisis; low or unstable self-esteem; low or unstable body image; labile behavior (mood swings); history of inability to plan solutions or see long-term consequences; use of manipulation to obtain nurturing relationship with others; chaotic/disturbed interpersonal relationships; emotionally disturbed, battered child; feels threatened with actual or potential loss of significant relationship (e.g., loss of parent/parental relationship); experiences dissociation or depersonalization; mounting tension that is intolerable; impulsivity; inadequate coping; irresistible urge to cut/damage self; needs quick reduction of stress; childhood illness or surgery; foster, group, or institutional care; incarceration; character disorder; borderline personality disorder; developmentally delayed or autistic individual; his-

S

• = Independent          ▲ = Collaborative

tory of self-injurious behavior; feelings of depression, rejection, self-hatred, separation anxiety, guilt, depersonalization; poor parent-adolescent communication; lack of family confidant

## Client Outcomes

### Client Will (Specify Time Frame):

- Have injuries treated.
- Refrain from further self-injury.
- State appropriate ways to cope with increased psychological or physiological tension.
- Express feelings.
- Seek help when having urges to self-mutilate.
- Maintain self-control without supervision.
- Use appropriate community agencies when caregivers are unable to attend to emotional needs.

## Nursing Interventions

NOTE: Prior to implementation of interventions in the face of self-mutilation, nurses should examine their own emotional responses to incidents of self-harm, to ensure that interventions will not be based on countertransference reactions.

- ▲ Provide medical treatment for injuries. Use careful aseptic technique when caring for wounds. Care for the wounds in a matter-of-fact manner.
- • Assess for risk of suicide.
- • Assess for signs of depression, anxiety, and impulsivity.
- • Assess for presence of hallucinations. Ask specific questions such as, "Do you hear voices that other people do not hear? Are they telling you to hurt yourself?"
- ▲ Assure the client that he or she will not be alone and will be safe during hallucinations. Provide referrals for medication.
- ▲ Assess for the presence of medical disorders, mental retardation, medication effects, or psychiatric disorders that may present with self-mutilation. Initiate referral for evaluation and treatment as appropriate.

• = Independent          ▲ = Collaborative

- Differentiate between self-mutilation due to other causes and Munchausen syndrome.
- Monitor the client's behavior using 15-minute checks at irregular times so that the client does not notice a pattern.
- Establish trust.
- Be extremely cautious about touching the client when he or she is experiencing an abreaction (reenactment of precipitating trauma). Sometimes physically holding a client is necessary to prevent self-injury.
- Assess the client's ability to enter into a no-suicide contract. Secure a written or verbal contract from the client to notify staff when experiencing the desire to self-mutilate.
- ▲ Use a collaborative approach for care.
- ▲ Refer for medication such as clozapine.
- ▲ Consider partial hospitalization with individual and group therapy.
- Refer to care plan for **Risk for Self-mutilation** for additional information.

## Home Care

- See care plan for **Risk for Self-mutilation.**

## Client/Family Teaching

- See care plan for **Risk for Self-mutilation.**

# Risk for Self-mutilation

S

## NANDA  Definition

At risk for deliberate self-injurious behavior causing tissue damage with the intent of causing nonfatal injury to attain relief of tension

## Risk Factors

Psychotic state (command hallucinations); inability to express tension verbally; childhood sexual abuse; violence between paren-

• = Independent          ▲ = Collaborative

tal figures; family divorce; family alcoholism; family history of self-destructive behaviors; adolescence; peers who self-mutilate; isolation from peers; perfectionism; substance abuse; eating disorders; sexual identity crisis; low or unstable self-esteem; low or unstable body image; history of inability to plan solutions or see long-term consequences; use of manipulation to obtain nurturing relationship with others; chaotic/disturbed interpersonal relationships; emotionally disturbed and/or battered child; feels threatened with actual or potential loss of significant relationship; loss of parent/parental relationships; experiences dissociation or depersonalization; experiences mounting tension that is intolerable; impulsivity; inadequate coping; experiences irresistible urge to cut/damage self; needs quick reduction of stress; childhood illness or surgery; foster, group, or institutional care; incarceration; character disorders; borderline personality disorders; loss of control of problem-solving situations; developmentally delayed or autistic individual; history of self-injurious behavior; feelings of depression, rejection, self-hatred, separation anxiety, guilt, and depersonalization

## Client Outcomes

### Client Will (Specify Time Frame):

- Refrain from self-injury.
- Identify triggers to self-mutilation.
- State appropriate ways to cope with increased psychological or physiological tension.
- Express feelings.
- Seek help when having urges to self-mutilate.
- Maintain self-control without supervision.
- Use appropriate community agencies when caregivers are unable to attend to emotional needs.

## Nursing Interventions

> NOTE: Prior to implementation of interventions in the face of self-mutilation, nurses should examine their own emotional responses to incidents of self-harm, to ensure that interventions will not be based on countertransference reactions.

• = Independent          ▲ = Collaborative

- Assessment data from the client and family members may have to be gathered at different times; allowing a family member or trusted friend with whom the client is comfortable to be present during the assessment may be helpful.
- Assess for risk factors of self-mutilation, including the categories of psychiatric disorders (particularly borderline personality disorder, psychosis, eating disorders, autism); psychological precursors (e.g., low tolerance for stress, impulsivity, perfectionism); psychosocial dysfunction (e.g., presence of sexual abuse, divorce, or alcoholism in the family; manipulative behavior to gain nurturing; chaotic interpersonal relationships), coping difficulties (e.g., inability to plan solutions or see long-term consequences of behavior), personal history (e.g., childhood illness or surgery, past self-injurious behavior), and peer influences (e.g., friends who mutilate, isolation from peers).
▲ Assess for the presence of medical disorders, mental retardation, medication effects, or psychiatric disorders that may present with self-mutilation. Initiate referral for evaluation and treatment as appropriate.
- Differentiate between self-mutilation due to other causes, such as Munchausen syndrome.
▲ Assess family dynamics and need for family therapy, community supports
- Assess for presence of hallucinations. Ask specific questions such as, "Do you hear voices that other people do not hear? Are they telling you to hurt yourself?"
▲ Assure the client that he or she will not be alone and will be safe during hallucinations. Provide referrals for medication. Hallucinations can be very frightening; therefore clients need reassurance that they will not be left alone. Significantly reduced rates of further self-harm were observed for depot flupentixol versus placebo in multiple repeaters.
- Be alert to other risk factors of self-mutilation in clients with psychosis, including acute intoxication, dramatic changes in body appearance, preoccupation with reli-

S

• = Independent          ▲ = Collaborative

gion and sexuality, and anticipated or perceived object loss.

- Monitor clients with obsessive-compulsive disorder for possible self-mutilation.
- Assess clients who have issues with gender identity or men who were molested as children for possible self-mutilation. Clients attending gender dysphoria clinics may be at risk for self-mutilation.
- Maintain ongoing surveillance of the client and environment. Monitor the client's behavior using 15-minute checks at irregular times so that the client does not notice a pattern.
- ▲ When the client is experiencing extreme anxiety, use one-to-one staffing. Offer activities that will serve as a distraction.
- Implement active listening and early intervention.
- ▲ Refer to mental health counseling.
- When working with self-mutilative clients with borderline personality disorder, develop an effective therapeutic relationship by avoiding labeling, seeking to understand the meaning of the self-mutilation, and advocating for adequate opportunities for care.
- When working with self-mutilative clients with a diagnosis of a Cluster B Personality Disorder (borderline, antisocial, narcissistic, or histrionic), carefully assess suicidal ideation.
- Maintain a consistent relational distance from the client with borderline personality disorder who self-mutilates: neither too close nor too distant, neither rewarding unacceptable behavior nor trying to control or avoid the client.
- Inform the client of unit expectations for appropriate behavior and consequences. Emphasize that the client must comply with the rules of the unit. Contract with the client for no self-harm. Give positive reinforcement for compliance and minimize attention paid to disruptive behavior while setting limits.
- Assess the client's ability to enter into a no-suicide contract. Secure a written or verbal contract from the cli-

• = Independent          ▲ = Collaborative

ent to notify staff when experiencing the desire to self-
mutilate.

- Clients need to learn to recognize distress as it occurs
  and express it verbally rather than as a physical action
  against the self.
- Assist the client to identify the motives/reasons for self-
  mutilation that have been perceived as positive.
- Help the client identify cues that precede impulsive behavior. Early recognition of triggers permits the client to
  initiate self-calming procedures, such as relaxation
  techniques.
- Give praise when the client identifies urges and delays
  self-destructive behavior.
- Assist clients to identify ways to soothe themselves and
  generate hopefulness when faced with painful emotions.
- Be extremely cautious about touching the client when he
  or she is experiencing an abreaction (reenactment of
  precipitating trauma). Sometimes physically holding a
  client is necessary to prevent self-injury.
- Reinforce alternative ways of dealing with depression and
  anxiety such as exercise, engaging in unit activities, or
  talking about feelings.
- Keep environment safe; remove all harmful objects from
  the area. Use of unbreakable glass is recommended for
  the client at risk for self-injury.
- Encourage the client to seek out care providers to talk as
  urge to harm self occurs. Develop positive therapeutic
  relationship.
- Anticipate trigger situations and intervene to assist the
  client in applying alternatives to self-mutilation.
- Reduce or eliminate use of caffeine, alcohol, and street
  drugs.
- If self-mutilation does occur, use a calm, nonpunitive approach. Whenever possible, assist the client to assume
  responsibility for consequences (e.g., dress self-inflicted
  wound). Refer to care plan for **Self-mutilation.**
- ▲ If the client is unable to control behavior, provide interactive supervision, not isolation. Isolation and deprivation take away individuals' coping abilities and place

● = Independent          ▲ = Collaborative

them at risk for self-harm. Implementing seclusion for clients who have injured themselves in the past may actually facilitate self-injury. Clients are extraordinarily resourceful at identifying environmental objects with which to self-mutilate.

▲ Refer for medication such as clozapine.

• Involve the client in planning of care and problem-solving, and emphasize that the client makes choices.

▲ Involve the client in group therapy.

▲ Use group therapy to exchange information about methods of coping with loneliness, self-destructive impulses, and interpersonal relationships, as well as housing, employment, and health care system issues directly and noninterpretively.

▲ Refer to protective services if there is evidence of abuse.

▲ Discharge planning: Provide follow-up to ensure clients attend mental health appointments.

• Monitor the client for self-harm impulses that may progress to suicidal ideation.

## Pediatric

• Be aware of increasing incidence of self-mutilation, especially among teens and young adults.

• Conduct a thorough physical examination, alert for superficial scars that may be patterned, although there is not usually scabbing or infection.

• Maintaining a therapeutic relationship with teens requires explicit assurances of confidentiality, consistency of clinical routines, and a nonjudgmental communication style.

• Attend to behavioral clues of self-mutilation; a brief self-report assessment can be useful.

• Assess for the presence of an eating disorder or substance abuse. Attend to the themes that preoccupy teens with eating disorders who self-mutilate.

• Evaluate for suicidal ideation/suicide risk. Refer to care plan for **Risk for Suicide** for additional information.

• Be aware that there is not complete overlap between self-

• = Independent          ▲ = Collaborative

mutilation and suicidal behavior. The motivation may be different (coping with difficult feelings rather than ending life), and the method is usually different

- Use treatment approaches detailed above, with modifications as appropriate for this age group.

## Geriatric

- Provide hand or back rubs and calming music when elderly client experiences symptoms of anxiety.
- Provide soft objects for elderly clients to hold and manipulate when self-mutilation occurs as a function of delirium or dementia. Apply mitts, splints, helmets, or restraints as appropriate.
- Older adults who show self-destructive behaviors should be evaluated for dementia.

## Home Care

- Communicate degree of risk to family/caregivers; assess the family and caregiving situation for ability to protect the client, and to understand the client's self-mutilative behavior. Provide family and caregivers with guidelines on how to manage self-harm behaviors in the home environment.
- Establish an emergency plan, including when to use hotlines and 911. Develop a contract with the client and family for use of the emergency plan. Role-play access to the emergency resources with the client and caregivers.
- Assess the home environment for harmful objects. Have family remove or lock objects as able.
▲ If client behaviors intensify, institute emergency plan for mental health intervention. The degree of disturbance and the ability to manage care safely at home determines the level of services needed to protect the client.
▲ Refer for homemaker or psychiatric home health care services for respite, client reassurance, and implementation of therapeutic regimen.
▲ If the client is on psychotropic medications, assess client

• = Independent          ▲ = Collaborative

and family knowledge of medication administration and side effects. Teach as necessary.

▲ Evaluate the effectiveness and side effects of medications.

## Client/Family Teaching

• Explain all relevant symptoms, procedures, treatments, and expected outcomes for self-mutilation that is illness-based (e.g., borderline personality disorder, autism).

• Assist family members to understand the complex issues of self-mutilation. Provide instruction on relevant developmental issues, and on actions parents can take to avoid media that glorify self-harm behaviors.

• Provide written instructions for treatments and procedures for which the client will be responsible.

• Instruct the client in coping strategies (assertiveness training, impulse control training, deep breathing, progressive muscle relaxation).

• Role play (e.g., say, "Tell me how you will respond if someone ignores you.").

• Teach cognitive-behavioral activities, such as active problem solving, reframing (reappraising the situation from a different perspective), or thought-stopping (in response to a negative thought, picture a large stop sign and replace the image with a prearranged positive alternative). Teach the client to confront his or her own negative thought patterns (or cognitive distortions), such as catastrophizing (expecting the very worst), dichotomous thinking (perceiving events in only one of two opposite categories), or magnification (placing distorted emphasis on a single event).

▲ Provide the client and family with phone numbers of appropriate community agencies for therapy and counseling.

▲ Give the client positive things on which to focus by referring to appropriate agencies for job-training skills or education.

• = Independent      ▲ = Collaborative

## Disturbed Sensory perception (specify: visual, auditory, kinesthetic, gustatory, tactile, olfactory)

### NANDA Definition

Change in the amount or patterning of incoming stimuli accompanied by a diminished, exaggerated, distorted, or impaired response to such stimuli

### Defining Characteristics

Poor concentration; auditory distortions; change in usual response to stimuli; restlessness; reported or measured change in sensory acuity; irritability; disoriented in time, in place, or with people; change in problem-solving abilities; change in behavior pattern; altered communication patterns; hallucinations; visual distortions

### Related Factors (r/t)

Altered sensory perception; excessive environmental stimuli; psychological stress; altered sensory reception, transmission, and/or integration/insufficient environmental stimuli; biochemical imbalances for sensory distortion (e.g., illusions, hallucinations); electrolyte imbalance; biochemical imbalance

### Client Outcomes

**Client Will (Specify Time Frame):**

- Demonstrate understanding by a verbal, written, or signed response.
- Demonstrate relaxed body movements and facial expressions.
- Explain plan to modify lifestyle to accommodate visual or hearing impairment.
- Remain free of physical harm resulting from decreased balance or a loss of vision, hearing, or tactile sensation.
- Maintain contact with appropriate community resources.

• = Independent        ▲ = Collaborative

## Nursing Interventions

### Visual—Loss of Vision

- Identify name and purpose when entering the client's room.
- Orient to time, place, person, and surroundings. Provide a radio or talking books.
- Keep doors completely open or closed. Keep furniture out of path to bathroom, and do not rearrange furniture.
- Feed the client at mealtimes if blindness is temporary.
- Keep side rails up using half rails, maintain bed in a low position, keep call light readily available, and designate client a Fall Risk.
- Converse with and touch the client frequently during care if frequent touch is within the client's cultural norm.
- Walk the client by having the client grasp nurse's elbow and walk partly behind nurse.
- Walk a frightened or confused client by having the client put both hands on nurse's shoulders; nurse backs up in desired direction while holding the client around the waist.
- Keep call light button within client's reach, and check location of call light button before leaving the room.
- ▲ For blind client, consider referring to a clinic for use of a blind mobility aid device that utilizes ultrasound.
- Ensure access to eyeglasses or magnifying devices as needed.
- Pay attention to the client's emotional needs. Encourage expression of feelings and expect grieving behavior.
- ▲ Refer to optometrist, ophthalmologist, or specialist in vision loss for vision care if needed.

### Auditory—Hearing Loss

- Keep background noise to a minimum. Turn off television and radio when communicating with the client. If noisy environment, take the client to a private room and shut the door.
- Stand or sit directly in front of the client when communicating. Make sure adequate light is on nurse's face, avoid chewing gum or covering mouth or face with

• = Independent          ▲ = Collaborative

hands while speaking, establish eye contact, and use non-verbal gestures.

- Speak distinctly in lower voice tones if possible. Do not over-enunciate or shout at the client.
- State the topic of conversation before begin the conversation, make it clear when you change conversation topics.
- Verify the client understands critical information by asking the client to repeat the information back.
- If necessary, provide a communication board or personnel who know sign language.
- ▲ Refer to appropriate resources such as a speech and hearing clinic; audiologist; or ear, nose, and throat physician. Refer children early for help.
- Encourage the client to wear hearing aid if available.
- ▲ Refer to hearing clinics.
- Observe emotional needs and encourage expression of feelings.
- For disturbed sensory perception: kinesthetic and tactile, see care plan for **Risk for Injury** or **Risk for Falls**. For disturbed sensory perception: olfactory and gustatory, see care plan for **Imbalanced Nutrition: less than body requirements.**

## Pediatric

- ▲ Test hearing of infants and begin treatment/therapy early as needed.
- For classroom learning, ensure that ambient noise is minimized and devices are used to decrease reverberation in the environment.
- ▲ Recommend the child utilize a frequency-modulated system along with a hearing aid in school.
- ▲ Refer the child to use of a language wizard player with Baldi, a computer-animated tutor for teaching vocabulary.

## Geriatric

- Keep environment quiet, soothing, and familiar. Use consistent caregivers.
- Avoid providing extremely hot or cold foods or using hot

• = Independent          ▲ = Collaborative

bath water if the client has decreased sensation in mouth, hands, or feet.

- If the client has a sensory deprivation, encourage family to provide sensory stimulation with music, voices, photographs, touch, and familiar smells.
- Increase the amount of light in the environment for elderly eyes; ensure it is nonglare lighting.
▲ Refer to low-vision clinics, or the Independent Living Program, which is designed for older individuals who are blind to help maintain independence.
- For a hearing impairment in the elderly, use the Hearing Handicap Inventory for the Elderly (HHIE-S) to determine how individuals perceive the emotional and social problems associated with a hearing loss.
- If the client has a hearing or vision loss, work with the client to ensure contact with others and to strengthen the social network.

## Home Care
- The listed interventions are applicable in the home care setting.

## Client/Family Teaching

### Low Vision
- Teach the client how to use a lighted magnification device to increase the ability to read text or see details.
- Teach the client to put a sheet of yellow acetate over text to make the text more visible. An alternative method is to highlight the text with a green or yellow highlighter.
- Put red or yellow identifiers on important items that need to be seen, such as a red strip at the edge of steps, red behind a light switch, or a red dot on a stove or washing machine to indicate how far to turn knob.
- Use a watch or clock that verbally tells time and a phone with large numbers and emergency numbers programmed in.
- Teach blind client how to feed self; associate food on plate with hours on a clock so that the client can identify location of food.

• = Independent            ▲ = Collaborative

- Use low-vision aids including magnifying devices for near vision and telescopes for seeing objects at a distance, a closed-circuit television that magnifies print, guides for writing checks and envelopes.
- Teach the client with vision loss:
  - Use a magnifying mirror to shave or apply makeup. Use electric razor only.
  - Put personal care products in brightly colored pump containers (red, yellow, or orange) for identification.
  - Use tactile clues such as safety pins or buttons placed in hems to help client match clothing.
  - Use prefilled medication organizer with large lettering or 3D markers.
- Increase lighting in the home to help vision in the following ways:
  - Ensure adequate illumination of entire home, adding light fixtures and increase wattage of existing bulbs as needed.
  - Decrease glare where light reflects on shiny surfaces, move or cover object.
  - Use nonglare wax on the floor.
  - Use motion lights that come on automatically when a person enters the room for nighttime use.
  - Add indoor strip or "runway" type of lighting to baseboards.

## Hearing Loss
- Suggest installation of devices such as ring signalers for the telephone and doorbell, sensors that detect an infant's cry, alarm clocks that vibrate the bed, and closed caption decoders for television sets. Other helpful devices include telephone amplifiers, speaker phones, pocket talker personal listening system, and FM and infrared amplification systems that connect directly to a TV or audio output jack. Also available is a telecommunication device—a typewriter keyboard with an alphanumeric display that allows the hearing impaired person to send typed messages over the telephone line, and software and modems are available that allow a home computer to be

S

• = Independent          ▲ = Collaborative

used in this fashion. Use of a hearing ear dog—a dog specially trained to alert its owner to specific sounds—may also be helpful.

- Teach client to avoid excessive noise at work or at home, wearing hearing protection when necessary. Any noise that hurts the ears or is above 90 decibels is excessive.
- Teach family how to provide appropriate stimuli in the home environment to prevent disturbed sensory perception.

# Sexual dysfunction

## NANDA Definition

Change in sexual function that is viewed as unsatisfying, unrewarding, or inadequate

## Defining Characteristics

Change of interest in self and others; conflicts involving values; inability to achieve desired satisfaction; verbalization of problem; alteration in relationship with significant other; alteration in achieving sexual satisfaction; actual or perceived limitation imposed by disease or therapy; seeking confirmation of desirability; alteration in achieving perceived sex role

## Related Factors (r/t)

Misinformation or lack of knowledge; vulnerability; values conflict; psychosocial abuse (e.g., harmful relationships); physical abuse; lack of privacy; ineffectual or absent role models; altered body structure of function (e.g., pregnancy, recent childbirth, drugs, surgery, anomalies, disease process, trauma, radiation); lack of significant other; biopsychosocial alterations of sexuality

## Client Outcomes

### Client Will (Specify Time Frame):

- Identify individual cause of sexual dysfunction.
- Identify stressors that contribute to dysfunction.

• = Independent          ▲ = Collaborative

- Discuss alternative, satisfying, and acceptable sexual practices for self and partner.
- Discuss with partner concerns about body image and sex role.

## Nursing Interventions

- Gather the client's sexual history, noting normal patterns of functioning and the client's vocabulary.
- Determine the client's and partner's current knowledge and understanding.
- ▲ Assess and provide treatment for erectile dysfunction. Involve the person's partner in the process. Consider pharmacologic and nonpharmacological interventions.
- Observe for stress, anxiety, and depression as possible causes of dysfunction.
- Observe for grief related to loss (e.g., amputation, mastectomy, ostomy).
- Explore physical causes such as diabetes, arteriosclerotic heart disease, arthritis, drug or medication side effects, or smoking (especially in males).
- Provide privacy and be verbally and nonverbally nonjudgmental.
- Provide privacy to allow sexual expression between the client and partner (e.g., private room, "Do Not Disturb" sign for a specified length of time).
- Explain the need for the client to share concerns with partner.
- Validate the client's feelings; let the client know that he or she is normal, and correct misinformation.
- ▲ Refer to appropriate medical providers for consideration of medication with premature ejaculation.
- ▲ Refer women for possible pharmacological intervention when sexual dysfunction is present.

## Geriatric

- ▲ Carefully assess the sexuality needs of the elderly client and refer for counseling if needed.
- Carefully assess sexual functioning needs of clients with dementia and provide privacy for them and their spouse.

S

• = Independent     ▲ = Collaborative

- Teach about normal changes that occur with aging: Female—reduction in vaginal lubrication, decrease in the degree and speed of vaginal expansion, reduction in duration and resolution of orgasm. Male—increase in time required for erection, increase in erection time without ejaculation, less firm erection, decrease in volume of seminal fluid, increase in time before another erection can occur (12 to 24 hours).
- Suggest the following to enhance sexual functioning: Female—use water-based vaginal lubricant, increase foreplay time, avoid direct stimulation of the clitoris if painful (clitoris may be exposed because of atrophy of the labia), practice Kegel exercises (alternately contracting and relaxing the muscles in the pelvic area), urinate immediately after coitus to prevent irritation of the urethra and bladder, and consult with a physician about use of systemic estrogen therapy or topical estrogen cream. Male—have female partner try a new coital position by bending her knees and placing a pillow under her hips to elevate pelvis (will more easily accommodate a partially erect penis); massage penis down using pressure at base, which puts pressure on major blood vessel and keeps blood in the penis; ask the female partner to push the penis into the vagina herself and flex her vaginal muscles that have been strengthened by Kegel exercises. If one of the partners has a protruding abdomen, experiment to find a position that allows the penis to reach the vagina (e.g., have woman lie on her back with legs apart and knees sharply bent while the man places himself over her with his hips under the angle formed by the raised knees).
- Explore with the client and partner various sexual gratification alternatives (e.g., caressing, sharing feelings).
- Discuss the difference between sexual function and sexuality.
- ▲ If prescribed, teach how to use nitroglycerin before sexual activity.
- See care plan for **Ineffective Sexuality pattern.**

S

• = Independent          ▲ = Collaborative

## Multicultural

- Assess for the influence of cultural beliefs, norms, and values on the client's perceptions of normal sexual functioning.
- Discuss with the client those aspects of sexual health/lifestyle that remain unchanged by his or her health status.
- Validate the client's feelings and emotions regarding the changes in sexual behavior.

## Home Care

- Above interventions may be adapted for home care use.
- Identify specific sources of concern over sexual activity. Provide reassurance and instruction on appropriate expectations as indicated.
- Help the client and significant other to identify a place and time in the home and daily living for privacy to share sexual or relationship activity. If necessary, help the client to communicate the need for privacy to other family members. Consider periodic escapes to desirable surroundings.
- ▲ Confirm that physical reasons for dysfunction have been addressed. Encourage participation in support groups or therapy if appropriate.
- Reinforce or teach the client about sexual functioning, alternative sexual practices, and necessary sexual precautions. Update teaching as the client status changes.

## Client/Family Teaching

- Provide accurate information for clients concerning sexual activity after a myocardial infarction consider use of a videotape.
- Teach the client to resume intimate physical contact by using mutual touching 3 to 6 weeks after a myocardial infarction.
- Teach the client to begin vigorous sexual activity after an MI when the client can walk rapidly for 10 minutes and then climb two flights of stairs in 10 seconds.

S

• = Independent          ▲ = Collaborative

▲ Provide written educational materials that address sexual issues for client and families of clients with implantable cardiac defibrillators.

▲ Refer to appropriate community resources, such as a clinical specialist, family counselor, or sexual counselor. If appropriate, include both partners in the discussion.

• Teach vaginal dilation to prevent stenosis. Inform the client to expect a bit of spotting after first session of intercourse.

• Teach how drug therapy affects sexual response (e.g., the possible side effects and the need to report them).

• Teach the importance of diabetic control and its effect on sexuality to clients with insulin-dependent diabetes.

▲ Refer for medical advice for erectile dysfunction that lasts longer than 2 months or is recurring.

• Teach the following interventions to decrease the likelihood of erectile dysfunction: limit or avoid the use of alcohol, stop smoking, exercise regularly, reduce stress, get enough sleep, deal with anxiety or depression, and see doctor for regular checkups and medical screening tests.

▲ Refer for medication to treat erectile dysfunction if necessary.

• Teach specifics if the client has a stoma: do not substitute the stoma for an anus.

• See geriatric interventions if there is a problem with erection associated with stoma surgery.

## S

# Ineffective Sexuality pattern

## NANDA Definition

Expressions of concern regarding own sexuality

## Defining Characteristics

Reported difficulties, limitations, or changes in sexual behaviors or activities

• = Independent          ▲ = Collaborative

## Related Factors (r/t)

Lack of significant other; conflicts with sexual orientation or variant preferences; fear of pregnancy or of acquiring a sexually transmitted disease; impaired relationship with significant other; ineffective or absent role models; knowledge/skill deficit about alternative responses to health-related transitions, altered body function or structure, illness, or medical treatment; lack of privacy

## Client Outcomes

### Client Will (Specify Time Frame):

- State knowledge of difficulties, limitations, or changes in sexual behaviors or activities.
- State knowledge of sexual anatomy and functioning.
- State acceptance of altered body structure or functioning.
- Describe acceptable alternative sexual practices.
- Identify importance of discussing sexual issues with significant other.
- Describe practice of safe sex with regard to pregnancy and avoidance of sexually transmitted diseases.

## Nursing Interventions

- After establishing rapport or therapeutic relationship, give the client permission to discuss issues dealing with sexuality. Ask the client specifically, "Have you been or are you concerned about functioning sexually because of your health status?"
- Determine the client's and partner's current knowledge and understanding.
- Encourage the client to discuss concerns with his or her partner.
- Discuss alternative sexual expressions for altered body functioning or structure. Closeness and touching are other forms of expression.
- Some clients choose masturbation for sexual release.
- If mutual masturbation is a choice of expression, provide latex gloves or nonlatex for latex-sensitive individuals.

S

• = Independent          ▲ = Collaborative

- The following are guidelines for sexual activity for clients who have had hip replacement:
  - Don't bend the affected leg more than 90 degrees at the hip.
  - When lying on your back, don't turn or roll your affected leg toward the other leg.
  - Don't turn the toes of the affected leg inward.
  - When lying on your side, keep both legs separated with pillows between them. Don't let your knees touch and don't let the toes of your affected leg turn downward.
- The following are recommended sexual positions for clients who have had hip replacement:
  - Bottom position for the male or female patient
    - Place one or two pillows under your affected thigh for support and comfort and to reduce friction on your skin, which may still be healing. Keep the toes of your affected leg pointed upward and slightly outward—but never inward.
  - Top position for male patients only
    - Do not bend your affected hip more than 90 degrees while getting into position. Keep your affected leg out to the side with your toes pointed slightly outward. (Female patients: Don't assume this position because it will require that you bend more than 90 degrees at the hip.)
  - Side-lying position for the male patient
    - Lie on your unaffected side. Both you and your partner should face the same direction. You should be behind your partner in a "spooning" position. Your partner should place at least two pillows between her legs and your affected leg should rest on top of hers during intercourse. Don't bend your affected leg more than 90 degrees, and don't let the toes of your affected leg dangle or turn downward.
  - Side-lying position for the female patient
    - Lie on your unaffected side and place enough pillows between your legs to support the affected leg.

• = Independent          ▲ = Collaborative

Make sure the affected leg doesn't drop off the pillows during intercourse. Your partner should assume the spooning position behind you. Don't bend your affected hip more than 90 degrees, and don't let the toes of your affected leg turn downward.

Caution: If you dislocate your hip during sexual intercourse, you will experience pain, your affected leg will appear shorter, and your foot will turn inward. Lie down, don't move, and tell your partner to call an ambulance.

- Provide client privacy for sexual expression (e.g., closed door when significant other visits, "Do Not Disturb" sign on door).

## Pediatric

- Provide age-appropriate information for adolescents regarding HIV/AIDS and sexual behavior.
- Provide support for the client's chosen ways to cope with HIV or AIDS.

## Geriatric

- ▲ Carefully assess the sexuality needs of the elderly client and refer for counseling if needed.
- Explore possible changes in sexuality related to menopause.
- Allow the client to verbalize feelings regarding loss of sexual partner or significant other. Acknowledge problems such as disapproval of children, lack of available partner for women, and environmental variables that make forming new relationships difficult.
- Provide a milieu that allows for discussion of sexual issues and a higher level of sexual satisfaction. Allow couples to room together and bring in double beds from home. Place signs on the door to ensure privacy.
- Provide clients with the following information:
  - Exercise, such as walking, swimming, cycling, and riding a stationary bike, will help control flabby thighs and weak musculature and make people feel more sexually attractive.

S

• = Independent          ▲ = Collaborative

- Overindulgence in food or alcohol can affect sexual activity (see care plan for **Imbalanced Nutrition: more than body requirements**).
- Resting and sleeping on a firm mattress may augment sexual desire.
- Femininity and masculinity are still important.
- Pay attention to cleanliness, skin care, and clothing.
- Change environment.
- Experiment with position changes.
- See care plan for **Sexual dysfunction.**

## Multicultural

- Assess for the influence of cultural beliefs, norms, and values on client's perceptions of normal sexual behavior.
- Discuss with the client those aspects of his or her sexual health/lifestyle that remain unchanged by their health status.
- Validate the client's feelings and emotions regarding the changes in sexuality patterns.

## Home Care

- Above interventions may be adapted for home care use.
- Help the client and significant other to identify a place and time in the home and daily living for privacy in sharing sexual or relationship activity. If necessary, help the client to communicate the need for privacy to other family members. Consider periodic escapes to desirable surroundings.
- ▲ Confirm that physical reasons for dysfunction have been addressed. Encourage participation in support groups or therapy if appropriate.
- Reinforce or teach about sexual functioning, alternative sexual practices, and necessary sexual precautions. Update teaching as client status changes.

## Client/Family Teaching

- ▲ Refer to appropriate community agencies (e.g., certified sex counselor, Reach to Recovery, Ostomy Association).
- Provide information regarding self-care and sexuality for the woman who has cancer and her partner.

● = Independent          ▲ = Collaborative

▲ Sexuality education is important to all populations, whether hearing or deaf, sighted or blind, disabled, or not disabled. Discuss contraceptive choices. Refer to appropriate health professional (e.g., gynecologist, nurse practitioner).

• Teach safe sex to all clients including the elderly, which includes using latex condoms (or nonlatex for latex-sensitive individuals), washing with soap immediately after sexual contact, not ingesting semen, avoiding oral-genital contact, not exchanging saliva, avoiding multiple partners, abstaining from sexual activity when ill, and avoiding recreational drugs and alcohol when engaging in sexual activity. Contrary to previously published information, the use of a spermicide containing nonoxynol-9 (N-9) should not be recommended as a preventative strategy for HIV infection.

# Impaired Skin integrity

## NANDA Definition

Altered epidermis and/or dermis

## Defining Characteristics

Invasion of body structures; destruction of skin layers (dermis); disruption of skin surface (epidermis)

## Related Factors (r/t)

### External

Hyperthermia; hypothermia; chemical substance (e.g., incontinence); mechanical factors (e.g., friction, shearing forces, pressure, restraint); physical immobilization; humidity; extremes in age; moisture; radiation; medications

### Internal

Altered metabolic state; altered nutritional state (e.g., obesity, emaciation); altered circulation; altered sensation; altered pig-

• = Independent          ▲ = Collaborative

mentation; skeletal prominence; developmental factors; immunological deficit; alterations in skin turgor (change in elasticity); altered fluid status

## Client Outcomes

### Client Will (Specify Time Frame):

- Regain integrity of skin surface.
- Report any altered sensation or pain at site of skin impairment.
- Demonstrate understanding of plan to heal skin and prevent reinjury.
- Describe measures to protect and heal the skin and to care for any skin lesion.

## Nursing Interventions

- Assess site of skin impairment and determine etiology (e.g., acute or chronic wound, burn, dermatological lesion, pressure ulcer, skin tear).
- Determine that skin impairment involves skin damage only (e.g., partial-thickness wound, stage I or stage II pressure ulcer). The following classification system is for pressure ulcers:
  - Stage I: Observable pressure-related alteration of intact skin with indicators as compared with the adjacent or opposite area on the body that may include changes in one or more of the following: skin temperature (warmth or coolness), tissue consistency (firm or boggy feel), and/or sensation (pain, itching). The ulcer appears as a defined area of persistent redness in lightly pigmented skin, whereas in darker skin tones, the ulcer may appear with persistent red, blue, or purple hues.
  - Stage II: Partial-thickness skin loss involving epidermis or dermis superficial ulcer that appears as an abrasion, blister, or shallow crater.

NOTE: For wounds deeper into subcutaneous tissue,

• = Independent          ▲ = Collaborative

muscle, or bone (stage III or stage IV pressure ulcers), see the care plan for **Impaired Tissue integrity.**

- Monitor site of skin impairment at least once a day for color changes, redness, swelling, warmth, pain, or other signs of infection. Determine whether the client is experiencing changes in sensation or pain. Pay special attention to high-risk areas such as bony prominences, skinfolds, the sacrum, and heels.
- Monitor the client's skin care practices, noting type of soap or other cleansing agents used, temperature of water, and frequency of skin cleansing.
- Individualize plan according to the client's skin condition, needs, and preferences.
- Monitor the client's continence status, and minimize exposure of skin impairment and other areas to moisture from incontinence, perspiration, or wound drainage.
▲ If the client is incontinent, implement an incontinence management plan to prevent exposure to chemicals in urine and stool that can strip or erode the skin. Refer to a continence care specialist, urologist, or gastroenterologist for incontinence assessment.
- For clients with limited mobility, use a risk-assessment tool to systematically assess immobility-related risk factors.
- Do not position the client on site of skin impairment. If consistent with overall client management goals, turn and position the client at least every 2 hours. Transfer the client with care to protect against the adverse effects of external mechanical forces such as pressure, friction, and shear.
- Evaluate for use of specialty mattresses, beds, or devices as appropriate. Maintain the head of the bed at the lowest possible degree of elevation to reduce shear and friction, and use lift devices, pillows, foam wedges, and pressure-reducing devices in the bed.
▲ Implement a written treatment plan for topical treatment of the site of skin impairment.

S

• = Independent         ▲ = Collaborative

▲ Select a topical treatment that will maintain a moist wound-healing environment and that is balanced with the need to absorb exudate.

• Avoid massaging around the site of skin impairment and over bony prominences.

▲ Assess the client's nutritional status. Refer for a nutritional consult, and/or institute dietary supplements as necessary.

• Identify the patient/client's phase of wound healing (inflammation, proliferation, maturation) and stage of injury.

## Home Care

• Some of the interventions described previously may be adapted for home care use.

• Instruct and assist the client and caregivers in understanding how to change dressings, and the importance of maintaining a clean environment. Provide written instructions and observe them completing the dressing change.

• Educate client and caregivers on proper nutrition, signs and symptoms of infection, and when to call the agency and or physician with concerns.

▲ It may be beneficial to initiate a consultation in a case assignment with a wound, ostomy, or continence nurse, or wound specialist to establish a comprehensive plan for complex wounds.

## Client/Family Teaching

S

• Teach skin and wound assessment and ways to monitor for signs and symptoms of infection, complications, and healing. Early assessment and intervention help prevent serious problems from developing.

▲ Teach the client why a topical treatment has been selected.

▲ If consistent with overall client management goals, teach how to turn and reposition at least every 2 hours.

• Teach the client to use pillows, foam wedges, and pressure-reducing devices to prevent pressure injury.

• = Independent        ▲ = Collaborative

# Risk for impaired Skin integrity

## NANDA Definition

At risk for skin being adversely altered

## Risk Factors

### External

Hypothermia; hyperthermia; chemical substance; excretions and/or secretions; mechanical factors (e.g., shearing forces, pressure, restraint); radiation; physical immobilization; humidity; moisture; extremes of age

### Internal

Medication; altered nutritional state (e.g., obesity, emaciation); altered metabolic state; altered circulation; altered sensation; altered pigmentation; skeletal prominence; developmental factors; immunological deficit; alterations in skin turgor (change in elasticity); psychogenetic, immunological factors
NOTE: Risk should be determined by the use of a risk assessment tool (e.g., Norton scale, Braden scale).

## Related Factors (r/t)

See Risk Factors.

## Client Outcomes

### Client Will (Specify Time Frame):

- Report altered sensation or pain at risk areas.
- Demonstrate understanding of personal risk factors for impaired skin integrity.
- Verbalize a personal plan for preventing impaired skin integrity.

## Nursing Interventions

- Monitor skin condition at least once a day for color or texture changes, dermatological conditions, or lesions. Determine whether the client is experiencing loss

• = Independent ▲ = Collaborative

of sensation or pain. Systematic inspection can identify impending problems early.

- Identify clients at risk for impaired skin integrity as a result of immobility, chronologic age, malnutrition, incontinence, compromised perfusion, immunocompromised status, or chronic medical condition such as diabetes mellitus, spinal cord injury or renal failure.
- Monitor the client's skin care practices, noting type of soap or other cleansing agents used, temperature of water, and frequency of skin cleansing.
- Avoid harsh cleansing agents, hot water, extreme friction or force, or too-frequent cleansing.
- ▲ Monitor the client's continence status, and minimize exposure of the site of skin impairment and other areas to moisture from incontinence, perspiration, or wound drainage. If the client is incontinent, implement an incontinence management plan to prevent exposure to chemicals in urine and stool that can strip or erode the skin; refer to a physician (e.g., continence care specialist, urologist, gastroenterologist) for an incontinence assessment.
- For clients with limited mobility, monitor condition of skin covering bony prominences.
- Use a risk-assessment tool to systematically assess immobility-related risk factors.
- Implement a written prevention plan.
- If consistent with overall client management goals, turn and position the client at least every 2 hours. Transfer the client with care to protect against the adverse effects of external mechanical forces (e.g., pressure, friction, shear).
- ▲ Evaluate for use of specialty mattresses, beds, or devices as appropriate.
- Avoid massaging over bony prominences.
- ▲ Assess the client's nutritional status; refer for a nutritional consult, and/or institute dietary supplements.

## Geriatric

- Limit number of complete baths to two or three per

• = Independent        ▲ = Collaborative

week, and alternate them with partial baths. Use a tepid
water temperature (between 90° and 105° F) for bathing.
- Use lotions and moisturizers to prevent skin from drying
  out, especially in the winter.
- Increase fluid intake within cardiac and renal limits to a
  minimum of 1500 mL per day.
- Increase humidity in the environment, especially during
  the winter, by using a humidifier or placing a container of water on a warm object.

## Home Care
- Assess caregiver vigilance and ability. In a limited study
  of the Braden scale, caregiver vigilance and ability were
  recognized as potentially significant variables for determining the risk of developing pressure sores.
- Initiate a consultation in a case assignment with a wound
  care specialist or wound, ostomy, continence nurse
  (WOC nurse) to establish a comprehensive plan as soon
  as possible.
- See the care plan for **Impaired Skin integrity**.

## Client/Family Teaching
- Teach the client skin assessment and ways to monitor for
  impending skin breakdown. Early assessment and intervention help prevent the development of serious problems.
- If consistent with overall client management goals, teach
  how to turn and reposition the client at least every 2 hours.
- Teach the client to use pillows, foam wedges, and
  pressure-reducing devices to prevent pressure injury.

S

# Sleep deprivation

## NANDA Definition

Prolonged periods without sleep (sustained natural, periodic
suspension of relative unconsciousness)

• = Independent             ▲ = Collaborative

## Defining Characteristics

Daytime drowsiness; decreased ability to function; malaise; tiredness; lethargy; restlessness; irritability; heightened sensitivity to pain; listlessness; apathy; slowed reaction; inability to concentrate; perceptual disorders (e.g., disturbed body sensation, delusions, feeling afloat); hallucinations; acute confusion; transient paranoia; agitated or combative; anxious; mild, fleeting nystagmus; hand tremors

## Related Factors (r/t)

Prolonged physical discomfort; prolonged psychological discomfort; sustained inadequate sleep hygiene; prolonged use of pharmacological or dietary antisoporifics; aging-related sleep stage shifts; sustained circadian asynchrony; inadequate daytime activity; sustained environmental stimulation; sustained unfamiliar or uncomfortable sleep environment; non-sleep-inducing parenting practices; sleep apnea; periodic limb movement (e.g., restless leg syndrome, nocturnal myoclonus); sundowner's syndrome; narcolepsy; idiopathic central nervous system hypersomnolence; sleep walking; sleep terror; sleep-related enuresis; nightmares; familiar sleep paralysis; sleep-related painful erections; dementia

## Client Outcomes

**Client Will (Specify Time Frame):**

- Wake up less frequently during night.
- Awaken refreshed and be less fatigued during day.
- Fall asleep without difficulty.
- Verbalize plan that provides adequate time for sleep.
- Identify actions that can be taken to improve quality of sleep.

## Nursing Interventions

- Obtain a sleep-wake history including work and other scheduled activities, history of sleep problems, changes in sleep with present illness, and use of medications and stimulants.
- Ask the client to keep a sleep-wake diary for several

• = Independent          ▲ = Collaborative

weeks, which includes bedtime, rise time, number of awakenings, naps, and scheduled daytime events that may be depriving the client of adequate sleep time.

- Observe for underlying physiological illnesses causing sleep loss (e.g., cardiovascular, pulmonary, gastrointestinal, hyperthyroidism, nocturia occurring with benign hypertrophic prostatitis or pain).

- Determine level of anxiety. If the client is anxious, utilize relaxation techniques. See care plan for **Anxiety.**

- Assess for signs of depression: depressed mood state, flat affect, statements of hopelessness, and poor appetite. Refer for counseling/treatment as appropriate.

▲ Assess the client for other symptoms of bipolar disorder (mania, hypomania). Refer for mental health services as indicated.

▲ Monitor for presence of nocturnal symptoms of restless leg syndrome with uncomfortable restless sensations in legs that occur before sleep onset or during the night. Also monitor for nocturnal panic attacks, presence of headaches, or gastroesophageal reflux disease. Refer for treatment as appropriate.

- Observe the client's medication, diet, and caffeine intake. Look for hidden sources of caffeine, such as over-the-counter medications.

▲ Monitor for presence of sleep disordered breathing as evidenced by loud snoring with periods of apnea, or other sleep disorders such as restless leg syndrome or periodic limb movement disorder. Refer to an accredited sleep disorder center.

- Keep environment quiet for sleeping (e.g., avoid use of intercoms, lower the volume on radio and television, keep beepers on nonaudio mode, anticipate alarms on IV pumps, talk quietly on unit).

- Use soothing sound generators with sounds of the ocean, rainfall, or waterfall to induce sleep, or use "white noise" such as a fan to block out other sounds. Also consider the use of earplugs.

- Encourage the client to use soothing music to facilitate sleep.

• = Independent          ▲ = Collaborative

## Geriatric

▲ Determine if the client has a physiological problem that could result in sleep loss such as pain, cardiovascular disease, pulmonary disease, neurological problems such as dementia, or urinary problems.

• Observe elimination patterns. Have the client decrease fluid intake in the evening, and ensure that diuretics are taken early in the morning.

▲ If the client is waking frequently during the night with periods of apnea or increased leg movement, consider the presence of sleep apnea problems or periodic leg movements disorder and refer to a sleep clinic for evaluation.

• Suggest light reading or TV viewing that does not excite as an evening activity.

• Help the client take a warm bath in the evening.

▲ If the client continues to have sleep loss despite developing good sleep hygiene habits, refer to a sleep clinic for further evaluation.

## Home Care

• Above interventions may be adapted for home care use.

• Obtain a full current assessment and history of sleep activity, sleep disturbance, and sleep disturbance–related behaviors.

• Instruct the client/family in expectations for normal sleep. Elicit expectations for sleep, previous sleep patterns; correct misconceptions that influence emotional responses to deviation from expectations.

• Have the client maintain a sleep diary, describing daily activity levels, use of stimulants, and activities and physical sensations around bedtime. Assess diary for potential areas of intervention.

• Assess environment for possible hazards to the client during period of deprivation (e.g., appliances, stairs). Ensure that, if client awakens during the night, there will be sufficient light (consider a nightlight), with passageways clear of obstruction between bed and bathroom.

• Obtain a listing of expected daily behaviors, before and

S

• = Independent          ▲ = Collaborative

since the onset of deprivation (e.g., mowing lawn, shaving, cooking). Identify tasks that may be delegated. Establish level of client participation in tasks. Use short task periods for the client.

- Assess client support system for availability of psychological and task-related support.
- ▲ Refer to chore, homemaker, or home health aide services as necessary.
- ▲ Assess family/caregiver response to client status. Provide nursing support; refer to medical social services or mental health services/support groups as necessary.
- ▲ If the client is taking medication, assess for effectiveness and safety in administration.
- ▲ Identify person administering medication if not the client.
- Assist the family to arrange for supervision if the client presents confusion or perceptual dysfunction.
- ▲ Refer the client to medical social services or mental health/group support services such as I Can Cope.
- ▲ In the presence of a psychiatric disorder, refer for psychiatric home health care services for client reassurance and implementation of therapeutic regimen.

## Client/Family Teaching

- Encourage the client to avoid coffee and other caffeinated foods and liquids and to avoid eating large high-protein or high-fat meals close to bedtime.
- Advise the client to avoid use of alcohol or hypnotics to induce sleep. Avoid alcohol ingestion 4 to 6 hours before bedtime.
- Encourage the client to develop a bedtime ritual that includes quiet activities such as reading, television, or crafts.
- Teach the following sleep hygiene guidelines for improving sleep habits:
  - Go to bed only when sleepy.
  - When awake in the middle of the night, go to another room, do quiet activities, and go back to bed only when sleepy.

S

• = Independent          ▲ = Collaborative

- Use the bed only for sleeping—not for reading or snoozing in front of the television.
- Avoid afternoon and evening naps.
- Get up at the same time every morning.
- Recognize that not everyone needs 8 hours of sleep.
- Do not associate lulls in performance with sleeplessness; sleeplessness should not be blamed for everything that goes wrong during the day.

# Disturbed Sleep pattern

## NANDA Definition

Time-limited disruption of sleep (natural periodic suspension of consciousness)

### Defining Characteristics

Prolonged awakenings; sleep maintenance insomnia; self-induced impairment of normal pattern; sleep onset greater than 30 minutes; early-morning insomnia; awakening earlier or later than desired; verbal complaints of difficulty falling asleep; verbal complaints of not feeling well-rested; increased proportion of Stage 1 sleep; dissatisfaction with sleep; less than age-norm total sleep time; three or more nighttime awakenings; decreased proportion of Stages 3 and 4 sleep (e.g., hyporesponsiveness, excess sleepiness, decreased motivation); decreased proportion of REM sleep (e.g., REM rebound, hyperactivity, emotional lability, agitation and impulsivity, atypical polysomnographic features); decreased ability to function

### Related Factors (r/t)

Ruminative presleep thoughts; daytime activity pattern; thinking about home; body temperature; temperament; dietary; childhood onset; inadequate sleep hygiene; sustained use of antisleep agents; circadian asynchrony; frequently changing sleep-wake schedule; depression; loneliness; frequent travel across time zones;

• = Independent          ▲ = Collaborative

daylight/darkness exposure; grief; anticipation; shift work; delayed or advanced sleep phase syndrome; loss of sleep partner, life change; preoccupation with trying to sleep; periodic gender-related hormonal shifts; biochemical agents; fear; separation from significant others; social schedule inconsistent with chronotype; aging-related sleep shifts; anxiety; medications; fear of insomnia; maladaptive conditioned wakefulness; fatigue; boredom

### Environmental

Noise; unfamiliar sleep furnishings; ambient temperature, humidity; lighting; other-generated awakening; excessive stimulation; physical restraint; lack of sleep privacy/control; interruptions for therapeutics, monitoring, lab tests; sleep partner; noxious odors

### Parental

Mother's sleep-wake pattern; parent-infant interaction; mother's emotional support

### Physiological

Urinary urgency, incontinence; fever; nausea; stasis of secretions; shortness of breath; position; gastroesophageal reflux

## Client Outcomes

### Client Will (Specify Time Frame):

- Wake up less frequently during night.
- Awaken refreshed and not be fatigued during day.
- Fall asleep without difficulty.
- Verbalize plan to implement sleep promoting routines.

## Nursing Interventions

- Obtain a sleep history including bedtime routines, history of sleep problems, changes in sleep with present illness, and use of medications and stimulants.
- Ask the client to keep a sleep diary for several weeks, which includes bedtime, rise time, number of awakenings, and record of naps.

• = Independent         ▲ = Collaborative

▲ Assess level of pain and use available pharmacological and non-pharmacological approaches to pain management.

▲ Determine level of anxiety. If the client is anxious, utilize relaxation techniques. See care plan for **Anxiety.**

▲ Assess for signs of new onset of depression: depressed mood state, statements of hopelessness, poor appetite. Refer for counseling as appropriate.

• Observe the client's medication, diet, and caffeine intake. Look for hidden sources of caffeine, such as over-the-counter medications.

• Provide measures to take before bedtime to assist with sleep (e.g., quiet time to allow the mind to slow down, carbohydrates such as crackers).

• Provide a back massage before bedtime.

• Provide pain relief shortly before bedtime and position the client comfortably for sleep.

• Keep environment quiet for sleeping (e.g., avoid use of intercoms, lower the volume on radio and television, keep beepers on nonaudio mode, anticipate alarms on IV pumps, talk quietly on unit).

• Use soothing sound generators with sounds of the ocean, rainfall, or waterfall to induce sleep, or use "white noise" such as a fan to block out other sounds. Also consider the use of earplugs.

• Encourage the client to use soothing music to facilitate sleep.

• For hospitalized stable clients, consider instituting the following sleep protocol to foster sleep:

  ■ Night shift: Give the client the opportunity for uninterrupted sleep from 1 AM to 5 AM. Keep environmental noise to a minimum.

  ■ Evening shift: Limit napping between 4 PM and 9 PM. At 10 PM turn lights off, provide sleep medication according to individual assessment, and keep noise and conversation on the unit to a minimum.

  ■ Day shift: Encourage short naps before 11 AM. Enforce a physical activity regimen as appropriate.

S

• = Independent          ▲ = Collaborative

Schedule newly ordered medications to avoid waking the client between 1 AM and 5 AM.

## Geriatric

▲ Determine if the client has new onset of a physiological problem that could result in insomnia, such as pain, cardiovascular disease, pulmonary disease, neurological problems such as dementia, or urinary problems.

• Observe elimination patterns. Have the client decrease fluid intake in the evening and ensure that diuretics are taken early in the morning unless contraindicated.

• Do a careful history of all medications including over-the-counter medications and alcohol intake.

▲ If the client is waking frequently during the night, consider the presence of sleep apnea problems and refer to a sleep clinic for evaluation.

▲ Evaluate the client for presence of depression or anxiety, which can result in insomnia. Refer for treatment as appropriate.

• Encourage social activities. Help elderly get outside for increased light exposure and to enjoy nature.

• Suggest light reading or TV viewing that does not excite as an evening activity.

• Increase daytime physical activity and social activities. Encourage walking as the client is able.

▲ Recommend avoidance of hypnotics and alcohol to induce sleep. Avoid alcohol ingestion 4 to 6 hours before bedtime.

• Reduce daytime napping in the late afternoon; limit naps to short intervals as early in the day as possible.

• Help the client take a warm bath in the evening.

• Help the client recognize that there are changes in length of sleep with aging. Client may not be able to sleep for 8 hours as when younger, and more frequent awakening is part of the aging process.

▲ If the client continues to have disturbed sleep despite developing good sleep hygiene habits, refer to a sleep clinic for further evaluation.

• = Independent          ▲ = Collaborative

## Home Care

- Above interventions may be adapted for home care use.
- Provide support to the family of the client with chronic sleep pattern disturbance.
- Instruct the client/family in expectations for normal sleep. Elicit expectations for sleep, previous sleep patterns; correct misconceptions that influence emotional responses to deviation from expectations.
- ▲ Assess the client for sleep apnea, particularly poststroke (e.g., interview partner regarding the client's sleep pattern and behaviors, have the client maintain sleep log).
- ▲ Assess the client for depression or other psychiatric disorder. Refer for mental health services as indicated.
- Have the client maintain a sleep diary, describing daily activity levels, use of stimulants, and activities and physical sensations around bedtime. Assess diary for potential areas of intervention.
- Assess environment for possible hazards to the client during periods of disturbance (e.g., appliances, stairs). Insure that, if client awakens during the night, there will be sufficient light (consider a nightlight), with passageways clear of obstruction between bed and bathroom.
- Initiate nonpharmacological interventions for insomnia: stimulus control, sleep restriction, relaxation techniques, increasing sunlight exposure, acupuncture, cognitive and educational interventions to address dysfunctional attitudes about sleep.
- In the presence of a cognitive disorder, reassure family regarding sleep expectations for the client, and address potential problems (e.g., enuresis will require frequent cleansing of client and changes of bed linens); procurement of a hospital bed with siderails may be necessary to prevent falling out of bed.
- ▲ In the presence of a psychiatric disorder, refer for psychiatric home health care services for client reassurance and implementation of therapeutic regimen.
- Provide support to the family of the client with chronic sleep pattern disturbance.

S

● = Independent          ▲ = Collaborative

## Client/Family Teaching

- Encourage the client to avoid coffee and other caffeinated foods and liquids and also to avoid eating large high-protein or high-fat meals close to bedtime.
- Advise the client to avoid use of alcohol or hypnotics to induce sleep. Avoid alcohol ingestion 4 to 6 hours before bedtime.
- Ask the client to keep a sleep diary for several weeks.
- Teach somatic and cognitive relaxation techniques to induce the relaxation response and facilitate sleep.
- Teach the client need for increased exercise. Encourage client to take a daily walk 5 to 6 hours before retiring.
- Encourage the client to develop a bedtime ritual that includes quiet activities such as reading, television, or crafts.
- Teach the following guidelines for good sleep hygiene to improve sleep habits:
  - Go to bed only when sleepy.
  - When awake in the middle of the night, go to another room, do quiet activities, and go back to bed only when sleepy.
  - Use the bed only for sleeping—not for reading or snoozing in front of the television.
  - Avoid afternoon and evening naps.
  - Get up at the same time every morning.
  - Recognize that not everyone needs 8 hours of sleep.
  - Move the alarm clock away from the bed so that it cannot be seen.
  - Do not associate lulls in performance with sleeplessness; sleeplessness should not be blamed for everything that goes wrong during the day.

S

# Readiness for enhanced Sleep

## NANDA Definition

A pattern of natural, periodic suspension of consciousness that provides adequate rest, sustains a desired lifestyle, and can be strengthened

• = Independent          ▲ = Collaborative

## Defining Characteristics

Expresses willingness to enhance sleep; amount of sleep and REM sleep is congruent with developmental needs; expresses a feeling of being rested after sleep; follows sleep routines that promote sleep habits; occasional or infrequent use of medications to induce sleep

## Related Factors (r/t)

Desire to improve sleep

## Client Outcomes

**Client Will (Specify Time Frame):**

- Awaken refreshed and not feel fatigued during day.
- Fall asleep without difficulty.
- Verbalize plan to implement sleep promotion routines.

## Nursing Interventions

- Obtain a sleep history including bedtime routines, sleep patterns, and use of medications and stimulants.
- Ask the client to keep a sleep diary for several weeks, which includes bedtime, rise time, number of awakenings, naps, and energy-using activities.
- Determine level of anxiety. If the client is anxious, use relaxation techniques. See care plan for **Anxiety.**
- Observe the client's medication, diet, and caffeine intake. Look for hidden sources of caffeine, such as over-the-counter medications.
- Provide measures to take before bedtime to assist with sleep (e.g., quiet time to allow the mind to slow down, carbohydrates such as crackers).
- Provide a back massage before bedtime.
- Initiate nonpharmacological interventions for improved sleep: stimulus control, sleep restriction, increasing sunlight exposure, acupuncture, cognitive and educational interventions to address dysfunctional attitudes about sleep.

S

• = Independent          ▲ = Collaborative

## Geriatric

- Encourage the client to develop a bedtime ritual that includes quiet activities such as reading, television, or crafts.
- Encourage the client take a warm bath in the evening.
- Observe elimination patterns. Have the client decrease fluid intake in the evening and ensure that diuretics are taken early in the morning unless contraindicated.
- Encourage social activities. Help elderly get outside for increased light exposure and to enjoy nature.
- Increase daytime physical activity. Encourage walking as the client is able.
- Recommend avoidance of hypnotics and alcohol to induce sleep. Avoid alcohol ingestion 4 to 6 hours before bedtime.
- Reduce daytime napping in the late afternoon; limit naps to short intervals as early in the day as possible.
- Help the client recognize that there are changes in length of sleep with aging.
- Teach somatic and cognitive relaxation techniques to induce the relaxation response and facilitate sleep.
- Teach the following guidelines for good sleep hygiene to improve sleep habits:
  - Go to bed only when sleepy.
  - When awake in the middle of the night, go to another room, do quiet activities, and go back to bed only when sleepy.
  - Use the bed only for sleeping—not for reading or snoozing in front of the television.
  - Avoid afternoon and evening naps.
  - Get up at the same time every morning.
  - Recognize that not everyone needs 8 hours of sleep.
  - Move the alarm clock away from the bed so that it cannot be seen.
  - Do not associate lulls in performance with sleeplessness; sleeplessness should not be blamed for everything that goes wrong during the day.

S

• = Independent          ▲ = Collaborative

• Encourage the client to use soothing music to facilitate sleep.

## Home Care

• Above interventions may be adapted for home care use.
• Obtain a full current assessment and history of sleep activity, sleep disturbance, and sleep disturbance–related behaviors.
• Instruct the client/family in expectations for normal sleep. Elicit expectations for sleep, previous sleep patterns; correct misconceptions that influence emotional responses to deviation from expectations.
• Have the client maintain a sleep diary, describing daily activity levels, use of stimulants, and activities and physical sensations around bedtime. Assess diary for potential areas of intervention.
• Assess environment for possible hazards to the client during period of deprivation (e.g., appliances, stairs). Insure that, if client awakens during the night, there will be sufficient light (consider a nightlight), with passageways clear of obstruction between bed and bathroom.
• Assess client support system for availability of psychological and task-related support. Refer to chore, homemaker, or home health aide services as necessary to relieve client of overexertion.
▲ Assess family/caregiver response to client status. Provide nursing support; refer to medical social services or mental health services/support groups as necessary.
• If the client is taking medication, assess for effectiveness and safety in administration. Identify person administering medication if not the client.
• Assist the family to arrange for supervision if the client presents confusion or perceptual dysfunction.
▲ Refer the client to medical social services or mental health/group support services such as I Can Cope.

• = Independent          ▲ = Collaborative

# Impaired Social interaction

## NANDA Definition

Insufficient or excessive quantity or ineffective quality of social exchange

## Defining Characteristics

Verbalized or observed inability to receive or communicate a satisfying sense of belonging, caring, interest, or shared history; verbalized or observed discomfort in social situations; observed use of unsuccessful social interaction behaviors; dysfunctional interaction with peers, family and/or others; family report of change of style or pattern of interaction

## Related Factors (r/t)

Knowledge/skill deficit regarding ways to enhance mutuality; therapeutic isolation; sociocultural dissonance; limited physical mobility; environmental barriers; communication barriers; altered thought processes; absence of available significant others or peers; self-concept disturbance

## Client Outcomes

### Client Will (Specify Time Frame):

- Identify barriers that cause impaired social interactions.
- Discuss feelings that accompany impaired and successful social interactions.
- Use available opportunities to practice interactions.
- Use successful social interaction behaviors.
- Report increased comfort in social situations.
- Communicate, state feelings of belonging, and demonstrate caring and interest in others.
- Report effective interactions with others.

## Nursing Interventions

- Observe for cause of discomfort in social situations; ask the client to explain when discomfort began and identify

S

• = Independent          ▲ = Collaborative

any losses (e.g., loss of health, job, or significant other; aging) and changes (e.g., marriage, birth or adoption of a child, change in body appearance).

- Assess the client's social support system.
- Spend time with the client.
- Use active listening skills including assessment and clarification of the client's verbal and nonverbal responses and interactions.
- Encourage social support for patients with visual impairments.
- Have the client list behaviors that are associated with being disconnected, and discuss alternative responses that may increase comfort.
- Monitor the client's use of defense mechanisms, and support healthy defenses (e.g., the client focuses on present and avoids placing blame on others for personal behavior).
- Have the client list behaviors that cause discomfort. Discuss alternative ways to alleviate discomfort (e.g., focusing on others and their interests, practicing making caring statements such as, "I understand you are feeling sad"). Encourage the client to express feelings to others (e.g., "I feel sad also").
- Identify client strengths. Have the client make a list of strengths and refer to it when experiencing negative feelings. He or she may find it helpful to put the list on a note card to carry at all times.
- Have group members identify each other's strengths in a group setting.
- Role-play comfortable and uncomfortable social interactions with the client and appropriate responses (e.g., acknowledging a friendly greeting, responding to rude remarks with an "I" statement, such as, "I understand you may feel that way, but this is how I feel").
- Model appropriate social interactions. Give positive verbal and nonverbal feedback for appropriate behavior (e.g., make statements such as, "I'm proud that you made it to work on time and did all the tasks assigned to you without saying that your supervisor was picking on you";

● = Independent          ▲ = Collaborative

make eye contact). If not contraindicated, touch the client's arm or hand when speaking. One way to learn social skills is to observe the productive interactions of others.
- Use humor as appropriate.
▲ Consider use of "animal" therapy; arrange for visitation.
- Consider using the Internet to promote socialization.

## Pediatric
- Provide computers and Internet access to children with chronic disabilities that limit socialization.
▲ Consider use of Rap Therapy in groups to advance social skills of urban adolescents.

## Geriatric
- Avoid assuming that social isolation is normal for elderly client.
▲ Assess the client's potential or actual sensory problems with hearing and vision and make appropriate referrals if a problem is identified.
- Monitor for depression, a particular risk in the elderly.
- Provide group situations for the client.
- Encourage physical activity such as aerobics or stretching and toning in a group.
- Have clients reminisce.

## Multicultural
- Acknowledge racial/ethnic differences at the onset of care.
- Assess for the influence of cultural beliefs, norms, and values on the client's perception of social activity and relationships.
- Approach individuals of color with respect, warmth, and professional courtesy.
- Assess the use of personal space needs, communication styles, acceptable body language, eye contact, perception of touch, and paraverbals when communicating with the client.
- Validate the client's feelings regarding social interaction.

S

• = Independent          ▲ = Collaborative

## Home Care

- Above interventions may be adapted for home care use.
- ▲ Assess family and living environment for social dynamics. Refer for medical social services to assist with family dynamics if appropriate.
- ▲ Assess the client for a psychiatric disorder. Refer for mental health services as indicated.
- Assess the client social skills; provide feedback regarding maladaptive skills, and opportunities to role play alternative communication styles.
- Suggest that the client avoid contact with negative persons.
- Identify activities that the client does alone and assist the client with balancing solitary and social activities.
- Establish pattern of care and daily activities that involve the client socially (e.g., Meals on Wheels, home health aide visits). Give supportive feedback for positive and appropriate interactions.
- ▲ Refer to or support involvement with supportive groups and counseling.
- ▲ In the presence of a psychiatric disorder, refer for psychiatric home health care services for the client reassurance and implementation of therapeutic regimen.

## Client/Family Teaching

- Help the client accept responsibility for own behavior. Have the client keep a journal, and review it together at prescheduled intervals. Give the client positive feedback for appropriate behaviors, and suggest alternative approaches for behaviors that do not enhance social interaction. Positive reinforcement perpetuates appropriate behaviors. Teach social interaction skills for use in actual situations the client is faced with daily.
- Practice social skills one-to-one and, when the client is ready, in group sessions.

• = Independent          ▲ = Collaborative

▲ Refer to appropriate social agencies for assistance (e.g., family therapy, self-help groups, crisis intervention).

## Social isolation

### NANDA Definition

Aloneness experienced by the individual and perceived as imposed by others and as a negative or threatened state

### Defining Characteristics

#### Objective

Absence of supportive significant others (e.g., family, friends, group); projection of hostility in voice and behavior; withdrawal; uncommunicativeness; demonstration of behavior unaccepted by dominant cultural group; desire to be alone or exist in a subculture; repetitive and meaningless actions; preoccupation with own thoughts; lack of eye contact; inappropriate or immature activities for developmental age/stage; evidence of physical/mental handicap or altered state of wellness; sad, dull affect

#### Subjective

Expression of feelings of aloneness imposed by others; expression of feelings of rejection; inappropriate or immature interests for developmental age/stage; inadequate or absent significant purpose in life; inability to meet expectations of others; expression of values acceptable to subculture but unacceptable to dominant cultural group; expression of interest inappropriate to developmental age/stage; feelings of differences from others; insecurity in public

### Related Factors (r/t)

Alterations in mental status; inability to engage in satisfying personal relationships; unacceptable social values; unacceptable social behavior; inadequate personal resources; immature

• = Independent     ▲ = Collaborative

interests; factors contributing to absence of satisfying personal relationships (e.g., delay in accomplishing developmental tasks); alterations in physical appearance; altered state of wellness

## Client Outcomes

### Client Will (Specify Time Frame):

- Identify feelings of isolation.
- Practice social and communication skills needed to interact with others.
- Initiate interactions with others; set and meet goals.
- Participate in activities and programs at level of ability and desire.
- Describe feelings of self-worth.

## Nursing Interventions

- Establish a therapeutic relationship by being emotionally present and authentic.
- Observe for barriers to social interaction (e.g., illness; incontinence; decreasing ability to form relationships; lack of transportation, money, support system, or knowledge).
- Note risk factors (e.g., membership in ethnic/cultural minority, chronic physiological or psychological illness or deformities, advanced age).
- Discuss causes of perceived or actual isolation.
- ▲ Promote social interactions. Support the expression of feelings. Consider the use of music therapy.
- Establish trust one on one and then gradually introduce the client to others. Allow the client opportunities to introduce issues and to describe his or her daily life.
- Involve clients in writing specific outcomes such as identifying what is most important from their viewpoint and lifestyle.
- Provide positive reinforcement when the client seeks out others.
- Help the client identify appropriate diversional activities to encourage socialization.

**S**

• = Independent          ▲ = Collaborative

- Encourage physical closeness (e.g., use touch) if appropriate.
- Identify available support systems and involve these individuals in the client's care.
▲ Refer clients to support groups.
- Encourage liberal visitation for a client who is hospitalized or in an extended care facility.
- Help the client identify role models and others with similar interests.
- See the care plan for **Risk for Loneliness.**

## Geriatric
- Assess physical and mental status to establish a firm basis for planning social activities.
- Assess for hearing deficit. Provide aids and use adaptive techniques such as facing the individual when speaking, speaking slowly, lowering the pitch of the voice, and enunciating clearly.
- Involve client in goal setting and planning activities. Have them write down 5 activities in which they would like to participate.
- If the client is in a health care facility, visit him or her for at least 10 minutes every 2 to 3 hours.
▲ Involve nonprofessionals in activities, projects, and goal setting with the client. Practice interdisciplinary management for unit-based activities: engaging in arts and crafts projects, sewing, watching videos, reading large-print books, reading magazines, playing games, playing musical instruments, and using assistive listening devices.
- Offer the client a choice of activities and persons with whom to sit and socialize. Introductions to strangers may need to be repeated several times.
- Put clients in groups according to activity preferences, abilities, age, life situations, personal and cultural characteristics, and social networks.
- Develop and display a seating chart for the common areas of each personal care unit and develop a process for

S

both identifying needed changes and executing them promptly.

- Provide physical activity, either aerobic or stretching and toning.
- Provide music with active participation; drumming, rhythm circle.
- Consider the use of simulated presence therapy (see the care plan for **Hopelessness**).
▲ Refer to programs such as Foster Grandparents and Senior Companions.
- Consider using computers and the Internet to alleviate or reduce loneliness and social isolation.

## Multicultural

- Acknowledge racial/ethnic differences at the onset of care.
- Approach individuals of color with respect, warmth, and professional courtesy.
- Assess personal space needs, communication styles, acceptable body language, attitude toward eye contact, perception of touch, and paraverbal messages when communicating with the client.
- Use a family-centered approach when working with Latino, Asian, African American, and Native American clients.
- Promote a sense of ethnic attachment.
- Validate the client's feelings regarding social isolation.

## Home Care

- The interventions described previously may be adapted for home care use.
▲ Assess the client for depression or other psychiatric disorder. Refer for mental health services as indicated.
▲ Confirm that the home setting has a telephone. Obtain one if necessary for medical safety. If the client lives alone, set up a Lifeline safety system that requires the client to answer the telephone.
- Consider the use of the computer and Internet to decrease isolation.

• = Independent          ▲ = Collaborative

- Encourage family involvement in daily life in small, non-threatening activities such as short outings, assistance with shopping, and solicitation of input from the isolated person in decision making.
▲ Establish a pattern of care and daily activities that involves the client socially (e.g., Meals on Wheels, home health aide visits).
- Have the client keep a diary of social experiences. Discuss the diary during visits.
- Identify activities that the client does alone. Assist the client with balancing solitary and social activities, keeping alone time to a minimum.
▲ Refer for visiting volunteer services.
- When the client is ready, encourage him or her to volunteer for short periods at community agencies in which contact is positive and nonthreatening (e.g., with hospitalized elders for 1 hr/wk).
▲ Assess options for living that allow the client privacy but not isolation (e.g., boarding home, congregate living, assertive community treatment programs).
▲ In the presence of a psychiatric disorder, refer for psychiatric home health care services for client reassurance and implementation of a therapeutic regimen.

## Client/Family Teaching

- Teach skills related to problem solving, communication, social interaction, activities of daily living, and positive self-esteem.
- Consider the use of telecommunication and group support via the Internet.
- Teach role playing (practicing communication skills in specific situations).
▲ Encourage the client to initiate contacts with self-help groups, counselors, and therapists.
- Provide information to the client about senior citizen services, house sharing, pets, day care centers, churches, and community resources.
▲ Refer socially isolated caregivers to appropriate support groups as well.

S

• = Independent          ▲ = Collaborative

- Teach caregivers methods to deal with troublesome behaviors related to memory disturbances, restlessness and agitation, catastrophic reactions, day/night disturbances, delusions, wandering, and physical violence.

# Chronic Sorrow

## NANDA Definition

Cyclical, recurring, and potentially progressive pattern of pervasive sadness that is experienced (by client, parent or caregiver, or individual with chronic illness or disability) in response to continual loss throughout the trajectory of an illness or disability

## Defining Characteristics

Feelings that vary in intensity, are periodic, may progress and intensify over time, and may interfere with client's ability to reach his or her highest level of personal and social well-being; expression of periodic, recurrent feelings of sadness; expression of one or more of the following feelings: anger, being misunderstood, confusion, depression, disappointment, emptiness, fear, frustration, guilt/self-blame, helplessness, hopelessness, loneliness, low self-esteem, recurring loss, being overwhelmed

## Related Factors (r/t)

Death of a loved one; experience of chronic physical or mental illness or disability such as mental retardation, multiple sclerosis, prematurity, spina bifida or other birth defects, chronic mental illness, infertility, cancer, Parkinson's disease; experience of one or more trigger events (e.g., crises in management of illness, crises related to developmental stages and missed opportunities or milestones that bring comparisons with developmental, social, or personal norms); unending caregiving as constant reminder of loss

## Client Outcomes

### Client Will (Specify Time Frame):

- Express appropriate feelings of guilt, fear, anger, or sadness.

• = Independent        ▲ = Collaborative

- Identify problems associated with sorrow (e.g., changes in appetite, insomnia, nightmares, loss of libido, decreased energy, alteration in activity levels).
- Seek help in dealing with grief-associated problems.
- Plan for future one day at a time.
- Function at normal developmental level.

## Nursing Interventions

- Assess the client's degree of sorrow. Use the Burke/NCRS Chronic Sorrow Questionnaire for the individual or caregiver as appropriate.
- Identify problems of eating and sleeping; ensure that basic human needs are being met.
- Spend time with the client and family.
- Develop a trusting relationship with the client by using empathetic therapeutic communication techniques.
- Help the client to understand that sorrow may be ongoing. There is no timetable for grieving, despite popular thought. After-loss life is characterized by good times and bad times when sorrow is triggered by events.
- Help the client recognize that, although sadness will occur at intervals for the rest of his or her life, it will become bearable. In time the client may develop a relationship with grief that is lifelong but livable, and as much filled with comfort as it is with sorrow.
- Encourage the use of positive coping techniques:
  - Taking action: Suggested strategies include keeping busy, keeping personal interests, going away, getting out of the house, doing something to gain a feeling of control over life.
  - Cognitive coping: Techniques include concentrating on the positive aspects of life, having a "can do" attitude, taking 1 day at a time, and taking responsibility for the quality of one's own life. Encourage the client to write about the experience.
  - Interpersonal coping: Techniques include talking to a close friend, a health care professional, or someone with the same condition or circumstance. Joining

**S**

• = Independent          ▲ = Collaborative

a support group can also help the sorrowful person to cope.

- ■ Emotional coping: Encourage the client to express feelings, cry as desired, give thanks, and pray if desired.
- Review past experiences, role changes, and coping skills. Use music if appropriate. One study revealed the theme of a need to remember and to hold onto the memory.
- Expect the client to meet responsibilities; give positive reinforcement.
- ▲ Refer the client to spiritual counseling if desired.
- ▲ Encourage the client to make time to talk to family members about the loss with the help of professional support as needed and without criticizing or belittling each other's feelings about the loss. Once these feelings are shared, family members can better begin to accept the chronic loss and develop coping strategies.
- Recognize that a stimulus for reactivation of sorrow in women is when a developmentally disabled child develops a health care crisis. In men, reactivation of sorrow is more associated with comparison with social norms.
- Help the client determine the best way and place to find social support.
- ▲ Identify available community resources, including grief counselors or support groups available for specific losses (e.g., Multiple Sclerosis Society).
- ▲ Encourage the client to become active in interests such as volunteer work, service projects, or church activities.
- ▲ Identify whether the client is experiencing depression, suicidal tendencies, or other emotional disorders. Refer for counseling as appropriate.

## Pediatric/Parent

- Treat the child with respect, give them the opportunity to talk about their concerns, and answer questions honestly.
- Listen to the child's expression of grief.
- Help parents recognize that the child does not have to be

● = Independent      ▲ = Collaborative

"fixed"; instead they need support going through an experience of grieving just as adults.

- Encourage children to listen to music that they enjoy.
- ▲ Consider the use of art for children in hospice care who are dying or dealing with the death of a parent, sibling, or other family member.
- ▲ Refer grieving children and parents to a program to help facilitate grieving if desired, especially if the death was traumatic.
- Help the adolescent determine sources of support and how to utilize them effectively.
- Encourage parents to seek mental health services as needed, learn stress reduction, and take good care of their health.

## Geriatric

- ▲ Use reminiscence therapy in conjunction with the expression of emotions. Refer to a reminiscence group if available.
- Identify previous losses and assess the client for depression.
- Evaluate the social support system of the elderly client. If the support system is minimal, help the client determine how to increase available support.

## Multicultural

- Assess for the influence of cultural beliefs, norms, and values on the client's expressions of sorrow.
- Identify whether the client had been notified of the health status of the deceased and was able to be present during death and illness.
- Validate the client's feelings regarding the loss.

## Home Care

- The interventions described previously may be adapted for home care use. Identify causes for chronic sorrow and observe the client's expression of this sorrow.
- ▲ Assess the client for depression. Refer for mental health services as indicated.

S

• = Independent          ▲ = Collaborative

▲ When sorrow is focused around loss of a pregnancy, encourage the client to follow through on a counseling referral.

• Encourage the client to participate in activities that are diversionary and uplifting as tolerated (e.g., outdoor activities, hobby groups, church-related activities, pet care).

• Encourage the client to participate in support groups appropriate to the area of loss or illness (e.g., Crohn's disease support group or Widow to Widow).

• Provide psychological support for family/caregivers.

▲ In the presence of a psychiatric disorder, refer for psychiatric home health care services for client reassurance and implementation of a therapeutic regimen.

▲ See the care plans for **Impaired Adjustment, Chronic low Self-esteem, Risk for Loneliness,** and **Hopelessness.**

## Spiritual distress

### NANDA Definition

Impaired ability to experience and integrate meaning and purpose in life through the individual's connectedness with self, others, art, music, literature, nature, or a power greater than oneself

### S Defining Characteristics

• Connections to self: Expresses lack of hope, meaning and purpose in life, peace/serenity, acceptance, love, forgiveness of self, courage; expresses anger, guilt, poor coping

• Connections with others: Refuses interactions with spiritual leaders; refuses interactions with friends and family; verbalizes being separated from their support system, expresses alienation

• Connections with art, music, literature, nature: Demon-

• = Independent          ▲ = Collaborative

strates inability to experience previous state of creativity (singing, listening to music, writing), disinterest in nature, and disinterest in reading spiritual literature

- Connections with power greater than oneself: Demonstrates inability to pray, inability to participate in religious activities, expressions of being abandoned by or having anger toward God; requests to see a religious leader; demonstrates sudden changes in spiritual practices, inability to be introspective/inward turning; expresses being hopeless and suffering

## Related Factors (r/t)

Self-alienation; loneliness/social isolation; anxiety; sociocultural deprivation; death and dying of self or others; pain; life change; chronic illness of self or others

## Client Outcomes

### Client Will (Specify Time Frame):

- Express sense of connectedness with self, others, arts, music, literature, or power greater than oneself.
- Express meaning and purpose in life.
- Express sense of hope in the future.
- Express ability to forgive.
- Express acceptance of health status.
- Discuss personal response to dying.
- Discuss personal response to grieving.

## Nursing Interventions

- Observe the client for loss of meaning, purpose, and hope in life.
- Respect the client's beliefs; avoid imposing your own spiritual beliefs on the client. Be aware of your own belief systems and accept the client's spirituality. Allow for self-disclosure. Promote a sense of love, caring, and compassion.
- Monitor and promote supportive social contacts.
- ▲ Refer the client to a support group.

• = Independent          ▲ = Collaborative

- Be physically present and actively listen to the client.
- Support meditation, guided imagery, therapeutic touch, journaling, relaxation, and involvement in art, music, or poetry. Support outdoor activities.
- Offer or suggest visits with spiritual and/or religious advisors.
- Help the client make a list of important and unimportant values.
- Assist the client in identifying and creating his or her own meaningful experiences. Help the client develop skills to deal with illness or lifestyle changes. Include the client in care planning.
- Ask how to be most helpful; encourage the client to look inward, look outward, reflect, and seek clarification.
- If the client is comfortable with touch, hold the client's hand or place a hand gently on the client's arm.
- Help the client find a reason for living and be available for support. Promote hope.
- Listen to the client's feelings about suffering and/or death. Be nonjudgmental and allow time for grieving.
- Provide appropriate religious materials, artifacts, or music as requested.
- Promote forgiveness.
- Provide privacy or a "sacred space."
- Allow time and a place for prayer.
- Encourage the use of humor, as appropriate, to promote spiritual well-being.

## Geriatric

- Discuss personal definitions of spiritual wellness with the client.
- Identify the client's past sources of spirituality. Help the client explore his or her life and identify those experiences that are noteworthy. Clients may want to read the Bible or other religious text or have it read to them.

## Multicultural

- Assess for the influence of cultural beliefs, norms, and

● = Independent          ▲ = Collaborative

values on the client's ability to cope with spiritual distress.
- Acknowledge the value conflicts from acculturation stresses that may contribute to spiritual distress.
- Encourage spirituality as a source of support.
- Validate the client's spiritual concerns and convey respect for his or her beliefs.

## Home Care
- All of the nursing interventions described previously apply in the home setting.
- Assist client to examine past and present risk factors, concentrating on the identification of capabilities, assets, and positive attributes, and how they relate to perceptions of the home setting.

# Risk for Spiritual distress

## NANDA Definition

At risk for impaired ability to experience and integrate meaning and purpose in life through the individual's connectedness with self, others, art, music, literature, nature, or a power greater than oneself

## Risk Factors

Physical: Physical illness, substance abuse/excessive drinking, chronic illness

Psychosocial: low self-esteem, depression, anxiety, stress, poor relationships, separate from support systems, blocks to experiencing love, inability to forgive, loss

Sociocultural: racial/cultural conflict, change in religious rituals

Spiritual: change in spiritual practices

Developmental: life transitions

Environmental: environmental changes, natural disasters

• = Independent          ▲ = Collaborative

## Client Outcomes

### Client Will (Specify Time Frame):

- Express sense of connectedness with self, others, arts, music, literature, or power greater than oneself.
- Express meaning and purpose in life.
- Express sense of optimism and hope in the future.
- Express ability to forgive.
- Express desire to discuss health state and integrate care in lifestyle.
- Discuss personal response to dying.
- Discuss personal response to grieving.
- Express satisfaction with life circumstances.

## Nursing Interventions

- Observe the client for loss of meaning, purpose, and hope in life.
- Respect the client's beliefs; avoid imposing your own spiritual beliefs on the client. Be aware of your own belief systems and accept the client's spirituality. Allow for self-disclosure. Promote a sense of love, caring, and compassion.
- Monitor and promote supportive social contacts.
- Inform the client about available support groups.
- Be physically present and actively listen to the client.
- Support meditation, guided imagery, therapeutic touch, journaling, relaxation, and involvement in art, music, or poetry. Support outdoor activities.
- Offer or suggest visits with spiritual and/or religious advisors.
- Help the client make a list of important and unimportant values.
- Assist the client in identifying and creating his or her own meaningful experiences. Help the client develop skills to deal with illness or lifestyle changes. Include the client in care planning.
- Ask how to be most helpful; encourage the client to look inward, look outward, reflect, and seek clarification.

S

• = Independent        ▲ = Collaborative

- If the client is comfortable with touch, hold the client's hand or place a hand gently on the client's arm.
- Help the client find a reason for living and be available for support. Promote hope.
- Listen to the client's feelings about suffering and/or death. Be nonjudgmental and allow time for grieving.
- Provide appropriate religious materials, artifacts, or music as requested.
- Promote forgiveness.
- Provide privacy or a "sacred space."
- Allow time and a place for prayer.
- Use humor, as appropriate, to promote spiritual well-being.

## Multicultural

- Assess for the influence of cultural beliefs, norms, and values on the client's ability to cope with spiritual distress.
- Acknowledge the value conflicts from acculturation stresses that may contribute to spiritual distress.
- Encourage spirituality as a source of support.
- Validate the client's spiritual concerns and convey respect for his or her beliefs.

## Home Care

- Interventions mentioned under other subheadings in this nursing diagnosis also apply to home care.

S

# Readiness for enhanced Spiritual well-being

## NANDA Definition

Ability to experience and integrate meaning and purpose in life through connectedness with self, others, art, music, literature, nature, or a power greater than oneself

• = Independent ▲ = Collaborative

## Defining Characteristics

- Connections to self: Desires enhanced connections; expresses hope, meaning, and purpose in life, peace and serenity, acceptance, surrender, love, forgiveness of self, satisfying philosophy of life, joy, courage, heightened coping, meditation
- Connections with others: Provides service to others, requests interaction with spiritual leaders, requests forgiveness of others, requests interaction with friends and family
- Connections with art, music, literature, nature: Displays creative energy (e.g., writing poetry), sings, listens to music, reads spiritual literature, spends time outdoors
- Connection with a power greater than self: Prays, reports mystical experiences, participates in religious activities, expresses reverence and awe

## Related Factors (r/t)

Health-seeking behaviors; empathy; self-care; self-awareness; desire for harmonious interconnectedness; desire to find meaning and purpose in life

## Client Outcomes

### Client Will (Specify Time Frame):

- Express hope.
- Express sense of meaning and purpose in life.
- Express peace and serenity.
- Express acceptance.
- Express surrender.
- Express forgiveness of self and others.
- Express satisfaction with philosophy of life.
- Express joy.
- Express courage.
- Describe being able to cope.
- Describe use of spiritual practices.
- Describe providing service to others.
- Describe interaction with spiritual leaders, friends, and family.
- Describe appreciation for art, music, literature, and nature.

• = Independent          ▲ = Collaborative

## Nursing Interventions

- Perform a spiritual assessment that includes the client's relationship with God, meaning and purpose in life, religious affiliation, and any other significant beliefs.
- Be present for the client.
- Listen actively to the client.
- Encourage the client to pray, setting the example by praying with and for the client.
- Encourage involvement in group religious practices.
- Encourage increased quality of life through social support.
- Assist the client in identifying religious or spiritual beliefs that encourage integration of meaning and purpose in the client's life.
- Encourage the client to use music as a means of reducing stress.
- Encourage the client to engage regularly in bibliotherapy.
- Encourage storytelling.
- Offer to read to the client.
- Support involvement in expressive art.
- Support the use of humor by the client.
- Encourage the client to use journal writing as a means of reflection on his or her life.
- Encourage the client to practice forgiveness.
- Support the client in contemplating, viewing, and/or experiencing nature.
- Encourage expressions of spirituality.
- Validate the client's spiritual concerns and convey respect for his or her beliefs.
- Help the client participate in religious rites or obtain spiritual guidance.
- Assist the client in developing spirituality. List the most valuable qualities he or she can bring from within, the circumstances most helpful for unfolding these qualities, and the ways of incorporating these circumstances into the client's lifestyle.

S

• = Independent        ▲ = Collaborative

## Pediatric

- Provide spiritual care for children based on developmental level.
    - **Infants:** Have the same nurse care for the child on a daily basis, hold, cuddle, rock play with, and sing to the infant.
    - **Toddlers:** Provide consistency in care and familiar toys, music, stories, clothing blankets, pillows, and any other individual object of contentment. Schedule home religious routines into the plan of care and support home routines regarding good and bad behavior.
    - **School-age children and adolescents**: Encourage both groups to express their feelings regarding spirituality. Ask them, "Do you wish to pray and what do want to pray about?" Children of all ages can express feelings in storytelling. Offer age-appropriate complimentary therapies such as music, art, videos, connectedness with peers through cards, letters, and visits.

## Geriatrics

- Discuss personal definitions of spiritual wellness with the client.
- Identify the client's past sources of spirituality. Help the client explore his or her life and identify those experiences that are noteworthy. Clients may want to read the Bible or other religious text or have it read to them.

## Multicultural

- Assess for the influence of cultural beliefs, norms, and values on the client's perceptions of spirituality.
- Encourage expressions of spirituality.
- Validate the client's spiritual concerns and convey respect for his or her beliefs.

## Home Care

- ▲ All of the nursing interventions mentioned previously

● = Independent          ▲ = Collaborative

apply in the home setting. Refer the client to parish nurses.

# Risk for Suffocation

## NANDA Definition

Accentuated risk of accidental suffocation (inadequate air available for inhalation)

## Risk Factors

### External

Vehicle warming in closed garage; use of fuel-burning heaters not vented to outside; smoking in bed; children's playing with plastic bags or inserting small objects into their mouths or noses; placement of propped bottle in infant's crib; placement of pillow in infant's crib; consumption of large mouthfuls of food; failure to remove doors on discarded or unused refrigerators or freezers; leaving children unattended in bathtubs or pools; household gas leaks; low-strung clothesline; hanging of pacifier around infant's neck

### Internal

Reduced olfactory sensation; reduced motor abilities; cognitive or emotional difficulties; disease or injury process; lack of safety education; lack of safety precautions

## Related Factors (r/t)

See Risk Factors.

## Client Outcomes

### Client Will (Specify Time Frame):

- Explain and undertake appropriate measures to prevent suffocation.
- Demonstrate correct techniques for emergency rescue maneuvers (e.g., Heimlich maneuver, rescue breathing, cardio-

• = Independent          ▲ = Collaborative

pulmonary resuscitation [CPR]) and describe situations that require them.

## Nursing Interventions

- Identify hospitalized clients at particular risk for suffocation, including the following:
    - Clients with altered levels of consciousness
    - Infants or young children
    - Clients with developmental delays
    - Clients with mental illness, especially schizophrenia

## Pediatric

- Counsel families on the following:
    - Following general safety practices such as not smoking in bed, properly disposing of large appliances, using properly functioning heating systems and ventilation, having functional smoke detectors, and opening garage doors when warming up a car
- Position infants on their back to sleep, do not position in the prone position.
- Avoid use of loose bedding such as blankets and sheets for sleeping. If blankets are used, they should be tucked in around the crib mattress so the infant's face is less likely to become covered by bedding. One strategy is to make up the bedding so that the infant's feet are able to reach the foot of the crib with the blankets tucked in around the crib mattress and reaching only the level of the infant's chest.
- Teach parents not to sleep with an infant, especially if alcohol or medications/illicit drugs are used by the parents.
- Conduct risk factor identification, noting special circumstances in which preventive or protective measures are indicated. Note the presence of environmental hazards, including the following:
    - Plastic bags (e.g., dry cleaner's bags, bags used for mattress protection)
    - Cribs with slats wider than $2^{3}/_{8}$ inches

• = Independent                    ▲ = Collaborative

- Ill-fitting crib mattresses that can allow the infant to become wedged between the mattress and crib
- Pillows in cribs
- Abandoned large appliances such as refrigerators, dishwashers, or freezers
- Clothing with cords or hoods that can become entangled
- Bibs, pacifiers on a string, drapery cords, pull-toy strings

- Counsel families to not serve these foods to the child younger than 4 years of age: Hotdogs, popcorn, nuts, pretzels, chips, peanut butter, chunks of meat, hard pieces of fruit or vegetables, raisins, whole grapes, hard candies, marshmallows.
- Provide information to parents about obtaining the "No-choke Test Tube," (No-choke tubes are sold at stores that sell baby items), or use of a toilet paper roll. If an object fits in the tube or the roll, it is too small to give to a child.
- Stress water and pool safety precautions, including vigilant, uninterrupted parental supervision.
- Underscore the necessity of not allowing children to play with or near electric garage doors and of keeping garage door openers out of the reach of young children.
- For adolescents, watch for signs of depression that could result in suicide by suffocation.

### Geriatric
- Assess the status of the swallow reflex. Offer appropriate foods and beverages accordingly.
- Observe the client for pocketing of food in the side of the mouth; remove food as needed.
- Position the client in high Fowler's position when eating and for 1 hour afterward.
- Use care in pillow placement when positioning frail elderly clients who are on bed rest.

### Home Care
- Assess the home for potential safety hazards in systems

that are not likely to be fixed (e.g., faulty pilot lights or gas leaks in gas stoves, carbon monoxide release from heating systems, kerosene fumes from portable heaters). Assist the family in having these areas assessed and making appropriate safety arrangements (e.g., installing detectors, making repairs).

## Client/Family Teaching

▲ Recommend that families who are seeking day care or in-home care for children, geriatric family members, or at-risk family members with developmental or functional disabilities inspect the environment for hazards and examine the first aid preparation and vigilance of providers.

▲ Involve family members in learning and practicing rescue techniques, including treatment of choking and lack of breathing, and CPR. Initiate referral to formal training classes.

# Risk for Suicide

## NANDA Definition

At risk for self-inflicted, life-threatening injury

## Related Factors (r/t)

### Behavioral

History of previous suicide attempt; impulsiveness; purchase of gun; stockpiling of medicines; making or changing of a will; giving away of possessions; sudden euphoric recovery from major depression; marked changes in behavior, attitude, or school performance

### Verbal

Threats of killing oneself; statement of desire to die/end it all

• = Independent          ▲ = Collaborative

## Situational

Living alone; retirement; relocation, institutionalization; economic instability; loss of autonomy/independence; presence of gun in home; residence of adolescent in nontraditional setting (e.g., juvenile detention center, prison, half-way house, group home)

## Psychological

Family history of suicide; alcohol and substance use/abuse; psychiatric illness/disorder (e.g., depression, schizophrenia, bipolar disorder); abuse in childhood; guilt; gay or lesbian orientation in youth

## Demographic

Age: elderly, young adult male, adolescent; race: white, Native American; gender: male; marital status: divorced, widowed

## Physical

Physical illness; terminal illness; chronic pain

## Social

Loss of important relationship; disrupted family life; grief, bereavement; poor support systems; loneliness; hopelessness; helplessness; social isolation; legal or disciplinary problems; cluster suicides

## Client Outcomes

### Client Will (Specify Time Frame):

- Not harm self.
- Maintain connectedness in relationships.
- Disclose and discuss suicidal ideas if present; seek help.
- Express decreased anxiety and control of impulses.
- Talk about feelings; express anger appropriately.
- Refrain from using mood-altering substances.
- Obtain no access to harmful objects.
- Yield access to harmful objects.
- Maintain self-control without supervision.

• = Independent          ▲ = Collaborative

## Nursing Interventions

NOTE: Prior to implementation of interventions in the face of suicidal behavior, nurses should examine their own emotional responses to incidents of suicide to ensure that interventions will not be based on countertransference reactions.

- Establish a therapeutic relationship with the client. Use a direct, nonjudgmental approach in discussing suicide.
- Monitor, document, and report the client's potential for suicide.
- Be alert for warning signs of suicide:
  - Making statements such as, "I can't go on," "Nothing matters anymore," "I wish I were dead"
  - Becoming depressed or withdrawn
  - Behaving recklessly
  - Getting affairs in order and giving away valued possessions
  - Showing a marked change in behavior, attitudes, or appearance
  - Abusing drugs or alcohol
  - Suffering a major loss or life change
- Pay particular attention to clients manifesting a psychiatric disorder associated with suicidal behavior, including depression, substance abuse, bipolar disorder, schizophrenia, panic disorder, dissociative disorder, antisocial personality disorder, or borderline personality disorder.
- Take suicide notes seriously. Consider themes of notes in determining appropriate interventions.
- Question family members regarding the preparatory actions mentioned.
- Assess for suicidal ideation when the history reveals the following:
  - Depression, substance abuse, or other psychiatric disorders
  - Attempted suicide, current or past
  - Recent stressful life events (divorce and/or separation, relocation, problems with children)
  - Recent unemployment

• = Independent          ▲ = Collaborative

- Recent bereavement
- Chronic pain or physical illness
- Childhood physical or sexual abuse
- Gay, lesbian, or bisexual gender orientation
- Family history of suicide

- Use brief self-report measures to improve clinical management of at-risk cases.
- Determine the presence and degree of suicidal risk. A number of questions will elicit the necessary information:
  - Have you been thinking about hurting or killing yourself?
  - How often do you have these thoughts and how long do they last?
  - Do you have a plan? What is it?
  - Do you have access to the means to carry out that plan?
  - How likely is it that you could carry out the plan?
  - Are there people or things that could prevent you from hurting yourself?
  - What do you see in your future a year from now? Five years from now?
  - What do you expect would happen if you died?
  - What has kept you alive up to now?
- ▲ Refer to mental health counseling and refer for possible hospitalization if there is evidence of suicidal intent, which may include evidence of preparatory actions (e.g., obtaining a weapon, making a plan, putting affairs in order, giving away prized possession, preparing a suicide note).
- Assign a hospitalized client to a room located near the nursing station.
- Search the newly hospitalized client and the client's personal belongings for weapons or potential weapons and hoarded medications during the inpatient admission procedure, as appropriate.
- ▲ Initiate suicide precautions (e.g., ongoing observation and monitoring of the client, provision of a protective environment) for a client who is at serious risk of suicide.
- Place the client in the least restrictive environment that

• = Independent          ▲ = Collaborative

allows for the necessary level of observation. Assess suicidal risk at least daily.

▲ Assess the client's ability to enter into a no-suicide contract. Contract (verbally or in writing) with the client for no self-harm; recontract at appropriate intervals.

▲ Increase surveillance of a hospitalized client at times when staffing is predictably low (e.g., staff meetings, change of shift report, periods of unit disruption).

▲ Consider strategies to decrease isolation and opportunity to act on harmful thoughts (e.g., use of a sitter).

▲ Observe, record, and report any changes in mood or behavior that may signify increasing suicide risk and document results of regular surveillance checks.

• Explain suicide precautions and relevant safety issues to the client and family (e.g., purpose, duration, behavioral expectations, and behavioral consequences).

▲ Refer for treatment and participate in the management of any psychiatric illness or symptoms that may be contributing to the client's suicidal ideation or behavior.

▲ Verify that the client has taken medications as ordered (e.g., conduct mouth checks following medication administration).

▲ Maintain increased surveillance of the client whenever use of an antidepressant has been initiated or the dosage increased.

• Search the environment routinely and remove dangerous items.

• Limit access to windows and exits unless locked and shatterproof, as appropriate.

• Monitor the client during the use of potential weapons (e.g., razor, scissors).

• Involve the client in treatment planning and self-care management of psychiatric disorders.

• Develop a positive therapeutic relationship with the client; *do not* make promises that may not be kept.

• Interact with the client at regular intervals to convey caring and openness, and to provide opportunities for the client to talk about feelings.

• = Independent          ▲ = Collaborative

- Explore with the client all circumstances and motivations related to the suicidality.
- Explore with the client all perceived consequences that could act as a barrier to suicide (e.g., impact on family, religious beliefs). Be aware that resources should not be assumed to be barriers to suicide without exploring the client's feelings toward them.
- Encourage the client to seek out care providers to talk whenever the urge to harm himself or herself occurs.
- Avoid repeated discussion of the client's suicide history by keeping discussion oriented to the present and future.
▲ Discuss plans for dealing with suicidal ideation in the future (e.g., how to identify precipitating factors, whom to contact, where to go for help, how to respond to desire for self-harm) and for dealing with questions from friends and others about the client's hospitalization/suicide attempt.
▲ Assist the client in identifying a network of supportive persons and resources (e.g., clergy, family, care providers).
▲ Refer family members and friends to local mental health agencies and crisis intervention centers if the client has suicidal ideation or there is a suspicion of suicidal thoughts.
▲ Consider outpatient commitment or an overnight psychiatric observation program for an actively suicidal client.
- Cognitive behavioral techniques help the client to modify thinking styles that promote depression, hopelessness, and a belief that suicide is a valid means of escaping the current situation.
- Group interventions can be useful to address recurrent suicide attempts.
▲ If imminent suicide is suspected or an attempt has occurred, call for assistance and do not leave the client alone.
▲ With the client's consent, facilitate family-oriented crisis intervention.

S

• = Independent          ▲ = Collaborative

▲ Involve the family in discharge planning (e.g., illness/ medication teaching, recognition of increasing suicidal risk, client's plan for dealing with recurring suicidal thoughts, community resources).

▲ Prior to discharge from the hospital, ensure that the client has a supply of ordered medications, has a plan for outpatient follow-up, understands the plan or has a caregiver able and willing to follow the plan, and has the ability to access outpatient treatment.

▲ In the event of successful suicide, refer the family to a therapy group for survivors of suicide.

• See the care plans for **Risk for self-directed Violence, Hopelessness,** and **Risk for Self-mutilation.**

## Multicultural

• Assess for the influence of cultural beliefs, norms, and values on the individual's perceptions of suicide.

• Support the implementation of suicide prevention and intervention programs for vulnerable populations.

• Facilitate modeling and role playing for the client and family regarding healthy ways to start a discussion about the client's suicide attempt.

• Identify and acknowledge the stresses unique to culturally diverse individuals.

• Identify and acknowledge unique cultural responses to stressors in determining sensitive interventions to prevent suicide.

• Encourage family members to demonstrate and offer caring and support to each other.

• Foster the client's use of available family and religious supports.

• Validate the individual's feelings regarding concerns about the current crisis and family functioning.

## Pediatric

• Determine the presence and degree of suicidal risk. A number of questions will elicit the necessary information:

■ "Did you ever feel so upset that you wished you were not alive or wanted to die?"

• = Independent             ▲ = Collaborative

- ■ "Did you ever do something that you knew was so dangerous that you could get hurt or killed by doing it?"
- ■ "Did you ever hurt yourself or try to hurt yourself?"
- ■ "Did you ever try to kill yourself?"
- ■ "Did you ever think about or try to commit suicide?"
- Use brief self-report measures to improve clinical management of at-risk cases.
- Assess for both medical and psychiatric disturbances that may contribute to suicidality.
- Recognize that the developmental issues of childhood and adolescence may heighten suicide risks and involve different issues from those with adults.
- Assess specific stressors for the adolescent client.
- Evaluate for the presence of self-mutilation. Refer to care plan for **Risk for Self-mutilation** for additional information.
- Be aware that there is not complete overlap between suicidal behavior and self-mutilation. The motivation may be different (ending life rather than coping with difficult feelings), and the method is usually different.
- Assess for the presence of an eating disorder. Attend to the themes that preoccupy teens with eating disorders who have suicidal ideations.
- Parental education groups can influence suicide risk factors.
- Support the implementation of school-based suicide prevention programs. School nurses can be key to early intervention.
- ▲ Prior to discharge from the hospital, ensure that the client's parent has a supply of ordered medications, has a plan for outpatient follow-up, has a caregiver who understands the plan or is able and willing to follow the plan, and has the ability to access outpatient treatment.

### Geriatric
- Perform careful assessment and ongoing evaluation of the potential for suicidal ideation in the older adult, particularly the older white man.

● = Independent          ▲ = Collaborative

- Evaluate the older client's mental and physical health status and financial stressors. The possibility of reversible/medical causes of depression, including medical or neurological disorders, as well as psychomimetic reactions to medications, should inform nursing observations.
- Explore with client any concerns or pressures (physical and financial) regarding ability to secure support of medical care, especially perceived pressures about being a burden on family.
- When assessing suicide risk factors, incorporate a higher degree of risk for older men and for some older adults who have lost a loved one in the previous year.
- Monitor the older adult for subtle signs of suicidal risk.
- Explore triggers of and barriers to suicidal behavior, with particular attention to real and perceived losses (e.g., professional role, health).
- An older adult who shows self-destructive behaviors should be evaluated for dementia.
- Anticipate overall responsiveness to treatment, but monitor for early relapse.
- ▲ Advocate for the older client with other professionals in securing treatment for suicidal states.
- Encourage physical activity in older adults. Benefits to mood have been found with exercise.
- Assist the older adult to identify protective factors that serve as resources to mitigate against suicidal ideation.
- Collaborative care management of older adults in primary care settings is a growing area for nursing intervention.

## Home Care

- Communicate the degree of risk to family/caregivers; assess the family and caregiving situation for ability to protect the client and to understand the client's suicidal behavior. Provide the family and caregivers with guidelines on how to manage self-harm behaviors in the home environment.

● = Independent          ▲ = Collaborative

▲ Establish an emergency plan, including when to use hotlines and 911. Develop a contract with the client and family for use of the emergency plan. Role play access to the emergency resources with the client and caregivers.

• Assess the home environment for harmful objects, especially guns. Have the family remove or lock up objects as possible.

• Counsel parents and homeowners to restrict unauthorized access to potentially lethal prescription drugs and firearms within the home.

• Identify the client's concerns and implement interventions to address the consequences of disability in a client with medical illness.

▲ If the client's suicidal ideation intensifies, or if a suicide plan with access to means becomes evident, institute an emergency plan for mental health intervention.

▲ Refer for homemaker or psychiatric home health care services for respite, client reassurance, and implementation of a therapeutic regimen.

• Telephone contacts can serve as an effective intervention for suicidal older adults.

▲ If the client is on psychotropic medications, assess the client's and family's knowledge of medication administration and side effects. Teach as necessary.

▲ Evaluate the effectiveness and side effects of medications, and adherence to the medication regimen. Review with the client and family all medications kept in the home; encourage discarding of old prescriptions. Monitor the amount of medications ordered/provided by the physician; limiting the amount of medications to which the client has access may be necessary.

## Client/Family Teaching

• Establish a supportive relationship with family members.

• Explain all relevant symptoms, procedures, treatments, and expected outcomes for suicidal ideation that is illness based (e.g., depression, bipolar disorder).

• Teach the family how to recognize that the client is at

• = Independent        ▲ = Collaborative

increased risk for suicide (changes in behavior and verbal and nonverbal communication, withdrawal, depression, or sudden lifting of depression).

- Provide written instructions for treatments and procedures for which the client will be responsible.
- Instruct the client in coping strategies (assertiveness training, impulse control training, deep breathing, progressive muscle relaxation).
- Role play (e.g., say, "Tell me how you will respond if a friend asks why you were in the hospital").
- Teach cognitive behavioral activities, such as active problem solving, reframing (reappraising the situation from a different perspective), or thought stopping (in response to a negative thought, picturing a large stop sign and replacing the image with a prearranged positive alternative). Teach the client to confront his or her own negative thought patterns (or cognitive distortions), such as catastrophizing (expecting the very worst), dichotomous thinking (perceiving events in only one of two opposite categories), or magnification (placing distorted emphasis on a single event).
- ▲ Provide the client and family with phone numbers of appropriate community agencies for therapy and counseling.

# Delayed Surgical recovery

S

## NANDA Definition

Extension in number of postoperative days required for individuals to initiate and perform on their own behalf activities that maintain life, health, and well-being

## Defining Characteristics

Evidence of interrupted healing of surgical area (e.g., redness, induration, draining, immobility); loss of appetite with or without nausea; difficulty in moving about; need for help to complete self-care; fatigue; report of pain or discomfort; postponement in resumption of employment activities; perception that more time is needed to recover

## Related Factors (r/t)

To be developed

## Client Outcomes

### Client Will (Specify Time Frame):

- Have surgical area that shows evidence of healing: no redness, induration, draining, or immobility.
- State that appetite is regained.
- State that no nausea is present.
- Demonstrate ability to move about.
- Demonstrate ability to complete self-care activities.
- State that no fatigue is present.
- State that pain is controlled or relieved after nursing interventions.
- Resume employment activities/ADLs.

## Nursing Interventions

- Perform a thorough assessment of the client, including risk factors. Allow time to be with the client.
- ▲ Assess for the presence of medical conditions and treat appropriately before surgery. If the client is diabetic, maintain normal blood glucose levels before surgery.
- ▲ Carefully assess client's use of dietary supplements such as feverfew, ginkgo biloba, garlic, ginseng, ginger, valerian, kava, St. John's wort, ephedra (Ma huang or Metabolite), and echinacea. It is recommended that all patients be advised to stop all dietary supplements at least 1 week prior to major surgical or diagnostic procedures.
- Provide preoperative teaching by a nurse to decrease postoperative problems of anxiety, pain, nausea, and lack of independence.

S

• = Independent          ▲ = Collaborative

- Provide preoperative information in verbal and written form.
- Play music of the client's choice preoperatively, intraoperatively, and postoperatively.
- Consider using healing touch in the perianesthesia setting and other mind body spirit interventions such as stress control and imagery.
- For female premenopausal clients, assess the date when the menstrual cycle is most likely to occur and schedule surgery on alternate dates if possible.
- Consider the use of preoperative reflective hats and jackets to reduce heat loss during surgery.
- Consider the use of an adjustable recliner if not contraindicated for recovery.
- Do not offer fluids in the immediate postoperative period.
- ▲ In a client with postoperative nausea and vomiting, consider the use of multiple antiemetic medications (double or triple combinations of antiemetic agents acting at different neuroreceptor sites), less emetogenic anesthesia techniques, and adequate intravenous hydration.
- The client should be provided with a complete, balanced therapeutic diet after the immediately postoperative period (24 to 48 hours).
- The client should have a nutritious diet with adequate protein intake that restores normal weight for the client.
- Use careful aseptic technique when caring for wounds.
- Suggest the use of a semipermeable dressing and suction drainage for selected orthopedic clients.
- ▲ Promote mobility and deep breathing with the use of a TENS (transcutaneous electrical nerve stimulation) unit for pain relief.
- ▲ Carefully consider the use of alternative therapy with a physician's order, such as application of aloe vera or aqueous cream to promote wound healing.
- Clients should be allowed to shower after surgery to maintain cleanliness if not contraindicated because of the presence of pacemaker wires, etc.
- Provide 20-minute foot and hand massage (5 minutes to

• = Independent          ▲ = Collaborative

each extremity), 1 to 4 hours after a dose of pain medication.
- Provide supportive telephone calls from nurse to client as a means of decreasing anxiety and providing the psychosocial support necessary for recovery from surgery.
- Assess and treat for depression and anxiety in a client complaining of continuing fatigue after surgery.
- Consider the use of alternative therapies: hypnosis, aromatherapy, music, guided imagery, and massage.
- Encourage the client to use prayer as a form of spiritual coping if this is comfortable for the client.
- See the care plans for **Anxiety, Acute Pain, Fatigue,** and **Impaired physical Mobility.**

## Pediatric
- Teach imagery and encourage distraction for children for post surgical pain relief.

## Geriatric
- Perform a thorough preoperative assessment including a cardiac assessment.
- ▲ Carefully assess the fluid and electrolyte status and glomerular filtration rate (GFR) of elderly clients before surgery. Provide fluid and electrolyte replacement per the physician's order.
- Carefully evaluate the client's temperature. Know what is normal and abnormal for each client. Check baseline temperature and monitor trends.
- To minimize risks, of hypothermia cover the patient with warmed forced-air blankets or blankets from a warmer, infuse only warm fluids and blood, and provide heated, humidified inspired gases.
- Teach guided imagery for pain relief.
- Offer spiritual support.

## Client/Family Teaching
- ▲ To decrease postoperative nausea and vomiting, the client should be instructed to fast before surgery, with the time frame to be determined by the physician.

• = Independent          ▲ = Collaborative

- Teach systematic muscle relaxation for pain relief.
- Provide individualized teaching plans for the client with an ostomy. Consider basic needs: (1) maintenance of a pouching seal for a consistent, predictable wear time; (2) maintenance of peristomal skin integrity; and (3) social and professional support of the patient.

# Impaired Swallowing

## NANDA Definition

Abnormal functioning of the swallowing mechanism associated with deficits in oral, pharyngeal, or esophageal structure or function

## Defining Characteristics

**Oral phase impairment:** Lack of tongue action to form bolus; weak suck resulting in inefficient nippling; incomplete lip closure; pushing of food out of mouth; slow bolus formation; falling of food from mouth; premature entry of bolus; nasal reflux; inability to clear oral cavity; long meals with little consumption; coughing, choking, or gagging before a swallow; abnormality in oral phase of swallow study; piecemeal deglutition; lack of chewing; pooling in lateral sulci; sialorrhea or drooling

**Pharyngeal phase impairment:** Altered head position; inadequate laryngeal elevation; food refusal; unexplained fever; delayed swallow; recurrent pulmonary infections; gurgly voice quality; nasal reflux; choking, coughing, or gagging; multiple swallows; abnormality in pharyngeal phase by swallowing study

**Esophageal phase impairment:** Heartburn or epigastric pain; acidic-smelling breath; unexplained irritability surrounding mealtime; vomitus on pillow; repetitive swallowing or ruminating; regurgitation of gastric contents or wet belches; bruxism; nighttime coughing or awakening; observed evi-

S

• = Independent    ▲ = Collaborative

dence of difficulty in swallowing (e.g., stasis of food in oral cavity, coughing, or choking); hyperextension of head, arching during or after meals; abnormality in esophageal phase by swallow study; odynophagia; food refusal or volume limiting; complaints of "something stuck"; hematemesis; vomiting

## Related Factors (r/t)

Congenital deficits; upper airway anomalies; failure to thrive; protein energy malnutrition; conditions with significant hypotonia; respiratory disorders; history of tube feeding; behavioral feeding problems; self-injurious behavior; neuromuscular impairment (e.g., decreased or absent gag reflex, decreased strength or excursion of muscles involved in mastication, perceptual impairment, or facial paralysis); mechanical obstruction (e.g., edema, tracheotomy tube, or tumor); congenital heart disease; cranial nerve involvement; neurological problems; upper airway anomalies; laryngeal abnormalities; achalasia; gastroesophageal reflux disease; acquired anatomic defects; cerebral palsy; internal or external traumas; tracheal, laryngeal, or esophageal defects; traumatic head injury; developmental delay; nasal or nasopharyngeal cavity defects; oral cavity or oropharynx abnormalities; prematurity

## Client Outcomes

### Client Will (Specify Time Frame):

- Demonstrate effective swallowing without choking or coughing.
- Remain free from aspiration (e.g., lungs clear, temperature within normal range).

## Nursing Interventions

- Determine the client's readiness to eat. The client needs to be alert, able to follow instructions, able to hold the head erect, and able to move the tongue in the mouth.
- ▲ If the swallowing impairment is of new onset, ensure that the client receives a diagnostic workup.
- Assess ability to swallow by positioning the thumb and

• = Independent          ▲ = Collaborative

index finger on the client's laryngeal protuberance. Ask
the client to swallow; feel the larynx elevate. Ask the client to cough; test for a gag reflex on both sides of the
posterior pharyngeal wall (lingual surface) with a tongue
blade. Do not rely on the presence of a gag reflex to
determine when to feed.

- Consider the use of the Massey Bedside Swallowing
Screen to screen for swallowing dysfunction.
- Observe for signs associated with swallowing problems
(e.g., coughing, choking, spitting of food, drooling, difficulty handling oral secretions, double swallowing or
major delay in swallowing, watering eyes, nasal discharge, wet or gurgly voice, decreased ability to move the
tongue and lips, decreased mastication of food, decreased ability to move food to the back of the pharynx,
slow or scanning speech).
- ▲ If the client has impaired swallowing, refer to a speech
pathologist for bedside evaluation as soon as possible. Ensure that the client is seen by a speech pathologist
within 48 hours after admission if the client has had
a CVA.
- ▲ To manage impaired swallowing, use a dysphagia team
composed of a rehabilitation nurse, speech pathologist, dietitian, physician, and radiologist who work
together.
- ▲ If the client has impaired swallowing, do not feed until
an appropriate diagnostic workup is completed. Ensure proper nutrition by consulting with a physician regarding enteral feedings, preferably using a percutaneous
endoscopic gastrostomy (PEG) tube in most cases.
- If client is not eating sufficient amount of food, recognize that the immune system may be impaired with
resultant increased risk of infection.
- If the client has an intact swallowing reflex, attempt to
feed. Observe the following feeding guidelines:
  - Position the client upright at a 90-degree angle with
  the chin tucked forward at a 45-degree angle.
  - Ensure that the client is awake, alert, and able to follow sequenced directions before attempting to feed.

• = Independent          ▲ = Collaborative

As the client becomes less alert, the swallowing response decreases, which increases the risk of aspiration.

- Begin by feeding the client one third of a teaspoon of applesauce. Provide sufficient time to masticate and swallow.
- Place the food on the unaffected side of the tongue.
- During feeding, give the client specific directions (e.g., "Open your mouth, chew the food completely, and when you are ready, tuck your chin to your chest and swallow").
- Ensure client is kept in an upright posture for an hour after eating.

▲ Watch for uncoordinated chewing or swallowing; coughing immediately after eating or delayed coughing, which may indicate silent aspiration; pocketing of food; wet-sounding voice; sneezing when eating; delay of more than 1 second in swallowing; or a change in respiratory patterns. If any of these signs is present, put on gloves, remove all food from the oral cavity, stop feedings, and consult with a speech and language pathologist and a dysphagia team.

· If the client tolerates single-textured foods such as pudding, hot cereal, or strained baby food, advance to a soft diet with guidance from the dysphagia team. Avoid foods such as hamburgers, corn, and pastas that are difficult to chew. Also avoid sticky foods such as peanut butter and white bread.

· Avoid providing liquids until the client is able to swallow effectively. Add a thickening agent to liquids to obtain a soft consistency that is similar to nectar, honey, or pudding, depending on the degree of swallowing problems.

· Preferably use prepackaged thickened liquids, or use a viscosimeter to ensure appropriate thickness.

▲ Work with the client on swallowing exercises prescribed by the dysphagia team (e.g., touching the palate with the tongue, stimulating the tonsillar arch and soft palate with a cold metal examination mirror [thermal stimulation], labial/lingual range-of-motion exercises).

S

• = Independent          ▲ = Collaborative

▲ For many adult clients, avoid the use of straws if recommended by the speech pathologist.

• Provide meals in a quiet environment away from excessive stimuli such as a community dining room.

• Ensure that there is adequate time for the client to eat. Clients with swallowing impairments often take two to four times longer than others to eat, if they are being fed.

▲ Have suction equipment available during feeding. If choking occurs and suctioning is necessary, discontinue oral feeding until the client is safely assessed with a videofluoroscopic swallow study.

• Check the oral cavity for proper emptying after the client swallows and after the client finishes the meal. Provide oral care at the end of the meal. It may be necessary to manually remove food from the client's mouth. If this is the case, use gloves and keep the client's teeth apart with a padded tongue blade.

• Praise the client for successfully following directions and swallowing appropriately.

• Keep the client in an upright position for 45 minutes to an hour after a meal. Maintaining an upright position ensures that food stays in the stomach until it has emptied and decreases the chance of aspiration following meals.

▲ Watch for signs of aspiration and pneumonia. Auscultate lung sounds after feeding. Note new crackles or wheezing, and note elevated temperature. Notify the physician as needed.

• Watch for signs of malnutrition and dehydration. Keep a record of food intake.

• Weigh the client weekly to help evaluate nutritional status. Evaluate nutritional status daily. If the client is not adequately nourished, work with the dysphagia team to determine whether the client needs to avoid oral intake with therapeutic feeding only or needs enteral feedings until the client can swallow adequately.

▲ If client has a tracheostomy, ask for referral to speech pathologist for swallowing studies before attempting to

• = Independent          ▲ = Collaborative

feed. After evaluation, decision should be made to have cuff either inflated or deflated when client eats.

## Pediatric

▲ Refer to a physician a child who has difficulty swallowing and symptoms such as difficulty manipulating food, delayed swallow response, and pocketing of a bolus of food.

• When feeding an infant or child, place the infant/child in a 90-degree position with the head slightly flexed. Change the consistency of the diet as needed, and use a curly straw for young children to facilitate tucking the chin, which helps improve swallowing ability.

• Give oral motor stimulation that increases oral-sensory awareness by waking the mouth using exercises that focus on temperature, taste, and texture.

• For infants with poor sucking and swallowing, do the following:

  ■ Support the cheeks and jaw to increase sucking skills.
  ■ Pace or rhythmically move the bottle, which encourages better suck-swallow-breath synchrony.

▲ Work with the dietitian. Some infants may need a high-calorie formula so that food volume can be decreased (which requires the infant to expend less energy) while still meeting nutritional requirements. Some infants may also need to have the tongue brushed, which provides tongue stimulation (tongue tip and tongue lateralization) and promotes lip seal and lip pursing.

• Watch for indicators of aspiration: coughing, a change in web vocal quality while feeding, perspiration and color changes during feeding, sneezing, and increased heart rate and breathing.

• Watch for warning signs of reflux: sour-smelling breath after eating, sneezing, lack of interest in feeding, crying and fussing extraordinarily when feeding, pained expressions when feeding, and excessive chewing and swallowing after eating.

## Geriatric

• Recognize that being elderly does not result in dysphagia, but having medical problems including such things as arthritis, hypertension, and other chronic medical problems can result in dysphagia.

▲ Evaluate medications the client is presently taking, especially if elderly. Consult with the pharmacist for assistance in monitoring for incorrect dosages and drug interactions that could result in dysphagia.

• Recognize that the elderly client with dementia needs a longer time to eat.

• Recognize that the loss of teeth can cause problems with chewing and swallowing. Without teeth, three to four times more effort may be required to chew food so that it is able to be swallowed.

## Home Care

▲ Refer to speech therapy.

## Client/Family Teaching

▲ Teach the client and family exercises prescribed by the dysphagia team.

• Teach the client a step-by-step method of swallowing effectively as prescribed by the dysphagia team.

• Educate the client, family, and all caregivers about rationales for food consistency and choices.

• Teach the family how to monitor the client to prevent and detect aspiration during eating.

T **Effective Therapeutic regimen management**

## NANDA Definition

Pattern of regulating and integrating into daily living a program for treatment of illness and its sequelae that is satisfactory for meeting specific health goals

• = Independent          ▲ = Collaborative

## Defining Characteristics

Appropriate choices of daily activities for meeting goals of a treatment or prevention program; illness symptoms within normal range of expectation; verbalization of desire to manage treatment of illness and prevention of sequelae; verbalization of intent to reduce risk factors for progression of illness and sequelae

## Related Factors (r/t)

None. Related factors are not relevant with strength diagnoses.

## Client Outcomes

### Client Will (Specify Time Frame):

- Acknowledge appropriateness of choices for meeting goals of treatment or prevention programs.
- Agree to continue making appropriate choices.
- Verbalize intent to contact health provider(s) for additional information, support, or resources as needed.

## Nursing Interventions

- Review self-management strategies and related outcomes, e.g., changes in function and/or relief of symptoms such as pain.
- Explore the meaning of the person's illness experience and identify uncertainties and needs through open-ended questions.
- Acknowledge the congruence of choices in activities of daily living (ADLs) with health-related goals.
- Support decisions regarding the person's methods of integrating therapeutic regimens into ADLs.
- Provide information on possible illness trajectories to allow planning for future management.
- Assist the person to resolve ambivalent feelings about the illness and management of therapeutic regimens.
- Review methods of contacting health provider(s) for changes in therapeutic regimen and/or methods of incorporating therapeutic regimens into ADLs.

T

• = Independent          ▲ = Collaborative

- Record the effectiveness of managing the therapeutic regimens.

**Multicultural**

- Assess for the influence of cultural beliefs, norms, and values on the individual's perceptions of the therapeutic regimen.
- Use a family-centered approach when working with Latino, Asian, African-American, and Native-American clients.
- Assist African Americans to integrate spirituality into their daily management routines.
- Discuss with the client those aspects of health and lifestyle that will remain unchanged by his or her health status.
- Validate the client's feelings regarding the ability to manage his or her own care and the impact on current lifestyle.

**Client/Family Teaching**

- Teach about the disease trajectory and ways to manage disease symptoms as the trajectory changes.

# Ineffective Therapeutic regimen management

## NANDA Definition

Pattern of regulating and integrating into daily living a program for treatment of illness and its sequelae that is unsatisfactory for meeting specific health goals

## Defining Characteristics

Choices of daily living ineffective for meeting goals of a treatment or prevention program; verbalization that client did not take action to reduce risk factors for progression of illness and sequelae; verbalization of desire to manage treatment of illness

• = Independent          ▲ = Collaborative

and prevention of sequelae; verbalization of difficulty with regulation of one or more prescribed regimens for prevention of complications and treatment of illness or its effects; verbalization that client did not take action to include treatment regimens in daily routines

## Related Factors (r/t)

Perceived barriers; social support deficits; powerlessness; perceived susceptibility; perceived benefits; mistrust of regimen and/or health care personnel; knowledge deficit; family patterns of health care; family conflict; excessive demands made on individual or family; economic difficulties; decisional conflicts; complexity of therapeutic regimen; complexity of health care system; faulty perception of illness seriousness; inadequate number and types of cues to action

## Client Outcomes

### Client Will (Specify Time Frame):

- Describe daily food and fluid intake that meets therapeutic goals.
- Describe activity/exercise patterns that meet therapeutic goals.
- Describe scheduling of medications that meets therapeutic goals.
- Verbalize ability to manage therapeutic regimens.
- Collaborate with health providers to decide on therapeutic regimen that is congruent with health goals and lifestyle.

## Nursing Interventions

NOTE: This diagnosis does not have the same meaning as the diagnosis **Noncompliance**. This diagnosis is made with the client, so if the client does not agree with the diagnosis, it should not be made. The emphasis is on helping the client to direct his or her own life and health, not on the client's compliance with the provider's instructions.

• = Independent          ▲ = Collaborative

- See the care plans for **Effective Therapeutic regimen management** and **Ineffective family Therapeutic regimen management.**
- Establish a collaborative partnership with the client for purposes of meeting health-related goals.
- Discuss all strategies with the client in the context of the client's culture.
- Involve family members in knowledge development, planning for self-management, and shared decision making.
- Explore the meaning of the person's illness experience and identify uncertainties and needs through open-ended questions.
- Review factors of the Health Belief Model with the client (i.e., individual perceptions of seriousness and susceptibility, demographic and other modifying factors, and perceived benefits and barriers).
- Identify the reasons for actions that are not therapeutic and discuss alternatives.
- Provide in-depth explanations of the therapeutic regimen to meet health-related goals, including pathophysiology and scientific rationales.
- Use various formats to provide information about the therapeutic regimen (e.g., brochures, videotapes, written instructions, computer-based programs).
- Help the client to develop a positive attitude toward the disease and therapeutic regimen management.
- Deliberate with the client on changes that are possible to meet therapeutic goals.
- Teach the client strategies for changing negative behaviors such as overeating, sedentary lifestyle, and smoking so that the client can self-manage his or her own health.
- Develop a contract with the client to maintain motivation for changes in behavior.
- Help the client to maintain consistency in therapeutic regimen management for optimal results.
- ▲ Review how to contact health providers as needed to

T

• = Independent        ▲ = Collaborative

address issues and concerns regarding self-management.
- Implement organizational changes to facilitate shared decision making for self-management of chronic illnesses.
- Use focus groups to evaluate the implementation of self-
management programs.

## Multicultural

- Conduct a self-assessment of the relation of culture to
ethically based care.
- Assess the influence of cultural beliefs, norms, values,
and attitudes on the client's ability to modify health
behavior.
- Discuss with the client those aspects of his or her health
behavior/lifestyle that will remain unchanged by the
therapeutic regimen.
- Assess temporal orientation and its relationship to the
management of the therapeutic regimen.
- Assess the effect of fatalism on the client's ability to
adopt the therapeutic regimen.
- Validate the client's feelings regarding the impact of the
therapeutic regimen on current lifestyle.

## Home Care

- Prepare and instruct clients/family members in the use of
a medication box. Set up an appropriate schedule for
filling the medication box, and post medication times/
doses in an accessible area (e.g., attached by magnet to a
refrigerator).
- Monitor adherence to the medical regimen.
- ▲ Consult with physician and/or pharmacist as questions
arise.

## Client/Family Teaching

- Identify what the client and/or family knows and adjust
teaching accordingly.
- Teach ways to adjust daily activities for inclusion of therapeutic regimens.

• = Independent          ▲ = Collaborative

- Teach safety in taking medications.
- Teach the client to act as a self-advocate with health providers who prescribe therapeutic regimens.

# Readiness for enhanced Therapeutic regimen management

## NANDA Definition

Pattern of regulating and integrating into daily living a program(s) for treatment of illness and its sequelae that is sufficient for meeting health-related goals and can be strengthened

## Defining Characteristics

Expression of desire to manage treatment of illness and prevention of sequelae; choices of daily living that are appropriate for meeting goals of treatment or prevention; expression of little to no difficulty with regulation/integration of one or more prescribed regimens for treatment of illness or prevention of complications; reduction of risk factors for progression of illness and sequelae; lack of unexpected acceleration of illness symptoms

## Client Outcomes

### Client Will (Specify Time Frame):

- Describe integration of therapeutic regimen into daily living.
- Demonstrate continued commitment to integration of therapeutic regimen into daily living routines.

## Nursing Interventions

- Acknowledge the expertise that the patient and family bring to self-management.
- Explore attitudes toward the illness/disease and the need for management of a therapeutic regimen.
- Review factors that contribute to the likelihood of health promotion and health protection. Use Pender's Health

• = Independent          ▲ = Collaborative

Promotion Model and Becker's Health Belief Model to identify contributing factors.
- Assess for depression.
- Facilitate the patient and family to obtain health insurance and drug payment plans whenever needed and possible.
- Further develop and reinforce contributing factors that might change with ongoing management of the therapeutic regimen, e.g., knowledge, self-efficacy, self-esteem, and perceived benefits.
- Support all efforts to self-manage therapeutic regimens.
- Review the client's strengths in the management of the therapeutic regimen.
- Collaborate with the client to identify strategies to maintain strengths and develop additional strengths as indicated.
- Identify contributing factors that may need to be improved now or in the future.
- Provide knowledge as needed related to the pathophysiology of the disease/illness, prescribed activities, prescribed medications, and nutrition.
- Use coaching strategies such as educational reinforcement, psychosocial support, and motivational guidance.
- Support positive health-promotion and health-protection behaviors.
- Help the client to maintain existing support and seek additional support as needed.

## Multicultural
- Acknowledge the cultural dimensions of health-promotion and health-protection behaviors.
- Assist the client in integrating cultural patterns with prescribed activities, prescribed medications, and prescribed diet.
- Manipulate community factors that may affect the management of the therapeutic regimen, e.g., barriers, support, insurance, education about the illness, and provider-client relationships.

T

• = Independent          ▲ = Collaborative

## Community Teaching

- Review therapeutic regimens and their optimal integration with daily living routines.
- Teach disease processes and therapeutic regimens for management of these disease processes.

# Ineffective community Therapeutic regimen management

### NANDA Definition

Pattern of regulating and integrating into community processes programs for the treatment of illness and its sequelae that are unsatisfactory for meeting health-related goals

### Defining Characteristics

Illness symptoms above norm expected for number and type of population; unexpected acceleration of illness(es); number of health care resources insufficient for incidence or prevalence of illness(es); deficits in aggregates for specific groups; deficits in people and programs to be accountable for illness care of specific groups; deficits in community activities for secondary and tertiary prevention; unavailability of health care resources for illness care

### Related Factors (r/t)

To be developed

### Community Outcomes

**T Community Members and Leaders Will (Specify Time Frame):**

- Secure community members and/or health providers who will be accountable for illness care of specific groups.
- Remain involved in advocacy for illness care and prevention programs.
- Develop health care plans for effective prevention and treatment of illnesses.

• = Independent          ▲ = Collaborative

- Make resources available for illness care and prevention.
- Initiate or improve strategies for prevention of sequelae of the illness.

## Nursing Interventions

NOTE: Nursing interventions are conducted in collaboration with community leaders, community and public health nurses, and members of other disciplines.

- Implement strategies to engage community members to be team members for health assessments and development of community programs.
- ▲ Request that a clinical nurse specialist (CNS) in community health nursing work with coalitions of health providers and community leaders.
- ▲ Recruit additional health providers as needed.
- Examine the perceptions of community members regarding service needs.
- Establish special action groups (SAGs) for specific problems and/or localities to address health policies and practices.
- Evaluate community infrastructures for adequacy in serving community illness-related needs.
- Apply the concept of caring to the community as client.
- Advocate for and with the community in multiple arenas (e.g., newspapers, television, legislative bodies, community boards).
- Provide information to public and private sources about community assessment, diagnosis, and plans of care.
- Mobilize support for the community to obtain the resources necessary for illness care and prevention.
- Establish culturally sensitive community health programs for self-management.
- Provide coaching interventions in programs for chronic disease self-management.
- Integrate the Internet with community health programs.
- Determine the cultural appropriateness of all programs.
- Support the population of family caregivers through implementation of the National Family Support Program.

● = Independent          ▲ = Collaborative

- Write grant proposals for the funding of new programs or the expansion of existing programs.
- Conduct research studies to convince others of the need to improve services or change policies.
- Avoid victim-blaming stances in efforts to promote community responsibility for health.

**Multicultural**

- Hire culturally diverse staff members for community agencies.
- Identify the health services and information resources that are currently available in the community.
- Identify cultural barriers such as acculturation issues, lack of community support, and lack of past experience with a health behavior.
- Work with members of the community to prioritize and target health goals specific to the community.
- Approach community leaders and members of color with respect, warmth, and professional courtesy.
- Establish and sustain partnerships with key individuals within the community in developing and implementing programs.
- Use community church settings as a forum for advocacy, teaching, and program implementation.

# Ineffective family Therapeutic regimen management

## NANDA Definition

Pattern of regulating and integrating into family processes a program for treatment of illness and its sequelae that is unsatisfactory for meeting specific health goals

## Defining Characteristics

Inappropriate family activities for meeting goals of treatment or prevention program; acceleration of illness symptoms of family

• = Independent          ▲ = Collaborative

member; lack of attention to illness and its sequelae; verbalization of difficulty with regulation/integration of one or more activities or prevention of complications; verbalization of desire to manage treatment of illness and prevention of its sequelae; verbalization that family did not take action to reduce risk factors for progression of illness and sequelae

## Related Factors (r/t)

Complexity of health care system; complexity of therapeutic regimen; decisional conflicts; economic difficulties; excessive demands on individual or family; family conflict

## Family Outcomes

### Family Will (Specify Time Frame):

- Make adjustments in usual activities (e.g., diet, activity, stress management) to incorporate therapeutic regimens of its members.
- Reduce illness symptoms of family members.
- Show desire to manage therapeutic regimens of its members.
- Describe a decrease in the difficulties of managing therapeutic regimens.
- Describe actions to reduce risk factors.

## Nursing Interventions

- Base family interventions on your knowledge of the family, family context, and family function.
- Use a family approach when helping an individual with a health problem that requires therapeutic management.
- Ensure that all strategies for working with the family are congruent with the culture of the family.
- Support religious beliefs and the comfort role of religion.
- Identify family interactions and their embedded contexts relative to specific health objectives.
- Review with family members the congruence and incongruence of family behaviors and health-related goals.
- Help family members make decisions regarding ways to integrate therapeutic regimens into daily living. Pro-

T

• = Independent          ▲ = Collaborative

vide advice or suggestions as solicited and accepted by
the family.

- Demonstrate respect for and trust in family decisions.
- Acknowledge the challenge of integrating therapeutic
  regimens with family behaviors.
- Review the symptoms of specific illness(es) and work
  with the family toward development of greater self-
  efficacy in relation to these symptoms.
- Selectively support family decisions to adjust therapeutic
  regimens as indicated.
- Advocate for the family in negotiating therapeutic regi-
  mens with health providers.
- Help the family to mobilize social supports.
- Help family members to modify perceptions as indicated.
- Use one or more theories of family dynamics to describe,
  explain, or predict family behaviors (e.g., theories of
  Bowen, Satir, Minuchin).
- Collaborate with expert nurses or other consultants re-
  garding strategies for working with families.

## Multicultural

- Acknowledge racial/ethnic differences at the onset of
  care.
- Approach families of color with respect, warmth, and
  professional courtesy.
- Assess for the influence of cultural beliefs, norms, and
  values on the family's perceptions of the therapeutic
  regimen.
- Give a rationale when assessing African-American
  families about sensitive issues.
- Use a family-centered approach when working with
  Latino, Asian, African-American, and Native-
  American clients.
- Facilitate modeling and role playing for the family
  regarding healthy ways to communicate and interact.
- Validate family members' feelings regarding the
  impact of the therapeutic regimen on the family
  lifestyle.

• = Independent          ▲ = Collaborative

## Client/Family Teaching

- Teach about all aspects of therapeutic regimens. Provide as much knowledge as family members will accept, adjust instruction to account for what the family already knows, and provide information in a culturally congruent manner.
- Teach ways to adjust family behaviors to include therapeutic regimens.
- ▲ Teach safety in taking medications.
- ▲ Teach family members to act as self-advocates with health providers who prescribe therapeutic regimens.

# Ineffective Thermoregulation

## NANDA Definition

Temperature fluctuation between hypothermia and hyperthermia

## Defining Characteristics

Fluctuations in body temperature above or below normal range; cool skin; cyanotic nailbeds; flushed skin; hypertension; increased respiratory rate; pallor (moderate); piloerection; reduction in body temperature below normal range; seizures/convulsions; shivering (mild); slow capillary refill; tachycardia; warmth to touch

## Related Factors (r/t)

Trauma; illness; immaturity; aging; fluctuating environmental temperature

T

## Client Outcomes

**Client Will (Specify Time Frame):**

- Maintain temperature within normal range.
- Explain measures needed to maintain normal temperature.
- Explain symptoms of hypothermia or hyperthermia.

• = Independent          ▲ = Collaborative

## Nursing Interventions

- Monitor temperature every 1 to 4 hours or use continuous temperature monitoring as appropriate.
- If the client is awake, measure the oral temperature, instead of the tympanic or axillary temperature.
- Take vital signs every 1 to 4 hours, noting changes associated with hypothermia: first, increased blood pressure, pulse rate, and respiratory rate; then, as hypothermia progresses, decreased blood pressure, pulse rate, and respiratory rate.
- ▲ Note, report, and treat changes in vital signs associated with hyperthermia: rapid, bounding pulse; increased respiratory rate; and decreased blood pressure accompanied by orthostatic hypotension.
- ▲ Monitor, report, and treat the client for signs of hyperthermia (e.g., headache, nausea and vomiting, weakness, absence of sweating, delirium, and coma).
- ▲ Note, report, and treat vital sign changes associated with hypothermia: first increased and then decreased blood pressure, pulse rate, and respiratory rate.
- ▲ Monitor, report, and treat the client for signs of hypothermia (e.g., shivering, cool skin, piloerection, pallor, slow capillary refill, cyanotic nailbeds, decreased mentation, dysrhythmias).
- Maintain a consistent room temperature (22.2° C [72° F]).
- Promote adequate nutrition and hydration.
- Adjust clothing to facilitate passive warming or cooling as appropriate.
- See the Nursing Interventions for **Hypothermia** or **Hyperthermia** as appropriate.

## Pediatric

- Recognize that pediatric clients have a decreased ability to adapt to temperature extremes. Take the following actions to maintain body temperature in the infant/child:
  - Keep the head covered.
  - Use blankets to keep the client warm.
  - Keep the client covered during procedures, transport, and diagnostic testing.

• = Independent          ▲ = Collaborative

- ■ Keep the room temperature at 22.2° C (72° F).
- • Recognize that the infant and small child are vulnerable to develop heat stroke in hot weather and ensure they receive sufficient fluids and are protected from hot environments.

## Geriatric

- • Do not allow an elderly client to become chilled or overheated. Keep the client covered when giving a bath and offer socks to wear in bed. Be aware of factors such as room temperature (heating/air conditioning), clothing (layered/loose), and fluid intake.
- • Ensure that elderly clients receive sufficient fluids during hot days and stay out of the sun.
- ▲ Assess the medication profile for the potential risk of drug-related altered body temperature.

## Home Care
### Prevention of Hypothermia in Cold Weather

- • Instruct the client to avoid prolonged exposure outdoors. When outdoors, the client should wear gloves and a cap on the head. Wool or fleece clothing can help to maintain body heat.
- • Keep the room temperature at 20° to 22.2 °C (68° to 72° F).
- ▲ Ensure an adequate source of heat. Refer to social services if the client/family has a low income and the heat could be turned off.
- • Help the elderly client locate a warm environment to which the client can go for safety in cold weather if the home environment is no longer warm.

### Prevention of Hyperthermia in Hot Weather

- • Encourage the client to wear lightweight cotton clothing. Help the elderly client remove the usual sweater.
- • Ensure that the client drinks adequate amounts of fluids—2000 mL/day—and avoids caffeine and alcohol.
- • Help the client obtain a fan or an air conditioner to increase evaporation, as needed.

• = Independent          ▲ = Collaborative

- Take the temperature of the elderly client in hot weather.
- Help the elderly client locate a cool environment to which the client can go for safety in hot weather.

### Client/Family Teaching

- Teach the client and family the signs of hypothermia and hyperthermia and appropriate actions to take if either condition develops.
- Teach the client and family an age-appropriate method for taking the temperature.
- Teach the client to avoid alcohol and medications that depress cerebral function.

## Disturbed Thought processes

### NANDA DEFINITION

Disruption in cognitive operations and activities

### Defining Characteristics

Cognitive dissonance; memory deficit/problems; inaccurate interpretation of environment; hypovigilance; hypervigilance; distractibility; egocentricity; inappropriate non–reality-based thinking

### Related Factors (r/t)

Organic brain changes (specify); changes in physical health (specify); mental illness (specify)

### Client Outcomes

#### Client Will (Specify Time Frame):

- Remain oriented to time, place, person, and circumstance; demonstrate improved cognitive function.
- Remain free from actual and potential harm by self or others.
- Perform activities of daily living (ADLs) adequately and independently.

• = Independent        ▲ = Collaborative

- Identify community resources for help after discharge.
- Understand the actions and side effects of medications.

## Nursing Interventions

- Observe for causes of altered thought processes (see Related Factors).
- Monitor, record, and report changes in client's neurological status (level of consciousness, increased intracranial pressure), mental status (memory, cognition, judgment, concentration), vital signs, laboratory results, and ability to follow commands.
- Obtain a medical history to rule out physical illness etiology for mental status changes.
- Complete a mental status examination of the client.
- Report any new onset or sudden increase in confusion.
- Adjust communication style to client. Speak slowly and calmly; use short phrases and concrete, nontechnical words; use writing if appropriate; allow time for thinking; use face-to-face communication; listen carefully; and seek clarification.
- Assess pain and promptly provide comfort measures.
- Identify and remove potentially dangerous items in the environment.
- ▲ Limit use of sedatives and drugs affecting the nervous system.
- ▲ Use soft restraints with discretion and per physician orders.
- Orient client and call client by name; introduce self on each contact; frequently mention time, date, and place; prominently display a clock and calendar that are easy to read in room and refer to them; and request family to bring in familiar pictures and articles from home.
- Provide validation of thoughts and feelings of client.
- Stay with clients if they are agitated and likely to be injured.
- Observe for therapeutic and side effects of psychotropic medications.
- Develop a therapeutic alliance to increase trust with the client.

T

• = Independent          ▲ = Collaborative

- Assess client's assault potential and maintain staff safety.
- Establish predictable care routines and maintain continuity of client's nursing staff.
- Frequently check on client and have brief interactions to prevent sensory deprivation.
- Assist client with daily hygiene as needed; encourage self-care.
- Observe for signs and symptoms of significant depression concomitant to altered thoughts.
- Provide support and education to family during client's period of cognitive change. Involve family in current care and in planning of postdischarge care, recognizing the family members' strengths and needs.
- Initiate a social service referral to find help for client following discharge.
- Observe for evidence of auditory and/or visual hallucination experiences. Teach management techniques.
- Ask empathic and direct questions such as, "What are you seeing (or hearing) now?" or "Do you sometimes hear or see things that other people don't hear or see?"
- Do not attempt to argue or change the client's beliefs. Without implying agreement, focus on feelings that accompany hallucinations and delusions rather than content of delusions (e.g., "You look frightened").
- Set limits on delusional conversations (e.g., "We discussed that; let's talk about what is happening on the unit").
- Ask for clarification when necessary.
- Help client state needs and ask for assistance.
- Involve client in short activities.
- See care plans for **Risk for self-directed Violence** and **Risk for other-directed Violence** for further nursing interventions.

### Geriatric

- Monitor for dementia, as evidenced by its gradual onset and progressive deterioration, or for delirium, as evidenced by its acute onset and generally reversible course.

• = Independent ▲ = Collaborative

- Focus on feelings associated with hallucinations and delusions rather than content.

## Multicultural

- Assess for the influence of cultural beliefs, norms, and values on the family's or caregiver's understanding of disturbed thought processes.
- Inform client's family or caregiver of the meaning of and reasons for common behaviors observed in client with disturbed thought processes.
- Validate the family members' feelings regarding the impact of client behavior on family lifestyle.

## Home Care

- The interventions described previously may be adapted for home care use.
- ▲ Assess the client for the presence of a psychiatric disorder. Refer for mental health services as indicated.
- Assess the family's knowledge of the disease process and plan of care; teach as necessary. Encourage participation.
- Identify the strengths of the caregiver and the caregiver's efforts to gain control of unpredictable situations. Help the caregiver to stay connected with a client who may be behaving differently than usual, to make life as routine as possible, to help the client set goals and sustain hope, and to allow the client space to experience progress.
- ▲ Assess the client's functional status as it relates to the ability for self-care; refer to a physician for evaluation of medication levels as indicated.
- Assess the home environment for the availability of distractions from hallucinations, such as playing music over headphones.
- ▲ If the client's condition deteriorates, seek acute medical or mental health intervention immediately, as appropriate.
- ▲ Identify an emergency plan and discuss criteria for its use with the family or caregivers.

T

• = Independent          ▲ = Collaborative

▲ Assess the client's ability to manage his or her own medications. If the client is unable, identify a responsible caregiver for medication administration. Teach the purpose, administration, and side effects of medications based on level of knowledge. Identify a plan for response to side effects if they occur.

• Assess and modify environmental stimuli that could be misinterpreted (e.g., use a night light, evaluate placement of mirrors).

• Allow the client control over aspects of his or her environment, as he or she is able. Control enhances self-esteem, although sometimes only for a short time. Refer to the care plan for **Powerlessness.**

• Identify the client's interests and skills. Provide an opportunity for the client to pursue interests and use skills without taxing the client's judgment and cognitive ability.

▲ Refer the client and family to community support groups (e.g., psychosocial rehabilitation programs for the client, National Alliance for the Mentally Ill for the client and family). Groups that include older adults with mental illness would be particularly useful.

▲ In the presence of chronic thought process disorder, institute case management of frail elderly to support continued independent living.

▲ When the client has a psychiatric disorder, pay special attention to the presence of comorbid medical conditions and the need for medical care.

▲ When the client has a psychiatric disorder, refer for psychiatric home health care services for client reassurance and implementation of a therapeutic regimen.

## Client/Family Teaching

• Teach family members reorientation techniques and about the need to frequently repeat instructions.

• Teach client distraction techniques to manage hallucinations.

• = Independent          ▲ = Collaborative

- Teach family members ways to support client without supporting delusional beliefs.
- Help family identify coping skills, environmental supports, and community services for dealing with chronically mentally ill clients.
- Discuss caregiver's need for respite. Offer support, encouragement, and information for meeting those needs.

# Impaired Tissue integrity

## NANDA Definition

Damage to mucous membrane, cornea, integumentary or subcutaneous tissues

## Defining Characteristics

Damaged or destroyed tissue (e.g., cornea, mucous membrane, integumentary or subcutaneous tissue)

## Related Factors (r/t)

Mechanical factors (e.g., pressure, shear, friction); radiation (including therapeutic radiation); nutritional deficit or excess; thermal factors (temperature extremes); knowledge deficit; chemical irritants (including body excretions, secretions, medications); impaired physical mobility; altered circulation; fluid deficit or excess

## Client Outcomes

### Client Will (Specify Time Frame):

- Report any altered sensation or pain at site of tissue impairment.
- Demonstrate understanding of plan to heal tissue and prevent injury.

• = Independent          ▲ = Collaborative

- Describe measures to protect and heal the tissue, including wound care.
- Experience a wound that decreases in size and has increased granulation tissue.

## Nursing Interventions

- Assess the site of impaired tissue integrity and determine the cause (e.g., acute or chronic wound, burn, dermatological lesion, pressure ulcer, leg ulcer).
- Determine the size and depth of the wound (e.g., full-thickness wound, stage III or stage IV pressure ulcer).
- Classify pressure ulcers in the following manner:
  - Stage III: Full-thickness skin loss involving damage to or necrosis of subcutaneous tissue that may extend down to but not through underlying fascia; ulcer appears as a deep crater with or without undermining of adjacent tissue
  - Stage IV: Full-thickness skin loss with extensive destruction; tissue necrosis; or damage to muscle, bone, or supporting structures (e.g., tendons, joint capsules)
- Monitor the site of impaired tissue integrity at least once daily for color changes, redness, swelling, warmth, pain, or other signs of infection. Determine whether the client is experiencing changes in sensation or pain. Pay special attention to all high-risk areas such as bony prominences, skin folds, sacrum, and heels. Systematic inspection can identify impending problems early.
- Monitor the status of the skin around the wound. Monitor the client's skin care practices, noting type of soap or other cleansing agents used, temperature of water, and frequency of skin cleansing.
- Monitor the client's continence status and minimize exposure of the skin impairment site and other areas to moisture from urine or stool, perspiration, or wound drainage.

T

• = Independent ▲ = Collaborative

- ▲ Refer to a continence care specialist, urologist, or gastro-enterologist for incontinence assessment.
- • Monitor for correct placement of tubes, catheters, and other devices. Assess the skin and tissue affected by the tape that secures these devices.
- • In an orthopedic client, check every 2 hours for correct placement of footboards, restraints, traction, casts, or other devices, and assess skin and tissue integrity. Be alert for symptoms of compartment syndrome (see the care plan for **Risk for Peripheral neurovascular dysfunction**).
- • For a client with limited mobility, use a risk assessment tool to systematically assess immobility-related risk factors.
- • Implement a written treatment plan for the topical treatment of the skin impairment site.
- • Identify a plan for debridement if necrotic tissue (eschar or slough) is present and if consistent with overall client management goals.
- • Select a topical treatment that maintains a moist wound-healing environment but that also allows absorption of exudate and filling of dead space. No single wound care product provides the optimal environment for healing all wounds.
- • Do not position the client on the site of impaired tissue integrity. If it is consistent with overall client management goals, turn and position the client at least every 2 hours and transfer the client carefully to avoid adverse effects of external mechanical forces (i.e., pressure, friction, and shear).
- • Evaluate for the use of specialty mattresses, beds, or devices as appropriate.
- • If the goal of care is to keep the client comfortable (e.g., for a terminally ill client), turning and repositioning may not be appropriate. Maintain the head of the bed at the lowest degree of elevation possible to reduce shear and friction, and use lift devices, pillows, foam wedges, and pressure-reducing devices in the bed.

T

• = Independent          ▲ = Collaborative

- Avoid massaging around the site of impaired tissue integrity and over bony prominences.
- Assess the client's nutritional status; refer for a nutritional consultation and/or institute use of dietary supplements.
- A comprehensive plan of care includes a thorough wound assessment, treatment interventions, support surfaces, nutritional products, adjunctive therapies, and evaluation of the outcome of care.

## Home Care

- Some of the interventions described previously may be adapted for home care use.
- Assess the client's current phase of wound healing (inflammation, proliferation, maturation) and stage of injury; initiate appropriate wound management.
- Instruct and assist the client and caregivers in understanding how to change dressings and the importance of maintaining a clean environment. Provide written instructions and observe the client or caregiver complete a dressing change.
- Initiate a consultation in a case assignment with a wound specialist or wound, ostomy, and continence nurse to establish a comprehensive plan as soon as possible. Plan case conferencing to promote optimal wound care.

## Client/Family Teaching

- Teach skin and wound assessment and ways to monitor for signs and symptoms of infection, complications, and healing. Early assessment and intervention help prevent serious problems from developing.
- Teach the client why a topical treatment has been selected. Explain wound bed changes that the caregiver can expect to see. Instruct on when the dressing needs to be changed.
- If it is consistent with overall client management goals, teach how to turn and reposition the client at least every 2 hours.

T

• = Independent          ▲ = Collaborative

• Teach the use of pillows, foam wedges, and pressure-reducing devices to prevent pressure injury.

# Ineffective Tissue perfusion (specify type: renal, cerebral, cardiopulmonary, gastrointestinal, peripheral)

## NANDA Definition

Decrease in oxygen resulting in failure to nourish tissues at capillary level

## Defining Characteristics

### Renal
Altered blood pressure outside of acceptable parameters; hematuria; oliguria or anuria; elevation in blood urea nitrogen/creatinine ratio

### Cerebral
Speech abnormalities; changes in pupillary reactions; extremity weakness or paralysis; altered mental status; difficulty in swallowing; changes in motor response; behavioral changes

### Cardiopulmonary
Altered respiratory rate outside of acceptable parameters; use of accessory muscles; capillary refill longer than 3 seconds; abnormal arterial blood gas levels; chest pain; sense of impending doom; bronchospasms; dyspnea; dysrhythmias; nasal flaring; chest retraction

### Gastrointestinal
Hypoactive or absent bowel sounds; nausea; abdominal distention; abdominal pain or tenderness

### Peripheral
Edema; positive Homans' sign; altered skin or nail characteristics (hair, moisture); weak or absent pulses; skin discolorations; skin

• = Independent          ▲ = Collaborative

temperature changes; altered sensations; diminished arterial pulsations; pale skin color upon elevation of leg with color not returning upon lowering of leg; slow healing of lesions; cold extremities; blue or purple skin color

## Related Factors (r/t)

Hypovolemia; interruption of arterial flow; hypervolemia; exchange problems; interruption of venous flow; mechanical reduction of venous and/or arterial blood flow; hypoventilation; impaired transport of oxygen across alveolar and/or capillary membrane; mismatch of ventilation with blood flow; decreased hemoglobin concentration in blood; enzyme poisoning; altered affinity of hemoglobin for oxygen

## Client Outcomes

### Client Will (Specify Time Frame):

- Demonstrate adequate tissue perfusion as evidenced by palpable peripheral pulses, warm and dry skin, adequate urinary output, and absence of respiratory distress.
- Verbalize knowledge of treatment regimen, including appropriate exercises and actions and possible side effects of medications.
- Identify changes in lifestyle that are needed to increase tissue perfusion.

## Nursing Interventions

### Cerebral Perfusion

- If the client experiences dizziness when getting up because of postural hypotension, teach methods to decrease dizziness, such as remaining seated for several minutes before standing, flexing feet upward several times while seated, rising slowly, sitting down immediately if feeling dizzy, and trying to have someone present when standing.
- ▲ Monitor neurological status; perform a neurological examination; if symptoms of a cerebrovascular accident occur (e.g., hemiparesis, hemiplegia, or dysphasia), call 911 and send the client to the emergency department.

• = Independent          ▲ = Collaborative

▲ If an ischemic stroke is present, consider keeping the head of the bed lower or flat as long as the airway is maintained, after consulting with the physician.

• See the care plans for **Decreased Intracranial adaptive capacity**, **Risk for Injury**, and **Acute Confusion**.

## Peripheral Perfusion

▲ Check the dorsalis pedis, posterior tibial, and popliteal pulses bilaterally. If unable to palpate a pulse, use a Doppler stethoscope; notify the physician immediately if new onset of pulse not present.

• Note skin color and feel the temperature of the skin.

• Check capillary refill.

• Note skin texture and the presence of hair, ulcers, or gangrenous areas on the legs or feet.

• Note the presence of edema in the extremities and rate it on a four-point scale. Measure the circumference of the ankle and calf at the same time each day in the early morning.

• Assess for pain in the extremities, noting severity, quality, timing, and exacerbating and alleviating factors. Differentiate venous from arterial disease.

## Arterial Insufficiency

▲ Monitor peripheral pulses. If there is new onset of loss of pulses concomitant with bluish, purple, or black skin discoloration and extreme pain, notify the physician immediately.

• Do not elevate the legs above the level of the heart.

▲ For early arterial insufficiency, encourage exercise such as walking or riding an exercise bicycle from 30 to 60 min/day as ordered by the physician.

• Keep the client warm and have the client wear socks and shoes or sheepskin-lined slippers when mobile. Do not apply heat to the client's feet.

▲ Pay meticulous attention to foot care. Refer to a podiatrist if the client has a foot or nail abnormality.

• If the client has ischemic arterial ulcers, see the care plan

T

● = Independent          ▲ = Collaborative

for **Impaired Tissue integrity** but avoid use of occlusive dressings.

▲ If the client smokes, aggressively counsel the client to stop smoking, refer to the physician for medications to support nicotine withdrawal, and recommend a smoking withdrawal program.

## Venous Insufficiency

• Elevate edematous leg(s) as ordered and ensure that there is no pressure under the knee(s) of the affected leg(s).

▲ Apply graduated compression stockings as ordered. Ensure proper fit by measuring accurately. Remove the stocking at least twice a day, in the morning with the bath and in the evening, to assess the condition of the extremity; then reapply.

• Encourage the client to walk while wearing compression stockings and perform toe-up and point-flex exercises.

• If the client is overweight, encourage weight loss to decrease venous disease.

• If the client has venous leg ulcers, encourage the client to avoid prolonged sitting, standing, and elevation of the involved leg.

• Discuss lifestyle with the client to determine if the client's occupation requires prolonged standing or sitting, which can result in chronic venous disease.

• Observe for signs of deep vein thrombosis, including pain, tenderness, swelling in the calf and thigh, and redness in the involved extremity. Take serial leg measurements of the thigh and calf circumferences. In some clients a tender venous cord can be felt in the popliteal fossa. Do not rely on Homans' sign.

▲ Note the results of a D-dimer test and ultrasounds.

• If deep vein thrombosis is present, observe for symptoms of a pulmonary embolism including dyspnea, tachypnea, and tachycardia, especially if there is history of trauma.

• If client is receiving heparin subcutaneously, do not change the needle after drawing up the dose.

• = Independent          ▲ = Collaborative

- If client develops deep vein thrombosis after treatment and hospital discharge, recommend that during the day the client wear below-the-knee elastic compression stockings on the involved extremity.

## Geriatric

- Change the client's position slowly when getting the client out of bed.
- Recognize that the elderly have an increased risk of developing pulmonary embolism and that, if it is present, the symptoms are nonspecific and often mimic those of heart failure or pneumonia.

## Home Care

- The interventions described previously may be adapted for home care use.
- Differentiate between arterial and venous insufficiency.
- If arterial disease is present and the client smokes, aggressively encourage smoking cessation. See the care plan for **Health-seeking behaviors.**
- Examine the client's feet carefully at frequent intervals for changes and new ulcerations.
- ▲ Assess the client's nutritional status, paying special attention to obesity, hyperlipidemia, and malnutrition. Refer to a dietitian if appropriate.
- Monitor for development of gangrene, venous ulceration, and symptoms of cellulitis (redness, pain, and increased swelling in an extremity).

## Client/Family Teaching

- Explain the importance of good foot care. Teach the client and family to wash and inspect the feet daily. Recommend that the diabetic client wear padded socks, special insoles, and jogging shoes.
- ▲ Teach the diabetic client that he or she should have a comprehensive foot examination at least annually, including assessment of sensation using the Semmes-Weinstein monofilaments. If good sensation is not pre-

T

sent, refer to a footwear professional for fitting of therapeutic shoes and inserts, the cost of which is covered
by Medicare.
- For arterial disease, stress the importance of not smoking, following a weight loss program (if the client is
obese), carefully controlling a diabetic condition, controlling hyperlipidemia and hypertension, maintaining intake of antiplatelet therapy, and reducing stress.
- Teach the client to avoid exposure to cold temperatures,
to limit exposure to brief periods if going out in cold
weather, and to wear warm clothing.
- For venous disease, teach the importance of wearing
compression stockings as ordered, elevating the legs at
intervals, and watching for skin breakdown on the legs.
- Teach the client to recognize the signs and symptoms
that should be reported to a physician (e.g., change in
skin temperature, color, or sensation; presence of a new
lesion on the foot).

NOTE: If the client is receiving anticoagulant therapy, see
the care plan for **Ineffective Protection.**

# Impaired Transfer ability

## NANDA Definition

Limitation of independent movement between two nearby surfaces

## Defining Characteristics

Impaired ability to transfer: from bed to chair and chair to bed/on
or off toilet or commode/between uneven levels/from chair to car
or car to chair/from chair to floor or floor to chair/from standing
to floor or floor to standing

## Related Factors (r/t)

Intolerance to activity; decreased strength and endurance; pain or
discomfort; perceptual or cognitive impairment; neuromuscular

• = Independent          ▲ = Collaborative

impairment; musculoskeletal impairment; depression; severe anxiety

Suggested functional level classifications may include the following:

0—Completely independent
1—Requires use of equipment or device
2—Requires help from another person for assistance, supervision, or teaching
3—Requires help from another person and equipment or device
4—Dependent: does not participate in activity

## Client Outcomes

### Client Will (Specify Time Frame):

- Transfer from bed to chair and back successfully.
- Transfer from chair to chair successfully.
- Transfer from chair to toilet and back successfully.
- Transfer from chair to car and back successfully.

## Nursing Interventions

▲ Request a consult for a physical therapist (PT) and/or occupational therapist (OT) to develop an exercise and strengthening program early in the client's recovery.
▲ Obtain a consult for a PT, OT, or orthotist to evaluate, measure, and fit the client with the proper orthoses, braces, splints, collars, and walking aids before sitting and standing clients.
▲ Ergonomically assess the client's dependence level, weight, strength, movement ability, balance, tolerance to position change, sensation, behavior, and cognition, as well as available equipment and staff ratio/experience, to decide whether to perform a manual transfer or device-assisted lift. (If PT has identified a specific transfer method and it is compatible with the nursing assessment, then use it.)
• Do not use the under-axilla method to transfer, move, or weigh a physically dependent client. Rather, use mechan-

T

• = Independent          ▲ = Collaborative

ical devices such as hydraulic or battery-operated mechanical lifts, stand-assist lifts, and bed or wheelchair ramp scales.

- Apply a gait or walking belt to a client's lower back, or under the axilla if an abdominal wound or tube is present, before transferring him or her. Keep the belt and client close to you during the transfer.
- Remind clients to comply with weight-bearing restrictions ordered by their physician.
- Assist the client to don/doff orthoses, braces, collars, prostheses, immobilizers, and abdominal binders while in bed.
- Adjust transfer surfaces so they are similar in height. For example, lower a hospital bed to equal the height of a commode.
- Help clients don shoes or socks with nonskid soles before transfers.
- Remove or swivel the wheelchair arm rests, leg rests, and footplates off to the side, especially if clients do a squat or slide board transfer.
- Place the wheelchair, commode, or shower chair at a slight angle toward the surface to which the client will be transferring.
- Teach the client to consistently lock the brakes on the wheelchair, commode, shower chair, or bed before transferring.
- Position walking aids logistically so that the client can grasp and use them once he or she is standing.
- Teach clients that when changing from a sitting to a standing position, they should place one hand on the walker and push off the surface on which they are sitting with the other hand.
- Give clear, simple instructions; allow time to process the information; and let the client do as much of the transfer as possible.
▲ Implement and document on the team plan of care the type of transfer (e.g., slide board, squat), weight-bearing status (e.g., none, partial, full), equipment (e.g., lift, walker), level of assistance (e.g., standby, moderate),

• = Independent          ▲ = Collaborative

and type of assistance to provide (e.g., manual guidance, balance control, verbal cueing).

- Incorporate set position before transferring clients (e.g., sitting on the edge of the bed/seat with bilateral weight bearing on the buttocks, hips and knees flexed, front [balls] of the feet aligned under the knees, and the head in midline).

- Recognize the normal sequence of movements for standing (e.g., hips and knees flex; back extends; trunk, head, and knees then lean well forward over the feet; the weight shifts to the feet, thus lifting up the hips and buttocks—standing occurs as the knees, hips, and trunk extend).

- Support and stabilize the client's knee(s) by placing one or both of your knees next to or encircling the client's knee(s), rather than "blocking" the client's knee(s).

  (1) Squat transfer—the client leans well forward and slightly raises flexed hips off the surface; then the client pivots and sits down on the new surface. Used for clients who have poor muscle control and slight weight-bearing ability.

  (2) Standing pivot transfer—the client leans forward with hips flexed and pushes up with hands from the seat surface or arms of the chair; then the client stands erect and pivots toward the new surface and sits down. Used for clients who have at least partial weight-bearing ability.

  (3) Slide board transfer—client should have on pants, or a pillowcase should be placed over the board. Remove arm and leg rests from the chair and slightly angle chair toward the new surface. Have client lean sideways, thus shifting his/her weight so the transfer board can be placed under the upper thigh of the leg next to the new surface. Make sure the board is safely angled across both surfaces. Instruct client to return to neutral alignment and place one hand on the board and the other hand on the seat surface. Remind the client to perform a series of push-ups with the arms while leaning forward and lifting (not

• = Independent          ▲ = Collaborative

T

sliding) the hips in small increments, with each push-up. One or more nurses may need to help the client by using the gait belt and lifting up the hips during each push-up. Used for clients who have little to no weight-bearing ability.

▲ Extra staff may be needed to transfer debilitated bariatric (extremely obese) clients. Place their beds against a corner wall and lock the brakes. Assist them to establish balance as they sit up onto the edge of the bed and help them get into the set position by placing both knees level with their thighs (feet may need to be placed up on a stool). Help or remind client to lean well forward during the transfer.

▲ Investigate and use devices and equipment to safely transfer the bariatric population. Transfer aids may include air mattress overlay, Gore-Tex or silicone transfer sheet, 60-inch-long gait belt or two regular gait belts strapped together, supine sliding or roller board, bedside sling-lift or standing-lift device, overhead ceiling-mounted lift, or overhead A-frame lift. Special equipment may include high-low chair, 1000-pound load limit manual or powered wheelchair, wide and durable commode and shower chair.

• Administer bilevel or continuous airway pressure therapy at night to bariatric clients, as ordered.

## Home Care

▲ Obtain referral for OT and PT to develop a home exercise program and safe transfer routine and to evaluate for needed modifications such as ramps, wide doorways, safe floor surfaces, grab bars, tub seats, commode, clutter elimination, adequate lighting, and proper chairs.

▲ Assess for optimal furniture placement for functional activities and maneuverability while using an assistive device, and for stability in getting up in case of a fall. Fitted bedspreads are necessary so clients do not trip over them.

▲ Involve a therapist, social worker, and/or nurse case manager to educate the client and family about assistive technology availability and costs, financial benefits, and

• = Independent          ▲ = Collaborative

regulations associated with Medicare, Medicaid, and third-party payers, as well as local community options for securing aids and home care services.

- Implement ergonomic approaches for home care staff and family to safely handle and transfer clients in their homes.
- For further information see the care plans for **Impaired physical Mobility** and **Impaired Walking.**

## Client/Family Teaching

▲ Begin discharge planning as soon as possible with a case manager or social worker to assess the need for home care services.

- Assess client and family readiness to learn and use teaching modalities conducive to their personal learning styles.

▲ Coordinate with therapists to reinforce client and family education on safe and effective transfer methods; application and skin checks associated with devices such as braces, splints, and immobilizers; and proper fit, use, and care of transfer devices.

- Schedule supervised practice sessions accordingly, where client and family use gait belts, do the specified transfer, or return demonstrate proper use of lifts or other devices.
- Teach, model, and then monitor client's and family's consistent performance of safety precautions for transfers, including, for example, wearing proper shoes, placing equipment and chairs correctly, locking brakes, and swiveling leg rests out of the way.

▲ Teach the client and family how to check brakes on chairs to make sure they engage and how to check wheelchair tires for adequate air pressure. Recommend routine inspection and annual tune-up of the wheelchair.

▲ Offer information on safe use of shower and commode chairs to prevent serious complications such as discomfort, pressure ulcers, falls during transfer or transport, and inaccessibility for bowel care and hygiene (bowel care may take 30 minutes to 3 hours for persons with neurogenic bowel).

• = Independent          ▲ = Collaborative

- For further information, see the care plans for **Impaired physical Mobility** and **Impaired Walking.**

# Risk for Trauma

## NANDA Definition

Accentuated risk of accidental tissue injury (e.g., wound, burn, fracture)

## Risk Factors

### External

High-crime neighborhood and client vulnerability; pot handles facing toward front of stove; knives stored uncovered; inappropriate call-for-aid mechanisms for bed-resting client; inadequately stored combustibles or corrosives (e.g., matches, oily rags, lye); highly flammable children's toys or clothing; obstructed passageways; high beds; large icicles hanging from roof; nonuse or misuse of seat restraints; overexposure to sun, sunlamps, or radiotherapy; overloaded electrical outlets; overloaded fuse boxes; play or work near vehicle pathways (e.g., driveways, lane ways, railroad tracks); playing with fireworks or gunpowder; unlocked storage of guns or ammunition; contact with rapidly moving machinery, industrial belts, or pulleys; litter or liquid spills on floors or stairways; defective appliances; bathing in very hot water (e.g., unsupervised bathing of young children); bathtub without hand grip or antislip equipment; children playing with matches, candles, cigarettes, or sharp-edged toys; children playing at top of stairs without gates; children riding in front seat of car; delayed lighting of gas burner or oven; contact with intense cold; collection of grease waste on stove; operation of mechanically unsafe vehicle; driving after use of alcoholic beverages or drugs; driving at excessive speeds; entry into unlighted rooms; experimentation with chemicals or gasoline; exposure to dangerous machinery; faulty electrical plugs; frayed wires; contact with acids or alkalis;

• = Independent          ▲ = Collaborative

unsturdy or absent stair rails; use of unsteady ladders or chairs; use of cracked dishware or glasses; wearing of plastic apron or flowing clothes around open flame; lack of screening on fires or heaters; unsafe window protection in homes with young children; sliding on coarse bed linen or struggling within bed restraints; use of thin or worn potholders; unanchored electric wires; misuse of necessary headgear for motor cyclists or young children carried on adult bicycles; gas leaks; unsafe road or road-crossing conditions; slippery floors (e.g., wet or highly waxed); smoking in bed or near oxygen-delivery system; snow or ice on stairs or walkways; unanchored rugs; driving without necessary visual aids

## Internal

Lack of safety education; insufficient finances to purchase safety equipment or effect repairs; history of trauma; lack of safety precautions; poor vision; reduced temperature and/or tactile sensation; balancing difficulties; cognitive or emotional difficulties; reduced large or small muscle coordination; weakness; reduced hand-eye coordination

## Related Factors (r/t)

See Risk Factors.

## Client Outcomes

### Client Will (Specify Time Frame):

- Remain free from trauma.
- Explain actions that can be taken to prevent trauma.

## Nursing Interventions

- Screen clients using a fall risk factor assessment tool to identify those at risk for falls.
- Provide vision aids for visually impaired clients.
- Assist the client with ambulation.
- Have a family member evaluate water temperature for the client.
- Assess the client for causes of impaired cognition.

• = Independent         ▲ = Collaborative

- Keep walkways clear of snow, debris, and household items.
- Provide assistive devices in bathrooms (e.g., handrails, nonslip decals on the floor of the shower and bathtub).
- Ensure that call-light systems are functioning and that the client is able to use them.
- Use a night light after dark.
- Teach the client to observe safety precautions in high-crime neighborhoods (e.g., lock doors, do not leave home at night without a companion, keep entryways well lighted).
▲ Instruct the client not to drive under the influence of alcohol or drugs. Assess for a substance abuse problem and refer to appropriate resources for drug and alcohol education.
- Review drug profile for potential side effects that may inhibit performance of ADLs.
- See Nursing Interventions in the care plans for **Risk for Aspiration, Impaired Home maintenance, Risk for Injury, Risk for Poisoning,** and **Risk for Suffocation.**

## Pediatric

- Assess the client's socioeconomic status.
- Never leave young children unsupervised around water or cooking areas.
- Keep flammable and potentially flammable articles out of the reach of young children.
- Lock up harmful objects such as guns.

## Geriatric

- Assess the geriatric client's level of functioning both at admission and periodically.
- Perform a home safety assessment and recommend the following preventive measures: keep electrical cords out of the flow of traffic; remove small rugs or make sure they are slip resistant; increase lighting in hallways and other dark areas; place a light in the bathroom; keep towels, curtains, and other items that might catch fire away

• = Independent          ▲ = Collaborative

from the stove; store harmful products away from food products; provide at least one grab bar in tubs and showers; check prescribed medications for appropriate labels; store medications in original containers or in a dispenser of some type (e.g., egg carton, seven-day plastic dispenser); if the client cannot administer medications according to directions, secure someone to administer medications.

- Mark stove knobs with bright colors (yellow or red), and outline the borders of steps.
- Discourage driving at night.
- Encourage the client to participate in resistance and impact exercise programs as tolerated.
- Implement fall and injury prevention strategies in residential care facilities.

## Client/Family Teaching

- Educate the family regarding age-appropriate child safety precautions, environmental safety precautions, and intervention in an emergency.
- Teach the family to assess the childcare provider's knowledge regarding child safety, environmental safety precautions, and assistance of a child in an emergency.
- Educate the client and family regarding helmet use during recreation and sports activities.
- Encourage the use of proper car seats and safety belts.
- Teach how to plan safe prom and graduation parties.
- Teach parents the importance of monitoring youths after school.
- Teach firearm safety. Encourage the family to keep firearms and ammunition in locked storage.
- Educate that the use of psychotropic medications may increase the risk of falls and that withdrawal of psychotropic medications should be considered.
- For further information, see the care plans for **Risk for Aspiration, Impaired Home maintenance, Risk for Injury, Risk for Poisoning,** and **Risk for Suffocation.**

T

• = Independent          ▲ = Collaborative

# Readiness for enhanced Urinary elimination

## NANDA Definition

A pattern of urinary functions that is sufficient for meeting eliminatory needs and can be strengthened

## Defining Characteristics

Expresses willingness to enhance urinary elimination; urine is straw colored with no odor; specific gravity is within normal limits; amount of output is within normal limits for age and other factors; positions self for emptying of bladder; fluid intake is adequate for daily needs

## Client Outcomes

### Client Will (Specify Time Frame):

- Eliminate or reduce incontinent episodes.
- Recognize sensory stimulus indicating readiness for urine elimination.
- Respond to prompts for toileting.

## Nursing Interventions

- Assess the client for readiness for improving urine elimination patterns, focusing on need for physical assistance to access toilet and cognitive awareness of sensations indicating readiness for urine elimination and current continence status (bladder management strategy, frequency of incontinent episodes).
- Complete a bladder diary of diurnal and nocturnal urine elimination patterns and patterns of urinary leakage.
- Begin a scheduled toileting program (usually every 2 to 3 hours) for the client who is normally continent (recognizes cues to toilet and expresses readiness to toilet) but requires physical assistance to access the toilet.
- Remove environmental barriers to toilet access.
- Provide a urinal or bedside toilet as indicated.
- Assist client to remove clothing, transfer to the toilet, cleanse the perineal skin, and redress as indicated.

U

• = Independent      ▲ = Collaborative

- Ensure that toileting opportunities are offered both during daytime hours and during hours of sleep.
- For the client experiencing urinary incontinence who has mild cognitive deficits, begin a prompted voiding program or patterned urge response toileting program. Begin a prompted toileting program based on the results of a bladder log over a period of 2 to 3 days, using a check and change system as indicated.
- Approach the client and briefly explain that it is time to toilet.
  - Assist the client to the toilet, provide assistance removing clothing and urine-containment devices (pads or adult urine-containment briefs), and check for urinary leakage since the last scheduled toileting.
  - Praise the client when toileting occurs with prompting.
  - If the client does not toilet or has evidence of an incontinence episode, refrain from praise, gently inform the client of the urine loss, remove and replace the soiled containment device, and assist the client to redress and rejoin activities or return to bed.
- Institute regular use of incontinence-containment devices combined with routine perineal skin care for the client with severe cognitive impairment, significant functional impairment, or no reduction in urinary incontinence frequency or severity with a scheduled or prompted toileting program. (Refer to care plan for **Total urinary Incontinence**.)

# Impaired Urinary elimination

## NANDA Definition

Disturbance in urine elimination
NOTE: This broad diagnosis may be used to describe many dysfunctional voiding conditions. Refer to care plans for **Functional urinary Incontinence, Reflex urinary Incontinence,**

• = Independent          ▲ = Collaborative

**Stress urinary Incontinence, Total urinary Incontinence, Urge urinary Incontinence,** and **Urinary retention** for information on these more specific diagnoses.

## Defining Characteristics

The term *lower urinary tract symptoms* (LUTS) is now used to describe the variety of complaints associated with disorders of bladder filling/storage or altered patterns of urine elimination. Bothersome bladder filling/storage symptoms include diurnal frequency (voiding more than every 2 hours), infrequent urination (voiding less than every 6 hours), and nocturia (arising from sleep more than twice to urinate). Our understanding of the physiological desire is incomplete, but the term urgency has been defined as "a sudden and strong desire to urinate that is not easily deferred." Lower urinary tract pain may present as dysuria (pain associated with micturition), burning, pressure, or cramping discomfort during bladder filling and storage. Voiding symptoms may include reduced force of the urinary stream, intermittency, hesitancy, and the need to strain to evacuate the bladder. Other voiding symptoms are postvoid dribbling, feelings of incomplete bladder emptying, or the total inability to urinate (acute urinary retention).

Urinary incontinence is the uncontrolled loss of urine of sufficient magnitude to constitute a problem for the client, family, or caregivers. Stress urinary incontinence is the loss of urine with physical exertion. Urge urinary incontinence is the loss of urine associated with overactive detrusor contractions and a precipitous desire to urinate. It is part of a larger symptom syndrome called overactive bladder. The overactive bladder is characterized by bothersome urgency and typically associated with frequent daytime voiding and nocturia. Approximately 37% of patients with overactive bladder dysfunction experience urge urinary incontinence.

Reflex urinary incontinence is urine loss associated with neurogenic detrusor overactivity, diminished or absent sensations of bladder filling, and dyssynergia between the detrusor and striated urethral sphincter muscles. Functional urinary incontinence is urine loss associated with deficits of mobility, dexterity, cognition, or environmental barriers to timely toileting. Urine

• = Independent          ▲ = Collaborative

loss from an extraurethral source can be defined as total incontinence, and urinary retention is the condition where the client is unable to completely evacuate urine from the bladder despite micturition. Chronic urinary retention is defined as the inability to completely evacuate urine from the bladder after voiding, and acute urinary retention is the inability to urinate.

### Related Factors (r/t)

Bothersome lower urinary tract symptoms (urological disorders, neurological lesions, gynecological conditions, dysfunction of bowel elimination); incontinence (refer to specific diagnosis); urinary retention (refer to specific diagnosis); acute urinary retention (refer to care plan for **Urinary retention**).

### Client Outcomes

**Client Will (Specify Time Frame):**

- Demonstrate diurnal frequency no more than every 2 hours.
- Demonstrate nocturia 2 times or less per night.
- Be able to postpone voiding until toileting facility is accessed and clothing is removed.
- Be able to perceive and recognize cues for toileting, move to toilet or use urinal or portable toileting apparatus, and remove clothing as necessary for toileting.
- Demonstrate postvoiding residual volumes less than 150–200 mL or 25% of total bladder capacity.
- State absence of pain or excessive urgency during bladder storage or during urination.

### Nursing Interventions

- Routinely screen all adult women and aging men for urinary incontinence or lower urinary tract symptoms including bothersome urgency.
- Assess bladder function using the following techniques:
  - Take a focused history including duration of bothersome LUTS, characteristics of symptoms, patterns of diurnal and nocturnal urination, frequency and volume of urine loss, alleviating and aggravating factors, and exploration of possible causative factors.

U

• = Independent          ▲ = Collaborative

- Perform a focused physical assessment of perineal skin integrity, evaluation of the vaginal vault, evaluation of urethral hypermobility, and neurological evaluation including bulbocavernosus reflex and perineal sensations.
- Review results of urinalysis for the presence of urinary infection, polyuria, hematuria, proteinuria, and other abnormalities, or obtain urine for analysis.

- Complete a more detailed assessment on selected clients including a bladder log and functional/cognitive assessment. (Refer to care plans for **Functional urinary Incontinence, Reflex urinary Incontinence, Stress urinary Incontinence, Total urinary Incontinence,** and **Urge urinary Incontinence.**)
- Assess the client for urinary retention. (Refer to care plan for **Urinary retention.**)
- Teach the client general guidelines for bladder health:
  - Clients should avoid dehydration and its irritative effects on the bladder; fluid consumption for the ambulatory, normally active adult should be approximately 30 mL/kg of body weight (0.5 oz/lb/day).
  - Clients with storage lower urinary tract symptoms, overactive bladder dysfunction, or urinary incontinence should reduce or eliminate caffeine intake.
  - Clients with lower urinary tract pain or interstitial cystitis should be encouraged to eliminate multiple potential bladder irritants including caffeine, alcohol, aspartame, carbonated beverages, alcohol, citrus juices, chocolate, vinegar, and highly spiced foods such as those flavored with curries or peppers. These foods should be reintroduced singly to the diet to determine their effect (if any) on bothersome lower urinary tract symptoms.
  - All clients should be counseled about measures to alleviate or prevent constipation including adequate consumption of dietary fluids and dietary fiber, exercise, and regular bowel elimination patterns.
  - All clients should be strongly advised to stop smoking.

• = Independent    ▲ = Collaborative

▲ Consult the physician for culture and sensitivity testing and antibiotic treatment in the individual with evidence of a urinary infection.

▲ Refer client with chronic lower urinary tract pain to a urologist or specialist in the management of pelvic pain.

▲ Teach the client to recognize symptoms of urinary tract infection (dysuria that crescendos as the bladder nears complete evacuation; urgency to urinate followed by micturition of only a few drops; suprapubic aching discomfort; malaise; voiding frequency; sudden exacerbation of urinary incontinence with or without fever, chills, and flank pain).

▲ Teach the client to recognize and to seek help promptly if hematuria occurs.

▲ Assist the individual with urinary leakage to select a product that adequately contains urine, avoids soiling clothing, is not apparent when worn under clothing, and protects the underlying skin. (Refer to care plan for **Total urinary Incontinence.**)

▲ Teach perineal care including judicious use of soaps and use of vaginal douches only under special circumstances. (Refer to care plan for **Total urinary Incontinence.**)

## Geriatric

• Provide an environment that encourages toileting for the elderly client cared for in the home or in acute care, long-term care, or critical care units.

• Encourage elderly women to drink at least 10 oz of cranberry juice daily, regularly consume one to two servings of fresh blueberries, or supplement the diet with cranberry concentrate capsules (usually taken in 500-mg doses with each meal).

## Client/Family Teaching

• Provide all clients with the basic principles for optimal bladder function.

• Teach the community and health care providers that uri-

U

● = Independent      ▲ = Collaborative

nary incontinence is not a normal part of aging and that incontinence can be corrected or managed with proper evaluation and care.

- Provide information to health care providers and the community about the signs, symptoms, and management of urinary tract infections and interstitial cystitis.
- Teach all persons the signs and symptoms of urinary tract infection and its management.
- Teach all persons to recognize hematuria and to promptly seek care if this symptom occurs.

# Urinary retention

## NANDA Definition

Incomplete emptying of the bladder

## Defining Characteristics

Measured urinary residual greater than 150 to 200 mL or 25% of total bladder capacity; obstructive lower urinary tract symptoms (poor force of stream, intermittency of stream, hesitancy of urination, postvoid dribbling, feelings of incomplete bladder emptying); often accompanied by storage lower urinary tract symptoms (urgency, day and nighttime voiding frequency); occasionally accompanied by overflow incontinence (dribbling urine loss caused when intravesical pressure overwhelms the sphincter mechanism)

## Related Factors (r/t)

Bladder outlet obstruction (benign prostatic hyperplasia, prostate cancer, prostatitis, acute prostatic congestion and inflammation following implantation of irradiated seeds, urethral stricture, bladder neck dyssynergia, bladder neck contracture, detrusor striated sphincter dyssynergia, pseudo-dyssynergia or high tone pelvic floor muscle dysfunction, obstructing cystocele or urethral distortion, urethral tumor, urethral polyp, posterior urethral valves, postoperative complication); deficient detrusor contraction strength (sacral level spinal lesions, cauda equina syndrome, peripheral polyneuropathies, herpes zoster or simplex affecting sacral nerve roots, injury or extensive surgery causing denervation of pelvic plexus, medication side effect, complication of illicit drug use, impaction of stool)

## Client Outcomes

### Client Will (Specify Time Frame):

- Demonstrate a consistent ability to urinate when desire to void is perceived or via a timed schedule; have a measured urinary residual volume less than 150 to 200 mL or 25% of total bladder capacity (voided volume plus urinary residual volume).
- Experience correction or relief from obstructive symptoms.
- Experience correction or alleviation of irritative symptoms.
- Be free of upper urinary tract distress (renal function remains sufficient; febrile urinary infections are absent).

## Nursing Interventions

- Obtain a focused urinary history emphasizing the character and duration of lower urinary symptoms. Query the client about episodes of acute urinary retention (complete inability to void) or chronic retention (documented elevated postvoid residual volumes).
- Question the client concerning specific risk factors for urinary retention including:
  - Disorders affecting the sacral spinal cord such as spinal cord injuries of vertebral levels T12 to L2, disk problems, cauda equina syndrome, tabes dorsalis
  - Acute neurological injury causing sudden loss of mobility such as spinal shock or ischemic stroke
  - Metabolic disorders such as diabetes mellitus, chronic alcoholism, and related conditions associated with polyuria and peripheral polyneuropathies
  - Herpetic infection involving the sacral skin and underlying spinal dermatomes
  - Heavy-metal poisoning (lead, mercury) causing peripheral polyneuropathies

U

• = Independent          ▲ = Collaborative

- Advanced stage HIV
- Medications including antispasmodics/parasympatholytics, alpha-adrenergic agonists, antidepressants, sedatives, narcotics, psychotropic medications, illicit drugs
- Recent surgery requiring general or spinal anesthesia
- Bowel elimination patterns, history of fecal impaction, encopresis
- Current or recent surgical procedures

▲ Perform a focused physical assessment or review results of a recent physical including perineal skin integrity; inspection, percussion, and palpation of the lower abdomen for obvious bladder distention; a neurological examination including perineal skin sensation and the bulbocavernosus reflex; and vaginal vault examination in women and digital rectal examination in men.

▲ Determine the urinary residual volume by catheterizing the client immediately after urination or by obtaining a bladder ultrasound after micturition.

· Complete a bladder log including patterns of urine elimination, urine loss (if present), nocturia, and volume and type of fluids consumed for a period of 3 to 7 days.

▲ Consult with the physician concerning eliminating or altering medications suspected of producing or exacerbating urinary retention.

· Teach the client with mild to moderate obstructive symptoms to double void by urinating, resting in the bathroom for 3 to 5 minutes, and then trying again to urinate.

· Teach the client with urinary retention and infrequent voiding to urinate by the clock.

· Advise the male client with urinary retention related to benign prostatic hyperplasia (BPH) to avoid risk factors associated with acute urinary retention as follows:

- Avoid over-the-counter cold remedies containing a decongestant (alpha-adrenergic agonists).
- Avoid taking over-the-counter dietary medications (frequently contain alpha-adrenergic agonists).

U

● = Independent          ▲ = Collaborative

- Discuss voiding problems with a health care provider before beginning new prescription medications.
- After prolonged exposure to cool weather, warm the body before attempting to urinate.
- Avoid overfilling the bladder by adopting regular urination patterns and refraining from excessive intake of alcohol.

- Teach the elderly male client with BPH to self-administer a 5α-reductase inhibitor such as finasteride or dutasteride or an alpha-adrenergic–blocking agent such as tamsulosin, alfuzosin, doxazosin, or terazosin as directed. Provide careful instructions concerning the dosage, administration schedule, and side effects of these drugs including possible adverse side effects (postural hypotension) when multiple doses are inadvertently missed.

- Teach the client who is unable to void specific strategies to manage this potential medical emergency as follows:
  - Attempt urination in complete privacy.
  - Place the feet solidly on the floor.
  - If unable to void using these strategies, take a warm sitz bath or shower and void (if possible) while still in the tub or shower.
  - Drink a warm cup of coffee or tea to stimulate the bladder, which may promote voiding.
  - If unable to void within 6 hours or if bladder distention is producing significant pain, seek urgent or emergency care.

▲ Remove the indwelling urethral catheter at midnight in the hospitalized client to reduce the risk of acute urinary retention.

▲ Consult the physician about bladder stimulation in the client with urinary retention caused by deficient detrusor contraction strength.

▲ Teach the client with significant urinary retention to perform self-intermittent catheterization as directed.

- Advise clients who undergo intermittent catheterization that bacteria are likely to colonize the urine but that this condition does not indicate a clinically significant urinary tract infection.

U

• = Independent          ▲ = Collaborative

- For the individual with urinary retention who is not a suitable candidate for intermittent catheterization, insert an indwelling catheter.
- Advise clients with indwelling catheters that the presence of bacteria in the urine is an almost universal finding after the catheter has remained in place for a period of 30 days or longer and that only symptomatic infections warrant treatment.
- Employ the following strategies to reduce the risk for catheter-associated urinary tract infection whenever feasible:
  - Insert a silver-impregnated catheter for short-term indwelling catheterization (less than 30 days).
  - Maintain a closed drainage system whenever feasible.
  - Change the catheter every 4 to 6 weeks whenever possible; more frequent catheter changes should be reserved for patients who experience catheter encrustation and blockage.
  - Patients with a catheter-associated urinary tract infection who are managed in an acute care or long-term care facility should be placed in a separate room from patients who have an indwelling catheter to reduce the risk of spreading the offending pathogen.
  - Educate staff about the risks of catheter-associated urinary tract infection and specific strategies to reduce this risk.

### Geriatric

- Aggressively assess elderly clients, particularly those with dribbling urinary incontinence, urinary tract infections, and related conditions for urinary retention.
- Assess elderly clients for impaction when urinary retention is documented or suspected.
- Assess elderly male clients for retention related to BPH or prostate cancer.

### Home Care

- The interventions listed previously may be adapted for home care use.

• = Independent          ▲ = Collaborative

- Encourage the client to report any inability to void.
▲ Maintain an up-to-date medication list; evaluate side-effect profiles for risk of urinary retention.
▲ Refer the client for physician evaluation if there is a new occurrence of urinary retention.

## Client/Family Teaching

- Teach techniques for intermittent catheterization including use of a clean rather than a sterile technique, use of soap and water or a microwave technique to wash the catheter, and reuse of the catheter.
- Teach the client with an indwelling catheter to assess the tube for patency, maintain the drainage system below the level of the symphysis pubis, and routinely cleanse the bedside bag.
- Teach the client with an indwelling catheter or undergoing intermittent catheterization the symptoms of a significant urinary infection including hematuria, acute-onset incontinence, dysuria, flank pain, or fever.

# Impaired spontaneous Ventilation

## NANDA Definition

Decreased energy reserves resulting in an individual's inability to maintain breathing adequate for supporting life

## Defining Characteristics

Dyspnea; increased metabolic rate; increased heart rate, decreased $Po_2$, increased $Pco_2$, decreased $Sao_2$; increased restlessness; apprehension; increased use of accessory muscles; decreased tidal volume; decreased cooperation

## Related Factors (r/t)

Metabolic factors; respiratory muscle fatigue

• = Independent          ▲ = Collaborative

## Client Outcomes

### Client Will (Specify Time Frame):

- Maintain arterial blood gases within safe parameters.
- Remain free of dyspnea or restlessness.
- Effectively maintain airway.
- Effectively mobilize secretions.

## Nursing Interventions

- ▲ Collaborate with the client, family, and physician regarding possible intubation and ventilation. Determine whether the client has advanced directives and, if so, integrate them into the plan of care in conjunction with clinical data regarding overall health and reversibility of the medical condition.
- • Assess and respond to changes in the client's respiratory status. Monitor the client for dyspnea, increasing respiratory rate, use of accessory muscles, intercostal retractions, flaring of nostrils, and subjective complaints.
- • Have the client use a numerical scale (0 to 10) to rate dyspnea before and after interventions.
- • Assess for history of chronic respiratory disorders when administering oxygen. With chronic obstructive pulmonary disease (COPD), the respiratory drive is primarily in response to hypoxia, not hypercarbia; oxygenating too aggressively can result in respiratory depression.
- ▲ Collaborate with the physician and respiratory therapists in determining the appropriateness of noninvasive positive pressure ventilation (NPPV) for the decompensated client with COPD.
- ▲ Assist with implementation, client support, and monitoring if NPPV is used.
- ▲ If the client has apnea, pH <7.25, $Paco_2$ >50 mm Hg, $Pao_2$ <50 mm Hg, respiratory muscle fatigue, or somnolence, prepare the client for intubation and placement on a ventilator.

### Ventilator Support

- ▲ Explain the intubation intervention to the client and

**V**

• = Independent          ▲ = Collaborative

family as appropriate and, during the procedure, administer sedation for client comfort according to the physician's orders.

▲ Secure the endotracheal tube in place using either tape or a device, auscultate bilateral breath sounds, use a $CO_2$ detector, and obtain a chest x-ray to confirm endotracheal tube placement.

▲ Suction as needed, and hyperoxygenate and hyperventilate according to policy. Refer to care plan for **Ineffective Airway clearance** for further information on suctioning.

• Ensure activation of all monitor alarms for each nursing shift.

• Respond to ventilator alarms promptly. If unable to rapidly locate the source of alarm, use a manual self-inflating resuscitation bag to ventilate the client while waiting for assistance.

• Prevent unplanned extubation by maintaining stability of endotracheal tube and using soft wrist restraints on the client if needed and ordered.

• Drain collected fluid from condensation out of ventilator tubing as needed.

• Note ventilator settings of flow of inspired oxygen, peak inspiratory pressure, tidal volume, and alarm activation at intervals and when removing the client from the ventilator for any reason.

▲ Administer analgesics and sedatives as needed with a defined protocol to facilitate client comfort and rest. Use pain and sedation scales to provide a consistent way of monitoring sedation levels and ensuring that therapeutic outcomes are being met.

• To decrease anxiety use music therapy with selections of client's choice played on headphones at intervals.

▲ Analyze and respond to arterial blood gas results, end-tidal $CO_2$ levels, and pulse oximetry values.

• Use an effective means of communication with the client. Use nonverbal communication, an electronic voice output communication aid, an alphabet board, a picture board, a computer, or a writing slate. Ask the client for

V

input into care as able. Ensure client's human rights are met.
- Move the endotracheal tube from side to side every 24 hours, and tape or secure it with a device. Assess and document client's skin condition, and ensure correct tube placement at lip line.
- Provide oral care every 4 hours and as needed.
▲ Use endotracheal tubes that allow for the continuous aspiration of subglottic secretions (CASS) (if available).
- Position the client in a semirecumbent position with the head of the bed at a 45-degree angle to decrease the aspiration of gastric secretions.
- Turn the client from side to side every 2 hours or more often if possible. Use rotational bed therapy in patients for whom side-to-side turning is contraindicated or difficult.
- Assess bilateral anterior and posterior breath sounds every 2 to 4 hours and as needed; respond to any relevant changes.
- Assess responsiveness to ventilator support; monitor for subjective complaints and sensation of dyspnea.
- Collaborate with the interdisciplinary team in treating patients with acute respiratory failure.

**Geriatric**
- Recognize that elderly have a high rate of morbidity when mechanically ventilated.

**Home Care**
▲ Some of the interventions listed previously may be adapted for home care use. Begin discharge planning as soon as possible with the case manager or social worker to assess the need for home support systems, assistive devices, and community or home health services.
▲ With help from a medical social worker, assist the client and family to determine the fiscal impact of home care versus an extended care facility.
- Assess the home setting during the discharge process to

• = Independent        ▲ = Collaborative

ensure the home can safely accommodate ventilator support (e.g., adequate space and electricity).

- Have the family contact the electric company and place the client residence on a high-risk list in case of a power outage.
- Assess the caregivers for commitment to support a ventilator-dependent client in the home.
- Be sure that the client and family or caregivers are familiar with operation of all ventilation devices, know how to suction if needed, are competent in doing tracheostomy care, and know schedules for cleaning equipment. Have the designated caregiver or caregivers demonstrate care before discharge.
- Assess client and caregiver knowledge of the disease, client needs, and medications to be administered via ventilation-assistive devices. Avoid analgesics. Assess knowledge of how to use equipment. Teach as necessary.
- Establish an emergency plan and criteria for use. Identify emergency procedures to be used until medical assistance arrives. Teach and role-play emergency care.
- ▲ Institute case management of frail elderly clients to support continued independent living.

## Client/Family Teaching

- Explain to the client the potential sensations that will be experienced including relief of dyspnea, the feeling of lung inflations, the noise of the ventilator, and the reality of alarms.
- Explain to the client and family about being unable to speak, and work out an alternative system of communication. See previous intervention.
- Demonstrate to the family how to perform simple procedures such as suctioning the mouth with a tonsil-tip catheter, providing range-of-motion exercises, and reconnecting the ventilator immediately if it becomes disconnected.
- Offer both the client and family explanations of how the ventilator works and answer any questions asked.

• = Independent          ▲ = Collaborative

## Dysfunctional Ventilatory weaning response

### NANDA Definition

Inability to adjust to lowered levels of mechanical ventilator support that interrupts and prolongs the weaning process

### Defining Characteristics

#### Severe

Deterioration in arterial blood gases from current baseline; significant increase in respiratory rate from baseline; increase in baseline blood pressure (20 mm Hg); agitation; increase in baseline heart rate (20 beats/min); paradoxical abdominal breathing; adventitious breath sounds, audible airway secretions; cyanosis; decreased level of consciousness; full respiratory accessory muscle use; shallow, gasping breaths; profuse diaphoresis; breathing uncoordinated with the ventilator

#### Moderate

Slight increase in baseline blood pressure (<20 mm Hg); baseline increase in respiratory rate (<5 breaths/min); slight increase in baseline heart rate (<20 beats/min); pale, slight cyanosis; slight respiratory accessory muscle use; inability to respond to coaching; inability to cooperate; apprehension; changes in skin color; decreased air entry on auscultation; diaphoresis; eye widening, wide-eyed look; hypervigilance to activities

#### Mild

Warmth; restlessness; slight increase of respiratory rate from baseline; queries about possible machine malfunction; expressed feelings of increased need for oxygen; fatigue; increased concentration on breathing

### Related Factors (r/t)

#### Physiological

Ineffective airway clearance; sleep pattern disturbance; inadequate nutrition; uncontrolled pain or discomfort

V

## Psychological

Knowledge deficit of the weaning process and client role; perceived inefficacy about the ability to wean; decreased motivation; decreased self-esteem; moderate or severe anxiety or fear; hopelessness; powerlessness; insufficient trust in nurse

## Situational

Uncontrolled episodic energy demands or problems; inappropriate pacing of diminished ventilator support; inadequate social support; adverse environment (e.g., noise, activity, negative events in the room); low nurse-client ratio; extended nurse absence from bedside; unfamiliar nursing staff; history of ventilator dependence for >4 days to 1 week; history of multiple unsuccessful weaning attempts

## Client Outcomes

### Client Will (Specify Time Frame):

- Wean from ventilator with adequate arterial blood gases.
- Remain free of unresolved dyspnea or restlessness.
- Effectively clear secretions.

## Nursing Interventions

- Assess client's readiness for weaning as evidenced by the following:
  - Physiological readiness
    - Resolution of initial medical problem that led to ventilator dependence
    - Hemodynamic stability
    - Normal hemoglobin levels
    - Absence of fever
    - Normal state of consciousness
    - Metabolic, fluid, and electrolyte balance
    - Adequate nutritional status with serum albumin levels >2.5 g/dl
    - Adequate sleep
  - Psychological readiness—There has been little re-

V

• = Independent          ▲ = Collaborative

search devoted to the study of psychological readiness to wean.

- For best results ensure that the client is in an optimal physiological and psychological state before introducing the stress of weaning.
- Use evidence-based weaning protocol if available.
- Identify reasons for previous unsuccessful weaning attempts, and include that information in development of the weaning plan.
▲ Collaborate with an interdisciplinary team (physician, nurse, respiratory therapist, physical therapist, and dietitian) to develop a weaning plan with a timeline and goals; revise this plan throughout the weaning period.
- Use a communication device such as a weaning board or flow sheet.
- Assist client to identify personal strategies that result in relaxation and comfort (e.g., music, visualization, relaxation techniques, reading, television, family visits). Support implementation of these strategies.
- Provide a safe and comfortable environment. Stay with the client during weaning if at all possible. If unable to stay, make the call light button readily available, and assure the client that needs will be met responsively.
▲ Coordinate pain and sedation medications to minimize sedative effects.
- Schedule weaning periods for the time of day when the client is most rested. Cluster care activities to promote successful weaning. Avoid other procedures during weaning: keep the environment quiet and promote restful activities between weaning periods.
- Promote a normal sleep-wake cycle, allowing uninterrupted periods of nighttime sleep.
- During weaning, monitor the client's physiological and psychological responses; acknowledge and respond to fears and subjective complaints. Validate that the client is doing the work of weaning.
- Monitor subjective and objective data (breath sounds, respiratory pattern, respiratory effort, heart rate, blood

V

• = Independent          ▲ = Collaborative

pressure, oxygen saturation per oximetry, amount and type of secretions, anxiety, and energy level) throughout weaning to determine client tolerance and responses.

- Coach the client through episodes of increased anxiety. Remain with client or place a supportive and calm significant other in this role. Give positive reinforcement, and with permission use touch to communicate support and concern.
- Terminate weaning when the client demonstrates predetermined criteria or when the following signs of weaning intolerance occur:
  - Tachypnea, dyspnea, or chest and abdominal asynchrony
  - Agitation or mental status changes
  - Decreased oxygen saturation: $Sao_2$ <90%
  - Increased or decreased pulse rate or blood pressure or presence of new onset of dysrhythmias
- ▲ If the dysfunctional weaning response is severe, consider slowing weaning to brief increments of time (e.g., 5 minutes). Continue to collaborate with the team to determine whether an untreated physiological cause for the dysfunctional weaning pattern remains. Consider an alternative care setting (subacute, rehabilitation facility, home) for clients with prolonged ventilator dependence as a strategy that can positively affect outcomes.

### Geriatric
- Recognize that older clients may require longer periods of time to wean.

### Home Care
NOTE: Weaning from a ventilator at home should be based on client stability and comfort of the client and caregivers under an intermittent care plan. The client and/or family may be more comfortable having the client rehospitalized for the process.

- Assess comfort and coping ability of the client and/or

family to wean at home, as well as fiscal implications and home care coverage.

- Establish an emergency plan and methods of implementation. Include emergency aeration and reestablishment of the ventilation-assistive device.
- ▲ Obtain orders for alternative routes of medication administration when medications have been administered via a ventilation device. Instruct the client and family in changes.

# Risk for other-directed Violence

## NANDA Definition

At risk for behaviors in which an individual demonstrates that he or she can be physically, emotionally, and/or sexually harmful to others

## Risk Factors

Body language (e.g., rigid posture, clenching of fists and jaw, hyperactivity, pacing, breathlessness, threatening stances); history of violence against others (e.g., hitting, kicking, scratching, or biting someone; spitting at someone; throwing objects at someone; attempted rape; rape; sexual molestation; urinating/defecating on someone); history of threats of violence (e.g., verbal threats against property, verbal threats against person, social threats, cursing, threatening notes/letters, threatening gestures, sexual threats); history of violent antisocial behavior (e.g., stealing, insistent borrowing, insistent demanding of privileges, insistent interrupting of meetings, refusing to eat, refusing to take medication, ignoring instructions); history of violence, indirect (e.g., tearing off clothes, ripping objects off walls, writing on walls, urinating on floor, defecating on floor, stomping feet, displaying temper tantrum, running in corridors, yelling, throwing objects, breaking a window, slamming doors, making sexual advances); neurological impairment (e.g., positive EEG, CAT, or MRI; head trauma; positive neurological findings; seizure

**V**

• = Independent        ▲ = Collaborative

disorders); cognitive impairment (e.g., learning disabilities, attention deficit/hyperactivity disorder, decreased intellectual functioning); history of childhood abuse; history of witnessing family violence; cruelty to animals; fire setting; prenatal/perinatal complications or abnormalities; history of drug or alcohol abuse; pathological intoxication; psychotic symptomatology (e.g., auditory, visual, command hallucinations; paranoid delusions; loose, rambling, or illogical thought processes); motor vehicle offenses (e.g., frequent traffic violations, use of a motor vehicle to release anger); suicidal behavior; impulsivity; availability/possession of weapon(s)

## Client Outcomes

### Client Will (Specify Time Frame):

- Stop all forms of abuse (physical, emotional, sexual; neglect; financial exploitation).
- Have cessation of abuse reported by victim.
- Display no aggressive activity.
- Refrain from verbal outbursts.
- Refrain from violating others' personal space.
- Refrain from antisocial behaviors.
- Maintain relaxed body language and decreased motor activity.
- Identify factors contributing to abusive/aggressive behavior.
- Demonstrate impulse control or state feelings of control.
- Identify impulsive behaviors.
- Identify feelings/behaviors that lead to impulsive actions.
- Identify consequences of impulsive actions to self or others.
- Avoid high-risk environments and situations.
- Identify and talk about feelings; express anger appropriately.
- Express decreased anxiety and control of hallucinations as applicable.
- Displace anger to meaningful activities.
- Communicate needs appropriately.
- Identify responsibility to maintain control.
- Express empathy for victim.
- Obtain no access or yield access to harmful objects.
- Use alternative coping mechanisms for stress.

V

• = Independent          ▲ = Collaborative

- Obtain and follow through with counseling.
- Demonstrate knowledge of correct role behaviors.

**Victim (and Children If Applicable) Will (Specify Time Frame):**

- Have safe plan for leaving situation or avoiding abuse.
- Resolve depression or traumatic response.

**Parent Will (Specify Time Frame):**

- Monitor social/play contacts.
- Provide supervision and nurturing environment.
- Intervene to prevent high-risk social behaviors.

## Nursing Interventions

### Client Violence

▲ Monitor the environment, evaluate situations that could become violent, and intervene early to deescalate the situation. Enlist support from other staff rather than attempting to handle the situation alone.

▲ Know and follow institution's policies and procedures concerning violence.

- Initiate client assessment by distinguishing the broadest categories of causes of aggression: social versus biological.

▲ Assess the client for risk factors of violence including those in the following categories: psychiatric disorders (particularly paranoid or bipolar disorders, substance abuse), neurological disorders (e.g., head injury, temporal lobe epilepsy), psychological precursors (e.g., low tolerance for stress, impulsivity), coping difficulties (e.g., inability to plan solutions or see long-term consequences of behavior), and personal history (e.g., past violent behavior).

▲ Assess for potential indicators of impending violence against others: frequent medication change, high use of sedative drugs, past violent behavior, a *Diagnostic and Statistical Manual of Mental Health IV* diagnosis of antisocial personality or borderline personality disorder, and long hospitalization. Other indicators include hyper-

V

• = Independent    ▲ = Collaborative

vigilance, hostility, substance abuse, and lack of adherence to medication regimen.

- Assess the client with history of previous assaults. Listen to and acknowledge feelings of anger, observe for increased motor activity, and prepare to intervene if the client becomes aggressive.
- Assess for the client's experience of physiological signs and for external signs of anger.
- A brief self-report from the client may aid in the assessment of violence risk.
- Assess for the presence of hallucinations.
- Determine the presence and degree of homicidal risk. A number of questions will elicit the necessary information:
  - Have you been thinking about harming someone? If yes, who?
  - How often do you have these thoughts, and how long do they last?
  - Do you have a plan? What is it?
  - Do you have access to the means to carry out that plan?
  - What has kept you from hurting the person until now?
- Take action to minimize personal risk:
  - Use nonthreatening body language.
  - Respect personal space and boundaries.
  - Do not allow the client to block access to an exit.
  - If speaking with the client alone, keep the door to the room open.
  - Be aware of where other staff are at all times.
  - Notify other staff of where you are at all times.
  - Take verbal threats seriously, and notify other staff.
  - Wear clothing and accessories that are not restricting and that will not be dangerous (e.g., sandals or shoes with heels can lead to twisted ankles; necklaces or dangling earrings could be grabbed).
- Maintain at least an arm's length distance from the client; do not touch the client without permission (unless physical restraint is the goal).
- Remove potential weapons from the environment. Be

**V**

• = Independent          ▲ = Collaborative

prepared to remove obstructions to staff response from the environment.

- Search the client and his or her belongings for weapons or potential weapons on admission to the hospital as appropriate.
- Inform the client of unit expectations for appropriate behavior and the consequences of not meeting these expectations. Emphasize that the client must comply with the rules of the unit. Give positive reinforcement for compliance.
- Increase surveillance of the hospitalized client at smoking, meal, and medication times.
- Assign a single room to the client with a potential for violence toward others.
- Maintain a secluded area for the client to be placed when violent. Ensure that staff are continuously present and available to client during seclusion.
- Maintain a calm attitude in response to the client.
- Provide a low level of stimulation in the client's environment; place the client in a safe, quiet place, and speak slowly and quietly.
- Redirect possible violent behaviors into physical activities (e.g., walking, jogging) if the client is physically able.
- Provide sufficient staff if a show of force is necessary to demonstrate control to the client.
- Protect other clients in the environment from harm. Remove other individuals from the vicinity of a violent or potentially violent client. Follow safety protocols of the department.
▲ Use chemical restraints as ordered. Obtain an order for medication, and administer it immediately.
▲ Use mechanical restraints if ordered and as necessary.
▲ Follow institution's protocol for releasing restraints. Observe client closely, remain calm, and provide positive feedback as client's behavior becomes controlled.
▲ If restraints are necessary, provide the client with musical tapes and a headset.
- Encourage clients to eat a healthy, balanced diet.

• = Independent          ▲ = Collaborative

- Form a therapeutic alliance with the client, identifying the source of anger as external to both nurse and client.
- Allow and encourage the client to verbalize feelings either one on one or in a group setting.
- Recognize that anger is generally purposeful and situation dependent. Actively listen to the client; explore the source of the client's anger, and negotiate resolution when possible.
- Teach the client healthy ways to express feelings/anger, appropriate gender roles to exhibit, and methods to communicate needs appropriately.
- Help the client identify when anger develops. Have the client keep an anger diary and discuss alternative responses. Teach cognitive-behavioral techniques.
- Identify stimuli that initiate violence and means of dealing with the stimuli.
- Emphasize that the client is responsible for his or her choices and behavior. Introduce descriptions of possible effects of client's aggressive/violent behavior on others.
- ▲ Always follow up a violent episode with a debriefing of clients and staff.

## Domestic Violence

NOTE: Before implementation of interventions in the face of domestic violence, nurses should examine their own emotional responses to abuse, their knowledge base about abuse, and systemic elements within the emergency department to ensure that interventions will be compassionate and appropriate. Particular attention to the influence of domestic violence on children and adolescents is warranted.

- Screen for possible abuse in women or children with a pattern of multiple injuries, particularly if there is any suspicion that the physical findings are inconsistent with the explanation of how the injuries were incurred.
- ▲ Report suspected child abuse to Child Protective Services. Refer women suspected of being in a spousal abuse

V

• = Independent          ▲ = Collaborative

situation to an area crisis center and provide phone number of area crisis hotline. Rapid screening tools are helpful to identify intimate partner violence.

- With women who repeatedly have injuries associated with domestic violence, maintain a nonjudgmental approach and continue to offer resources/referrals. If the woman voices a willingness to leave her situation, assist with developing an emergency plan that will consider all contingencies possible (e.g., safe location, financial resources, care of children, when to leave safely).

▲ In cases where spouse or child abuse accompanies substance abuse, refer the abusive client to a substance abuse treatment program and the spouse being abused to Al-Anon (children to Alateen).

▲ In cases where an adult reveals a history of unresolved/untreated sexual abuse as a child, referral to a local Adults Molested as Children (AMAC) group may be helpful.

▲ In dealing with abused wives, maintain a nonjudgmental response when clients return to husbands or refuse to leave them.

- Women with physical or mental disabilities require extended assessment if abuse is suspected or present to determine unique ways in which they may experience abuse. In addition to an assessment of the usual power and control concerns, a comprehensive functional assessment should be conducted along with attention to cultural issues and the nature of the disability.

▲ Women with disabilities who experience abuse may require referral to disability service providers, along with domestic violence services.

- Women with disabilities may experience abuse from multiple sources, and may have fewer resources and options to use. Particular attention should be paid to needs for resource referrals and the additional emotional stresses for these women.

▲ In cases of potential child abuse, refer the parent to parenting classes or a parental counseling support group. Early intervention may prevent abuse from occurring.

• = Independent          ▲ = Collaborative

Young parents in particular may have difficulty dealing with the stresses of parenthood combined with other life stresses; sharing their concerns with others can help normalize the stress. Support from others can help prevent the need to displace anger and frustration.

## Social Violence

- ▲ Assess the support network of women who become victims of violent crime, and refer for appropriate levels of assistance.
- • Be aware that there is a growing amount of hate crime, particularly toward transgendered individuals, requiring support and advocacy for victims.
- ▲ Victims of violence seen in the emergency department should receive an assessment for needed services and assignment to case management. Establishment of linkages with social service agencies can provide important services for referral.

## Pediatric

- • Assess for dating violence among adolescent girls. Additional assessments may be required for sexually transmitted diseases and pregnancy.
- • Pregnant teens should be assessed for abuse, particularly if they are with an older partner.
- • When physical abuse by parents is present, parent-child interaction therapy (PCIT) may be helpful.
- ▲ In the case of child abuse or neglect, refer for early childhood home visitation.

## Geriatric

- • Be alert to the potential for elder abuse in clients.
- • Assess for changes in physiological functions (e.g., constipation, dehydration) or impairment of the ability to meet basic needs (e.g., inadequate toileting, decreased mobility).
- • Observe for dementia and delirium.
- • Assess sensory impairments and the influence they may have on the client's behavior.

V

• = Independent          ▲ = Collaborative

- Observe for signs of fear, anxiety, anger, and agitation, and intervene immediately.
▲ Monitor for paradoxical drug reactions, and report any to the physician.
▲ Assess for brain insults such as recent falls or injuries, strokes, or transient ischemic attacks.
- Decrease environmental stimuli if violence is directed at others.
- Provide hand or back rubs and calming music when elderly client experiences agitation.
▲ If abuse or neglect of an elderly client is suspected, report the suspicion to a local Adult Protective Services agency.

## Home Care

- Be alert to the potential for violent behavior in the home setting. Respond to verbal aggression with interventions to deescalate negative emotional states.
- Assess family members or caregivers for their ability to protect the client and themselves.
- Include an initial and ongoing assessment and evaluation of potential abuse and neglect. Photograph evidence of abuse or neglect when possible.
▲ If neglect or abuse is suspected, identify an emergency plan that addresses the problem immediately, ensures client safety, and includes a report to the appropriate authorities. Discuss when to use hotlines and 911. Role-play access to emergency resources with the client and caregivers.
- Encourage appropriate safety behaviors in abused women; call the client at intervals during a 6-month period to determine whether safety behaviors are being carried out.
- Assess the home environment for harmful objects. Have the family remove or lock up objects as able.
▲ Refer for homemaker or psychiatric home health care services for respite, client reassurance, and implementation of a therapeutic regimen.
▲ If the client is taking psychotropic medications, assess

V

• = Independent ▲ = Collaborative

client and family knowledge of medication and its administration and side effects. Teach as necessary.

▲ Evaluate effectiveness and side effects of medications.

• If client displays mildly intensifying aggressive behavior, attempt to diffuse anger or violence (e.g., ask for a glass of water to distract client). Later in the visit explain that aggressive behavior is not acceptable and present consequences of continued aggressive behavior (i.e., right of agency to discontinue services).

• Document all acts or verbalizations of aggression.

▲ If client verbalizes or displays threatening behavior, notify supervisor and plan to make joint visits with another staff person or a security escort.

▲ If the client behaves in such a manner as to make the nurse uncomfortable without overt threat, a meeting may be held outside the home in sight of others (e.g., front porch).

▲ Never enter a home or remain in a home if aggression threatens your well-being.

▲ Never challenge a show of force such as a gun threat. Leave and notify your supervisor and the appropriate authorities. Document the incident.

▲ If client behaviors intensify, refer for immediate mental health intervention.

## Client/Family Teaching

• Teach relaxation and exercise as ways to release anger.

• Teach cognitive-behavioral activities such as active problem solving, reframing (reappraising the situation from a different perspective), or thought stopping (in response to a negative thought, picture a large stop sign and replace the image with a prearranged positive alternative). Teach the client to confront his or her own negative thought patterns (or cognitive distortions) such as catastrophizing (expecting the very worst), dichotomous thinking (perceiving events in only one of two opposite categories), magnification (placing distorted emphasis on a single event), or unrealistic

V

expectations (e.g., "I should get what I want when I want it").

- For religious couples, encourage the use of prayer.
▲ Refer to individual or group therapy.
- Teach the adolescent client violence prevention and encourage him or her to become involved in community service activities.
- Teach caregivers and family members of clients with dementia to use expressive physical touch and verbalization (EPT/V) when caring for these clients.
▲ Teach the use of appropriate community resources in emergency situations (e.g., hotline, community mental health agency, emergency department, 911 in most places in the United States, the toll-free National Domestic Violence Hotline [1-800-799-SAFE]).
▲ Encourage the use of self-help groups in nonemergency situations.
▲ Inform the client and family about medication actions, side effects, target symptoms, and toxic reactions.

# Risk for self-directed Violence

## NANDA Definition

At risk for behaviors in which an individual demonstrates that he or she can be physically, emotionally, and/or sexually harmful to self

## Risk Factors

Body language (e.g., rigid posture, clenching of fists and jaw, hyperactivity, pacing, breathlessness, threatening stances); history of violence against others (e.g., hitting, kicking, scratching, or biting someone; spitting at someone; throwing objects at someone; attempted rape; rape; sexual molestation; urinating/defecating on someone); history of threats of violence (e.g., verbal threats against property, verbal threats against person, social

**V**

• = Independent        ▲ = Collaborative

threats, cursing, threatening notes/letters, threatening gestures, sexual threats); history of violent antisocial behavior (e.g., stealing, insistent borrowing, insistent demanding of privileges, insistent interrupting of meetings, refusing to eat, refusing to take medication, ignoring instructions); history of violence, indirect (e.g., tearing off clothes, ripping objects off walls, writing on walls, urinating on floor, defecating on floor, stomping feet, displaying temper tantrum, running in corridors, yelling, throwing objects, breaking a window, slamming doors, making sexual advances); neurological impairment (e.g., positive EEG, CAT, or MRI; head trauma; positive neurological findings; seizure disorders); cognitive impairment (e.g., learning disabilities, attention deficit/hyperactivity disorder, decreased intellectual functioning); history of childhood abuse; history of witnessing family violence; cruelty to animals; fire setting; prenatal/perinatal complications or abnormalities; history of drug or alcohol abuse; pathological intoxication; psychotic symptomatology (e.g., auditory, visual, command hallucinations; paranoid delusions; loose, rambling, or illogical thought processes); motor vehicle offenses (e.g., frequent traffic violations, use of a motor vehicle to release anger); suicidal behavior; impulsivity; availability/possession of weapon(s)

## Client Outcomes

### Client Will (Specify Time Frame):

- Refrain from self-injury.
- State appropriate ways to cope with increased psychological or physiological tension.
- Talk about feelings; express anger appropriately.
- Seek help when feeling self-destructive or having urges to self-mutilate.
- Maintain self-control without supervision.
- Use appropriate community agencies when caregivers are unable to attend to emotional needs.
- Maintain connectedness in relationships.
- Express decreased anxiety and control of impulses.
- Refrain from using mood-altering substances.
- Obtain no access to harmful objects.

• = Independent          ▲ = Collaborative

- Yield access to harmful objects.
- Maintain self-control without supervision.

## Nursing Interventions

- Refer to care plan for **Risk for Suicide**.
- Refer to care plans for **Self-mutilation** and **Risk for Self-mutilation**.

# Impaired Walking

## NANDA Definition

Limitation of independent movement within the environment on foot (or artificial limb)

## Defining Characteristics

Impaired ability to climb stairs; walk on uneven surfaces; walk required distances; walk on even surfaces; walk on an incline or decline; navigate curbs

## Related Factors (r/t)

Intolerance to activity; decreased strength and endurance; pain or discomfort; perceptual or cognitive impairment; neuromuscular impairment; musculoskeletal impairment; depression; severe anxiety

NOTE: These are the same as the etiologies for **Impaired physical Mobility** with the addition of lower extremity amputation.

Suggested functional level classifications follow:

0—Completely independent
1—Requires use of equipment or device
2—Requires help from another person for assistance, supervision, or teaching
3—Requires help from another person and equipment device
4—Dependent (does not participate in activity)

W

• = Independent          ▲ = Collaborative

## Client Outcomes/Goals

### Client Will (Specify Time Frame):

* Demonstrate optimal independence and safety in walking.
* Demonstrate the ability to direct others on how to assist with walking.
* Demonstrate the ability to properly and safely use and care for assistive walking devices.

## Nursing Interventions

▲ Reinforce or request physical therapy (PT) consult to teach "bridging" (lifting the hips up); have client use the technique to move side to side in bed and to raise buttocks off bed.

▲ Explain progressive mobilization (gradual elevation of head of bed, tilt table, reclined chair, sitting, standing) to immobilized clients.

• Apply antiembolic stockings, elastic wraps, and abdominal binders; raise head of bed in small increments; teach client to sit up and change positions slowly and sit on the edge of the bed a few minutes before standing to prevent orthostatic hypotension.

▲ If suspected, monitor for orthostatic hypotension by comparing lying, sitting, and standing blood pressures and pulses. If systolic blood pressure falls 20 mm Hg or diastolic pressure decreases 10 mm Hg from the lying to standing position within 3 minutes, and/or if lightheadedness, weakness, syncope, or unexplained falls occur, consult physician.

▲ Administer oral water and medications as prescribed by physician to treat orthostatic hypotension.

• Place clients supine and elevate legs to oppose postprandial syncope.

▲ Employ prophylaxis for deep vein thrombosis (DVT) and pulmonary emboli (PE) in clients with prolonged immobility, recent lower extremity surgery or major surgery, and stroke, and in the aged. Refer to care plan for **Impaired Tissue perfusion.**

W

• = Independent          ▲ = Collaborative

- Vigilantly apply antiembolic or elastic stockings and intermittent pneumatic compression devices on persons at risk for DVT and PE.
▲ Follow physician orders for activity and ambulation in persons diagnosed with DVT and PE since early ambulation versus bed rest may be recommended.
▲ Remind clients of physician's orders for weight-bearing limitations during walking (e.g., non–weight-bearing on left foot).
▲ As weight bearing resumes after prolonged bed rest, teach clients to ingest protein, avoid nonsteroidal anti-inflammatory drugs (NSAIDs) for 7 days, prevent exposure to infections, and realize that depression is possible.
- Encourage patients to stand and walk frequently.
- Assist clients to properly apply orthoses, immobilizers, splints, and braces before walking.
- Teach clients with leg amputations to correctly don sheath, stump socks, liner, and prosthesis before walking.
- Use individualized assistive devices (as recommended by PT) when walking a client, including gait belts, walkers, crutches, and canes.
- Obtain the appropriate number of assistants to walk clients. One team member should give short, simple instructions (e.g., ask client to raise the head).
- Ask the PT where to stand in relation to the client. Assistants commonly stand slightly behind and to the side of the client, holding onto the gait belt with one supinated hand. The other hand rests on the client's closest shoulder.
- Strategically place obstacles in the walking path as the client's balance, gait, endurance, and concentration improve.
- Document on the care plan how many assistants are needed to walk the client, level of assistance needed (e.g., maximum, standby), type of assistance needed (e.g., physical support, verbal cues, balance control), and assistive devices used.
- Collect a baseline pulse rate and rhythm before walking the client, and reassess it 5 minutes after walking. If

W

• = Independent        ▲ = Collaborative

abnormal, let the client sit and rest 5 minutes before taking the pulse again. If still abnormal, walking may need to be done more slowly, with more help, or for a shorter time period.

▲ Monitor the client's tolerance for walking. Initiate a 5-minute rest period if any of the following are noted: shortness of breath, use of accessory muscles to breathe, chest pain, nausea, cold sweat, pale or flushed skin, dizziness, syncope, or mental confusion. If signs persist, notify the physician. For more information, refer to the care plan for **Activity intolerance.**

▲ Perform initial and subsequent screening to detect clients at high risk for falls.

• Individualize interventions to prevent falls and overuse of restraints and bedrails, including scheduled toileting, lower extremity balance and strength training, sleep hygiene, education on risk of medication and alcohol's relationship to falls, removal of hazards, and detection and treatment of underlying medical problems.

### Geriatric

• Monitor pulse, respirations, and blood pressure before and 5 minutes after a new activity. Stop activity if any of the following occur: resting heart rate >100 beats/min, exercise heart rate 35% greater than resting rate, exercise systolic blood pressure >25 to 35 mm Hg above resting pressure, or a decrease in systolic blood pressure of >20 mm Hg.

• Recognize that use of a walking aid increases energy and therefore may raise pulse and blood pressure.

▲ Implement safety and fall precautions, such as visual identification (arm bands) of clients at high risk for falling; call system placed within reach and repeated reminders given to call for help before standing; bed/chair alarm or one-to-one observation, obstacle clearance; assistive devices that are specifically chosen and measured for clients; side rails of bed in down position.

• Assess for swaying, poor balance, and short first step length during standing and walking of elders.

• = Independent          ▲ = Collaborative

- If the client experiences dizziness from orthostatic hypotension when arising, teach compensatory methods mentioned previously. Have someone present or a stable support surface to hold onto while arising.
- Emphasize the importance of wearing firm, low-heeled shoes with nonskid and nonfriction soles and seeking medical care for foot pain, foot problems, and diabetes.
- ▲ Introduce and reinforce positive perceptions of old age.

## Home Care

- Assess the client and obtain a complete history with reference to reasons for walking impairments.
- Explain the importance of adequate lighting both day and night; tacking carpet edges down, removing throw rugs from traffic flow areas, and having nonskid backings on those rugs that are used; applying nonskid wax on floors; and removing clutter from the floor.
- Assess the home environment for all barriers to walking.
- Assess client's support system for emergency and contingency care (e.g., Lifeline).
- ▲ Refer clients at risk for falls to PT and OT for skill and strength building, resistive training, and stretching and exercise programs (especially those with osteoporosis and postural problems).
- ▲ Refer to home health aide services as appropriate for assistance with activities of daily living.
- ▲ Provide support to the client and caregivers. Refer to case manager/medical social services or mental health/support group services as necessary.
- ▲ Ensure that the client has information on advocacy, environmental accessibility, assistive technology, and related issues under the Americans with Disabilities Act.
- Teach client and family to check assistive devices to keep them in safe working order; for example, replace rubber tips if worn and remove dirt in grooves of walkers, crutches, and canes; otherwise they will not grip the floor. Check push button locks on walkers with telescoping legs. Inspect and repair prostheses for cracks, rough

W

• = Independent          ▲ = Collaborative

spots inside the socket, and odd noises or movement at the joints or foot.

▲ Recommend daily weight-bearing activities, walking, calcium and vitamin D supplementation, and avoidance of smoking to men and women with osteoporosis and hip fractures. Strongly encourage clients to drink milk at mealtime. Estrogen-replacement therapy and antiresorptive therapy are also therapeutic; therefore clients should consult their physicians.

# Wandering

## NANDA Definition

Meandering; aimless or repetitive locomotion that exposes the individual to harm; frequently incongruent with boundaries, limits, or obstacles

## Defining Characteristics

Frequent or continuous movement from place to place, often revisiting the same destinations; persistent locomotion in search of "missing" or unattainable people or places; haphazard locomotion; locomotion in unauthorized or private spaces; locomotion resulting in unintended leaving of a premise; long periods of locomotion without an apparent destination; fretful locomotion or pacing; inability to locate significant landmarks in a familiar setting; locomotion that cannot be easily dissuaded or redirected; following behind or shadowing a caregiver's locomotion; trespassing; hyperactivity; scanning, seeking, or searching behaviors; periods of locomotion interspersed with periods of nonlocomotion (e.g., sitting, standing, sleeping); getting lost

## Related Factors (r/t)

Cognitive impairment, specifically memory and recall deficits, disorientation, poor visuoconstructive (or visuospatial) ability, and language (primarily expressive) defects; cortical atrophy;

W

• = Independent          ▲ = Collaborative

premorbid behavior (e.g., outgoing, sociable personality); premorbid dementia; separation from familiar people and places; sedation; emotional state, especially frustration, anxiety, boredom, or depression (agitation); overstimulating/understimulating social or physical environment; physiological state or need (e.g., hunger/thirst, pain, urination, constipation); time of day

## Client Outcomes

### Client Will (Specify Time Frame):

- Decrease incidence of falls (preferably free of falls).
- Decrease incidence of elopements.
- Maintain appropriate body weight.

### Caregiver Will (Specify Time Frame):

- Be able to explain interventions he or she can use to provide a safe environment for a care receiver who displays wandering behavior.

## Nursing Interventions

- Assess and document the amount (frequency and duration), pattern (random, lapping, or pacing), and 24-hour distribution of wandering behavior over a 3-day interval.
- Document particular aspects of wandering that are troubling.
- Obtain a history of personality characteristics and behavioral responses to stress.
- Evaluate for neurocognitive strengths and limitations, particularly language, attention, visuospatial skills, and perseveration.
- Assess for physical distress or needs such as hunger, thirst, pain, discomfort, or elimination.
- Assess for emotional or psychological distress such as anxiety, fear, or feeling lost.
- Observe wandering episodes for antecedents and consequences.
- Apply observed consequences of wandering, such as personal attention and obtaining food, at times when the

W

•  = Independent          ▲ = Collaborative

person is *not* wandering, and withhold them while the person is wandering.

- Assess regularly for the presence of or potential for negative outcomes of wandering such as declining social skills, falls, and elopement.
- Weigh client at defined intervals to detect onset of weight loss and watch for symptoms associated with inadequate food intake including constipation, dehydration, muscle wasting, and starvation.
- For the client who displays wandering behavior during mealtimes, use behavioral interventions to shape behavior including verbal statements, nonverbal social behavior, and systematic extinguishing of undesirable client behavior.
- Provide for safe ambulation with comfortable and well-fitting clothes, shoes with nonskid soles and foot support, and any necessary walking aids (such as a cane, walker, or Merry-Walker).
- Provide safe and secure surroundings that deter accidental elopements by using perimeter control devices, camouflage, or electronic tracking systems.
- During periods of inactivity, position the wanderer so that desirable destinations (such as the bathroom) are within the client's line of vision and undesirable destinations (such as exits or stairwells) are out of sight.
- If wandering takes a random or haphazard route, reduce environmental distractions and increase relevant environmental cues. Note and eliminate stimuli that distract the wanderer while in route. Provide afternoon rest periods if assessment reveals that random-pattern wandering worsens as the day progresses.
- Enhance institutional settings with areas that provide interesting views and opportunities to sit.
- Engage wanderers in social interaction and structured activity, especially when wanderers appear distressed or otherwise uncomfortable or their wandering presents a challenge to others in the setting.
- If wandering has a pacing quality, attempt to identify and

• = Independent          ▲ = Collaborative

address any underlying problems or concerns. Offer stress-reducing approaches such as music, massage, or rocking. Attempts to distract or redirect the pacing wanderer may worsen wandering.

- If wandering is a new or recently acquired behavior or if it increases in intensity over previous levels, evaluate for constipation, pneumonia, or acute physical problems.
- If wandering has a lapping or circuitous pattern, signs or labels may be effective. Substitute another repetitive activity such as folding or rocking if lapping becomes problematic or excessive.
- Provide a regularly scheduled and supervised exercise or walking program, particularly if wandering occurs excessively during the night or at times that are inconvenient in the setting.
- Use slow-stroke, hand, or foot massage before the times of day or events that induce wandering.

## Multicultural

- Assess for the influence of cultural beliefs, norms, and values on the family's understanding of wandering behavior.
- ▲ Refer the family to social services or other supportive services to assist with the impact of caregiving for the wandering client.
- ▲ Encourage the family to use support groups or other service programs.
- Validate the family's feelings regarding the impact of client wandering on family lifestyle.

## Home Care

- Help the caregiver set up a plan to deal with wandering behavior using the interventions mentioned in Nursing Interventions.
- Assess the home environment for modifications that will protect the client and prevent elopement.
- Assist the family to set up a plan of exercise for the client, including safe walking.

W

• = Independent          ▲ = Collaborative

▲ Enroll wanderers in the Safe Return Program of the Alzheimer's Association, and help the caregiver develop a
  plan of action to use if the client elopes.
• Help the caregiver develop a plan of action to use if the
  client elopes.
▲ Institute case management of frail elderly clients to support continued independent living.
▲ Refer for homemaker or psychiatric home health care
  services for respite, client reassurance, and implementation of a therapeutic regimen. Refer to the care plan
  for **Caregiver role strain.**

## Client/Family Teaching

• Inform the client and family of the meaning of and reasons for wandering behavior.
• Teach the caregiver/family methods to deal with wandering behavior using the interventions mentioned in
  Nursing Interventions.

• = Independent          ▲ = Collaborative

# INDEX

Page numbers followed by *b* indicate boxes; *t*, tables.

## A

Abdomen, 2
  acute, 5
  aneurysm of, surgery for, 14
  dehiscence, of, 50-51
Abortion, 2-3
Abruptio placentae, 3
Abscess(es)
  anorectal, 15
  formation of, 3
Absent bowel sounds, 26
Absent corneal reflex, 46
Absent gag reflex, 68
Absent peripheral pulse, 143
Abuse
  of children, 36, 169-170
  of cocaine, 40
  of drugs, 57
  of laxatives, 95
  of spouse, parent, or significant other,
      3-4
  of substances, 166-167
Accessory muscle, use in breathing, 4
Accident(s)
  cerebrovascular, 48
  proneness to, 4
Achalasia, 4
Acidosis, 4
Acne, 4
Acquired immunodeficiency syndrome,
    9-10
Acromegaly, 5
Activity(ies)
  deficient diversional, 56, 372-376
  intolerance of, 5, 188-194
Acute abdomen, 5
Acute respiratory distress syndrome, 18
Adams-Stokes syndrome, 5
Adaptive capacity, decreased intracranial,
    89, 571-574
Addiction, nicotine, 116
Addison's disease, 5
Adenoidectomy, 5-6
Adjustment impairment, 195-198
Adolescent(s)
  maturational issues in, 102
  sexuality in, 159
  terminally ill, 172
Adoption, giving child up for, 7
Adrenal crisis, 7

Adult(s)
  failure to thrive in, 64, 381-386
  seizure disorders in, 155-156
  terminally ill, 172
Advance directives, 7
Affect, flat, 66
Affective disorders, 7
  seasonal, 152
Aggressive behavior, 8
Aging, 8
Agitation, 8-9
Agoraphobia, 9
Agranulocytosis, 9
AIDS. *See* Acquired immunodeficiency
    syndrome.
Airway
  ineffective clearance of, 198-203
  obstruction of, 10
  secretions of, 10
Alcohol, acute intoxication from, 5
Alcoholism, 10-11, 392-399
Alkalosis, metabolic, 104
Allergy, latex, 11, 95, 204-211,
    207-209b
Alopecia, 11
ALS. *See* Amyotrophic lateral
    sclerosis.
Alterations
  body temperature, 25
  breathing pattern, 28
  consciousness level, 43-44
  protection, 142
  role performance, 151-152
  sensory/perceptual, 158
  urinary elimination, 180
Alzheimer's type dementia,11-12
Amenorrhea, 12
Amnesia, 12
Amniocentesis, 12
Amputation, 12-13
Amyotrophic lateral sclerosis, 13
Analgesia, patient-controlled,
    127
Anaphylactic shock, 13
Anasarca, 13
Anemia, 13
  aplastic, 17
  pernicious, 129
  sickle cell, 160
Anencephaly, 115-116

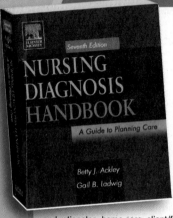